SYSTEM FOR OPHTHALMIC DISPENSING

SYSTEM FOR OPHTHALMIC DISPENSING

Third Edition

Clifford W. Brooks, OD
Professor of Optometry
Indiana University School of Optometry
Bloomington, Indiana

Irvin M. Borish, OD, DOS, LLD, DSc
Professor Emeritus, Indiana University School of Optometry
Bloomington, Indiana

Former Benedict Professor
University of Houston School of Optometry
Houston, Texas

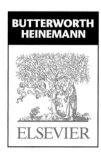

BUTTERWORTH
HEINEMANN

ELSEVIER

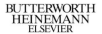

BUTTERWORTH
HEINEMANN
ELSEVIER

11830 Westline Industrial Drive
St. Louis, Missouri 63146

SYSTEM FOR OPHTHALMIC DISPENSING, THIRD EDITION

ISBN-13: 978-0-7506-7480-5
ISBN-10: 0-7506-7480-6

Notice

Neither the Publisher nor the Authors assume any responsibility for any loss or injury and/or damage to persons or property arising out of or related to any use of the material contained in this book. It is the responsibility of the treating practitioner, relying on independent expertise and knowledge of the patient, to determine the best treatment and method of application for the patient.

The Publisher

Previous edition copyrighted 1996

ISBN-13: 978-0-7506-7480-5
ISBN-10: 0-7506-7480-6

Publishing Director: Linda Duncan
Senior Editor: Kathy Falk
Senior Developmental Editor: Christie M. Hart
Publishing Services Manager: Pat Joiner
Senior Project Manager: Karen M. Rehwinkel
Designer: Amy Buxton

Working together to grow
libraries in developing countries

www.elsevier.com | www.bookaid.org | www.sabre.org

ELSEVIER   BOOK AID International   Sabre Foundation

Printed in China

Last digit is the print number: 9 8 7 6

*This book is dedicated to our students, whose interest and desire
to master the subject prompted its writing.*

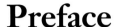

Preface

The original goal for creating *System for Ophthalmic Dispensing* was not to create a comprehensive textbook. Rather, we envisioned a student manual to aid in the teaching of how to dispense prescription eyewear. As the "manual" developed, Professional Press learned of the project, expressed an interest, and requested sample chapters. It became evident that such a publication might be useful beyond the confines of teaching at Indiana University.

Once a preliminary manuscript copy was available, it was sent out for review. This resulted in a request for the addition of material on the optics of lenses. Thus the second section of the book was added. Perhaps because of the large number of photographs and illustrations, the first edition was found to be useful in both educational programs and in ophthalmic practices.

Ophthalmic dispensing of eyewear is basic throughout the eye care world. And so is an understanding of how ophthalmic lenses perform. Both are essential for a new employee in an optical dispensary who is learning on the job and for an experienced eye care practitioner. Knowing the varied backgrounds of the reading audience, an attempt was made to write in a manner that would be understandable to someone new to the field, but would also include the type of information needed by those with years of ophthalmic experience.

The second edition built upon and updated the original edition, adding sections on lens material and lens design. The second edition contained large numbers of photos—all in black and white. For the third edition the decision was made to start all over again, with color photos throughout. Hundreds of photos were taken, each from the point of view of the eye care provider. There are major changes in the second half of the book concerning ophthalmic lenses. All of these chapters have been extensively reorganized and rewritten. Included are large amounts of new material on progressive lenses, occupational progressive lenses, aspheric and atoric lenses, and absorptive lenses. There are also two completely new chapters—one on the optical aspects of aniseikonia, the other on how lenses are edged.

All of these changes have been made in an attempt to address the needs of two groups of professionals. The first group consists of eye care providers who must stay current themselves, but also must individually train new personnel. The second group is made up of ophthalmic educators and students in formalized educational programs. Both groups need well-illustrated, comprehensive educational resources.

The process of attempting to fulfill these needs has been both time consuming and painstaking. You now see the results. We hope that you will find the new third edition of *System for Ophthalmic Dispensing* to be informative, easy to use, and personally beneficial.

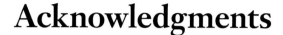

Acknowledgments

For help in preparing the first edition, the authors would especially like to thank Jacque Kubley for the original photography and many of the illustrations; Sandra Corns Pickel and Sue Howard for serving as models; and Dr. Linda Dejmek, Kyu-Sun Rhee, Dennis Conway, and Steve Weiss for the artwork and illustrations. For all the help received for the first edition, we continue to be very grateful.

For the second edition, again thanks to Jacque Kubley for his continued assistance in photography and a number of the graphics. In the second and now the third edition, thanks to Glenn Herringshaw, who manages Indiana University's optical laboratory, for many helpful ideas and suggestions; and to Glenn and Regina Herringshaw for serving as models for a number of the photographs. Also thanks to Pam Gondry and Dr. Eric Reinhard for joining in the "modeling team" for the third edition. A specific word of appreciation goes to Robert Woyton of Hilco for reviewing the chapter on repairs and supplying a number of photographs for both the second and third editions.

Thanks to Ric Cradick of IU Photographic Services for taking the multitude of new color photos for the third edition. His professional expertise is much appreciated.

To our students, we owe a debt of gratitude. They suffered through preliminary manuscripts, yet were exceedingly helpful in pointing out omissions, making valuable suggestions, and asking just the right questions.

Finally, special thanks to our many friends within the profession for offering suggestions and supplying ideas for improving the text. Without your advice and the information you provided, it would have been impossible to complete the task.

Contents in Brief

Contents

SYSTEM FOR OPHTHALMIC DISPENSING

PART I

Ophthalmic Dispensing

CHAPTER 1

Frame Types and Parts

The purpose of this chapter is to acquaint the reader with the basic terminology used in eyewear. This knowledge is essential to avoid misunderstanding the terms used later in the text to describe in detail the actual dispensing procedures.

BASIC PARTS

The frame is that portion of the spectacles that holds the lenses containing the ophthalmic prescription in their proper position in front of the eyes.

A frame generally consists of the *front*, which in one form or another contains the lenses, and the *temples*, which attach to the front and hook over the ears to help hold the spectacles in place. Frames occasionally do not have temples and are instead held in place by pressure on the sides of the nose (pince-nez), by attachment to another frame (clip-ons), or by being held in the hand (lorgnettes).

Frame Fronts

That area of the frame front between the lenses that rests on the nose is the *bridge*. The rim going around the lenses is known as the *eyewire* or *rim*. The outer areas of the frame front, to the extreme left and right where the temples attach, are known as the *endpieces*. A few plastic frames may still have a metal *shield* on the front of the endpiece to which rivets are attached to hold the hinge in place (Figure 1-1).

The *hinges* hold the temples to the front, and consist of an odd number of interfitting *barrels*, the total number being three, five, or seven. Hinges may vary in construction, but for simplicity are usually classified by the total number of barrels they have when assembled, such as a three-barrel hinge.

Some frames have *nose pads*, which are plastic pieces that rest on the nose to support the frame. These may be directly attached to the frame or to connecting metal pieces known as *guard arms* or *pad arms*.

Temples

The portion of the temple that is nearest its attachment to the front is known as the *butt portion* or *butt end*. The place on the temple where it first bends down to go over the ear is called the *bend*. The portion of the temple

between the butt end and the bend is called the *shank* or *shaft*, and that portion beyond the bend and behind the ear is referred to as the *earpiece, bent-down portion*, or *curl* (Figure 1-2).

CONSTRUCTION

Frames

Frames without an eyewire going completely around the lens are called *mountings*. Lenses are "inserted" into frames, but "mounted" into mountings. Frames themselves can be classified in a simplified manner by one of the following categories of frames or mountings.

Plastic

Plastic frames are made of some type of plastic material. Plastic frames were occasionally referred to as *shell* frames, dating back to the time when eyeglass frames were made of tortoise shell. This term has fallen into disuse. Another general term that many still use for certain plastic frames is *zyl*, since at one time zylonite (cellulose nitrate) was a commonly used material. Zylonite is highly flammable and no longer used for spectacle frames. The name "zyl" continues to be used, but usually refers to the most commonly used plastic material-cellulose acetate. Now, with the emergence of many new materials, either the exact name of the plastic material is used or the frame is simply referred to as *plastic* (Figure 1-3).

Metal

Metal frames are those made of all metal parts, except for the nose pads and the posterior temple sections, which are plastic covered. The eyewire runs completely around the lens (Figure 1-4).

Nylon cord frames

Nylon cord frames, sometimes called *string mounted frames* or *nylon supras* hold the lenses in place by means of a nylon cord that fits around the edge of the lens. This gives the glasses the appearance of being rimless. Usually the top of the lens is fitted into the upper rim of the frames. The rest of the lens has a small groove cut into an otherwise flat edge (Figure 1-5).

3

Combination

Combination frames are commonly frames having a metal *chassis* and plastic top rims and temples (Figure 1-6). The chassis includes the eyewire and center or bridge section. Although this is the most common construction, technically any frame with a combination of metal and plastic could be included in this category, as in the case of a

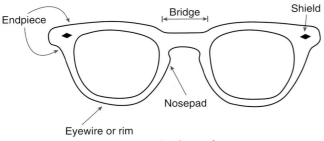

Figure 1-1. The frame front.

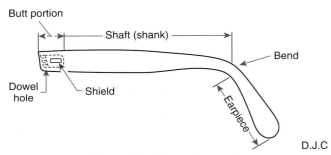

Figure 1-2. Parts of a temple.

frame with plastic eye-wires and metal bridge and temples.

Half-eye

Half-eyes are frames made especially for those who need a reading correction but no correction for distance. They are constructed to sit lower on the nose than normal, and are only half as high as normal glasses. This allows the wearer to look over the top of the glasses. They may be of plastic, metal, or even nylon cord construction (Figure 1-7). Less common are half-eyes for distant vision, which allow the wearer to look under the lenses for reading.

Rimless, Semirimless, and Numont

Rimless mountings hold the lenses in place by some method other than eyewires or nylon cords. Often screws are used, but cement, clamps, and plastic posts have been used. Most rimless mountings have two areas of attachment per lens, one nasally and one temporally (Figure 1-8). Rimless mountings are sometimes referred to as *3-piece mountings*.

Semirimless mountings are similar to the rimless except for a metal reinforcing *arm*, which follows the upper posterior surface of the lens and joins the *centerpiece* of the frame to the endpiece. The centerpiece of a mounting consists of bridge, pad arms, and pads (Figure 1-9).

Numont mountings hold the lenses in place only at their nasal edge. They are seldom seen today. The lenses are attached at the bridge area and the temples are attached to a metal arm that extends along the posterior

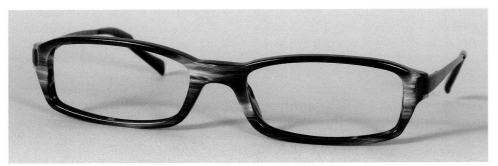

Figure 1-3. An example of a plastic frame.

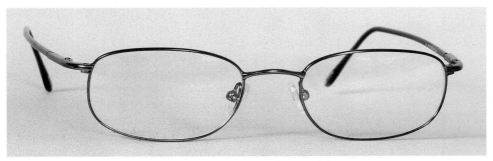

Figure 1-4. One version of a metal frame.

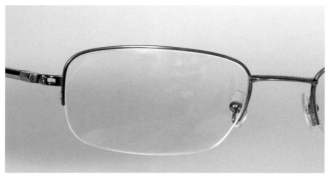

Figure 1-5. A nylon cord frame or "string mount" holds the lens in place with a cord that fits around the edge of the grooved lens.

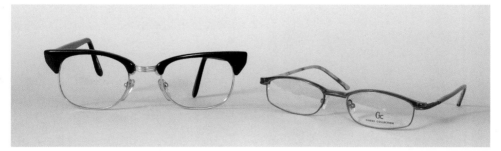

Figure 1-6. Examples of combination frames.

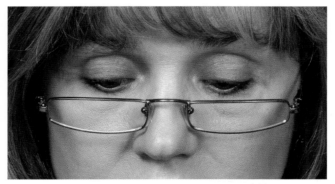

Figure 1-7. Half-eye frames in use. Half-eyes are made especially for those who need a reading correction but no correction for distance vision.

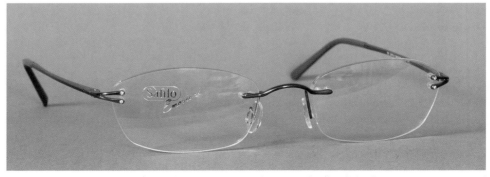

Figure 1-8. An example of a rimless mounting. The central area of the frame is not connected to the endpieces. The only connecting points are the lenses themselves.

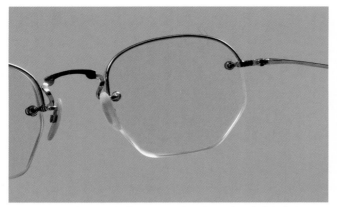

Figure 1-9. A semirimless mounting has a bar behind the top of the lens connecting the endpieces to the bridge area.

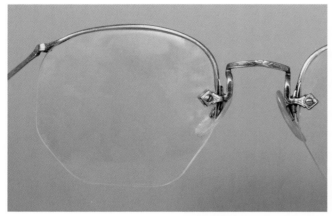

Figure 1-10. A Numont mounting has only one nasal point of attachment per lens.

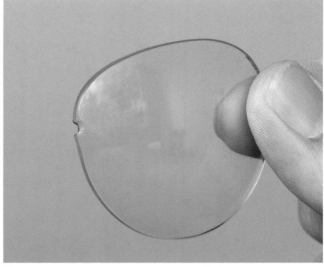

A

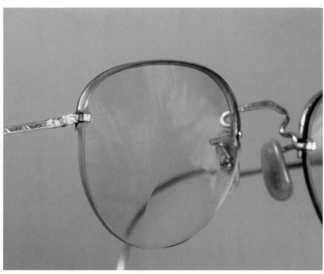

B

Figure 1-11. A balgrip mounting. In this form of rimless mounting, the slotted lenses (**A**) are held in place with clips (**B**).

surface temporally. Thus there is only one point of attachment per lens (Figure 1-10).

Currently most dispensers refer to any of these three variations of a rimless mounting as "rimless." They do not differentiate between the three.

Other Mountings

Balgrip mountings secure the lens in place with clips attached to a bar of tensile steel that fits into a nasal and a temporal notch on each side of the lens. The lens can be easily removed by pulling the clips back from the lens. For this reason, this type of mounting can be used with more than one pair of lenses for the same frame. Sunlenses, special purpose lenses, or tinted lenses could then be used interchangeably with the patient's regular lenses (Figure 1-11). Notches are now more often used in combination with drilled holes in rimless mountings to lend stability to the mounting.

Bridge Area

The bridge area of a frame can be constructed of either plastic or metal. Because of the variety of nose shapes,

there is also quite an assortment of bridge constructions in both materials.

Plastic Bridges

The bridge area of a plastic frame is preformed and sits directly on the bridge of the nose. It is important, then, in picking out a plastic frame that the frame fit the nose well, since adjustments to this part of the frame are extremely difficult. Bridge adjustments for certain plastics, such as nylon, carbon fiber and polyamide, are not possible.

The *saddle bridge* is shaped like a saddle in a smooth curve and follows the bridge of the nose (Figure 1-12). This spreads the weight of the frame evenly over the sides and crest of the nose.

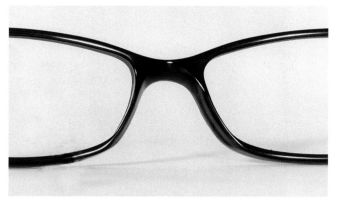

Figure 1-12. The saddle bridge closely follows the contour of the nose, evenly spreading the weight of the frame.

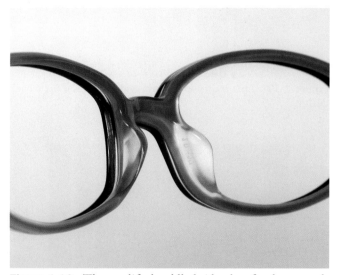

Figure 1-13. The modified saddle bridge has fixed nose pads attached at the back to increase the weight-bearing area of the frame.

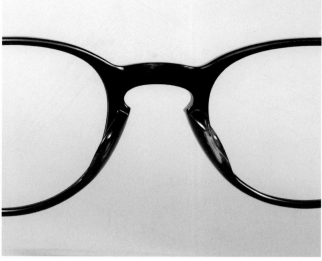

Figure 1-14. Besides having an identifying shape, the keyhole bridge supports the frame weight upon pads.

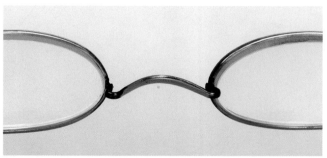

Figure 1-15. Metal saddle bridges were originally designed to rest directly on the crest of the nose. They may still be used as originally designed shown in the frame pictured. Often a metal saddle bridge is just for decorative purposes and is used in conjunction with nosepads.

In the *modified saddle*, the bridge area looks much the same as the saddle bridge does when viewed from the front. The difference is that there are nose pads that are part of the back of the bridge. These pads help to carry some of the weight of the frame (Figure 1-13).

The *keyhole* bridge is shaped like an old-fashioned keyhole. At the top, the bridge flares out slightly. The bridge rests on the sides of the nose, but not on the crest (Figure 1-14).

Metal Bridges

The bridge commonly used in metal frames is the *pad bridge* (see Figure 1-8). In the pad bridge, nose pads are attached to the frame by metal pad arms. In this case, the pads alone support the weight of the glasses.

When a metal frame is equipped with a clear plastic saddle-type bridge, the bridge type is referred to as a *comfort bridge.*

Metal and rimless frames were, and sometimes still are, constructed with a *metal saddle bridge** (Figure 1-15) and enjoyed widespread use for a period of history. It may yet appear exactly as before or decoratively in conjunction with nosepads.

With rimless mountings, the *crest* of the bridge does not include the pads or straps, but is the center most area.

Endpiece Construction

Endpiece construction, like the bridge area construction, can be of either plastic or metal.

Plastic Endpieces Construction

There are three general types of endpiece construction in plastic frames (Figure 1-16). The most common

---

*Historically the metal saddle bridge was called a *W bridge.*

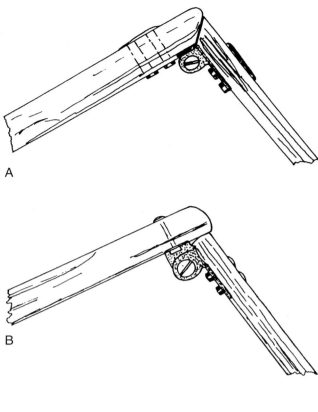

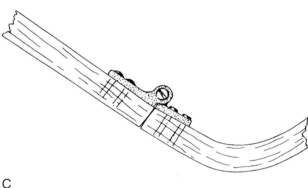

Figure 1-16. Endpieces of plastic frames classified as mitre **(A)**, butt **(B)**, and turn-back **(C)**.

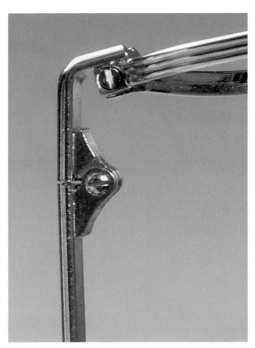

Figure 1-17. This traditional metal endpiece has a turn-back design.

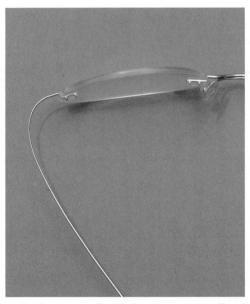

Figure 1-18. Some metal endpieces are not really endpieces at all. The endpiece and temple are one continuous piece of material as in this "wrap" endpiece design.

endpiece construction is the *butt* type, in which the front is straight and the temple butt is flat, and both meet at a 90-degree angle. The *mitre* endpiece causes the frame front contact area and temple butt to meet at a 45-degree angle. In the *turn-back* type, the frame front bends around and meets the temple end to end.

Metal Endpiece Construction

The traditional metal endpiece has a construction similar to the turn-back endpiece of the plastic frame (Figure 1-17). There are now a wide variety of metal endpiece designs.

Endpieces are also noticeable by their absence. Instead of an endpiece, some frame fronts and temples are made as one *continuous piece* (Figure 1-18).

Temple Construction

Temples also vary greatly in their construction. In general, there are five major categories (Figure 1-19).

1. *Skull temples* bend down behind the ear and follow the contour of the skull, resting evenly against it. The bent-down portion is narrower at the top of the ear and widens toward the end.

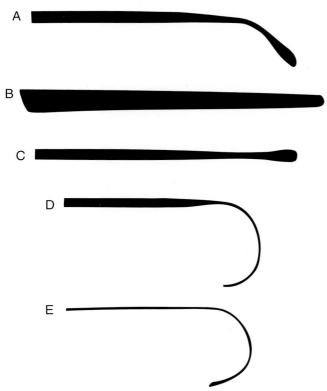

Figure 1-19. Categories of temples are: **A,** Skull; **B,** Library; **C,** Convertible; **D,** Riding bow (in plastic); **E,** Comfort cable (in metal).

2. *Library temples* usually begin with an average width at the butt and increase in width posteriorly. They are practically straight and hold the glasses on primarily by pressure against the side of the head. They are also known as *straight-back temples.*
3. *Convertible temples* were originally designed so they could be bent down to take on the form of skull temples, and "converted" from the straight-back to the skull design. Because this temple is versatile and can be made to fit people with a variety of temple length requirements, it is commonly used. However, it now comes already bent down for a certain temple fit. If the bend is in the wrong location, the temple may be easily straightened out and then re-bent to fit the wearer.
4. *Riding bow temples* curve around the ear, following the crotch of the ear where the ear and the head meet and extend to the level of the earlobe. They are sometimes used in children's and safety frames.
5. *Comfort cable temples* are shaped the same as riding bow temples, but are of metal construction with the curl, or behind the ear portion, constructed from a flexible coiled cable.

"Classic" Rimless Fronts

The centerpiece of a rimless front consists of the bridge, pad arms, and pads. These parts are the same as for metal frames. Rimless construction varies considerably. The "classic" rimless point of lens attachment contains a *strap* or *straps*. This is the part of the mounting that contacts the front and back surfaces and the edge of the lens, holding the lens in place. The traditional strap consists of the shoe and the ear.

The *shoe*, also known as the *shoulder* or *collar*, contacts the edge of the lens, bracing it and keeping it from rocking back and forth in its mounting. On some traditional mountings, there is a small metal *spring* between the shoe and the lens, which helps keep the lens tight in the mounting.

The *ear*, or *tongue*, is that portion of the strap that extends from the shoe, contacting the surface of the lens. There are sometimes two ears per strap, one on each lens surface, with a screw passing through both ears and the lens to hold the lens in place. The term *straps* is sometimes used to refer only to the ears (Figure 1-20).

The *arm* is that part of a *semirimless* mounting that extends posteriorly along the top edge of the lens (see Figure 1-9). The arm is not to be confused with the pad arm, which is part of the nose pad assembly. This arm is sometimes referred to as a *bar* or *brow-bar*.

The endpieces of rimless fronts are the same as those listed for metal frames. In addition, rimless endpieces also have straps to hold the lenses, as well as hinges for temples.

Coloration

Plastic frames may be partially classified by coloration. A *solid* frame is all one color. A *vertically gradient* frame is darker all the way across the top, including the bridge, and is lighter across the bottom. A *horizontally gradient* frame is darker at the temporal portions and lightens toward the central area. *Clear bridge* frames somewhat resemble the horizontal gradient, but are dark at the top, except for the bridge area. The bridge, along with the lower half of the frame, is clear plastic. The multitude of color combinations available now makes categorization beyond this difficult.

FRAME MATERIALS

Plastic Frame Materials

The first classification of a frame is by the material used in its construction: either plastic or metal. Several types of both are used to make frames.

The first plastics used for spectacle frames were made from *bakelite* and *galalith*.[1] These did not perform well in cold weather because of their brittleness. Later *cellulose nitrate (zylonite)* was widely used. Cellulose nitrate accepts a good polish, but is flammable if brought to a sufficiently high temperature. Because of the danger posed, cellulose nitrate has been banned by the FDA and is no longer used for spectacle frames. However, because these zylonite frames were the only plastic frames commonly used for a period of time, plastic frames were known as

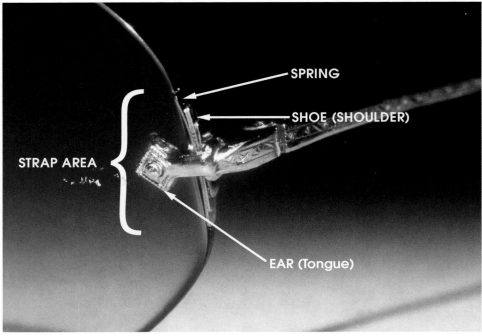

Figure 1-20. The strap area in a classic-style rimless mounting has the same construction at both center and endpiece locations. Contemporary rimless mountings do not necessarily have this classic-style construction.

"zyl" frames. In spite of zylonite disappearing from the market, the "zyl" nickname for plastic frames remained. Now that nickname is primarily used to refer to cellulose acetate material.

Cellulose Acetate

A material used extensively for spectacle frames is *cellulose acetate*. The basic cellulose material may be extracted from cotton or wood pulp and then further processed.[1] When derived from cotton, the material used is the fiber that adheres to the cottonseed after ginning and is too short to be used for making textiles. These fibers are called cotton linters.[2] This cotton or wood material is treated with a mixture of anhydride and acetic acid using sulfuric acid as a catalyst. Plasticizers and aging stabilizers are then added to this material.[2] Nevertheless, cellulose acetate does become brittle with age.

Some allergies are attributed to wearing cellulose acetate frames, though this is rare. More often skin problems are not so much allergic reactions to the material itself, but to those things which can be absorbed by the material. Higher quality cellulose acetate frames are coated in order to seal the surface. When left uncoated, cellulose acetate may absorb materials which might be allergen producing. A good frame coating will contain a UV inhibitor.* This inhibitor in the coating keeps frame color from fading.

Cellulose acetate can be formed into sheets of plastic from which frame parts can be cut, or it can be made into acetate granules that are used for injection molding. For spectacle frames, cellulose acetate is generally made into sheets and milled (Figure 1-21).

Propionate

Cellulose aceto-propionate, more commonly referred to as *propionate*, has many of the same characteristics as cellulose acetate and works better for injection molding. Propionate has less color stability than cellulose acetate and, unless it is covered with a high quality frame-coating material containing UV absorbers, will fade within a relatively short period of time. Propionate frames are made beginning with granules of the material that are heated until liquid, then injection molded to the desired frame shape. Granules may initially be colorless, allowing the frame parts to be dyed to the desired color after they have been molded. Propionate has a slight weight advantage over acetate, in that it is about three quarters of the weight.

Optyl

Epoxy resin is used for spectacle frames and is known under the trade name of Optyl. A liquid resin and a hardener are mixed together and drawn into the frame molds using a vacuum process. The material is *thermoelastic*. This means that it will bend when heated and will return to its original shape when reheated. (Cellulose acetate is *thermoplastic*. This means that it will bend when

---

*A "UV inhibitor" blocks out the sun's ultraviolet rays.

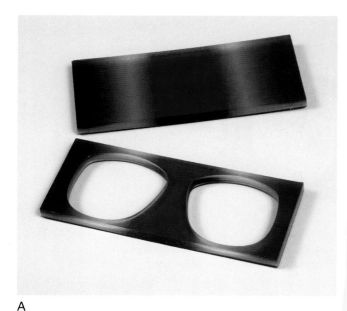

A

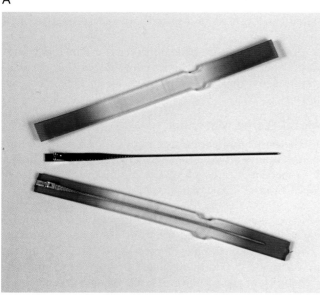

B

Figure 1-21. Frame fronts and temples can be milled from slabs of cellulose acetate. They are finished in steps until being polished, and usually coated to protect the frame material from sunlight and to decrease the possibility of allergic reactions in sensitive wearers. **A,** The frame front is being milled from a slab of plastic. **B,** One method for making temples. First the cellulose acetate is formed (*top*). Then the metal hinge and core (*middle*) is injected into the plastic (*bottom*). From this point, the temple is milled to the desired form and shaped.

heated but does not return to its original shape when reheated because it does not have a "plastic memory.") Optyl is approximately 30% lighter than cellulose acetate.[2] Because of its stability, Optyl is appropriate for those who might be allergic to other types of frame materials. (For more information on working with Optyl material, see Chapter 7, Insertion into an Optyl Frame.)

Nylon and Nylon-Based Materials

Nylon. Nylon is a material of high flexibility. When used alone in spectacle frames, nylon will lose that flexibility unless periodically soaked in water overnight. Otherwise, over time, it will become brittle. "Pure" nylon was previously used extensively for sports eyewear. It has also been used for over-the-counter sunglasses.[3] It is now being combined with other material for added strength and stability, remaining a part of the array of frame materials in use. (See Chapter 7, Insertion into a Nylon Frame.)

Polyamide/Copolyamide. Polyamide is a nylon-based material that is quite strong. Because it can be made thinner and is only 72% of the weight of cellulose acetate, polyamide has a real weight advantage. Polyamide frames can be made opaque or translucent. Frames made from polyamide are resistant to chemicals and solvents, and are also hypoallergenic.[3] (For more on polyamide frames, see Chapter 7, Insertion into a Polyamide Frame.)

Grilamid. Grilamid is a nylon-based material used in sports and performance type of eyewear. Unlike plain nylon frame material, grilamid has a large variety of color possibilities. Some manufacturers have fused Grilamid with titanium to create a strong, comfortable variation of this frame material.

Carbon Fiber

Carbon fiber material is used to create a thin, strong frame. This material is made from strands of carbon fibers combined with nylon. It is not adjustable and is consequently used mainly for frame fronts. The temples are generally made from another material. In other words, if a carbon fiber frame does not fit well in frame selection, do not plan on making it fit well later on. The principle advantage is the light weight that can be achieved. Carbon fiber is 60% the weight of cellulose acetate. Not only is the material light weight, but because of its strength, it can also be made thinner. Since carbon is black, frame colors will be opaque and are limited.

Some problems may be encountered with breakage in cold weather. Because of the thermal problems, it is imperative that the material not be directly worked with right after it has been outside. (For more information on working with carbon fiber material, see Chapter 7, Insertion into a Carbon Fiber Frame.)

Polycarbonate

Polycarbonate is a material usually associated with lenses, but can be molded into frames. Frames made from polycarbonate are primarily for sport or safety purposes. When made for nonprescription purposes, the lenses and frame are molded as one unit.

Frames (and lenses) made from polycarbonate are very impact resistant. Unfortunately, polycarbonate frames do not work well for conventional eyeglasses because of their resistance to adjustment. They are better suited for

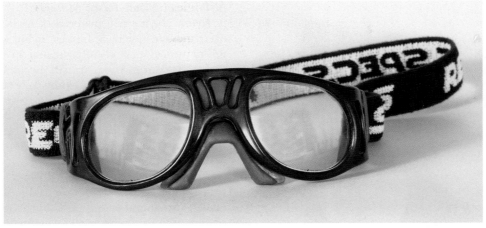

Figure 1-22. Polycarbonate sports frames can be ordered from the manufacturer with plano lenses already in place. They can also be ordered without lenses for prescription use.

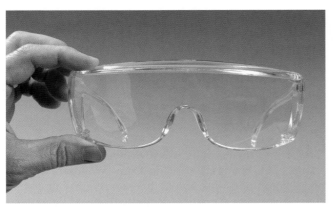

Figure 1-23. Safety frames with plano lenses can be molded as one unit. In the sample shown, both the frames and lenses are molded together from polycarbonate material.

the type of sports glasses that are held in place with elastic straps (Figure 1-22) or for shield types of glasses that may be used either alone or worn over conventional glasses (Figure 1-23).

Kevlar
Kevlar is a material that is also mixed with nylon. It, too, is a strong, lightweight ophthalmic frame material. Kevlar will remain stable over a large temperature range, but is difficult to adjust. Although it becomes pliable with heat, it will not shrink or stretch.

Rubber
Some sports eyewear and sunglass frames may be made from a combination of nylon and rubber. As would be expected, these frames are flexible and will return to their original shape, but are not adjustable.[4]

Combinations of Plastic Materials
There are numerous possible combinations of plastic materials. These include materials sometimes called

memory plastics. Memory plastics are tough and flexible. They can be bent or twisted and still return to their original shape.

Not all composite plastic materials are memory plastics. Other composite plastics combine various materials to produce frames and frame parts for specific needs and purposes.

Metal Frame Materials
In the past, gold-containing alloys were the more predominant metals used for spectacle frames. (See Chapter 2, Gold Classifications for Metal Frames with Substantial Gold Content.) Today few frames contain any gold.

Great progress has been made in metal frames because of the electrolytic treatment techniques, which allow for corrosion resistance and finished beauty. Any nostalgia over the disappearance of gold alloy frames from the marketplace should be dispelled by the beauty and serviceability of the product that has taken its place.

It is also common for frames to be made with more than one material. The temples may be from one material for flexibility, the frame front from another, and the connecting pieces something different still.

Nickel-Based Materials
Nickel is a material that is often used for eyeglass frames. It is strong and malleable. The main disadvantage is the number of people who may have an allergic reaction to nickel. It is reported that 10% of the population may be allergic to nickel.[5] Fortunately high-quality ophthalmic frames are coated with a protective material that both prevents corrosion and keeps the metal from coming in direct contact with the skin while the coating remains on the frame.

Pure Nickel. Nickel resists corrosion. Because of malleability, pure nickel frames are easily adjusted. Nickel's characteristic of accepting color well makes these frames versatile.

Nickel Silvers. Nickel silvers contain more than 50% copper, 25% nickel, and the rest zinc. But "nickel silver" contains no silver. Copper gives the material its pliability, zinc adds strength, and nickel gives the alloy a whitish appearance. When the nickel content of nickel silver exceeds 12%, the copper color no longer shows through.[1] Another name for nickel silver is *German silver*.

Monel Metal. Monel is whitish in color, is pliable for good adjustment, resists corrosion, and accepts a high polish. It is made from nickel, copper, iron, and traces of other elements. The largest component of the material (63% to 70%) is nickel. The second largest component is copper. Iron constitutes only 2.5%, and there are traces of silicium, carbon, and sulfur.[1] Monel is used quite often as a frame material.

Aluminum

Aluminum is both strong and extremely lightweight. It can be finished in a wide variety of colors and does not corrode. Aluminum does not solder or weld well, so must be made such that its parts are assembled with screws or rivets.[6] It holds the adjustment well, but has no flexibility. If it bends, it stays that way.

Stainless Steel

In the nineteenth century, some frames were made from regular (nonstainless) steel material. Stainless steel was developed in the early 20th century. It is made mainly from iron and chrome and is highly resistant to corrosion. Stainless steel is strong. When made very thin, it has an element of springiness and flexibility that makes it well suited for temples. Yet that very springiness means that "adjustments are difficult and often do not hold.[7]" Stainless steel is one of the more nonallergenic materials.

Titanium

Titanium is a versatile and abundant material that has become increasingly common for use in ophthalmic frames. The *advantages* include the following:

- Titanium is extremely light in weight. When compared with conventional metal frame materials, titanium is 48% lighter.[8]
- Titanium is very strong, which allows titanium frames to be designed exceedingly thin. Thinness also contributes to still more weight reduction.
- Titanium is very corrosion resistant. This makes titanium an excellent choice for people in hot climates or those working in conditions where they would be perspiring a great deal.
- Titanium is hypoallergenic. It should be noted that titanium is often used in combination with other metals. If the wearer is allergic to another of the metals in the alloy, then, unless the frame is appropriately coated, allergic reactions could still occur. But when titanium is not mixed with other metals, it is the metal of choice for those with skin allergies related to frame wear. This makes titanium a very attractive frame material for those with skin allergies.
- When used in combination with other metals, titanium allows frames to be made so that they are very flexible. It should be noted that some frames use titanium in combination with nickel to increase flexibility. Without an appropriate coating on the frame, this would increase the likelihood of an allergic response for some.

The *disadvantages* of titanium are fewer. These include the following:

- Titanium is hard to solder or weld.
- Because the manufacturing process is more demanding, titanium is more expensive than conventional materials.

Titanium Marking Guidelines and Classifications. The Vision Council of America (VCA) has established voluntary marking guidelines for frames containing titanium. The reason for these guidelines was "to end some of the confusion that arises when frames are labeled 'titanium' but are actually only part titanium—or do not contain titanium at all.[9]" Because these are voluntary guidelines, this means that there may still be some confusion in marking. However, if frames are marked according to VCA standards, then the buyer should know what that particular frame contains. To be certified, the titanium content of the frame must be tested by an independent accredited laboratory. Here are the guidelines:[10]

- *Certified 100% Titanium*—All major components of the frame are at least 90% titanium by weight and, to assure there will be no problems with wearer allergy, the frame must not contain any nickel (Figure 1-24, *A*).
- *Certified Beta Titanium*—All major components of the frame are at least 70% titanium by weight, and there must be no nickel content (Figure 1-24, *B*).

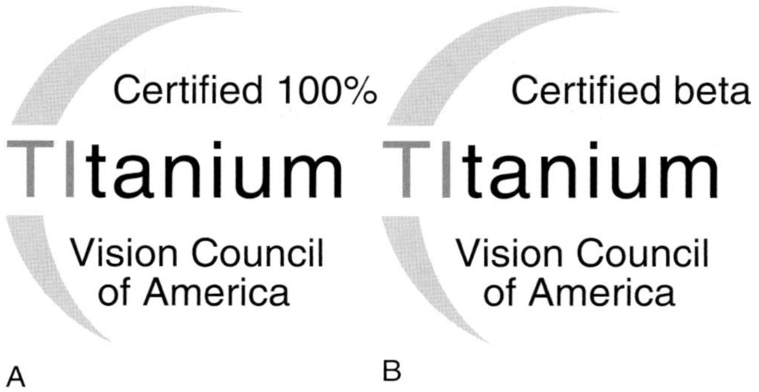

Certified 100% TItanium — Vision Council of America

A

Certified beta TItanium — Vision Council of America

B

Figure 1-24. The Vision Council of America marking guidelines for titanium uses a symbol that would normally appear on the demonstration lens of the display frame. **A,** Certified 100% Titanium means 90% titanium and there is no nickel contained in the frame. **B,** Certified Beta Titanium means 70% minimum titanium with no nickel content.

Not included in the Vision Council of American classification is what has been called *combination titanium*—a name applied to frames with titanium for the major parts of the frame and trim pieces made from other metals.[8] The name *nickel titanium* or *shape memory alloy (SMA)* is applied to a titanium alloy made with 40% to 50% titanium and the rest nickel.[11] Sometimes simply called *memory metal*,[12] this material is extremely flexible and returns to its original shape after being twisted or flexed. (It should be noted that there will be other types of metal frame materials that will also function like a "memory metal.")

Bronze
Bronze is a metal alloy traditionally made from copper and tin. It is suited for spectacle frames because it is corrosion-resistant, lightweight, and takes color well.

Magnesium
Magnesium is even lighter in weight than titanium. Frames made from magnesium are extremely lightweight and exceptionally durable. The exterior of the frame is normally sealed because of the corrosiveness of raw magnesium. Magnesium is also used as part of an alloy in combination with other metals.

Other Materials and Alloys
There are other materials that are also suitable for frames, including cobalt, palladium, ruthenium, and beryllium.

As would be expected, there are many different possible combinations of the previously listed metals that may be combined to optimize certain characteristics. Some have trade names applied especially for a particular combination used by a given frame manufacturer. One, for example, called FX9 is a combination of copper, manganese, tin, and aluminum engineered to yield a hypoallergenic, lightweight, and malleable material.[13] Another, referred to as Genium, combines 12% carbon, 17.5% to 20% manganese, 1% silicone, 17.5% to 20% chrome, and 58.9% to 63.9% steel. These materials are combined to create a hypoallergenic frame that is thin, strong, lightweight, flexible, and durable.[14] As frame designs change, metal alloy combinations will vary to meet these new design demands.

ALLERGIC REACTIONS TO FRAME MATERIALS

As previously noted, most frame manufacturers will use a coating on their plastic frames to protect the frames and also to reduce any possibility of allergic reactions. However, sometimes this is not enough.

To reduce the possibility of a reaction for people who have a history of skin reactions to wearing frames, use frame materials that are known to be hypoallergenic. Here are some that are reported to be hypoallergenic:

- Optyl material
- Polyamide/Copolyamide
- Titanium
- Stainless steel

If a person is already having a reaction to their frame, here are some things that may be done to the frame to reduce allergic reactions:

- Have a clear coat finish applied to a frame. Companies that specialize in frame repairs may offer this service. (Incidentally, some dispensers have tried to just coat the inside of the temples with clear nail polish to solve the problem. Unfortunately, this does not work for very long.)
- Use ultrathin, clear heat-shrink tubing over the temples. Optical shrink tubing is available from optical suppliers of spare pairs, pliers, and accessories.

If a person has an allergic reaction to nosepads, there are replacement pads available that will eliminate the problem. These pads are:

- Gold-plated metal nosepads
- Titanium nosepads
- Crystal nosepads

(See also the section in Chapter 10 on Hypoallergenic Nosepad Materials.)

For allergic reactions to metal cable temples, use a temple cover to cover the temple. Temple covers come in plastic, vinyl, and silicone materials. There is also "heat shrink" tubing sold for this purpose, which reportedly takes care of eliminating allergic reactions. (For more on this see the section in Chapter 10 on Adding Covers to Cable Temple Earpieces.)

An additional note on allergies: There is a liquid lens liner sometimes used in the groove of a frame to make a loose lens more secure. This material contains latex and should not be used on frames whose wearers have latex allergies.

REFERENCES

1. Ophthalmic optics files: 8. Spectacle Frames, Paris, undated, Essilor International.
2. Today's frame material for tomorrow, Munich, Germany, undated, Optyl Holding GmbH & Co.
3. August EC: Professional selling skills and frame materials, Eye Quest Magazine, 2:40, 42, 1992.
4. Bruneni JL: Perspective on lenses 1995, Merrifield, Va, Optical Laboratories Association.
5. Parker L: Titanium tactics—part 2: translating titanium into sales, Eyewear, 1999.
6. Barnett D: What's in a frame? Eyecare Business, September, p.76, 1988.
7. DiSanto M: Rimless eyewear: making the right choice, 20/20, New York, NY, 2004, Jobson Publishing.
8. Szczerbiak M: The ABCs of titanium frames, Visioncare-products.com, vol 2, no 1, January/February 2002.
9. OMA debuts titanium guideline, Eyecare Business, August, p. 22, 1999.

10. Vision Council of America, Titanium marking guidelines, http://www.visionsite.org/s_vision/sec.asp?TRACKID=&CID=266&DID=397, February 2006.

11. Hohnstine, Nicola, Spina: Make it a lite...a titanium lite, 20/20 Online, 30:11, 2003.

12. What are the different frame materials? Essilor website: Http://www.essilorha.com/frames.htm, excerpted from

"OLA Perspective on Lenses," Optical Laboratory Association, 1997.

13. O'Keefe J: Make mine metal, Visioncareproducts.com, vol 4, April 2004.

14. O'Keefe J: Frame materials go beyond zyl and monel, Visioncareproducts.com, vol 3, May 2003.

Proficiency Test

(Answers can be found in the back of the book.)

Match the name of the frame with its description:

1. ___C___ Commonly has a metal chassis and plastic top rims.

2. ___D___ Has two holes per lens and a metal reinforcing arm that follows the upper posterior surface of the lens.

3. ___E___ Holds the lenses in place only at their nasal edge.

    a. Balgrip
    b. Half-eyes
    c. Combination
    d. Semirimless
    e. Numont

Match the name of the frame with its description:

4. ___B___ Made especially for those needing a reading correction but no distance correction

5. ___A___ Secures the lenses in place with clips attached to a bar of tensile steel that fits into a slot on each side of the lenses

6. ___D___ Secures the lenses in place by means of a small string that goes around the lenses

    a. balgrip
    b. half-eyes
    c. semirimless
    d. nylon cord

Match the following terms:

7. ___h___ Optyl

8. ___A___ lorgnettes

9. ___f___ aluminum

10. ___C___ half-eyes

11. ___B___ "shell"

12. ___G___ convertible

13. ___i___ nylon cord

14. ___e___ Numont

15. ___d___ earpiece

    a. hand-held
    b. "zyl"
    c. reading
    d. curl
    e. only nasal
    f. anodized
    g. straight back
    h. has memory
    i. string mount

16. Which type of temple curves around the ear following the crotch of the ear where ear and head meet, extending to the level of the earlobe? This type of temple is usually plastic, and is often used in children's and safety frames.
    a. library
    b. skull
    c. riding bow
    d. convertible

17. This follows the bridge of the nose smoothly, spreading the weight of the frame and using nose pads attached to the back of the bridge.
    a. keyhole bridge
    b. modified saddle bridge
    c. saddle bridge
    d. pad bridge
    e. none of the above

Match the description with the correct frame material:

18. _E_ A frame material that is generally made into sheets and milled to make frames.

19. _A_ A material of high flexibility that will maintain that flexibility when soaked overnight periodically.

20. _B_ Frames from this material can be made thin and are lightweight. Frame colors are primarily opaque and some problems may be encountered with breakage in cold weather.

21. _F_ Used primarily for sport or safety purposes. Does not adjust well. Does not work well for conventional eyeglasses.

22. _G_ Frames made from these materials are made beginning with granules that are heated until liquid, then injection molded to the desired frame shape.

23. _C_ A nylon-based material that can be made translucent, not just opaque.

24. _H_ This material is made from a liquid resin and a hardener that are mixed together and drawn into the frame molds using a vacuum process.

a. nylon
b. carbon fiber
c. polyamide
d. Kevlar
e. cellulose acetate
f. polycarbonate
g. propionate
h. optyl

Match the description with the correct frame material so that all answers are used and no answer is used more than once:

25. _E_ Is often used for temples because of its strength and flexibility.

26. _D_ Extremely light in weight and will not rust. Can be made thin.

27. _B_ Is lightweight and can be finished in a variety of colors.

28. _F_ A synonym for nickel silver.

29. _A_ Is whitish in color, pliable, resists corrosion, and accepts a high polish.

30. _C_ Resists corrosion, malleable, accepts color well.

a. Monel metal
b. aluminum
c. pure nickel
d. titanium
e. stainless steel
f. German silver

Match the following titanium frame material classifications with the most appropriate answer:

31. _B_ Shape memory alloy

32. _C_ Certified 100% titanium

33. _A_ Certified Beta titanium

a. All major components at least 70% titanium by weight. No nickel.
b. Combination of titanium and nickel.
c. All major components at least 90% titanium by weight. No nickel.
d. All titanium and no other metal present.
e. All major components at least 70% titanium by weight and remainder nickel.

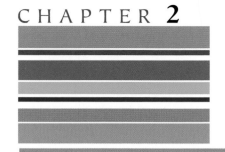

CHAPTER 2

Frame Measurements and Markings

Familiarity with frame measurements and how they are marked is essential to proper ordering of prescription glasses. Knowledge of measurement procedures assures receipt of the proper size when ordering a replacement for a broken part. The purpose of this chapter is to give the reader a complete understanding of frame dimensional properties. The confidence and capability achieved as a result of this is the base on which to develop skill in frame selection.

THE OLDER DATUM SYSTEM

The previously used datum system for measuring lenses was established as a system of reference points for frames and lenses so that placement of lens optical centers and bifocal segment heights would be consistent.

With the lens placed as it should sit in the frame, horizontal lines were drawn at the highest and lowest edges of the lens (Figure 2-1). A line drawn halfway between the two horizontal lines and parallel to them was known as the *datum line*. The width of the lens along this line was called the *datum length* or eye size. The point along the datum line halfway between the edges of the lens is the *datum center*. The depth of the lens, measured as the vertical depth through the datum center, was the *mid-datum depth*.

The datum system preceded the currently used boxing system.

THE BOXING SYSTEM

The boxing system improved on the foundation provided by the datum system. The datum system used two horizontal lines—one against the top and the other against the bottom of the lens. The boxing system kept these two horizontal lines and added two vertical lines. These vertical lines are placed against right and left edges of the lens. All four lines form a box around the lens (Figure 2-2).

Horizontal Midline

There is a horizontal line halfway between the top and bottom of the lens. In the datum system, this was called the datum line. This name continues to be used. However, in the boxing system, this line is more commonly referred to as the *horizontal midline* or *the 180-degree line*.

Geometric Center

The center of the lens is the point on the horizontal midline halfway between the two lens-bordering vertical lines. It is known as the *geometric center* or *boxing center* of the edged lens. This term does not imply anything about the optical positioning of the lens.

Size

The size of the lens then is the length and depth of the box containing the lens. The horizontal length is now commonly referred to as the *eye size* when referring to the frame and the *lens size* when referring to the lenses. Both are measured in millimeters.

When most practitioners speak of lens size or eye size, they are referring primarily to the horizontal measure of the lens, denoted by the letter "A" in Figure 2-2. Some frames list an eye size value that is different from and unrelated to the frame A dimension. Such procedures attempt to relate this eye size number to a "fitting value." This is not a recommended practice and leads to confusion, but is so commonplace that frame reference materials will usually list both an A dimension and an eye size, even if they are the same value.

The letter "B" denotes the vertical measure of the box enclosing the lens. Both "A" and "B" are in a sense independent of lens shape. The letter "C" refers to the width of the lens itself along the horizontal midline.[1] (This can vary considerably from the A dimension.) The C dimension of a lens is seldom used. In the older datum system, this was the eye size of the frame. Some people still mistakenly measure the eye size this way.

The C dimension of a lens should not be confused with the "C-size" of a lens. *C-size* is the circumference of the edged lens and is sometimes used to increase accuracy when duplicating an old lens size when edging.

Measurement

In determining the horizontal boxing dimensions of a *frame*, the measurement begins at the inside of the groove on the left side of the imaginary enclosing box and extends horizontally across the lens opening to the farthest part of the groove on the right side of the box (Figure 2-3). Do not tilt the box.

In measuring a *lens*, the measurement begins at the apex, or point, of the bevel on the left side of the box enclosing the lens and extends to the apex of the bevel on the right side of the box. Remember, the A dimension is the width of the enclosing box. It is not the width of the lens at the middle of the shape.

Effective Diameter

The effective diameter of a lens is found by doubling the distance from the geometric center of the lens to the apex of the lens bevel farthest from it (see Figure 2-2).

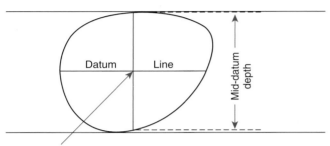

Figure 2-1. In the datum system, the middatum depth may not always be equal to the distance between the horizontal tangents. The datum eye size is the width of the lens at the level of the datum line. The datum system eye size and the boxing system eye size are not the same. Some measure the eye size according to the datum system, thinking they are using the boxing system. The two eye size measures are not the same.

This measurement helps determine the smallest lens blank from which the lens can be cut. (See Chapter 5: Determining Lens Blank Size.)

Frame Difference

The difference between the horizontal and the vertical measurements is known as the *frame difference* and is measured in millimeters. The larger the difference, the more rectangular the enclosing box appears (Figure 2-4). Frame difference is sometimes referred to as *lens difference*.

Distance Between Lenses (DBL) or Bridge Size

The boxing system also makes it possible to define the distance between lenses (DBL). The DBL is the distance between the two boxes when both lenses are boxed off in the frame. This is usually synonymous with bridge size, although it is important to note that manufacturers not adhering to the boxing system may mark a bridge size that does not correspond to the distance between lenses.

Bridge size or DBL is measured on the frame as the distance from the inside nasal eyewire grooves across the bridge area at the narrowest point (Figure 2-5). This distance is measured in millimeters. Naturally, two frames having the same DBL will not necessarily fit the same person in the same manner because of variations in lens shapes.

Geometric Center Distance (GCD)

The distance between the two geometric centers of the lenses is known as the geometric center distance (GCD).

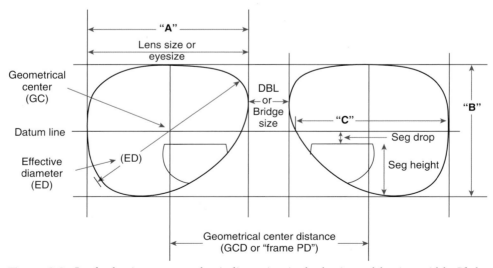

Figure 2-2. In the boxing system, the A dimension is the horizontal boxing width. If the frame is properly marked, the eye size will be equal to the A dimension of the frame. The B dimension is the vertical boxing length. The C dimension is the width of the lens along the horizontal midline. This dimension is seldom used today. The C dimension should not be confused with the "C-size" of a lens. The C-size of a lens is the distance around the lens (i.e., its circumference). The dispenser uses the C-size to ensure that a lens ordered by itself (without the frame) will be exactly sized for that frame.

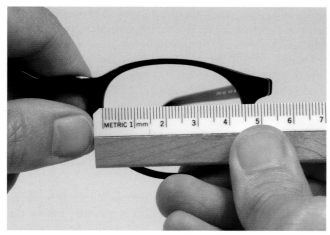

Figure 2-3. To measure the horizontal dimension of a frame, the measurement begins at the inside of the groove on one side and extends across the lens opening to the farthest part of the groove on the other. We cannot see the inside of the groove when looking from the front. This means we can estimate where it will be and hold the ruler so that the zero point is at the position of the left-hand side of the groove. Then we need to read the ruler at the position where the groove will be on the right. If the opening itself is measured, then about ½ mm per side needs to be added to the measure to allow for the depth of the groove. This may vary somewhat, depending upon the depth of the groove.

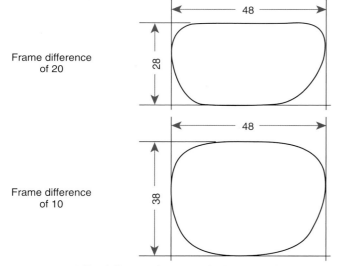

Frame difference of 20

Frame difference of 10

Figure 2-4. The difference between the horizontal and vertical measurements of a frame is known as the frame difference.

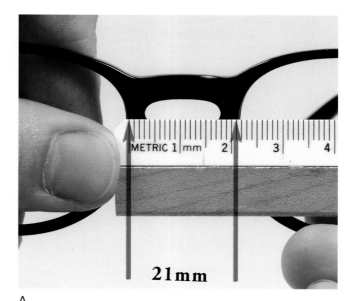

21mm

A

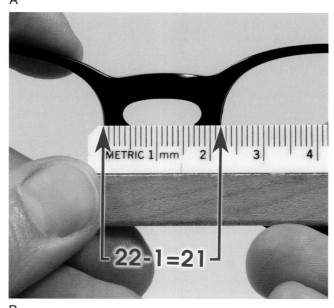

22−1=21

B

Figure 2-5. A, The DBL or bridge size is measured on the frame as the distance from the inside nasal eyewire grooves across the bridge area at its narrowest point. When measuring the bridge size, we cannot see the inside of the groove and must estimate its location. **B,** If the measurement is made from lens opening to lens opening, then approximately ½ mm per groove must be *subtracted* from the measure depending upon the depth of the groove.

It can be measured more easily as the distance from the far left side of one lens opening to the far left side of the other (i.e., from the left side of one "box" to the left side of the other "box.") Or the geometric center distance can be calculated by simply adding the eye size to the DBL. The result is the same.

The GCD is also known by three other names:
1. *Distance between centers* (DBC)
2. *Frame center distance*
3. *Frame PD*

The term frame PD is commonly used in dispensing, but has no relationship to the wearer's

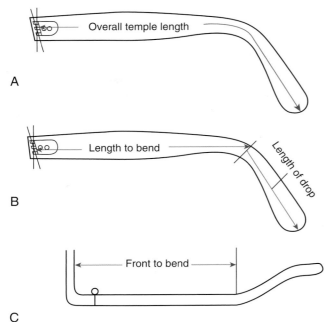

Figure 2-6. A-C, Various methods used in specifying temple lengths.

interpupillary distance or distance between pupil centers.*

Seg Height

When specifying bifocal or trifocal segment height, the reference points are given in millimeters as either (l) the distance below or above the horizontal midline (called *seg drop* or *seg raise*), or (2) the distance from the lower line of the boxing system rectangle enclosing the lens shape (called *seg height*). In the actual measuring process, the level of the lower line of the box corresponds to the lowest point in the eyewire groove. *This level may be different from the depth of the point on the lens edge found directly below the pupil* as can be seen by looking carefully at Figure 2-2.

TEMPLE LENGTH

Most temples are currently marked with the total, or overall, temple length. Temple lengths are expressed in millimeters. Temple length may be measured in one of the following ways.

Overall Temple Length

The overall temple length is the distance from the center of the center barrel screw hole to the posterior end of the temple, measured along the center of the temple (Figure 2-6, *A*). Many times the center of the barrel

*The term "Frame PD" may have originated when frame size was determined by selecting the correctly fitting bridge size, then choosing an eye size so that the wearer's pupils would be at the geometric centers of the frame's lens openings.

screw hole will match the position of the butt end of the temple. But this is not always the case. Also, when measuring the overall temple length, it is necessary to measure around the bend and not in a straight line, unless of course the temple is straight. The easiest way to do this is shown in Figure 2-7, *A* through *D*.

Comfort cable temples are measured in terms of overall length. The actual measurement is done by grasping the tip and extending the temple along the ruler (Figure 2-8).

Length to Bend (LTB)

An older method of measuring temple length is in terms of the length to bend (LTB). This is measured from the center of the barrel to the middle of the bend (Figure 2-6, *B*). The distance from the middle of the temple bend to the end of the temple is known as the *length of drop* (see Figure 2-6, *B*).

Front to Bend (FTB)

If the endpieces wrap around in a swept-back manner, there is a distance between the plane of the frame front and the actual beginning of the temple. In this case, the temple length could be specified as frame to bend (FTB) (Figure 2-6, *C*), which would be slightly longer than LTB. This measurement method is seldom used.

FRAME MARKINGS

Most frames are marked according to size with three measurements: eye size, DBL, and temple length. Metal frames that are manufactured from "rolled gold" are also marked as to the amount of gold found in the frame. Rolled gold frames were used regularly a good while ago. Any new rolled gold frames are very expensive.

Eye Size and DBL

When a frame marking such as 50□20 is seen, it means that the eye size is 50 mm and the distance between lenses is 20 mm. The box between the numbers means that the eye size is measured according to the boxing method; it also serves to separate the two numbers and prevent confusion. The eye size and DBL are sometimes simply marked 50-20 or 50/20.

Location of Markings

On a *plastic frame* the marking may be found in any of several places. It may be printed on the inside of the nosepad, or it may be found on the upper outer section of the eyewire. Some frames had the size printed on the back side of the endpiece, and the temple must be folded closed to find it. Sometimes the eye size is printed on one endpiece and the DBL on the other. As it should be, temple length is printed on the inner side of the temples. Some manufacturers put all three measurements on the temple. This is done because most frames are sold as a complete unit rather than a frame front with a matching

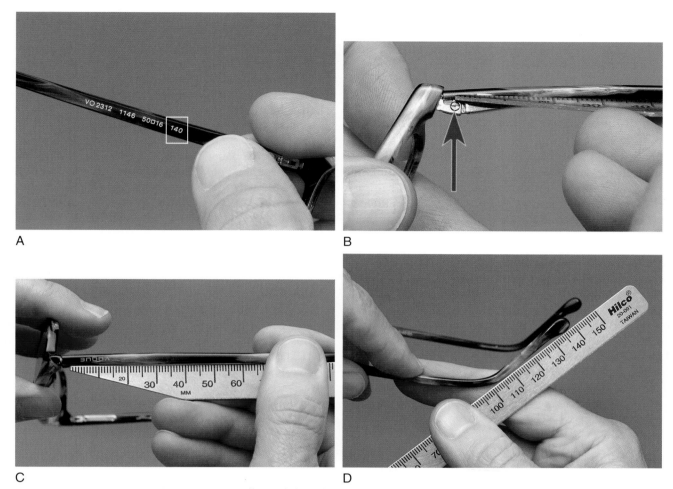

Figure 2-7. Measuring overall temple length. **A,** Here is a temple marked with a temple length of 140. We will be measuring this temple and comparing our results with what is marked. **B,** Begin the measurement by placing the zero on the ruler at the center of the hinge barrel, as seen in this measuring view. **C,** Looking at the temple from the side it is evident that the zero point is not at the butt end of the temple. Often times the position of the center of the barrel and the butt end of the temple are at the same location. It is obvious from the photo that in this case they are not and the beginning point for measuring does not start at the end of the temple. **D,** Turn the ruler around the temple bend and note where the end of the temple falls on the ruler scale. This is the overall temple length.

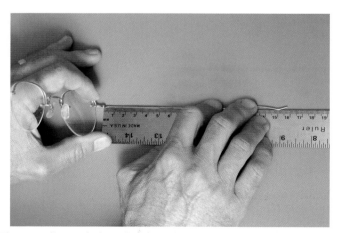

Figure 2-8. The overall temple length for a cable temple is obtained by stretching the cable temple along the ruler.

set of temples. Unfortunately this leads to confusion when temples are exchanged.

On *metal frames* and frames with metal chassis, the eye size and DBL are usually on the inside of the bridge, although occasionally they are printed on the underside of a top reinforcing bar, or again, on the temples.

Frame Manufacturer Name, Color, and Country of Origin

Frames should also be marked as to country of origin, manufacturer, and frame name. Many frame manufacturers use a number rather than a name. This can be confusing if the frame color is also specified by number and both numbers are stamped on the frame. Consulting a frame reference catalog or database will help.

Safety Frame Markings

Frames that are suitable for use as safety glasses must have "Z87" or "Z87-2" and the name or logo of the manufacturer stamped on the frame front and on both temples. This is as specified by the American National Standards Institute (ANSI) in their standard called *American National Standard Practice for Occupational and Educational Eye and Face Protection*. The standard is numbered as Z87.1. If a pair of glasses has safety lenses, but is not in a frame marked "Z87" or "Z87-2," the glasses are not safety glasses. (For more on safety eyewear, see Chapter 23.)

Gold Classifications for Metal Frames With Substantial Gold Content

Metal frames may not have any gold or any significant amount of gold in the frame. This does not imply anything about the quality of the frame. (See Chapter 1 for more on frame materials.) When a frame has a substantial gold content, numbers other than those indicating the size of the frame are printed on the frame to indicate the nature of the gold content. Gold or part-gold articles can be classified as fine gold, solid gold, gold filled, or having gold plating or gold flashing (Table 2-1).

The color of a frame with gold content has nothing to do with its quality. The color depends on what type of metal is used in combination with gold to make the gold alloy.

The karat system is used to determine the amount of gold present. The number marked on the article is the amount of gold by weight in comparison to a total of 24 units: an article marked 12k is an alloy made up of one-half gold and one-half another metal.

Fine Gold

Fine gold is the name used for an article that has no metal in it other than gold. The gold found in it is chemically pure. Although this is the purest form, it is not always the most practical, as is the case in spectacle frames. Frames of fine gold would be too malleable and would bend and dent too easily to be practical. Using the karat system, fine gold is 24 karats fine, which means that by weight, 24 parts out of 24 are gold.

Solid Gold

Solid gold articles are actually an alloy of gold and another metal, a mixture of gold and a base metal. Thus the term is misleading, as it does not mean all gold. The solid gold article is made entirely of the gold alloy. It maintains its luster regardless of how far down it is worn through use.

The symbol θ is used to denote a 10k solid gold bridge; the symbol $\square$ to denote a 12k solid gold bridge.

Gold Filled

Gold-filled articles are made of a metal other than gold and then covered with a gold alloy. The term does not indicate that the article is "filled with gold," but rather the opposite: an outer wrapper of gold alloy is "filled" with a baser metal. To be classified as gold filled, a minimum of one twentieth of the article's total weight must be gold.

Articles in this classification are marked with a fraction, a karat rating, and the abbreviation for gold filled. The fraction shows what part of the total weight of the article is represented by the gold alloy covering. The karat rating shows, as always, the amount of gold by weight in the gold alloy in comparison to a total of 24 units. The GF classifies the article as gold filled. For example:

- 1/10—10% of the total weight of the article is alloy.
- 12k—12 parts out of 24 parts of the covering alloy by weight are gold.
- GF—The article is classified as gold filled.

Thus the article would bear the marking of 1/10 12k GF.

A gold-filled article retains its luster until the gold covering eventually wears through.

If a frame is made from parts having different percents of gold, the frame must be marked according to the part containing the least amount of gold. If, for example, the temples are 1/8 12k GF and the front is 1/10 12k GF, the frame must be marked 1/10 12k GF.

TABLE 2-1 Gold Classifications	
Name	**Meaning**
Fine gold	100% pure gold
Solid gold	Gold plus base metal evenly mixed throughout
Gold filled	Base metal inside a "solid gold" coating
Gold plating	A base metal thinly plated with gold
Gold flashing	A base metal with gold thinly and quickly applied in a manner similar to that of gold plating

Gold Plating

Gold plate articles are made of some other metal, the surface of which is plated with gold, usually by an electrolytic process. Articles classified as gold plate have no minimum requirement as to the total amount of gold used. Gold plate articles maintain luster only until the thin plating is worn through and the base metal is exposed.

Gold Flashing

Gold flashing is a method of gold application that is done in almost the same way that gold plating is done, only faster. Gold flashing is applied using a cyanide-based bath instead of an acid-based bath.[2] It produces an extremely thin layer of gold. If it were not for the protective coating, which works very well, the gold would not be very durable. A large percentage of spectacle frames have gold flashing and because of the coating are very serviceable.

For a summary of gold classifications, see Table 2-1.

REFERENCES

1. Fry G: The boxing system of lens and frame measurement, part IV, Optical J and Rev Optom 98(17):32-38, 1961.
2. Sipe J: As good as gold, Eyewear Feb:44, 1998.

Proficiency Test

(Answers can be found in the back of the book.)

There may be more than one correct response to some of the multiple choice questions found below.

1. True or false? In the boxing system, the effective diameter is the diagonal of the box.

2. True or false? The frame difference for a frame with a circular lens shape is always zero.

3. Answer yes or no to each of the following: Is the geometric center distance the same as:
   a. the eye size plus the bridge size?   (yes/no)
   b. the wearer's PD?   (yes/no)
   c. the "frame PD"?   (yes/no)

4. Would the above GCD change if the lenses were decentered in 3 mm each?

5. A frame has the following dimensions:
   A = 51
   B = 47
   C = 49.5
   DBL = 19
   Seg drop (distance below the horizontal midline) = 4 mm
   What is the seg height?
   a. 19.5 mm
   b. 20 mm
   c. 21.5 mm
   d. 23.5 mm
   e. none of the above

6. The larger the frame difference, the _____ the lens shape.
   a. rounder
   b. more squared off
   c. narrower
   d. wider (i.e., deeper)

7. If a frame's dimensions are A = 50 and C = 48, with a frame difference of 8, what is B?
   a. 58 mm
   b. 56 mm
   c. 52 mm
   d. 46 mm
   e. 42 mm

8. A frame is marked 52□18. The lens shape is round. What is the effective diameter of the lens?
   a. 70 mm
   b. 61 mm
   c. 58 mm
   d. 52 mm
   e. 18 mm

9. What is the geometric center distance of a frame marked 52□17?
   a. 52
   b. 60.5
   c. 69
   d. 72
   e. equal to the person's PD

10. What gold classification(s) has/have no minimum requirement as to the total amount of gold used?
   a. fine gold
   b. solid gold
   c. gold filled
   d. gold plated
   e. gold flash

11. The color of a frame with gold in it depends on:
   a. the quality of gold used.
   b. the quantity of gold used.
   c. the kind of metal used to make the alloy.
   d. the kind of base metal used in the frame.
   e. none of the above

12. An article made out of a metal other than gold and then covered with a gold alloy may be:
   a. fine gold.
   b. gold filled.
   c. gold plated.
   d. rolled gold.
   e. gold flash.

13. What is the name used for an article that has no metal in it other than chemically pure gold?
   a. fine gold
   b. gold filled
   c. gold plated
   d. gold flash

14. A frame marked θ 1/10 12k GF
   a. has 10% gold by weight.
   b. has a 12k solid gold bridge.
   c. has a 10k solid gold bridge.
   d. is 50% gold by weight.
   e. is 10% gold by volume.

Matching

15. ____ A   a. 2 × (longest radius)

16. ____ B   b. vertical boxing dimension

17. ____ ED   c. A + DBL

18. ____ GCD   d. eye size

                          e. C

19. Safety frames must be marked with
   a. The manufacturer's name on both of the temples and the frame front.
   b. "Z80" or "Z80-2" on both of the temples and the frame front.
   c. "Z87" or "Z87-2" on both of the temples and the frame front.
   d. The manufacturer's name and "Z80" or "Z80-2" on both of the temples and the frame front.
   e. The manufacturer's name and "Z87" or "Z87-2" on both of the temples and the frame front.

CHAPTER 3

Measuring the Interpupillary Distance

This chapter provides the methodology for measuring the interpupillary distance (PD). Failure to accurately determine the interpupillary distance results in a misplacement of the optical center of the lenses. This induces unwanted prismatic effects, requiring the wearer to turn his eyes inward, or even outward, to keep from experiencing double vision. Over time, this effort causes visual discomfort and can result in a decreased ability of the eyes to work together in binocular vision.

DEFINITION

The *anatomic PD* is the distance from the center of one pupil to the center of the other pupil, measured in millimeters. Before ordering prescription glasses or even before doing a visual examination, the distance between the pupils must be determined. It can be measured in a variety of ways.

DISTANCE PD

Binocular PD

The most common method used to measure the PD also requires the least amount of equipment. The technique uses a simple millimeter ruler, commonly referred to as a *PD rule.*

Technique

When the PD is to be measured, the dispenser should be positioned at a distance of 40 cm (16 inches) directly in front of the subject, with his or her eyes at the same vertical level as those of the subject. The PD rule is positioned across the subject's nose with the measuring edge tilted back so that it rests on the most recessed part of the nose. The dispenser holds the PD rule between thumb and forefinger and steadies the hand by placing the remaining three fingers against the subject's head.

The dispenser closes the right eye and sights with the left (Figure 3-1). The subject is instructed to look at the dispenser's open eye while the dispenser lines up the zero mark of the rule with the center of the subject's pupil.

When the zero mark is lined up correctly, the dispenser closes the left eye and opens the right. The subject

is instructed to look at the dispenser's open eye. The PD for the distance prescription is read off as that mark falling in the center of the subject's left pupil (Figure 3-2).

The dispenser now closes the right eye and opens the left. The subject is again instructed to look at the dispenser's open eye. This step is primarily a recheck to make sure the zero mark is still properly aligned. (This technique is summarized in Box 3-1.)

When difficulty is experienced in determining the exact center of the pupil, the edge of the pupil may be used as a measuring point if both pupils are the same size. Measurement is read from the left side of one pupil to the left side of the other. Measuring from the inside edge of one pupil to the inside edge of the other would give an artificially low reading; from the outside edge of one pupil to the outside edge of the other, an artificially high reading.

When a person has dark irises or unequally sized pupils, it may be difficult to use either the center or the edge of the pupil. In this case, the dispenser may use the limbus edge—the sharp demarcation between white sclera and dark iris (Figure 3-3). (Because the pupil is displaced 0.3 mm nasal ward from the center of the limbal ring,[1] a limbal measure will be approximately 0.5 mm greater than the measure found using pupil centers.) The same rule must be applied when using the limbus edge as when using the pupil edge: the same sides of the limbus (both left or both right) must be used, or an extremely large error is induced.

Common Difficulties and Their Solutions

Dispenser Cannot Close One Eye. Occasionally the person doing the measuring is unable to close one eye independent of the other. This can be remedied by occluding (covering) the eye with the free hand. The practice of holding the lid down with one finger gives an unprofessional appearance, especially when wearing glasses. Occluding the eye with the hand held flat appears to be a natural part of the test and does not reveal a person's inability to close only one eye.

Dispenser Visually Impaired in One Eye. If the dispenser is blind in one eye, or has visual acuity too poor to allow the ruler to be read accurately, then the technique is modified. The dispenser places the good eye directly in front of the subject's right eye and at the normal distance. The zero mark is lined up as usual. The dispenser then moves sideways until the good eye is positioned in front of the subject's left eye and the measurement is read. Unfortunately this method can easily lead to parallax errors. The most desirable solution for someone with this difficulty is to use another type of instrument that only requires the use of one eye.

Subject Is Strabismic. The strabismic subject, whose eyes are in a tropic position (i.e., with one eye pointing in a different direction from the other) presents a special problem, since the PD rule method of measurement may then give an artificially high or low reading. To determine a true reading, simply cover the subject's eye not

being observed. This ensures that the subject is fixating with the eye under observation and ensures that it is not turned unless eccentric fixation is present. Even if eccentric fixation is present, the PD measurement is still correct, since the subject never uses this eye in any other position relative to the dominant eye.

In some instances where one eye turns out constantly, the prescribing doctor may determine that the wearer is better served if the lenses are centered in front of the pupils, even for the eye that is turned. This will require that a separate measure be taken for each eye. One measurement will then be considerably larger than the other.

Subject Is an Uncooperative Child. If the subject is young or uncooperative, making normal PD measurements impossible, the dispenser may have to take a canthus-to-canthus measurement. (The canthus is the corner of the eye where the upper and lower lids meet.) This is done by measuring from the outer canthus of one eye to the inner canthus of the other eye. Unfortunately,

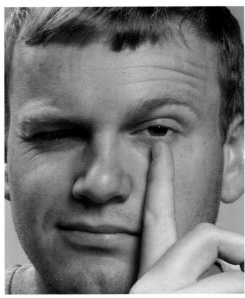

Figure 3-1. Position of the dispenser for beginning the PD measurement using just a PD ruler.

BOX 3-1

Steps in Measuring the Binocular Distance PD

1. Dispenser positions at 40 cm (16 in).
2. Dispenser closes right eye, subject fixates on dispenser's left eye.
3. Dispenser lines up zero point on subject's right eye at the pupil center, left pupillary border, or left limbus.
4. Dispenser closes left eye, opens right eye; subject fixates right eye.
5. Dispenser reads off scale directly in line with left pupil center, left pupillary border, or left limbus.
6. Dispenser closes right eye, opens left; subject fixates left eye.
7. Dispenser checks to make sure zero point is still correct.

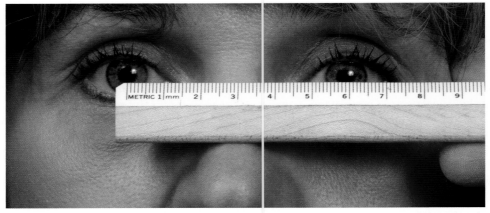

Figure 3-2. The dispenser uses his or her left eye to establish the zero point of the PD rule in the center of the pupil of the subject's right eye as shown here. The subject is looking at the dispenser's left eye. Next the subject looks at the dispenser's right eye. The dispenser uses his or her right to read the pupillary distance at the center of the subject's left eye. (This is not what is seen in this photo.)

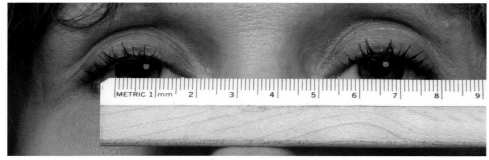

Figure 3-3. When the subject has dark irises, the outside edge of the limbus may be used as the zero reference point and the inside limbal edge of the other eye as the measuring point.

this measurement is not entirely exact, since the inner canthi of the eyes encroach farther across the sclera with younger children.

Common Causes of Errors

There are several common causes of errors inherent in using a PD rule.[2]

1. There will be an error in measurement if the measurer's PD differs significantly from the subject's because the lines of sight are not parallel. For example, if the measurer's PD is 16 mm larger than the subject's, the reading will be 1 mm too high because of this parallactic error.
2. The above error will be increased if the PD rule is not tilted on the subject's nose so that the scale is in the most recessed area. The most recessed area corresponds to the approximate position where the spectacles will be worn.
3. Just as error will be increased when the measurer's PD is significantly different from the subject's, the parallactic error will also be increased even more if the dispenser is too close to the subject. Too close is closer than the normal 40 cm (16 inch) distance.
4. A significant error will be induced if the subject is strabismic (one eye turns in or out) or if the subject does not fixate binocularly* during the PD measurement.
5. An error can result if the subject's head moves.
6. An error can result if the person measuring moves his or her head.
7. An error will result if the person measuring does not close or occlude one eye at a time to ensure sighting from directly in front of the subject's eye under observation.
8. The subject may not look directly at the measurer's pupil during the test, as he or she should, which will result in an error.

---

*What does "not fixating binocularly" mean? It means that one eye may have a tendency to turn in or out when the subject is not concentrating. In simple terms, they will only be using one eye to see instead of both eyes. When this does happen, one eye usually turns outward somewhat and the measurement is then too large.

Monocular PD

Since faces are not always symmetrical, it is often necessary to specify the PD for each eye independently. The main goal in taking the PD is to eventually place the optical centers of the lenses directly in front of the subject's eyes to prevent any undesired prismatic effect.

If one eye is set closer to a person's nose than is the other and the optical centers of the lenses are placed symmetrically in the frames, the wearer's lines of sight will not pass through the optical centers of the lenses. The error is not too serious if the lenses are of the same power and are not strong. If, however, one lens is very different from the other, the centers must be placed accurately to prevent unwanted binocular prismatic effects (Figure 3-4). Monocular PDs are also important when using aspheric lenses or high index lenses, including polycarbonate lenses. High index lenses have more chromatic aberration than crown glass or regular (CR-39) plastic lenses. The negative effect of chromatic aberration on vision is increased if the eye is not looking through the optical center of the lens. (For more information on high index lenses, see Chapter 23. For more information on aspheric lenses, see Chapter 18.)

Procedure for Measuring Monocular PDs Using a Ruler

The monocular PD is best taken using a pupillometer. When a pupillometer is not available, monocular PDs are taken by measuring from the center of the nose to the center of the pupils. The procedure consists of the following three steps:

1. Measure the binocular PD as described earlier in the chapter. Use the center of the pupil as the reference point.
2. Before moving the ruler, note the scale reading on the ruler at the center of the nose. This is the right monocular PD.
3. Subtract this reading from the binocular reading to obtain the left monocular PD.

For example, the binocular PD is 66. The scale reading at the center of the nose is 32. The monocular PD for the right eye is then 32. To calculate the monocular PD

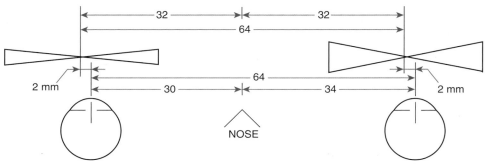

Figure 3-4. Here the PD has been measured binocularly as shown on the top measurements. However, the wearer has very different monocular PDs. Even though the distance PD is 64, the monocular PDs are not 32 and 32. Instead they are 30 and 34. When the lenses are made as if the wearer had 32/32 monocular PDs, in this case there will be unintended Base Out prism caused by the misplaced lenses.

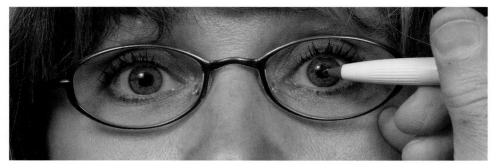

Figure 3-5. To measure monocular PDs using a marking pen and a frame with lenses in the frame, the same procedure is followed as would be used with a ruler. It is essential that the wearer be looking at the dispenser's eye that is directly in front of the eye being measured. In other words, to mark the location of the wearer's right pupil center, the wearer looks at the dispenser's open, left eye. (The dispenser's right eye is closed.) To mark the location of the wearer's left pupil center, the wearer looks at the dispenser's open right eye. (The dispenser's left eye is closed.)

for the left eye, subtract 32 from 66, to get a reading of 34. The procedure is the same as in taking a binocular PD measurement, except that the two readings are independent of one another and, for purposes of measuring, the center of the pupil is always used. (There are other methods that are considerably more dependable than this method in their ability to yield consistently accurate results.)

Procedure for Measuring Monocular PDs Using the Frame

One error inherent in using a ruler alone appears when a person has an asymmetrical nose. An asymmetrical nose often occurs when a nose has been broken. In this case, the frame positions itself somewhat to the left or right. For the lenses to be accurately placed, this factor must be taken into account. It is possible to use an overhead transparency marking pen and the glazed* lenses

in the sample frame. If the sample frame does not have glazed lenses, clear tape may be placed over the lens opening of the empty frame.

The procedure for measuring monocular PDs begins by adjusting the frame. The frame should occupy the exact position it will have with the lenses in place. The dispenser should be at the same level as the wearer and approximately 40 cm away. The dispenser closes the right eye. The wearer is instructed to look at the dispenser's open left eye. Since there is no ruler used, the dispenser uses an overhead transparency marking pen and marks a cross on the right glazed lens. If there is no lens in the frame, the clear tape placed over the lens opening is marked instead, directly over the center of the wearer's right pupil (Figure 3-5).

Next the dispenser closes the left eye and opens the right eye. The subject is instructed to look at the dispenser's open eye. The dispenser then marks a cross on the lens or tape directly over the left pupil center.

Because of the movement involved in marking pupil centers and the ease with which unintentional head

---

*Glazed lenses are also called "coquilles," "dummy lenses," or "demo lenses."

BOX 3-2

Steps in Measuring Monocular PDs Using the Sample Frame

1. The selected frame is adjusted in exactly the same manner as it will be when worn.
2. Dispenser positions at 40 cm from the wearer and at the same level.
3. Dispenser opens left eye, closes right eye, and instructs wearer to look at dispenser's open (left) eye.
4. Dispenser marks location of wearer's right pupil center on glazed lens.
5. Dispenser opens right eye, closes left eye, and instructs wearer to look at dispenser's open (right) eye.
6. Dispenser marks location of wearer's left pupil center on glazed lens.
7. Dispenser rechecks the locations of the marked crosses by repeating steps 3 and 5 and notes the positions of the marked crosses.
8. If one or both crosses are wrong, the frames are removed and the cross(es) erased using a damp cloth.
9. When crosses are accurate, monocular PDs are measured from frame center to cross center.

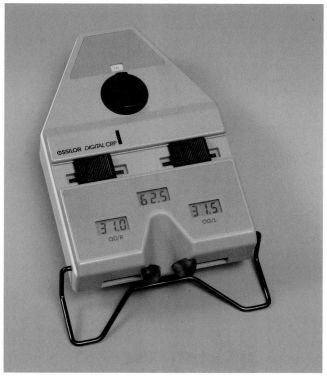

Figure 3-6. The digital version of Essilor's pupillometer displays monocular PDs for the right and left eyes, as well as the binocular PD. It can be set to measure distance or near PDs.

movement can occur, it is important that these markings be carefully rechecked.

When the dispenser is confident that pupil centers are accurately marked, the frames are removed and the distances from the center of the bridge to the center of each cross are measured and recorded. (These steps are summarized in Box 3-2.)

PD Measuring Instruments

The interpupillary distance is most easily measured by using an instrument especially designed for this purpose. Readings taken using this instrument are not nearly as subject to parallax errors as those taken using a PD rule. Such a device also solves the problems caused when the person doing the measuring is monocular or is amblyopic in one eye.

Most instruments have an occlusion system, which allows for individual monocular measurements, with each eye fixating alternately in cases of strabismus.

A well-designed PD measuring instrument should rest against the bridge of the subject's nose exactly as a frame would. This most accurately approximates the way the glasses will position themselves. It should also position the measuring plane at the approximate spectacle plane.

The subject will see a ring of white or colored light around a dark, central dot within the instrument. The dispenser will see the subject's eye and a scale appearing on it, from which a direct measure is read. Alternately, in some instruments, a split image of the pupil may be seen.

Instruments Using Corneal Reflexes

Although some instruments use a method of taking the PD where the reference point is the geometric center of the pupil itself, the popular alternate corneal-reflex method is used in instruments such as the Essilor pupillometer (Figure 3-6) or the Topcon PD-5, PD Meter. The instruments are supported by means of pads positioned so as to cause the instrument to rest on the nose where the average frame would rest. This is superior to a forehead support system used alone.

The dispenser asks the subject to hold his or her end of the pupillometer so that the pads rest on the nose (Figure 3-7). The forehead support should be against the forehead. The dispenser uses one eye to look into the instrument. (A real advantage for dispensers with good vision in only one eye.)

An internal light produces an image by reflection on each cornea, and the hairline within the device is moved until coincident with this corneal reflection (Figure 3-8). The measurement is assumed to correspond with the subject's line of sight, but is an objective measurement of the position of the corneal reflection rather than the position of the line of sight. In addition to a distance PD, near PD may be measured for near points from 30 or 35 cms to infinity.

The line of sight is defined as a line passing from the center of the pupil to the object of regard. This is the line that desirably passes through the optical center of

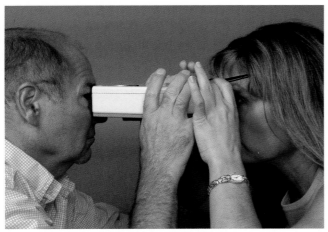

Figure 3-7. To use a pupillometer, the subject (on the right) holds the pupillometer so that the pads rest on the nose in the manner of normal eyeglasses. The dispenser views the subject's eyes through the instrument.

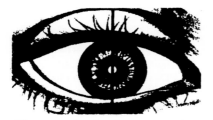

Figure 3-8. The corneal reflection as seen through Essilor's pupillometer. The hair line is adjusted to the center of the corneal reflex. (Courtesy of Essilor, Inc.)

the lenses and is the basis upon which the measurement of interpupillary distance rests.

Corneal reflections are observed along a line which intersects perpendicularly the center of curvature of the anterior surface of the cornea. (Technically this line is referred to as the pupillary axis.) This line intersects the line of sight at the entrance pupil of the eye. It varies in its orientation by an angle,* which for the average eye is approximately 1.6 degrees.[1] This places the corneal reflection somewhat toward the nose. Thus a PD determined on the basis of corneal reflections will vary slightly from that determined by the centers of the pupils.

It is possible to use a corneal-reflection-style instrument to measure a PD based on pupil center distances. To do this, the hairline within the device is moved to the center of the pupil rather than the center of the corneal reflection. The corneal reflection method is definitely the method of choice when measuring a PD for someone with pupils dilated from a recent eye examination.

---

*This angle is angle lambda, but is often commonly designated as angle kappa.

Using Corneal Reflections to Measure the PD without a Pupillometer

It is possible to use corneal reflections to measure interpupillary distance with even a PD ruler, or by using the frame with glazed lenses. Procedures need only be slightly modified. The dispenser should be positioned at the near working distance. The dispenser holds a pen light directly below his or her eye and shines it into the eye of the subject. The subject looks either at the pen light or the dispenser's eye. The reflection of the pen light on the cornea is used as the reference point instead of the geometric center of the pupil. The sequence of measurements is followed exactly as outlined in Boxes 3-1 and 3-2, except that the dispenser must position the pen light directly below his or her "open eye" throughout the sequence.

Photographic Instruments for Measuring PD

There are instruments available for taking a wearer's interpupillary distance that make use of a photograph of the wearer's eyes with the frame in place. The frames are adjusted as they are to be worn. The wearer fixates a light in the instrument, and the photo is taken. PD and segment height measurements are determined using the picture. Up to this point, no photography-based PD measuring system has successfully penetrated the U.S. ophthalmic market.

NEAR PD

The near PD is required for single vision reading glasses or for multifocals.

For *single vision reading glasses*, the lenses are set so that their optical centers will be in the lines of sight of the eyes when the eyes are converged for reading.

For *multifocals*, the distance portion is ground to correspond to the distance PD, while the bifocal or trifocal portion is decentered inward to be properly situated for near vision. The near PD can be either measured or calculated.

Measuring Near PD With a PD Rule

To measure the near PD with the PD rule, the dispenser is positioned at the subject's working distance; that is, at the distance for which the reading portion is prescribed.

Closing his or her poorer eye, the dispenser aligns his or her better eye directly before the subject's nose and instructs the subject to look into that open eye.

The PD rule is lined up with the zero point corresponding to the center of the subject's right pupil. It should also be held in the same place that the subject's new frames will rest because this will also affect the reading.

The dispenser then notes the mark corresponding to the center of the subject's left pupil. This is the near PD (Figure 3-9). The subject is not required to shift gaze,

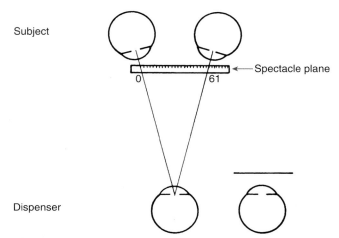

Figure 3-9. Using a PD rule, near PD may be taken with the dispenser positioned as shown. The distance between dispenser and subject is equal to the subject's working distance.

BOX 3-3

Steps in Measuring the Near PD

1. Dispenser places his or her dominant eye in front of subject's nose at the subject's near working distance. This is the distance for which the near prescription is intended—normally 40 cm (16 in).
2. Dispenser closes the nondominant eye.
3. Subject fixates dispenser's open eye.
4. Dispenser places zero point of PD rule at center of subject's right pupil.
5. Dispenser reads scale marking at center of subject's left pupil.

---

and the dispenser is not required to change eyes during the procedure. (See Box 3-3 for a summary of this technique.)

It should be added that it is also possible to use the edge of the pupil or the limbus for reference points in taking the near PD, as long as only the right or only the left edges are used, and not both outer or both inner edges.

In practice, many who use a PD rule to measure the binocular distance PD, measure the near PD at the same time. This is done as follows:

(The first three steps are how binocular distance PD measures begin.)

1. Dispenser is positioned at 40 cm.
2. The dispenser closes his or her right eye and the subject, using both eyes, fixates on dispenser's left eye.
3. Dispenser lines up zero point of ruler on center of subject's right pupil. (This next step allows for the near PD measurement.)
3A. The dispenser looks over at the subject's left eye and reads the scale on the ruler at the location of the left pupil center. This is a measure of the near

PD for the distance from the subject to the dispenser.

The dispenser now continues the steps for finding the binocular distance PD as listed in Box 3-1.

Taking Near PD Using a Pupillometer

Usually a PD measuring instrument will allow both distance and near PD to be measured. This is done through the use of a movable internal lens that changes the image distance and convergence for the subject. The near readings are carried out in the same manner as the distance readings.

USING THE NEAR PD FOR BIFOCAL INSET

For the near "reading" area of a pair of glasses to be used most comfortably, it must be positioned accurately in the lens. Horizontal placement of the near segment viewing area is determined by the near PD. (Vertical placement depends on frame depth and the individual's visual need and will be covered extensively in Chapter 5.)

The horizontal position of bifocal segments is specified as the distance from the farpoint PD that the segments are set in toward the bridge.

Because of the possibility of unequal monocular PDs, segment inset is usually specified individually for each eye. Ordinarily segment inset is the difference between the distance PD and the near PD, divided by 2:

$$\text{Segment Inset} = \frac{(\text{distance PD}) - (\text{near PD})}{2}$$

For example, if the distance PD is 68 and the near PD is 64, then the segment (seg) inset for each eye is 2 mm.

Where inequality of the monocular PDs exists, this rule may result in errors, since both eyes may not be required to converge equal angular amounts for near fixation. The actual amount of error is usually so slight, however, that it is usually ignored. The exceptions would be cases of very marked differences in monocular PD or very strong lenses.

If there is a large difference in monocular PDs, insetting the bifocal segments accordingly may result in a rather unusual-looking pair of glasses (Figure 3-10). This effect can be made less noticeable by using a bifocal with a wider segment.

Calculating the Near PD

There are several other factors to be considered when calculating the near interpupillary distance, most notably those that cause differences in segment inset.

Calculation

The most logical way to calculate the interpupillary distance is to draw a triangle with the center of rotation of

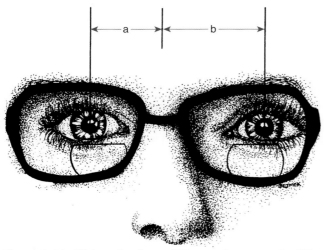

Figure 3-10. If there is a large difference in monocular PDs, insetting the bifocal segments from these points may result in a rather unusual-looking pair of glasses. Using a wider segment size or changing to a progressive addition lens is a better choice.

the eyes being two points of the triangle and the near point of fixation being the third. A similar triangle is then constructed by drawing a line corresponding to the spectacle plane.

By similar triangles, the monocular near PD can be calculated from the monocular distance PD (Figure 3-11).

When using a prewritten prescription, the working distance will normally never exceed the reciprocal of the power of the near addition. For example, a +2.00 diopter near addition will indicate a working distance no further than 50 cm.

$$\frac{1}{+2.00} = 0.50 \text{ meters} = 50 \text{ cms}$$

Unless the professional situation or physical build of the wearer indicates otherwise, the customary near working distance can be assumed to be 40 cm. If, however, the power of the near addition (add power) is greater than +2.50 diopters, then the working distance

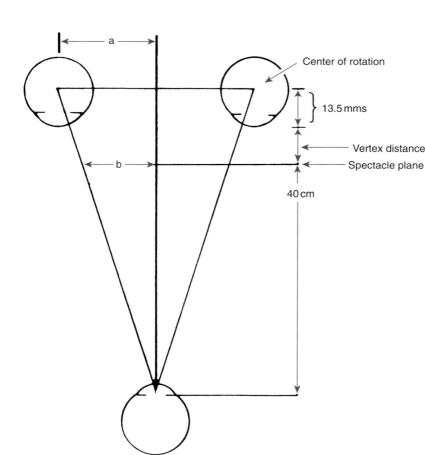

Figure 3-11. a = monocular distance PD; b = calculated monocular near PD. The distance from the front surface of the cornea to the center of rotation of the eye is normally considered to be 13.5 mm. (The diagram is, for clarity, not drawn to scale.)

TABLE 3-1
Segment Inset as Determined by the Wearer's Distance PD and Near Working Distance

For PD (mm)	Near Working Distance (cm)										
	100.0	**50.0**	**40.0**	**33.3**	**25.0**	**20.0**	**16.7**	**14.3**	**12.5**	**11.1**	**10.0**
50.0	0.7	1.4	1.7	2.0	2.6	3.1	3.7	4.2	4.7	5.2	5.6
55.0	0.8	1.5	1.8	2.2	2.8	3.4	4.0	4.6	5.1	5.6	6.1
60.0	0.8	1.6	2.0	2.4	3.1	3.8	4.4	5.0	5.6	6.1	6.7
65.0	0.9	1.8	2.2	2.6	3.3	4.1	4.8	5.4	6.1	6.7	7.2
70.0	1.0	1.9	2.3	2.8	3.6	4.4	5.1	5.8	6.5	7.2	7.8
75.0	1.0	2.0	2.5	3.0	3.8	4.7	5.5	6.3	7.0	7.7	8.3
	1.00	**2.00**	**2.50**	**3.00**	**4.00**	**5.00**	**6.00**	**7.00**	**8.00**	**9.00**	**10.00**

Dioptric Demand*

*The dioptric demand is the reciprocal of the working distance expressed in meters.

will be the reciprocal of the add power. For example, a +3.00 diopter add indicates a working distance of $33\frac{1}{3}$ cm.

$$\frac{1}{+3.00 \text{ D}} = 0.33\frac{1}{3} \text{ meters} = 33\frac{1}{3} \text{ cms}$$

Gerstman[3] has simplified the calculation of the near inset with a rule which he calls the *three-quarter rule*. The three-quarter rule states that for every diopter of *dioptric demand*, the optical center of each reading lens, or the geometric center of each bifocal addition, should be inset 0.75 (three-quarters) mm. Dioptric demand is the inverse of the reading distance in meters and is independent of the actual bifocal addition power.

Example **3-1**

For a reading distance of 40 cm, and an add power of +1.00 D, what is the inset per lens?

Solution

To find the answer, we first need to know the dioptric demand. The dioptric demand is the inverse of the working distance, *not* the inverse of the +1.00 add power. Therefore since the working distance is 40 cm or 0.40 m, the dioptric demand is

$$\frac{1}{0.40} = 2.50 \text{ D}$$

Having found the dioptric demand, we can find the inset per lens by multiplying by three-quarters, as the rule name implies. Therefore the inset per lens is

$$2.50 \times \frac{3}{4} = 1.9 \text{ mm}$$

The three-quarter rule tends to give the appropriate inset at all reading distances for the typical adult. Gerstman defines the typical adult as one whose interpupillary distance is between 62 and 68 mm. For those whose PDs do not fall within this range, it becomes necessary to refer to an inset table (Table 3-1). This table is a quick reference for determining the segment inset when reading distance (working distance) and distance PD are known.

The Influence of Distance Lens Power on Segment Inset

The power of the distance prescription has an effect on bifocal inset. When a person looks at a near object, the eyes turn inward and are no longer looking through the optical centers of the lenses. Negative power, or minus lenses, keep the eyes from converging as much as they normally would because of the Base In prismatic effect at this point on the lens. Positive power, or plus lenses, cause the eyes to converge slightly more than they normally would because of their Base Out prismatic effect.

For positive lenses then both the measured or the Gerstman-calculated near PD would need to be reduced (i.e., the segment inset of the bifocal increased). For minus lenses, the near PD would need to be increased (i.e., the inset of the segment reduced).

The position of the near reading area becomes more important when the reading area is small. This means that for progressive addition lenses, the position of the intermediate and near readings areas is very important. Progressive addition lens designers are now taking distance power into consideration when determining how much inset the near viewing area should have.

Segment Inset Formula. There have been several factors listed as having an effect on segment inset. These were:

- The distance the lenses are from the eyes
- The distance PD
- The near working distance
- The power of the distance lens

Taking all these factors into consideration, Ellerbrock[4] derived the following formula for segment inset.

$$i = \frac{P}{1 + \omega\left(\dfrac{1}{s} - \dfrac{1}{f}\right)}$$

where P is one half the distance PD, ω is the distance of the lens from the working nearpoint, s is the distance from the lens to the center of rotation of the eye, and f is the focal length of the lens in the 180-degree meridian. All measurements are expressed in millimeters.

Example **3-2**

What would the segment inset be for a person with a 70 mm distance PD who is wearing a prescription of +6.50D? Assume they are wearing a +2.50 add, but are working at a near working distance of 20 cm. The spectacle lenses are 25 mm from the center of rotation of the eye to the back of the lens.

Solution

We are using Ellerbrock's formula. In Ellerbrock's formula P is half the distance PD, so

$$P = \frac{70}{2} = 35 \text{ mm.}$$

The value of ω is the distance from the lens to the near working point in millimeters. This distance is given as 20 cm, which is the same as 200 mm.

The focal length of the lens is the reciprocal of the power of the lens. This is

$$\frac{1}{6.50} = 0.1538 \text{ Meters}$$
$$= 153.5 \text{ mm}$$

Since the lens is a sphere, the power in the 180-degree meridian is the same as the power in any other meridian.

The distance from the lens to the center of rotation of the eye is given as 25 mm, so s = 25 mm.

Inserting all of this into Ellerbrock's formula results in

$$i = \frac{P}{1 + \omega\left(\dfrac{1}{s} - \dfrac{1}{f}\right)}$$
$$= \frac{35}{1 + 200 \cdot \left(\dfrac{1}{25} - \dfrac{1}{153.5}\right)}$$
$$= 4.5 \text{ mm}$$

So the inset per lens for this wearing situation is 4.5 mm per eye.

Summary of Factors

Fortunately the variations in segment inset caused by all these factors are not radically different from that found using the measured near PD. This assumes, of course, that the near PD is measured at the appropriate working distance.

Table 3-2 summarizes the effect of distance lens power on segment inset for the normal working distance (40 cm or 16 in).[5]

Recommendations For Finding The Near PD

After all of these possibilities, what is the most appropriate way to determine segment inset? Here are some recommendations for different situations. The idea is to provide the best accuracy without making it too difficult. Keep in mind that just using a PD ruler may not be the most reliable method.

Recommendations for Finding the Correct Segment Inset

- When the working distance is normal (40 cm)
  1. Measure the near PD with a pupillometer or a PD ruler.
  2. If the distance lens powers are high, use Table 3-2.
- When the working distance is less than 40 cm
  1. Again, measure the near PD with a pupillometer or PD ruler. Be certain to set the correct working distance in the pupillometer before measuring. When measuring with a PD ruler, the dispenser must be at the shorter working distance.
  2. If the working distance is less than that allowed for in the pupillometer, use Gerstman's three-quarter rule (assuming adult PDs between 62 and 68 mm), or use Table 3-1.
- When the distance lens powers are especially high
  1. If the working distance is normal (40 cm), use Table 3-2.
  2. If the working distance is closer than 40 cm, use Ellerbrock's formula. (Ellerbrock's formula could actually be used in any of the above circumstances, but it is unhandy to work with.)

Examples for Finding the Near PD

Here are some examples. Both the power of the prescription and the distance PD are known. Use the most appropriate method to find the segment inset and then the near PD.

Example **3-3**

A spectacle lens wearer has the following prescription

R: −1.00 D sphere
L: −1.00 D sphere
add: +2.00

TABLE 3-2
Insets to Make Reading Fields Coincide at 16 Inches

Power of distance lens in 180th	Distance from Nose to Center of Pupil									
	27	28	29	30	31	32	33	34	35	36
+15	2.5	2.5	2.5	2.5	3	3	3	3	3	3
+14	2.5	2.5	2.5	2.5	2.5	3	3	3	3	3
+12	2	2.5	2.5	2.5	2.5	2.5	2.5	3	3	3
+10	2	2	2	2.5	2.5	2.5	2.5	2.5	2.5	3
+9	2	2	2	2	2.5	2.5	2.5	2.5	2.5	2.5
+8	2	2	2	2	2	2.5	2.5	2.5	2.5	2.5
+7	2	2	2	2	2	2.5	2.5	2.5	2.5	2.5
+6	2	2	2	2	2	2	2.5	2.5	2.5	2.5
+5	2	2	2	2	2	2	2	2.5	2.5	2.5
+4	2	2	2	2	2	2	2	2	2.5	2.5
+3	1.5	2	2	2	2	2	2	2	2	2.5
+2	1.5	1.5	2	2	2	2	2	2	2	2
+1	1.5	1.5	1.5	2	2	2	2	2	2	2
0	1.5	1.5	1.5	2	2	2	2	2	2	2
−1	1.5	1.5	1.5	1.5	2	2	2	2	2	2
−2	1.5	1.5	1.5	1.5	2	2	2	2	2	2
−3	1.5	1.5	1.5	1.5	1.5	2	2	2	2	2
−4	1.5	1.5	1.5	1.5	1.5	1.5	2	2	2	2
−5	1.5	1.5	1.5	1.5	1.5	1.5	1.5	2	2	2
−6	1.5	1.5	1.5	1.5	1.5	1.5	1.5	2	2	2
−7	1.5	1.5	1.5	1.5	1.5	1.5	1.5	1.5	2	2
−8	1.5	1.5	1.5	1.5	1.5	1.5	1.5	1.5	1.5	2
−9	1.5	1.5	1.5	1.5	1.5	1.5	1.5	1.5	1.5	1.5
−10	1.5	1.5	1.5	1.5	1.5	1.5	1.5	1.5	1.5	1.5
−12	1	1.5	1.5	1.5	1.5	1.5	1.5	1.5	1.5	1.5
−14	1	1	1.5	1.5	1.5	1.5	1.5	1.5	1.5	1.5
−16	1	1	1	1.5	1.5	1.5	1.5	1.5	1.5	1.5
−18	1	1	1	1	1.5	1.5	1.5	1.5	1.5	1.5
−20										

The distance PD is measured as 64 mm. For a 40 cm working distance, what is the expected near PD?

Solution

Since the working distance is 40 cm, simply measure the near PD with a pupillometer (or PD ruler). If a pupillometer is not available, use Table 3-2. In the table, we find the inset for a 32 mm monocular distance PD with a −1.00 D power to be 2 mm. Therefore the binocular near PD would be 4 mm less than the distance PD. Since 64 − 4 = 60 mm, then the near PD equals 60 mm.

Example **3-4**

Suppose an individual has a distance PD of 64 mm, a distance prescription of −1.00 D sphere for both eyes, and a bifocal add of +2.00. (These are the same lens powers as given in the previous example.) What would the near PD be if the near working distance was 25 cm instead of 40 cm?

Solution

Since the working distance is less than 40 cm, we would find the near PD either by a direct measurement using a pupillometer (or PD ruler) or by using the three-quarter rule. To find the near PD by measurement, the best option would be to use a pupillometer. Unfortunately, most pupillometers only measure up to 33 cm. However, it is possible to use a PD ruler. If a ruler is used, the dispenser's face must be at the subject's near working distance.

If the near PD is to be calculated, it is possible to do these calculations with Gerstman's three-quarter rule. To use the three-quarter rule, begin by the finding the dioptric demand. Dioptric demand is the reciprocal of the working distance in meters. In this example, the working distance is 25 centimeters or 0.25 meters. Therefore

$$\text{Dioptric demand} = \frac{1}{0.25 \text{ meters}} = 4\,D$$

Next, to find the inset per eye, the dioptric demand is multiplied by 3/4.

$$\frac{3}{4} \times 4 = 3 \text{ mm per eye}$$

Thus the near PD will be

Distance PD − (segment inset × 2)

Or

64 − 6 or 58 mm.

This means that a prescription for a person with a bifocal add and a 25 cm working distance should have the distance optical centers set for a far PD of 64 mm and the segments set for a near PD of 58 mm.

Using Table 3-1 would have yielded an inset of 3.3 mm per eye and a near PD of 57.4 mm. Remember that the three-quarter rule is a close approximation and because the table does not list every PD and working distance, it may also be a close approximation.

Example **3-5**

A prescription reads as follows:

R: +1.50 − 1.00 × 180
L: +1.50 − 1.00 × 180
add +3.50

The distance PD is found to be 61 mm. What should the near PD be?

Solution

A near addition with a power greater than +2.50 D should be a red flag to the dispenser. An add greater than +2.50 D means that the working distance will be less than 40 cm. The near PD is best found by direct measurement with a pupillometer or PD ruler. The three-quarter rule is not as accurate because the PD is smaller than the normal 62 to 68 mm range. The next best thing is to use Table 3-1.

To measure directly with pupillometer or PD ruler, the working distance must be known. When an add power is greater than +2.50 D, unless another distance is specified the working distance is found by taking the reciprocal of the add power.

$$\text{Working Distance} = \frac{1}{3.5} = 0.29 \text{ M or 29 cms}$$

Now the near PD may be measured for this 29 cm working distance with the pupillometer or at this 29 mm working distance with a PD ruler.

Table 3-1 is not ideal, because neither the distance PD nor the "working distance" can be found directly and must be interpolated, choosing a number in between those given in the table. If the number halfway between is chosen, this makes the closest seg inset to be 2.75 mm per lens. This makes the near PD

Near PD = 61 − (2 × 2.75)
= 61 − 5.5
= 55.5 mm

The other way to find the near PD would be to use the three-quarter rule. This is done by multiplying the dioptric demand (3.5 D) by 0.75.

Which is:

$$(0.75) \times (3.5) = 2.625 \text{ mm per lens}$$

Now the near PD is

Near PD = distance PD − (2 × seg inset)
= 61 − (2 × 2.625)
= 61 − 5.25
= 55.75

Either inset number will yield a similar answer and both answers will round to 56 mm for the near PD.

Example **3-6**

A prescription reads as follows:

R: −8.50 D sphere
L: −8.50 D sphere
add = +1.50

For this prescription, we will assume that the distance monocular PDs have been measured. The right monocular distance PD was measured as 28 mm and the left as 31 mm. For a 40 cm working distance, find the near monocular PDs.

Solution

For high-powered lenses, calculated near PDs will be more accurate than measured near PDs. This is because measured near PDs do not take the prismatic effects of high plus or high minus spectacle lenses into consideration. (Looking nasally through high minus lenses causes a base-in prismatic effect and reduces the amount the eyes converge for near viewing.) However, there is one situation for high-powered lens prescriptions where measured near PDs are as accurate as calculated near PDs. This occurs if the near PDs are measured while the prescribed distance lenses are being worn. So if the wearer has the same existing prescription in single vision lenses or multifocals, a PD ruler may be used while the person is wearing their existing frame and lenses.

This prescription is for the normal working distance. The easiest method to find the near PD for this high-powered prescription is to consult Table 3-2. For the right and the left lens, Table 3-2 shows segment inset to be 1.5 mm per lens. Therefore the monocular near PDs are

R: 28 mm − 1.5 mm or 26.5 mm
L: 31 mm − 1.5 mm or 29.5 mm

REFERENCES

1. Loper LR: The relationship between angle lambda and residual astigmatism of the eye, master's thesis, Bloomington, Ind, 1956, Indiana University.
2. Hofstetter HW: Parallactic P.D. pitfalls: the refraction letter, Rochester, NY, 1973, Bausch & Lomb Inc.
3. Gerstman DR: Ophthalmic lens decentration as a function of reading distance, Brit J Physical Optics, 28 (1), 1973.
4. Ellerbrock LR: A clinical evaluation of compensation for vertical imbalances, Arch Amer Acad Optom, 25:7, 1948.
5. Borish IM: Clinical Refraction, ed 3, vol 2, Stoneham, Mass, 1975, Butterworth/Heinemann.

Proficiency Test

(Answers can be found in the back of the book.)

1. True or false? When taking PD measurements, the person measuring covers or closes one of his eyes at a time. He *never* covers one of his subject's eyes.

2. When is it especially important to use monocular PD measurements? (There may be more than one correct response.)
   a. When eyes are asymmetrically placed.
   b. When the prescription lenses are of high power.
   c. When the lenses are aspheric.
   d. When the two lenses are considerably different in power from one another.
   e. When progressive addition lenses are used.

3. For bifocal lenses with a high plus correction, the near PD should be:
   a. increased slightly over the measured value.
   b. decreased slightly over the measured value.
   c. left the same as the measured value.

4. True or false? The Essilor pupillometer measures the PD using a corneal reflex.

5. True or false? Because of optical considerations, it is always best to decenter bifocal segments asymmetrically if there are high amounts of difference in the measured monocular PD positions. This is true even if the cosmetic result of the oddly-placed segment appears to be somewhat unusual.

6. To measure monocular PDs using the glazed lenses in the frame and an overhead transparency pen:
   a. the dispenser should mark the glazed lenses on the horizontal midline, directly below the pupil center.
   b. the wearer should look at the bridge of the dispenser's nose. The dispenser should view the wearer's right eye with his or her left eye and the wearer's left eye with his or her right eye.
   c. the dispenser should spot the glazed lenses at the center of the wearer's pupils. The wearer can view either the bridge of the dispenser's nose or a distant object, as long as the gaze is held fixed.
   d. the dispenser should spot the glazed lenses at the center of the wearer's pupils. The distance between the marked dots is measured. This distance divided by 2 will yield the right and left monocular PDs.
   e. There is a flaw in every one of the above answers. None of them are true.

7. May the limbal edge be used as a reference point in taking monocular PDs?

8. The distance PD measures out to be 64 mm, and the near PD calculates out at 59 mm. What is the seg inset per lens?

9. A person has a prescription that calls for a +4.00 add power. For what distance would you measure the near PD?
   a. 40 cm
   b. 30 cm
   c. 25 cm
   d. 20 cm
   e. arm's length

10. A prescription reads:

    OD: +1.00 sph
    OS: +1.00 sph
    +5.00 add

    According to Gerstman's three-quarter rule, how much must each lens be decentered?

11. Near PD can either be measured or calculated. When measured, the distance from the dispenser's eye to the subject's eye should be:
    a. the proposed working distance.
    b. the near point of accommodation.
    c. 40 cm.
    d. 33 cm.
    e. arm's length.

12. Given the following specifications for a pair of glasses, what should the binocular near PD be when calculated using Ellerbrock's formula?
    — Monocular PDs for right and left eyes are 32 mm each
    — Distance from the back of lens surface to the center of rotation of the eye is 33 mm
    — Lens power for both right and left lenses is +4.00 +2.00 × 90
    — Add power is +2.50

13. A person has a distance PD of 66, a low distance prescription, and a bifocal add that requires the reading material be held at 25 cm. Rounded to the nearest 0.5 mm, what should the seg inset be for each lens?
    a. 1.5 mm per lens
    b. 2.0 mm per lens
    c. 3.0 mm per lens
    d. 4.0 mm per lens

14. Suppose an individual has a distance PD of 64 mm, a distance prescription of −1.50 D sphere for both eyes, and a bifocal add of +3.00. What would the near PD be if the near working distance was 20 cm instead of either 33 or 40 cm?

15. A spectacle lens wearer has the following prescription

    R: −1.00 D sphere
    L: −1.00 D sphere
    add: +2.50

    The distance PD is measured as 58 mm. For a 40 cm working distance, what is the expected near PD?

16. Suppose an individual has a distance PD of 64 mm, a distance prescription of −1.00 D sphere for both eyes, and a bifocal add of +2.50. (These are the same lens powers as given in the previous problem.) What would the near PD be if the near working distance was 30 cm instead of 40 cm?

17. A prescription reads as follows:

    R: −6.00 D sphere
    L: −6.00 D sphere
    add = +2.50

    For this prescription we will assume that the distance monocular PDs have been measured. The right monocular PD was measured as 32 mm and the left as 34 mm. For a 40 cm working distance, find the near monocular PDs.

CHAPTER **4**

Frame Selection

rame selection entails considerably more than just helping a person try on frames. At the very least, a working knowledge of basic facial shapes is necessary. The person aiding in selection must have the ability to know what the frame will look like with lenses, and how it will perform in fulfilling the wearer's needs. This chapter provides the knowledge necessary to acquire basic competency in frame selection.

USING THE WEARER'S OLD FRAME

Sometimes a person wants to use their old frames instead of selecting something new. This may or may not be appropriate.

There are a number of valid reasons for wanting to use the old frame and not purchase a new one. These include cost, comfort of the old frames, and sometimes the inability of the wearer to look in the mirror with any other frame and still have what they see look right to them. Even though any of these could be considered valid, there are other factors that could outweigh keeping the old frame. If none of these others are overriding factors and the frames are in good condition, then there is no reason not to use the old frames. However, even if there are valid reasons not to use the old frames, if the wearer has been fully informed of the pitfalls and still persists, their desires should be respected.

Factors to Consider Before Using the Wearer's Old Frames*

There are certain precautions that must be considered before using the old frame for the new prescription. These are the most common:

- Putting new lenses in an old frame may involve putting additional stress on the frame. Older frames may not withstand that stress very well, particularly older plastic frames that have become brittle with age. Sometimes frames will withstand the stresses of the new lenses, but be weakened, only to break shortly thereafter.

---

*Many of the factors listed in this section are from the following brochure: Cook P: Should I use my old frames, Item No. BRO011, 1999, Diversified Ophthalmics.

- It is hard to predict how long an old frame will last. Will it last the life of the new lens prescription? If the frame breaks, it is not a simple task to find another frame into which those new lenses will fit.
- If the old frame needs repairing in the future, will there be parts available? A used frame may already be discontinued. If it has been and there are no parts available, any savings could be lost when both frames and lenses need to be repurchased.
- Usually people keep their old glasses as a backup spare pair in case they lose or break their new pair. Using the old frames eliminates the emergency backup.
- Sometimes old lenses can be tinted and the older pair be transformed into prescription sunglasses. This is particularly true if the only change in a multifocal prescription is in the near vision portion. A person could get a second pair of prescription eyeglasses for the cost of tinting the old lenses.
- If the existing frames have not been discontinued and the wearer decides to get exactly the same frame, there is an advantage to having interchangeability of parts should the new frame break.
- Does the lab need the old frames to make the new lenses correctly? If so, can the wearer do without their current glasses while the frames are at the laboratory?
- Are the old frames out of style or nearly out of style? If they are nearly out of style, what will these older frames look like by the time the wearer is ready for the next prescription change?

In summary, there are a number of reasons why a person may not be well-served in keeping their old frames. These reasons have to be logically and carefully explained; otherwise the wearer will conclude that the dispenser is only interested in their own financial gain.

COSMETIC CONSIDERATIONS

From an aesthetic point of view, glasses are of no small importance to the person wearing them. Each individual expects and should receive help, not only with sizing, but also with the cosmetic aspects of a frame.

The habitual wearer often needs just as much help in frame selection as the nonwearer because individuals are used to seeing themselves in the frame style they are presently wearing. Any new frame will represent a change and will look strange. The wearer who is forced to change frames because the style has been discontinued will be especially dependent on the advice of the person fitting the frames.

Despite continuous changes in frame styles, there are still certain basics that can be used to arrive at an aesthetically pleasing and comfortable frame. The wearer ultimately has the final choice of what will be worn, but should not be allowed free rein in selecting a frame.

Frame selection is often a process of trial and error, can be time consuming and is frequently frustrating. An experienced fitter aware of the basics of frame selection can save considerable time and earn the wearer's gratitude by being able to readily select several frames that are obviously suitable.

Proper assistance in frame selection is especially important for the type of person who may be inclined to accept the first frame presented. Unless such a frame consists of a good bridge fit, proper eye size, and an acceptable shape, the fitter may inherit the almost impossible task of attempting to adapt a frame to a face for which it was not designed.

At the same time, what is cosmetically correct for a given face must be related to whatever styles are in vogue. At a time when narrow frames are in fashion, a person whose face requires a deep frame will not wear one quite as deep as when larger, deeper frames are in style. The person with a narrow interpupillary distance can wear a wide frame more acceptably when everyone is wearing large frames than when everyone is wearing smaller frames. Just as changes in styles of clothing—longer or shorter hemlines, wider or narrower neckties—become customary by repetitious display, so do variations in spectacle designs. Thus when basics in frame selection are noted, it is understood that they are applied within the framework of current eyewear trends.

Frame Shape and Face Shape

Since frames are exceedingly obvious on the face, their shape tends to emphasize or deemphasize characteristics of the face. A good frame selection can be simplified by considering first which facial lines are complimentary to the person. Those lines should be emphasized through repetition, usually by the upper and lower eyewires. On the other hand, uncomplimentary lines should not be repeated by the frame line.

Because a hairstyle can also alter the apparent shape of the face, frames are generally chosen to compliment the face as it appears with the hairstyle being worn at the time of frame selection. A radical change in hairstyle may also radically change the effect that the frame has on the face.

Few faces meet the artistic ideal in bone structure and conformity. A well-selected frame can increase the attractiveness of a face by emphasizing those planes and lines more closely approaching the "ideal" and by drawing attention away from those most contradicting it. Conversely, a frame that tends to overemphasize or repeat the less desirable aspects of a face can make that face more unattractive.

In most instances, the lines of the frame selected should create the effect of balancing facial planes that are not components of idealized proportions. The idea is the same as using vertical stripes to enhance the appearance of a short or an obese person.

Facial Types

Knowledge of basic facial shapes is not essential for appropriate frame selection, but it is a valuable aid in making a quicker and more accurate decision about a specific frame. The average fitter can tell how appropriate a frame looks after it has been placed on the face. The accomplished fitter who has an understanding of facial shapes will know how a frame will look before placing it on the face.

The awareness of the considerable influence that spectacle frames can have on the basic facial shape, either positively or negatively, is essential to competent selection of the ultimate frame for each specific face.

Generally, there are seven basic facial shapes:
1. *Oval*—considered to be the ideal type
2. *Oblong*—thinner and longer than usual, with the sides of the head being more parallel to one another than in the oval type
3. *Round*—more circular than the oval
4. *Square*—again, the sides of the face are more parallel than in the oval, with the face being wider and shorter than usual
5. *Triangular*—the lower part of the face is wider than the upper part
6. *Inverted triangular*—the upper part of the face, the temple area, is wider than the lower jaw area
7. *Diamond*—the central section of the face is wider, with the upper and lower extremities of the face narrowing down considerably (Table 4-1)

To simplify the face shapes to help choose frame width and depth, the seven shapes can be condensed to the following five shapes.[1] The oval face is considered *normal* and can wear almost any frame, so only the general rules apply. The oblong face is simply referred to as *long*. Both the round and the square face fall into the category of the *wide* face. The *erect* or base-down triangular face is a category that does not lend itself to condensation. For fitting purposes, the diamond face is included in the *inverted* or base-up triangular classification, since these shapes are all fit in basically the same manner. Using this simplified system, a face may deviate from the normal in four essential ways: it may be either too long, too wide, or too triangular, with the base of the triangle up or down.

TABLE 4-1
Fitting By Face Shape

Basic Facial Shapes	Fitting Shapes		Fitting Suggestions
Oval	Normal		May wear most any type
Oblong	Long face	*Contrasting shapes*	Deep frame Low temple attachment
Round Square }	Wide Face		Narrow frame High temple attachment
Base down triangular	Erect (base down) triangular face	*Contrasting shapes*	Fit size to largest part of lower facial area Dark colors or bolder look are in order
Inverted triangle } Diamond }	Inverted (base up) Triangular face		Unobtrusive frame (metal or rimless works well) Light or medium weight frame Lighter color is in order Rounded lens shape Delicate characteristics of frame for women

Affecting the Length of the Face

For purposes of frame selection, we are concerned with the vertical and horizontal *dimensions* of the frame, the roundness or squareness of the frame *shape*, and the *coloration* of the frame front.

For simplification, discussion of the shape of frame suitability can be broken down into two categories. The first concerns the width and depth of the frame (dimensions) and whether the emphasis should be in the upper portion of the frame, as with a gradient frame, or across the entire frame, as with a frame that is solid in color (emphasis/coloration). These considerations all relate to the length and breadth of the face. The second category deals with the angularity or roundness of the frame line (shape) as related to the angularity or roundness of the face and the eyebrow line.

The proper *width* of the frame* can be gauged as approximately equal to the widest part of the skull's

*The width of the frame is taken as the outer width of the frame itself, and not simply the outer edges of the lenses.

facial bone structure. This "rule" is subject to modification with style changes, but the widest bony part of the face is always used as the reference point.

The bone structure is used instead of the actual width because excess body and face weight may cause the wearer's features to appear to be set in toward the center of the face; a frame based on the width of the actual face rather than structure would cause the person to appear cross-eyed.

As a general rule, the longer the face, the greater the vertical *depth* (distance from the upper to the lower rim) should be to keep the frame proportional to the face. The shorter the face, the smaller the vertical depth. In other words, a deeper frame is more complimentary to a long face, while a narrower frame lends itself more easily to a wide face. In a sense, the frame "covers" part of the face and covering more of a long face gives the illusion of reducing its length.

Frame fronts may be vertically gradient, horizontally gradient, or a solid color. A darker, solid-colored frame will aid the effect of shortening a long face more readily than a vertically gradient frame. Included in the "vertically gradient" category is any frame that draws the viewer's attention to the upper part of the frame. For example, a nylon cord frame with a dark upper portion would fall into this category. A solid frame seems to curtail the length of the face in the area extending from the dark lower rim to the chin.

On a frame with a dark upper rim section and a lower rimless or nylon cord section, the reference point for face length is from the dark part of the frame at eyebrow level (the part that immediately catches our eye) to the bottom of the chin. Thus these frames have a face-lengthening effect, making them more compatible to the wide face.

The *outer areas* of the frame may also be used to advantage in giving the illusion of shortening or lengthening the face. The eyes are actually set very close to the vertical center of the head, although they are usually assumed to be at the top because the visual reference is from the hairline to the eyes and from the eyes to the bottom of the chin.

Spectacle *temples* interject an artificial dividing line. The lower the line, the shorter the face appears; the higher the line, the longer it appears. Thus for long faces, frame fronts with lower endpieces shorten the face. For wide faces, temples with high endpieces add length to the face.

When the face is viewed from the side, it is divided by the location of the spectacle temple, which interposes an artificial dividing line.

If the temple attaches high on the frame front, there is more facial area below this line, and the face appears lengthened (Figure 4-1, *A*). If the temple is attached lower on the frame, there is less distance from this line to the bottom of the chin, and the face appears shorter (Figure 4-1, *B*). If the face is too long, lower endpieces

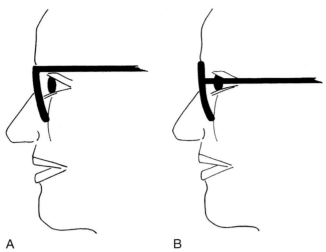

A   B

Figure 4-1. **A,** If the temple attaches high on the frame front, there is more facial area below this line, and the face appears lengthened. **B,** If the temple attaches lower, there is less distance from this line, and the face appears shorter.

will help give the appearance of less length; if the face is wide and short, higher endpieces are desirable.

An extreme case of the wide face would be one with smallish features that appear to be bunched centrally in the middle of a large face.[1] Actually, as the person gains weight, head size increases but features remain stationary, giving the face a "bunched-up" look. The width of the frame should be gauged by the bone structure of the face and not by the actual widest part of the head. Otherwise the person's face will be overpowered by the frame or the eyes will appear abnormally close together.

The same rules that apply to fitting the wide face also apply to the pudgy face, but must be adhered to more strictly. The less obvious the frame, the better. In a plastic frame, a medium to lightweight plastic would be appropriate, but a better alternative is the thin metal, nylon cord, or even rimless frame. Attention also must be given to the vertical dimension of the frame.

Affecting Facial Balance
With faces somewhat wider in one area than in another, frames can be used to balance out a wider area and to shift the facial emphasis.

The widest part of the *base-down triangular face* is the lower area. Simply wearing glasses often enhances the appearance of the face because the frames lend balance. The frames themselves should be approximately the same width as the lower facial area. The actual width will vary somewhat, depending on current frame styles.

An oval or upswept shape is preferable, as opposed to one of rectangular design. This is particularly true of the lower rim, which, if it is a straight line paralleling the jawline, tends to emphasize the width of the base of the triangle. Frames for men in these cases may appear satisfactory with somewhat squared-off shapes because the lower line is not continuous and angular lines in a man's face are not considered uncomplimentary. For women, a frame with rounded lines will give a softer, more feminine look and squared-off lines a more assertive look.

The frame should be a dark color for emphasis to further balance the overall facial shape: solid if the face is long, vertically gradient or with emphasis on the upper part of the frame if the face is short.

The *base-up triangular face* is somewhat more difficult to fit. It is not possible to use the mere location of the frames to counterbalance the wider part of the face. Obviously a prominent frame on this type of face draws attention to the wider facial area.

To avoid undue emphasis, the frame should be as unobtrusive as possible. The frame should be the minimal width that still stays within current fashion lines. Keep in mind that the farther out the frames extend from the side of the head, the more pointed the chin will look.

The frame should be of light or medium weight and of a lighter color when possible. Metal or rimlesslike varieties lend themselves well to this type of face.

A heavy lower line sometimes helps to counterbalance. A rounded lens shape will soften the triangularity of the face, but a squared-off frame will emphasize it. This type of face on a woman usually has a certain delicateness to it; thus the frame should also have delicate characteristics.

Frame Lines
Repeating a facial line through the line of the frame emphasizes the facial line. This can be used to advantage provided the line being repeated is complementary or used to achieve a desired effect. Inadvertently repeating an uncomplimentary line can, by the same principle, have an undesirable effect.

The lines of the frame are determined by the curve or squareness of the upper and lower rims—in other words, by the basic shape of the lens. At this point, the depth and width of the desired frame should be fairly well known, depending on the length, width, or triangularity of the face.

As a general rule, when using the frame shape for cosmetic emphasis, the upper areas of the frame are determined by the eyebrow line, while the lower frame areas are determined by the lines of the cheek and jaw. The lower eyewire area near the nose should follow the nasal contour of the face, as discussed previously.

The *upper frame area*, or upper rim, should have the same basic shape as the eyebrow itself. Too much deviation from this line creates a disharmonious look to the face, roughly similar to the confused effect of wearing stripes with plaids. Ideally the upper rim should follow the lower edge of the eyebrow, leaving it visible. At its highest possible position, the upper rim bisects the eyebrow. This is not always possible or desirable. Some even prefer an above-the-eyebrow position.[2] In any case, the most important thing to be kept in mind when dispensing conventional eyewear is to follow the basic line of the eyebrow with the upper line of the frame.

Balding males may benefit from a frame with a straight browbar.[3] The theory underlying this is that the browbar takes away some of the forehead area, detracting from the appearance of a large forehead.

As far as the *lower frame area* is concerned, apart from a squared or rounded effect, which is determined by the squared or rounded aspects of the face, the most important thing a lower rim can do is add a lift to a face that has begun to sag with age. Using an upsweep on either upper or lower rim of a frame tends to counteract the downward lines of the face. In general, a frame with a downward line, which emphasizes the undesirable characteristic, should be avoided.

Frame lines can somewhat alter the mood expression of the face, causing the wearer to have a happier, sadder, more stern, or even a somewhat surprised look, depending on the interaction of the frame lines with the background facial configuration.

Another important effect that may be accomplished through the use of lower rims is to help conceal the bags that many people have under their eyes. Helpful camouflage is attained by choosing a frame with fairly thick lower rims of a dark color, properly positioned to cover the lowest part of the bags.

Frame Color

Up to this point, frame color has been noted essentially in regard to how certain effects can be emphasized through the use of a darker color or deemphasized through the use of a lighter color. Although the actual color chosen may be left to the wearers, the dispenser has a responsibility to guide them toward the final choice.

Hair color, skin color, feature size, and eye color can all give valuable clues to the suitability of eyewear color. With all the possible shades and degrees of translucence in available frames, plus innovative uses of color combinations, firm rules to guide color selection are difficult.

Clothing and Accessories. The common sense rules that apply to clothing and accessories also apply to the proper choice of eyewear. Certainly the favorite or dominate color that the individual regularly wears ought not be overlooked. Choosing a frame color should not be done based on skin, eye, and hair color at the exclusion of habitual dress. Eyeglasses are considered to be accessories and, as Dowaliby states, "It is traditional... that the best dressed are identified by accessories repeating tones in the ensemble.[4]"

Considering that most people do not wear the same colors continually, it should be understood that one single frame cannot be expected to coordinate with every possible mode of dress—both in color and in effect. Those who choose one pair of glasses to serve in every work or recreational situation, with every style and color of clothing, should be aware of the limitations this imposes.

Hair. Frames in pale tints of blue or rose benefit gray hair. People with thicker, darker hair are able to wear heavier, darker, bolder frames than individuals with lighter, finer hair. A lighter-colored, more delicately styled frame is recommended for the person with light, fine hair. A bold dark frame on a person with light, fine hair draws attention to itself much more emphatically than it would on someone with thicker, darker hair.

When a metal frame is to be dispensed, those with blond, light brown, or red hair can wear gold well; those with gray hair can wear silver well. Those with black or extremely dark hair can wear either color well. Individuals with salt-and-pepper hair, or hair that is just starting to gray will find that choosing a silver frame will make the "salt" component of their salt-and-pepper hair more noticeable.[3] It should be kept in mind that not everyone may consider choosing a frame color that will emphasize beginning grayness to be a detrimental choice. Much depends upon the image the individual wishes to project. Therefore the role of the dispenser becomes that of an aide in helping a person find a frame that produces the desired effect, while avoiding any unintentional changes the wearer may consider unpleasant.

Facial Features. As far as facial feature size is concerned, the smaller and more delicate the features, the lighter the frame color can be; the heavier the features, the darker the frame color allowable.

Narrow and Wide-Set Eyes. A person whose eyes are set close together in comparison to the total width of the face will want to choose eyewear that does not draw attention to the center of the frame. Low-set, thick, dark-bridged frames will make such an individual look as though the eyes are so close together there is hardly room for the frame to sit on the nose. Instead, this person should choose a frame with a clear bridge (little central emphasis) but with distinctive upper temporal areas. In this way the observer's attention is drawn outward and away from the close-set eyes.[5]

An individual with extremely wide-set eyes needs the exact opposite. The best choice is the frame with a low-set, dark, thick bridge. The space between the eyes is "filled in" and the eyes do not appear as widely spaced.

Frame Color by Season. In spite of suggestions given on frame color up to this point, it is very difficult to determine rules that work consistently. It is true that some people can wear certain colors better than others. The difficulty lies in finding which colors are best suited for each individual.

In an attempt to facilitate finding the colors that are most complimentary for a given individual, one approach divides individuals into one of four basic groups. Each group is identified by one of the four seasons. "For just as nature has divided herself into four distinct seasons, Autumn, Spring, Winter, and Summer, each with its unique and harmonious colors, your genes have given you a type of coloring that is most complimented by one of the seasonal palettes.[6]"

To determine which "season" a person is, skin tone, hair color, and sometimes eye color are evaluated. Finding the correct "season" is reportedly best done by trial and error using colored fabric drapings to discover those that are most complimentary to a person's skin and hair color. All individuals, regardless of season "...can wear almost any color; it is the shade and intensity that count.[6]" If someone already knows which "shades and intensities" of color he or she looks best in, frame color selection may be simplified. If not, trying on one frame after another while looking for the best effect is certainly simpler than first trying to determine season, *then* selecting frame color.

In summary, although it may be possible to find a few starting points for frame color selection, the process does not lend itself to simple answers. Most probably, in the end, personal tastes in color combined with trial and error will prevail.

Lens Tint

There are many purposes for a tint in prescription eyewear—so many, in fact, that a complete chapter in this book is devoted to the subject. Yet sometimes the only reason a person wants tinted lenses is to make the glasses look better. When this is the case, the color of the tint is usually coordinated with the frame.

Frame Thickness

Many of the effects caused by the lightness or darkness of a frame go hand in hand with frame color. As with frame color, the smaller and more delicate the features, the lighter (thinner) the frame should be. The larger and broader the features, the heavier (thicker) the frame should be.

One exception is a man with large, broad facial features who is smaller in stature than would be expected for the ruggedness of the face. To help neutralize the effect of a head out of proportion to the body, a frame weight lighter than normal might be used.[7] The size must not be too small for the face, however, because a frame that is too small for the face is still too small, whatever the size of the body. A bold frame look can be created by using a dark color in spite of the reduction in frame thickness (Table 4-2).

Children and women with childlike features are especially complimented by a thin frame. Using a frame too thick for these features will easily overpower the face and create a puny appearance rather than add a complimentary facet to the face.[7]

Occasionally the fitter will encounter a person whose features are not strong enough for a heavy frame but who

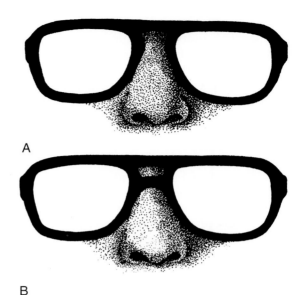

Figure 4-2. To "lengthen" the nose, a frame is chosen that exposes as much of the nose as possible. The frame in **A** is correct; the frame in **B** is incorrect.

TABLE 4-2	
Fitting By Frame Weight	
Frame Weight	**Indicated for**
Heavy	Large, broad features
Medium	Normal features, large features, and small stature
Light	Small, delicate features, women with childlike features, children

wants the heavy frame look. The answer is to use a frame of medium thickness in a very dark color. The dark color makes the frame appear heavier. Similarly, a frame with clear lower rims makes the weight appear less than it really is.

When in doubt as to which frame weight to choose, always select the lighter weight.

Bridge Design

Frame selection can cause the nose to appear longer or shorter than it really is, depending on the frame bridge chosen. Apparent nose length depends on the extent of nose visible beneath the frame bridge, just as apparent face length depends on the area of face observed below the frame.

To "lengthen" the nose, choose a frame that exposes as much of the nose as possible (Figure 4-2). An open-bridged frame allows most of the nose to be seen because it rests on the sides and not on the crest of the bridge.

Dark frame colors draw attention to the surrounding facial area and tend to emphasize whatever characteristics are created by the fit of the frame. In the case of the

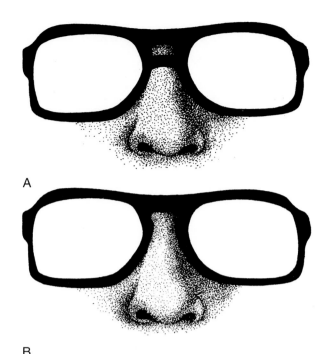

A

B

Figure 4-3. The lower the bridge, the greater the impression of shortening the nose. The bridge in **A** is correct; the bridge in **B** is incorrect.

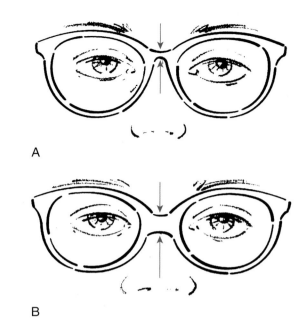

A

B

Figure 4-4. A, If the base of the nose is narrow, choose a frame with a high, thin bridge style. **B,** If the base of the nose is wide, choose a frame with a low-set, vertically wide bridge. (Reprinted with permission from Wylie S: Eyewear Beauty Guide: Don't Choose Your Eyewear Blindfolded! Oldsmar, Fla, 1986, Varilux Press.)

keyhole bridge, using a dark frame color will increase the illusion of nose length. If for reasons of physical fit the keyhole bridge must be used on a person with a long nose, the lengthening effect will not be as emphasized if the bridge is clear or light-colored or if a frame with darker endpieces is used.

The saddle bridge is designed to cut across the crest of the nose. The lower the bridge, the greater the effect of shortening the nose (Figure 4-3). A darker color will give a sharper demarcation and make the nose look shorter still, while a lighter color has a tendency to reverse the effect.

Up to this point, the discussion has been on how frame bridge design affects the apparent length of the nose. Yet with some individuals the length of the nose may not be of primary importance, but rather the width of the base of the nose may matter most. (The base of the nose refers to the lowest point of attachment at the sides of the nostrils.) If the base of the nose is narrow, the bridge of choice is one that is relatively high and thin. Whereas if the base of the nose is wide, the best bridge design will be one that is low-set and vertically wide (Figure 4-4).

FITTING CONSIDERATIONS

Many difficulties associated with adjusting a pair of spectacles appropriately rest with errors in the initial fitting or selection of the frame. Once the lens size and shape have been selected, the essence of the well-fitted frame rests in the choice of the proper bridge and the proper temple style and length. The spread of weight or force over the largest surface is the objective for both pads of the bridge and the behind-the-ear portion of the temple.

The Bridge

When the bridge is fixed, as in most plastic frames, the choice of the appropriate bridge is determined by how well the weight of the frame is borne on the nose. If the bridge is not properly selected, attempts to adjust the frame and the bridge to secure wearer comfort are exceedingly difficult and essentially hopeless.

The appropriate bridge is determined by its width, the position of its pads, the frontal angle of the bridge at the pads, the flare or splay angle of the pads, and the vertical angle of the pads. The bridge selected should not allow the eyewires to ride on the cheeks.

The Significant Nasal Angles for Fitting

If the nose is observed from the front, it will be noted that the two sides form a *frontal angle* with each other, which if projected, would have its apex somewhere on the forehead and its base across the nostrils and tip of the nose. The angle with which each side deviates from the vertical is called the frontal angle (Figure 4-5).

The *splay angle* is seen as the nose widens from front to back. It can be best visualized as if viewed from above and is at the level where the nosepads of the frame will rest (Figure 4-6).

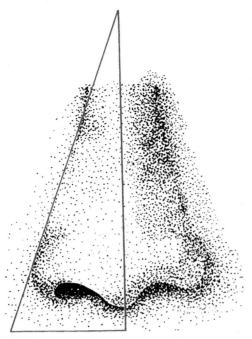

Figure 4-5. The angle with which each side of the nose deviates from the vertical is called the frontal angle.

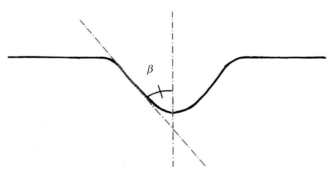

Figure 4-6. The splay angle (β) of the nose is the angle formed by the side of the nose as viewed from the top. The drawing shows a cross section of the nose at the level where the nose-pads will rest.

Both of these angles are of prime importance to the proper fit of the frame. These frontal and splay angles may vary greatly among individuals.

The Frontal Angle. If a frame has a frontal angle which does not parallel the sides of the frontal triangle of the nose, either the inner bottom rims of the frame front or the top of the bridge crest will rest on the nose rather than the pads which should support the frame (Figures 4-7 and 4-8). Matching the angle becomes particularly important if the bridge is fixed and unadjustable.

It should be remembered that the pads will lie on the side of the nose only if the width of the bridge (or DBL) is proper, even after the angle has been matched. If the bridge is too wide, even if the angle is correct the frame will still either rest on the bridge crest or will rest low

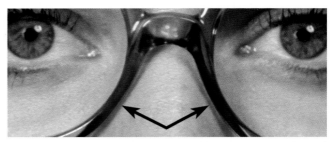

Figure 4-7. With the frame pictured here, the frame frontal angle is too vertical for the angle of the nose. As a result, the frame has a tendency to rest on the bottom rims.

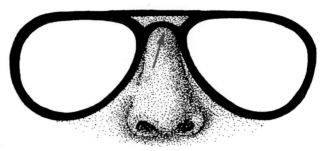

Figure 4-8. With the frame pictured here, the bridge area is too flared for the nose. Since the nose and frame frontal angles do not correspond, the top of the bridge crest is the only part supporting the weight of the frame.

on the nose with the lenses too low. The lines of sight will then be close to the upper rim, or the lower rim may touch the cheeks. A keyhole bridge that is too large may fit like a saddle bridge.

If the bridge is too narrow, the upper rim may be above the eyebrows, the lines of sight may pass through the lenses near the lower rim or in the bifocal, and the lower rims may carry the weight on the side of the nose rather than on the pads.

To check *bridge size*, lift the frame very slightly from the nose and move it to the left or right. There should be about 1 mm of clearance between the nose and free side of the bridge.

With noses that exhibit very broad frontal angles, rather flat crests, and wide splay angles, it is recommended that a bridge design at least somewhat lower than others be used.[8] This type of frame is depicted in Figure 4-4, *B*. Despite the wide area of the crest, a rather narrow bridge is recommended so that the actual pads can be bent back enough to place their flat surfaces on the sides of the nose.

If the bridge is adjustable, it is possible to align the pads to the matching angle by bending the pad arms. If it is not adjustable, the frontal angle of the pads (corresponding to the frontal angle of the nose) can be altered within limits by changing the shape of the lenses.

When the wearer has a nose that flares out too much for the frame selected and there is no suitable alternative frame available, it is possible to reshape the lenses using

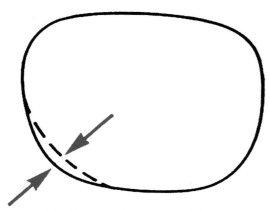

Figure 4-9. The drawing shows the position and amount of material removed from the lens when using a "nasal cut" technique. Unless the dispenser specifies otherwise, the amount usually removed is approximately 1.5 mm.

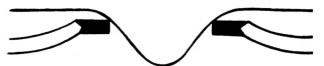

Figure 4-10. If the frame is such that its bridge area does not flare enough when the wearer's nose exhibits a wide splay angle, the back of the bridge area will cut into the side of the nose. The drawing is a top view in cross section and has been exaggerated for clarity.

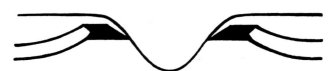

Figure 4-11. If the frame is such that the flare of the nose area exceeds the splay angle of the nose, the fronts of the bridge area may cut into the sides of the nose. The drawing is a top view in cross section and has been exaggerated for clarity.

a *nasal cut* technique (Figure 4-9). With rimless mountings, this is extremely simple; some of the lower nasal corner of the lens is cut away (hence the name *nasal cut*).* An alternative for plastic frames consists of heating the empty frame eyewire and *reshaping the eyewire* to conform to the wearer's facial requirements. A pattern may then be made from this modified shape, or the shape may be traced with a frame tracer. Both lenses are cut to the new configuration.

The Splay Angle. The nose becomes wider as it approaches the inner corners of the eyes, therefore the pads must not only have an appropriate frontal angle, but must also exhibit an appropriate splay angle so that the weight of the spectacles is distributed over the entire *flat* surface of the pad.

If the angle of the pads is such that the backs of the pads are about the same distance apart as are the fronts, but the nose exhibits a wide splay angle, the backs of the pads will cut into the sides of the nose. With a heavy frame this will produce painful and obvious grooves in that area of the nose (Figure 4-10).

If the angle of the pads is such that the backs are farther apart than are the fronts and the amount exceeds the splay angle of the nose, the fronts of the pads or eyewires will cut into the sides of the nose (Figure 4-11).

The Crest Angle

Observing the face from the side reveals the crest angle of the nose: the angle from base to top compared with a vertical plane roughly parallel to the brows and cheeks (Figure 4-12).

This angle is not of great concern in bridge selection unless a saddle or contoured bridge is used. Then the angle of the inside of the contour should parallel the

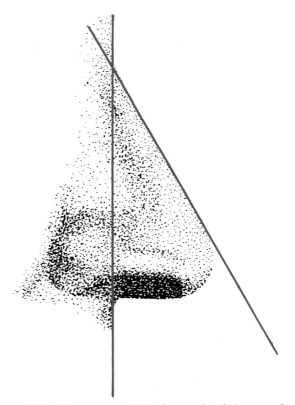

Figure 4-12. The crest angle is that angle of the nose from the base to the top compared with a vertical plane roughly parallel to the brows and cheeks.

---

*If lenses are edged "in-house" an extra pattern for the selected frame can be reshaped. When the altered pattern is used, left-right lens shape symmetry is assured.

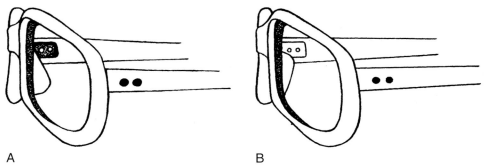

A   B

Figure 4-13. A, Notice how there is more support at the bottom of this nosepad, making it more suitable for children. **B,** Compare the nosepad in **(A)** with an adult-style nosepad.

crest angle so the bridge contacts the nose with its full expanse.

Adjustable Pads

The position of the pads on the nose is of utmost importance. The essential objective is that the *full flat* surfaces of the pads rest on the sides of the nose. Since the pad arms that carry the pads are malleable, the pads can be adjusted individually for each side of the nose. In selecting a frame with adjustable pads, the principal criteria therefore are:

1. The DBL should be such that the pads can be easily set to rest on the sides of the nose without either stretching the pad arms a great deal laterally or compressing them together.
2. When heavy frames or lenses are being selected, the following factors influence pad comfort.
   a. The inclination of the frontal angle of the nose on which the pad surface will rest. The closer to vertical the pad is, the greater will be the pressure on the nose to hold the frame in place.[10]
   b. If the surface of the pad is almost vertical, it is best to use lightweight lenses. Pads made from silicone material do not tend to slip as much as regular plastic pads.
3. The questions of proper vertical angle, splay angle, and full contact of the broad side of the pad are usually handled by bending the pad arms. (Refer to Chapters 8 and 9 for detailed descriptions.)

   In selecting a frame with an adjustable bridge, however, care must also be given to the type of pad arm and its attachment to the eyewire. Certain frames carry the pads via practically straight, very short, vertically attached pad arms. Such arms allow only very limited adjustment of the pads. Any attempt to raise and lower pads with these pad arms is almost impossible. Selection of frames with this type of pad arm requires that the DBL and the lens position be correct almost from the beginning and that adjustment of the pads be minimal. (For more on adjustable pads, see Chapter 9.)
4. The center of gravity of a heavy frame is closer to the front. If the pads are set closer to the frame

front, the frame moves closer to the face. This places the center of gravity farther back, resulting in the frame staying in place more easily. Thus it is desirable to set the pads as close to the front as facial construction, lash length, and so forth, will allow.

Larger pads, which distribute the weight over a larger area on the nose, can also be used as the mass of the spectacles is increased.

Children's Bridges

It has been found that in children between the ages of 3 and 18 years there is only a slight change in the crest angle of the nose (the slope from the crest to the tip of the nose).[11] The main change is in the splay angle (the slope from the crest of the nose to the cheek) and in the depth of the nasal bridge.

What this means in terms of fitting children is that there needs to be (1) more support at the bottom of the nose pad area, and (2) a larger pad splay angle (more flare to the pad). A larger pad or contact surface area helps the frame sit better (Figure 4-13).

Temples

The distribution of forces necessary to hold a frame in place on the face generally shifts from the nose to the ears as the head is bent forward. Thus the activity of the wearer and the intended use of the spectacles should be considered to determine the temple style ordered. Because temple style is greatly dependent on wearer preference, these considerations should be pointed out.

Spectacles with flat, straight-back, or library temples are suitable when their removal and replacement without altering adjustment is desired. This situation would arise when the spectacles are to be worn only occasionally or mainly for reading or desk work.

A skull temple is applicable if the wearer's activity requires the normal amount of movement or constant wear. If the head is to be lowered markedly or the individual is physically active, riding bows or comfort cable temples are preferable.

All temples help hold the lenses in place primarily by the area of contact with the side of the head and not by

TABLE 4-3
Fitting Temple Styles

Temple Style	Indicated for	Contraindicated for
Comfort cable or riding bow	Active people Jobs requiring unusual head positions Young children Especially heavy frames and/or lenses	Off and on wear
Straight back	Off and on wear	Heavy lenses Persons with parallel-sided noses Persons with flat noses Frames with weak fronts
Skull	Normal, everyday wear	Jobs requiring unusual head positions

pressure at the tip of the temple or against the upper crease in the ear. The choice of proper length is therefore important in frame selection. The temple should be long enough so that the bend of the temple takes place just barely past the top of the ear (see Figure 9-12). The exact fit of the bent-down portion or earpiece against the head can be achieved during adjustment of the frame.

Table 4-3 summarizes the temple styles suitable when considering both the activity of the wearer and the intended use of the spectacles.

Selecting Frames for the Progressive Addition Lens Wearer

A progressive addition lens wearer needs a frame with:
1. A minimal vertex distance.
2. An adequate pantoscopic tilt.
3. Sufficient vertical depth in the nasal portion of the frame shape.

A *minimal vertex distance** is required because of the relatively narrow viewing areas afforded by the progressive optics of the lens for intermediate and near distances (see Chapter 20). The closer the progressive viewing zone is brought to the eye, the wider the intermediate and near viewing areas will be.

Using a frame with an *adequate pantoscopic tilt* will also help bring the lower (reading) half of the lens closer to the eyes. When the eyes are turned downward for near viewing, the reading width will be increased.

The shape of the frame is important with progressive addition lenses. If the lens has too much of the lower nasal area cut away, as with the classic aviator shape, the reading area is reduced (Figure 4-14, *A*). Also, when the lens is narrow vertically, much of the near viewing area will be lost. This loss may be prevented if a progressive lens specifically designed for frames with narrow vertical dimensions is chosen (Figure 14-14, *B*). However, frames with an extremely narrow vertical dimension will not

work well for progressive addition lenses. A good frame shape for a progressive lens has a *sufficient vertical depth and not much nasal cut* (Figure 4-14, *C*). The best design for a progressive addition lens is one that has extra vertical depth in the inferior, nasal portion of the shape (Figure 4-14, *D*). Unfortunately, style and function do not always agree.

Selecting Frames for the High Minus Wearer

Although lenses are usually chosen for optical appropriateness, the cosmetic effects of certain types of lenses also should be considered. These are usually lenses at extreme powers of minus or plus, which notably minify or magnify the eyes and face behind them. Several cosmetic factors must be taken into account when fitting the high minus correction wearer (Box 4-1).

Size

Size considerations include avoiding frames with lenses that are very large, since the lens edge gets thicker farther away from the center. Frames with rounded corners should be used when possible for this same reason.

A frame wider than the wearer's face at the temple area should also be avoided, since high minus lenses make the side of the wearer's head look narrower through the lenses (Figure 4-15).

Excessive *decentration* should be avoided or the outer lens edge will be much thicker than the inner edge. An alternative is to use a wider bridge and smaller eye size. The nose pads can be brought closer together, if necessary, rather than decentering too much. For example, a 48□20 can be used instead of a 50□18. (For −12.00 D lenses, this will also reduce the weight of the lenses by a considerable amount.)

Lens Material

Lens edges are thicker with low-index CR-39 plastic. Using a lens of a higher index material will reduce the edge thickness. High index plastic lenses are chosen over high index glass because of the weight factor. High index

---

*Vertex distance is the distance from the back surface of the lens to the front surface of the eye.

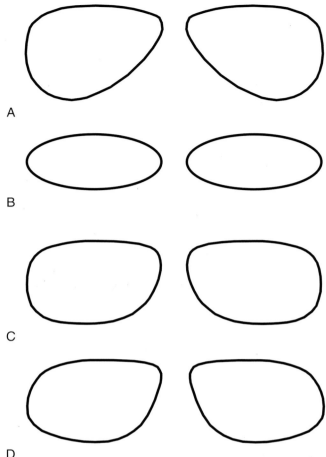

A

B

C

D

Figure 4-14. The best shapes for progressive addition lens wear have sufficient vertical depth and are not restricted in the inferior nasal lens area. **A,** This frame choice is not a good choice for progressive lenses. The area nasally where the progressive lens near zone is located is cut away by the aviator-style shape of the frame. **B,** This frame shape will work for a progressive if the progressive lens style chosen is designed for frames with a narrow vertical dimension. A frame with a narrow vertical dimension should not be used with standard-style progressive lenses. **C,** The best frame style for progressive lenses is one that has enough vertical depth to allow full use of both intermediate and near viewing areas of the progressive lens. **D,** Though not always cosmetically appropriate, a frame with a generous inferior-nasal lens area is optically ideal for a progressive addition lens.

plastic lenses are an excellent choice for high minus lenses.

Polycarbonate lenses offer both a weight and edge thickness advantage. Polycarbonate lenses can be made with a thinner center thickness because of their high impact resistance. This translates into a thinner edge. Even if a polycarbonate lens has the same center thickness as a regular plastic CR-39 lens, the edge of the polycarbonate lens will still be thinner than the CR-39. This is because the polycarbonate lens has a higher index of refraction (1.586) than the CR-39 lens

---

BOX 4-1

Fitting the High Minus Wearer

Use	Avoid
Smaller eye size	Large lenses
If in between sizes, use the smaller indicated eye size and larger indicated bridge size	Excessive decentration
Rounded corners	Squared-off corners
Low density (light weight) lenses if weight reduction is important	Crown glass lenses
Midindex or high index lenses, such as polycarbonate or high index plastic	Low index lenses, such as CR-39 plastic lenses
Flatter or "hidden" bevels	Full V bevels
Polished or rolled and polished edges	Nonpolished, frosted-looking edges causing a concentric-ring appearance
Without rolled and/or polished edges, use frames with rims that hide lens edges combined with bevel placement that balances	Thin rims in combination with lenses having unpolished edges
Antireflection coating or a light tint (AR coating is preferred over a light tint)	Frames that extend beyond the side of the wearer's head
Aspheric or atoric lenses	Flat, non-AR-coated front curves
For exceptionally high minus—biconcave or minus lenticular lenses	

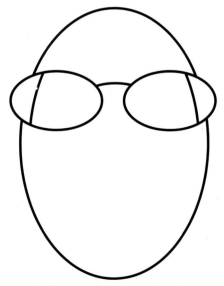

Figure 4-15. High minus lenses minify objects. When high minus lenses are worn in a frame that is too large, the observer sees the wearer's face minified through the lenses. This makes the head look narrow in the area behind the lenses compared with the rest of the face.

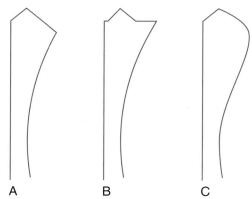

Figure 4-16. **A,** A regular 40-degree bevel is inappropriate for a high minus lens. Fortunately, it is almost never used. **B,** A flat bevel reduces some of the internal reflections and concentric rings that would otherwise be seen with a regular 40-degree bevel. However, the edge will still appear thick. **C,** A rolled and polished bevel reduces edge thickness.

(1.498). (For more information on lens materials see Chapter 23.)

Reflections, Base Curve, and Lens Bevel

Reflections, curve, and *bevel* are additional considerations. The larger the bevel, the more reflection rings will be noticeable because these rings are a reflection of the lens edge. Using a now-standard hidden bevel as shown in Figure 4-16, *B* (rather than the older 40-degree bevel as shown in Figure 4-16, *A*) reduces the problem.

The edge of a high minus lens can be made less noticeable by *rolling the edge.* This is especially true for metal or thin plastic frames. Rolling the edge changes it from flat to rounded, as shown in Figure 4-16, *C,* giving a nice appearance to the lens when polished and often reducing measured edge thickness by as much as 2 mm. *Polishing the edges* will make the lens look better to an observer, but unless an antireflection (AR) coating is used, such polishing will introduce internal reflections, which are disturbing to many wearers. Thus the combination of *roll and polish* looks very good. Some recommend using a roll and polish with caution because of the possibility of wearer dissatisfaction because of the distortion caused by the rolled area in the periphery of the lens. An edge does not have to be rolled to be polished. A conventionally beveled lens edge can also be polished. With better manufacturing techniques, polish edges are much easier to produce and are coming to be expected on lenses with visible bevels.

Unless antireflection coated, a *front curve* reduced below +2.00 D will result in a high reflection of light from the front. Unfortunately, high minus lenses made with ordinary spherical curves require a fairly flat front curve to give good optics. It is possible to use an aspheric design to allow for a different front curve and to slightly thin the edge of the lens by steepening the lens in the periphery. An aspheric high minus lens may have a better

cosmetic appearance than a conventional, spherically based lens of the same power. (For more information on lens design and aspherics, see Chapter 18.)

Even though a light tint will reduce internal lens reflections, an antireflection (AR) coating does a much better job. Even lenses with flat front curves will lose their mirrorlike reflective appearances with an AR coating. Antireflection coatings also eliminate the concentric rings, which are frequently seen with high minus lens prescriptions.

For wearers with excessively high minus lenses, a minus lenticular design is an option. (For more on the subject see Chapter 18.)

Miscellaneous Factors

An interesting consideration is that high minus lenses tend to cause eye *makeup* to show up less, whereas high plus lenses cause any type of makeup to be more noticeable.

Selecting Frames for the High Plus Wearer

Size and Thickness

Size and *thickness* are considerations with high plus lenses (Box 4-2). Large lenses should be avoided because of excessive weight and the increase in center thickness. High plus lenses magnify the wearer's eyes. When lens size increases, so does center thickness, causing an even greater magnification problem.

Because of differences in frame shapes, eye size is not the only influence on lens thickness. The effective

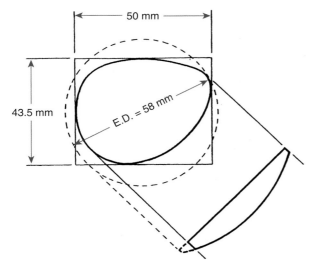

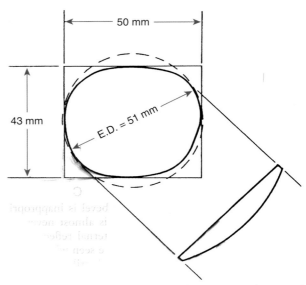

Figure 4-17. The larger the effective diameter of a plus lens for a given eye size, the thicker the edge appearance will be in certain meridians. Because a larger lens blank size is required, the center thickness will also be greater.

Figure 4-18. When the effective diameter is close to the frame eye size, the edge thickness will be more uniform and held to a minimum. Small effective diameters also make possible a lens of minimal center thickness. (For a further explanation of effective diameter, see Chapters 2 and 5.)

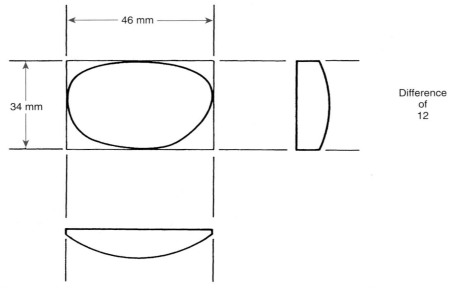

Figure 4-19. In the case of the high plus lens, the larger the frame difference, the thicker the lens will appear on the top and bottom. The case is reversed with the high minus lens, however, since the thicker edges will then be in the horizontal meridian.

diameter of a lens is increased whenever a lens deviates from a round or oval shape. The more the lens deviates from round or oval, the larger and thicker the lens will be (Figures 4-17 and 4-18). A good rule of thumb for very high plus lenses, such as the older cataract lenses, is to avoid frames with an effective diameter more than 2 mm larger than the eye size.

Frame Difference
The "frame difference" is an additional factor when selecting a proper frame shape for the high plus wearer

(see Chapter 2). Frames with narrow lens openings (where the difference between horizontal and vertical measurements is large) cause a high plus lens to be thick on the top and bottom edges (Figure 4-19). This causes the strong plus lens to look even stronger. For the high plus lens wearer, frame differences greater than 9 mm should be avoided.

Cataract Lenses and UV Protection
Cataract lenses are very high plus lenses that were used after cataract surgery before the advent of intraocular

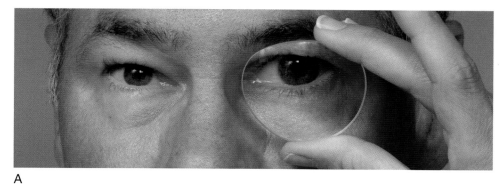

A

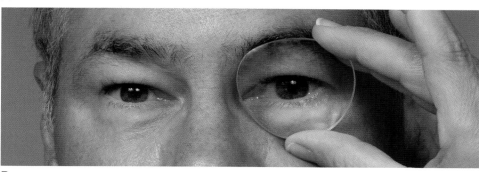

B

Figure 4-20. The lens in **A** is positioned with a large vertex distance, whereas in **B** the vertex distance is minimal. The same lens was used in both photographs, which were taken under circumstances that were as identical as possible. The only difference between the two photographs is the distance from lens to eye. In both cases the eye is magnified, as can readily be seen by comparing the eye behind the lens with the eye without the lens. However, the eye behind the lens in **B** shows less magnification than the eye behind the lens in **A**.

lens implants. They are now uncommon. Cataract lenses usually range in power from +9.00 D to +22.00 D, depending upon the wearer's lens prescription before surgery. The prescription was this high because it had to replace the power of the crystalline lens of the eye that was removed during surgery. Fortunately the crystalline lens is now replaced with a small lens implanted into the eye. People who have had cataract surgery and have not received an intraocular lens implant are aphakic (which means "without lens"). They are referred to as *aphakes*. Aphakes must either wear contact lenses or high plus cataract spectacle lenses. Fortunately intraocular lens implants are now the standard for cataract surgery and such situations are rare.

Aphakes are often more light-sensitive than other individuals as a result of crystalline lens removal. To prevent damage to the retina of an aphakic individual caused by *ultraviolet (UV) light*, protection is essential. Only lenses with UV inhibiting properties should be used for aphakes. (For more information on UV protection see Chapter 22, Absorptive Lenses.)

Frame Characteristics

There are certain frame characteristics that are absolutely necessary for properly fitting high plus lenses. With medium power plus lenses, these characteristics can be considered as suggested guidelines, but with high plus or cataract lenses they are mandatory prerequisites.

Frames should be chosen for their ability to hold their *alignment*. Flimsy construction allows the lenses to slide down the nose. This is not only irritating to the wearer, but also has some rather serious optical side effects. These include:

1. The blurring of distance vision as a result of an increased effective lens power.
2. A smaller field of view.
3. An increase in the magnification of objects viewed by the wearer.
4. An increase in the apparent size of the wearer's eyes to an observer (Figure 4-20); as the vertex distance decreases for plus lenses, the wearer's eyes look less magnified when viewed by an observer.

A frame should be chosen that allows the distance optical center of the lenses to be positioned properly before the eyes. See Figures 4-21 and 4-22 for further explanations.

Because field of view is increased and magnification decreased as plus lenses are moved closer to the eyes, the frame selected should hold the lenses as close as possible to the eyes. The wearer's eyelashes should just clear the back surfaces of the lenses.

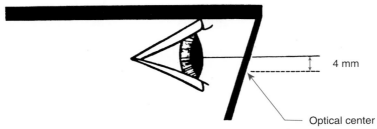

4 mm

Optical center

Figure 4-21. To avoid adversely affecting the optical performance of the lens, for every millimeter that the optical center is below the wearer's line of sight, there must be 2 degrees of pantoscopic tilt. For example, as pictured here, the optical center falls 4 mm below the lenses, requiring 8 degrees of pantoscopic tilt in relationship to the plane of the face.

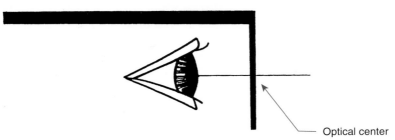

Optical center

Figure 4-22. When the pupil corresponds to the optical center of the lens, there should be no pantoscopic tilt. Any lens tilt added will change the sphere power of the lens and cause an unwanted cylinder component to be manifested. For low power lenses, the power effect is negligible, but with a higher power lens it can be quite evident. (For further explanation see Chapters 5 and 18.)

Adjustable nosepads become more of a necessity as the power of the lenses increases. They offer the advantage of versatility in allowing modification of the vertical position of the frame. This allows the major reference point height, bifocal height, or progressive lens fitting cross height to be exactly adjusted.

Adjustable nosepads also allow the lenses to be positioned at varying distances from the eyes. This allows more precision in the refractive power of the correction. Unless a high-powered lens is fitted at the refracting distance used during the eye examination, an error in power will result. Unless a compensation for the vertex distance change is made, significant error results. For example, if a +15.00 D lens is intended for a 12 mm vertex distance between the cornea and rear lens surface, but is fitted at 17 mm, the lens will be almost +1.25 D too strong. It is obvious then that with high-powered lenses, power compensation for variations in vertex distance is a necessity for bridge designs not using adjustable pads. (For how vertex distance power compensations are done, see the *Effective Power* section in Chapter 14.)

Serious consideration should be given to using *comfort cable temples* when the anatomic features of the nose do not lend themselves to keeping the glasses in place or if the prescribed glasses tend to be somewhat heavy. Cable temples help keep the glasses from slipping down the nose and thus help avoid the difficulties listed above.

Selecting Frames for Children

When selecting frames for children, safety should be the first concern. Children are always doing things that are unexpectedly hazardous, and children's eyeglasses can be expected to endure much abuse. The main concern is not so much that the frames and lenses hold up to such abuse, but rather that the child is not put at risk because of a poorly chosen frame.

Remember, a frame that is small and sold for children may not necessarily be the best design for children. Because style is important to children, too, children's frames often mimic adult styles.

Children's frames should be sturdy. Look for solidly built frames, be they plastic or metal. The lens grooves should be deep so that the lenses are more securely seated in the frame.

It is advisable to avoid nylon cord frames because the thin cord does not hold the lenses in place securely enough for rough-and-tumble play.

When available, high quality spring temples are a good option. When hit from the side, the spring takes much of the shock, instead of transferring all of it to the side of the nose. In addition, spring temples will save trips back to the dispensary to have the frames realigned.

Although not directly related to the subject of frame selection, it is important to note that polycarbonate

Frame Selection for Children

Use	Avoid
Sturdy frames	Lightly constructed copies of adult frames
Deeply grooved frame fronts	Frames with shallow grooves
Quality spring temples	Nylon cord frames
Bridges that give support in the area of the lower portion of the nosepad	
High impact lenses such as polycarbonate or Trivex	Any lenses that are not highly impact resistant, especially glass lenses
Sports protection when applicable	

lenses or Trivex lenses are the lenses of choice for children. The increased safety far outweighs any considerations given to the tendency for a polycarbonate lens to scratch. In short, children need high-impact-resistant lenses and dispensers have a responsibility to make sure that parents know why.

Both polycarbonate and Trivex lenses have the added benefit of giving children ultraviolet (UV) protection at no additional cost. The crystalline lens of a child's eye will let more light through than will the lens of an adult. UV light can begin to take its toll early in life, and with the increased radiation because of the earth's decreased ozone layer, it is never too early to begin protection.

If a child leaves the dispensary with lenses other than high impact lenses, the record should contain a dated statement noting that the parents were informed of the advisability of using such lenses and refused that option. A form to that effect signed by a parent is a further precaution against liability, but is not a legal requirement. (For more on the issue of liability, see Chapter 23.)

With an increased emphasis on sports for children, specialty sports glasses should not be overlooked. Children who participate in sports such as baseball may be at greater risk than adults who play the same sport. Not all children can react quickly enough to avoid a ball in the eye. Carelessness by other children when throwing balls or swinging bats also adds to the risks. A conscientious dispenser will be aware of options in sports eyewear for children and make them available. (For more on sports eyewear, see Chapter 23.)

See Box 4-3 for a summary of factors in selecting frames for children.

Selecting Frames for Older Wearers

When selecting frames for older wearers, perhaps the most important factor to consider is weight. With age, the skin looses its elasticity. This causes nosepads to depress the skin and underlying tissue, leaving marks that do not rebound easily. When the eyeglasses are heavy, red marks on the nose and ears can easily develop into sores that are slow to heal. Therefore choosing a frame that is lightweight and combining that selection with a lightweight lens material will do much to prevent problems.

The bridge of the frame must fit correctly. If the bridge fitting principles that were explained earlier in the chapter are exactly applied, the frame will be comfortable. Remember, with older wearers there is less room for error. The bridge must seat itself over the largest area possible to evenly spread the weight of the glasses. For this reason, when selecting a frame with adjustable pads, it is helpful to use a frame with larger pads when available.

Unless the wearer has no distance prescription, the shape of the frame must leave enough room for the type of multifocal design selected. (See the section in this chapter on selecting frames for progressive addition lens wearers.)

It should not be assumed that the older wearer will be unconcerned with style, or will only be interested in the same type of frame as they have been wearing. Older individuals appreciate being accorded the same frame styling options given everyone else.

Selecting Frames for Safety Eyewear

Safety frames are no longer limited to drab colors and "S7" safety frame shapes, but are available in a large variety of styles. In many cases they are not easily distinguished from regular "dress" eyewear. Although function is paramount, rules for selecting a well-fitting, nice-looking frame do not change dramatically when selecting safety eyewear.

Remember that a safety frame is not just a sturdy frame with thick lenses. A safety frame must comply with specific standards and be identified with the mark "Z87" or "Z87-2" on both the temples and frame front.

Metal frames should be avoided when electrical hazards are present, and side shields are necessary when eye injuries from the side are possible.

There are several factors other than the fit of the frame and the few obvious considerations listed here that must be taken into account when dispensing safety eyewear. Therefore before ordering it would be advisable to review the appropriate section on the subject found in Chapter 23.

Devices That Help in the Frame Selection Process

One problem in selecting frames occurs when uncorrected visual acuity is so poor that the frames cannot be seen without glasses. There are several possible solutions.

1. *Bring a friend*
   People who have been in the awkward situation of not being able to see the new frame on themselves

often bring a friend along to help them chose something suitable. Bringing a friend, however, does not really deal with the root problem.

2. *Use a trial lens*

If there is a trial lens set available, choose the spherical equivalent for the preferred eye. The spherical equivalent of a lens is one half of the cylinder power added to the sphere power. (Incidentally, if the wearer requires a near addition, it may be helpful to add about one half of the prescribed near addition power to the spherical equivalent.) With the frame on, the wearer holds the lens in front of the preferred eye and looks in the mirror. Although sometimes helpful, this solution does not win high praise.

3. *Use a Visiochoix*

One system that addresses the problem of not being able to see the frame on the wearer consists of using a set of lenses mounted in a clear plastic panel. Each plastic panel has a handle and can be held in front of the eyes. The person selecting their frames can see the frames he or she is wearing behind the lenses because the entire mounting is made of clear plastic. The lens pair closest to the prescription is chosen from the Visiochoix set,* and the wearer is able to use both eyes. This solution is usually much preferred over the single trial lens method.

4. *Use a video system.*

Just using a standard video camera will make it easier for someone to see themselves clearly with a new frame. An individual can put on a number of frames, one after the other. Each time a frame is tried on, the wearer can turn his or her head first one way, then the other, so that the frames in place can be seen from the side as well. Once a series of frames have been tried, the tape is rewound and the person can view the tape while wearing his or her own prescription. However, there is a better video system for aiding in this process that offers much more than just a video camera. This makes use of a computerized image-capturing system.

Computerized Image-Capturing Systems

Imaging systems that are made especially for the dispensary will offer several advantages over a standard video camera and VCR. A computerized imaging system can display an image faster and easier. Here are some of the other features available at the time of this writing. Not all features are available on all systems.

- Shows images of the same frame from different angles of view (Figure 4-23).
- Permits side-by-side comparisons of different frames on the same screen (Figure 4-24).
- May allow certain measurements to be calculated by the system, such as PD and multifocal segment

---

* Available from Bernell Corp., South Bend, IN.

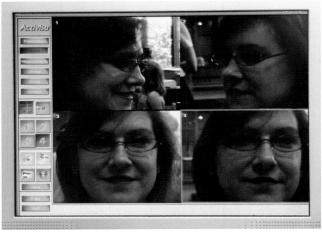

Figure 4-23. Computerized image-capturing systems can show images of the same frame from different angles of view.

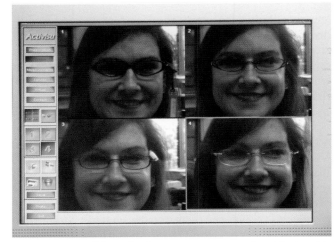

Figure 4-24. Here the image system permits side-by-side comparisons of different frames on the same screen.

heights after the frame shape has been outlined (Figure 4-25).

- May show the thickness of certain lens prescriptions from a side view of the lens, (Figure 4-26). An accompanying on-screen table comparing two lens materials for thicknesses and weight may be present.
- It may also be possible to take the image of the wearer with the prospective frames being worn and show what the lenses would look like:
  1. If AR coated.
  2. If tinted to a certain solid or gradient transmission.
  3. If made from a photochromic material.
- Included in some systems are simulations of how different scenes might appear to the wearer with and without an AR coating on the lenses.

In addition to the spectacle lens applications, some systems show an individual what they would look like if they were wearing tinted contact lenses of different colors.

A few systems allow web access by the wearer. This would include:
- Web access to previously recorded images of what certain frames look like while being worn. A password is required.

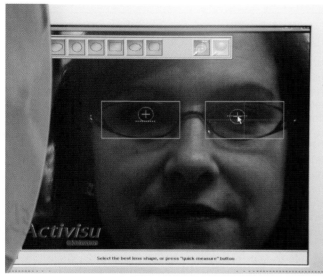

Figure 4-25. Some computer-based systems allow certain measurements to be calculated by the system after the frame shape has been outlined, such as PD and multifocal segment heights.

- Web access to a virtual frame try-on service from a home computer. This requires the wearer to have a previously recorded image of their face placed in a database at the optical dispensary. Then any frame in a data bank of possibilities can be superimposed to scale on the image of the wearer's face. This means a person could check later on to see if there were any new frame styles available that they might like.

Closing the Frame Selection Process

Selecting a frame is a decision-making process. And making decisions is difficult. A good dispenser can help in making that process easier. Here are a few suggestions.

1. Do not prejudge a person's financial situation by only showing less expensive frames. Let each person make his or her own decision on how much to spend.
2. Do not voluntarily categorize a person's face as being a certain shape for them. They may not agree with you. Be diplomatic.
3. Do not insist on a certain frame if the wearer does not like it, even though it may look best and be optically sound.
4. Do not allow the wearer to select a frame or lens style that you know would be unsafe or optically unsound.
5. Do not have a large number of frames spread out at any one time. People forget what they have looked

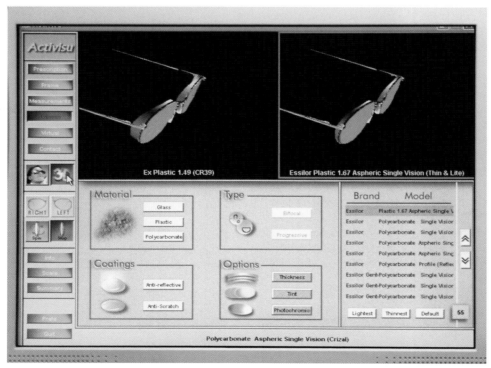

Figure 4-26. This image-capturing system shows the expected thickness of a lens prescription as seen from a side view of the lens. An accompanying on-screen table comparing two lens materials for thicknesses and weight may also be possible.

at and rejected. Too many frames out at once may cause a person to become confused or overwhelmed. If a frame choice is unsatisfactory, return the frame to the display or put it out of sight. Try and keep the number of frame styles being considered at three or less at any given time.

6. Do not ask "if;" ask "which." Presenting procrastination as a possible alternative is a disservice to those who find the decision-making process difficult. Helping to narrow the choice to two possibilities simplifies matters.

7. Do not overlook the possibility of more than one pair. In many cases one pair is not enough. Some people want or need more than one pair because:
   a. They like both and can afford both.
   b. They need a back-up pair and know it.
   c. Their visual needs vary in different work situations.

8. Be sure to point out the positive aspects of the frames that are being considered. People want to know they are buying an appropriate, quality product. The typical wearer of eyeglasses usually knows very little about frames and lenses. Telling the wearer why these frames and lenses are good will help them to feel confident in their decision.

A WORD ON FRAME MANAGEMENT

Good frame selection is based on the availability of a variety of quality frames in the dispensary. No matter how many frames are on the frame boards, if those frames are all the same style, the frame selection process will not lead to a successful outcome. The person responsible for buying frames needs to be aware of the various types of individuals who will be selecting frames and choose frames to buy with that in mind.

Left alone, frame inventory will most certainly obey the Second Law of Thermodynamics and go from order to disorder. Below are a few examples of what can happen with frame inventory in the dispensary. The solutions given are not limited just to the example stated, but are generally applicable to the dispensary.

Example **4-1:** *TOO MANY "DOGS"*

People seem to be having an increasing hard time finding frames they like. The staff has trouble helping them. It seems that most of the frames are just not very appealing. What went wrong?

Solution

The person buying frames buys a logical selection of frames. Some frames sell immediately. Unfortunately, they are not reordered. The ones that were not popular do not sell and stay on the board. Another frame representative arrives and the same scenario is repeated. Before long the dispensary has an overwhelming number of frames that nobody really wants.

To prevent this from happening, keep a log of which frames are selling and replace those frames immediately. If a frame requires a long time to sell, do not replace that frame when you sell it unless it is in the dispensary to serve a certain type of clientele. It is advisable to consult with your frame representatives as they know what frames are selling in your area.

Example **4-2:** *SOME FIND FRAMES EASILY; OTHERS CANNOT EVEN GET STARTED*

Unlike the previous situation where it is difficult to find the right frame, in this situation frame selection is frustrating with some people, but not everybody. It is not just wearer indecision. The staff has trouble helping certain individuals find something that looks right for them, too.

Solution

When a frame representative comes into the office, there are one or two of the staff that looks over the new available frames trying to decide what to buy. In the process, the staff tries on the frames to see what looks good. As a result, over time the dispensary is filled with frames that look great on the staff, who may have one facial type or one particular taste in style. People with other fitting characteristics are unable to find frames that are appropriate for them.

To keep the inventory balanced, the buyer needs to think about what is necessary for different facial types and different tastes in frames, such as conservative versus trendy.

Example **4-3:** *BACK-STOCK DRAWERS AND CABINETS ARE FULL*

Every dispensary has some place where extra frames are stored. There should be a limited number of frames in back stock. In this case, however, every drawer is full. What happened?

Solution

There is more than one reason why this situation could occur. The proper contents of these storage areas are backups for frames that are moving very quickly. If all of the stored frames are discontinued or frames that just will not move, then Example 4-1 above has been "solved" by removing the "dogs" from the board and ordering new frames. Here is an example of what can be happening if backups are not in this category.

Frame companies often have promotionals. With a certain sized order, the company may give away a "premium." This could include such things as trips, watches, or computer-related prizes. If the buyer finds these things desirable, it does not take long to end up with too much stock. Do not buy frames just because they come with rewards.

Example **4-4:** *EVERYTHING IS DISCONTINUED*

You have picked out just the right frame, but the color is wrong. You try to order the needed color, but the frame has been discontinued. Unfortunately, this is becoming a regularly occurring problem. What is wrong?

Solution

Some discontinued stock is unavoidable. But when the issue just keeps growing, there is a problem somewhere. Here are some typical causes and/or solutions. Most of them are just generally good practices for responsible frame management.

1. You may be buying frames from too many places. Having too many companies will make it difficult to track what is really happening with frame sales. Use a limited number of frame companies and know your representatives well. If you are not a large account for anybody, then your individual frame representatives do not have much of an interest in seeing that your frames are up-to-date. If you know your frame representatives and they know you, it should be in their best interest to work with you for the long-term benefit of your dispensary.

2. If you receive a notice that a frame is to be discontinued, act now. You have a limited time to return it for credit. Do not miss that time. If you miss the cut-off, how to get rid of the frame is your problem.

3. Be careful of "deals" where you can get a large number of frames for a very low price. Those frames may be scheduled to be discontinued or already be discontinued.

4. Before you bring a new frame company "on board," ask about their return policy. Tell the representative of that company that you expect them to keep you informed of frames that are to be discontinued.

5. Allocate a frame representative from a certain company a certain given number of spaces on your frame board. Let them know that it is their responsibility to work with you to keep those frames current and moving. It will be in their best interest to determine which frames sell best in your practice and which do not. They will not want any discontinued frames taking up space in their area.

6. Although it is good practice to immediately re-order frames that are selling quickly, it is not good practice to automatically re-order everything. If a frame is not selling, do not re-order when it does sell. If you notice that a frame is not moving, do not wait to exchange it.

7. If the problem exists already, try to recover without just moving mountains of discontinued frames into a "spare parts" box. Figure out ways to move stock that has not sold, is not returnable, and may still have value. Here are some ideas: Mark it down. Put plano sunglass lenses in the frame and sell them at an attractive price. If there are some frames that still will not move, donate them to a charitable organization for a tax write-off.

REFERENCES

1. Drew R: Professional ophthalmic dispensing, Stoneham, Mass, 1970, Butterworth/Heinemann.
2. Wilson C: Frame dynamics, nine ways to fit the perfect frame every time, Eye Talk, May/June, p. 33, 1983.
3. Dispensing Fashion Eyewear: The eye-glassery, Melville, NY, 1990, Marchon Eyewear, Inc.
4. Dowaliby M: Dr. Margaret Dowaliby's guide to the art of eyewear dispensing, Fullerton, Calif, 1987, Southern California College of Optometry.
5. Wyllie S: Eyewear beauty guide: don't choose your eyewear blindfolded, Oldsmann, Fla, 1986, Varilux Press.
6. Jackson C: Color me beautiful, New York, 1980, Ballatine Books.
7. Dowaliby M: The fundamentals of cosmetic dispensing, Stoneham, Mass, 1966, The Professional Press, Butterworth/Heinemann.
8. Wirz JR: Styling for blacks: follow the four 'Cs', Eye Talk, p.53, 1980.
9. Brooks C: Essentials of ophthalmic lens finishing, St. Louis, MO, 2003, Butterworth/Heinemann.
10. Fleck H, Mutze S: Sehhilfenanpassung, Berlin, 1970, VEB Verlag Technikpp.
11. Marks R: An investigation of the anatomical changes in the shape of children's noses, Rochester, NY, 1959, Shuron Division of Textron.

Proficiency Test

(Answers can be found in the back of the book.)

Match the correct frame characteristics with the face shape. (There may be up to two correct answers for each.)

1. ____ Oblong
2. ____ Round
3. ____ Inverted triangular (base-up)
4. ____ Triangular (base-down)

   a. darker colors or bolder look
   b. narrow frame
   c. rimless
   d. deep frame
   e. low temple attachment
   f. high temple attachment

5. Which of the following is indicated and should be used when fitting the high minus lens wearer?
   a. rounded corners
   b. large lenses
   c. 40-degree V-bevels
   d. crown glass lenses
   e. excessive decentration

6. Which face shape most lends itself to wearing glasses?
   a. the wide face
   b. the long face
   c. the base-down triangular face
   d. the base-up triangular face
   e. the diamond face

7. Which of the following would be examples of a frame appropriate for a wide face?
   a. a frame with a large difference between horizontal and vertical measurements
   b. a frame where the temples attach high on the frame
   c. a frame where the temples attach low on the frame
   d. a frame where the lenses are deep, covering a larger facial area

8. In fitting the base-up (inverted) triangular face, choose a frame that is:
   a. fairly heavy to add necessary emphasis to the upper facial area
   b. somewhat wider than normal
   c. a dark color
   d. medium to lightweight to be as unobtrusive as possible
   e. none of the above

9. When deciding upon the upper frame line design,
   a. it is desirable to choose an upper eyewire line that follows the basic line of the eyebrow.
   b. it is best to choose an upper eyewire line that contrasts with the eyebrow line somewhat.
   c. the best design is one that starts below the eyebrow, crosses the eyebrow at the midpoint, and continues on above the eyebrow.

10. Using an upsweep on either the upper or lower rim of a frame:
    a. always results in a surprised look and should be avoided.
    b. can add lift to a face that has begun to sag with age.
    c. brands the wearer as being out-of-date.

11. True or false? Choosing the favorite or dominant color a person wears for their frame color should be avoided, since the color repetition calls too much attention to the glasses.

12. True or false? A lighter-colored, more delicately styled frame is recommended for the person with light, fine hair.

13. True or false? Individuals with salt-and-pepper hair, or hair that is just starting to gray will find that choosing a silver frame will make the "salt" component of their salt-and-pepper hair more noticeable and should be routinely avoided.

14. True or false? When in doubt as to which frame weight to choose, select the heavier weight frame.

15. The lower the frame bridge, the greater the effect of:
    a. shortening of the nose.
    b. lengthening of the nose.

Match the following meases types with the indicated temple style.

16. ____ Active people
17. ____ On-and-off wear
18. ____ Normal, everyday wear
19. ____ Jobs requiring unusual head positions
20. ____ Especially heavy frame

   a. straight back
   b. comfort cable or riding bow
   c. skull

21. The frontal angle is:
    a. the angle from which the front crest of the nose deviates from the vertical when viewed from the side.
    b. the angle from which the side of the nose deviates from the horizontal when viewed from above.
    c. the angle from which the side of the nose deviates from the vertical when viewed from straight ahead.

22. When part of the lower, nasal portion of a lens shape is removed to allow for a better fit, it is called a _____.

23. Which of the following is *not* an important criterion in choosing a frame for a progressive addition lens wearer?
    a. a minimal vertex distance
    b. adequate pantoscopic tilt
    c. sufficient vertical depth in the nasal portion of the frame shape
    d. All of the above are important criterion when choosing a frame for a progressive addition lens wearer.

24. Which of the following should be *avoided* when fitting a high minus wearer?
    a. a high index lens material
    b. squared-off corners
    c. aspheric lenses
    d. smaller eye size
    e. an antireflection coating

25. Which of the following is *not* a good frame characteristic for a person having a high plus lens prescription?
    a. small lens size
    b. adjustable bridge
    c. library temples
    d. high index lenses
    e. as regular a lens shape as possible

26. With high plus lenses, should **more** or **less** eye makeup than average be used for an equal cosmetic effect compared with what would be worn without spectacle lenses?

27. To check bridge size, lift the frame very slightly from the nose and move it to the left or right. There should be about _____ millimeter(s) of clearance between the nose and free side of the bridge.
    a. 0.5
    b. 1.0
    c. 1.5
    d. 2.0

28. True or false? All metal pad arms and pad bridges lend themselves to versatility in adjusting the nose pads.

29. What is the best way to reduce ring reflections in a high minus prescription?

30. List at least four characteristics of frames that you could choose to keep the frame of a high plus lens wearer from sliding down the nose.

31. Of the frame characteristics listed below, which is the *least* desirable for children?
    a. deeply grooved frame fronts
    b. nylon cord frame construction
    c. bridges that give support in the area of the lower portion of the nosepad
    d. spring temples

32. True or false? Rules for selecting a well-fitting, nice looking frame change dramatically when selecting safety eyewear.

33. True or false? When buying frames for the office, one of the fastest and best ways to select appropriate frames is for the staff to try them on.

34. It becomes evident that there are a great many frames on the board that are discontinued. Which of the following is *least* likely to be a contributing factor to this situation?
    a. All frames are automatically re-ordered when they have been sold from the board.
    b. Large numbers of frames are being purchased at low-cost special prices.
    c. Frames are being purchased from a large number of sources.
    d. Frame representatives have been allocated a given number of board spaces and come in on a regular basis to check on how their frame product is moving.

CHAPTER 5

Reference Point Placement, Multifocal Height, and Blank Size Determination

No matter how accurate the visual examination has been, if the lenses, either single vision or multifocal, are improperly positioned before the eyes, the finished product is of inferior quality. The purpose of this chapter is to present the many "fine points" in lens positioning. A dispenser must master these fine points in addition to the general fitting rules to achieve consistency in excellence. Failure to put these points into practice can result in genuine visual hardship to wearers.

POSITION OF THE FRAME

If the frame is not properly positioned on the face for the initial measurements, both the frame and the lenses may not be in the correct positions when the frame is dispensed and properly adjusted.

With metal frames, the best policy is to adjust the nose pads to a correct angle and position before any measuring is done. This ensures a more correct bifocal height and bridge size evaluation.

With plastic frames, it is fairly simple to evaluate the bridge size. If the bridge of the sample frame is too small, the frame will sit too high; if it is too large, it will sit too low.

OPTICAL CENTERING FOR SINGLE VISION LENSES

Horizontal Placement of the Lenses in the Frame

Normally when spectacles are made, the lenses are positioned so that the *optical center (OC)* of the lens will line up with the pupil of the eye. Therefore the optical center becomes the major point of reference for the lens. When light goes through the optical center of the lens, it does not bend, but travels straight through. If the light did not travel straight through, but was bent, there would be a prismatic effect at that point. At the optical center of a lens there is no prismatic effect. Prism in spectacles is undesirable unless prescribed.

Prismatic Effect

To avoid undesired prismatic effects, the optical centers (OCs) of the lenses are placed the same distance apart as the wearer's lines of sight. The measurement techniques for finding the interpupillary distance (PD) are covered in Chapter 3.

In some cases, a lens prescription calls for a certain amount of prism. The optical center of the lens has no prism, so it will not be placed in front of the wearer's pupil. Instead a point on the lens where the amount of prism equals that called for in the prescription is chosen. This new point on the lens is now the point of major importance. This major reference point where the prismatic effect equals the prescribed amount of prism is called just that—the Major Reference Point (MRP). Succinctly stated, *the point on the lens where the prism is equal to that called for by the prescription is called the major reference point* (MRP).

Note that when there is no prism called for in the prescription, the OC and the MRP are at exactly the same point on the lens. But when there is prism in the prescription, the eye no longer looks through the OC. In other words, with prescribed prism the OC and MRP are in two different locations. The MRP is in front of the line of sight of the eye, whereas the OC is somewhere else.

If the wearer's eyes are at different distances from the nose, and if the two lenses are different in power, then the MRPs of the lenses must be placed according to the monocular PD rather than the binocular PD, to avoid inducing unwanted prism (see Figure 3-4).

Prentice's Rule

The amount of prism induced by improper lens placement depends on the power of the lens and the distance the OC is displaced. It is calculated according to *Prentice's rule*, which states:

$$\Delta = cF$$

where Δ is prism diopters of displacement, F is the dioptric power of the lens, and c is the distance from the OC in centimeters.

For example, if the lens power is +2.00 D and the OC varies from the wearer's interpupillary reference point (usually the center of the pupil) by 6 mm, the induced prism will be:

$$\Delta = 0.6 \times 2.00 = 1.2$$

The base direction for plus lenses is toward the center of the lens, and the base direction for minus lenses is toward the margin of the lens.

"Face Form"

There is also a relationship between the placement of the OCs in the frame and the extent to which the curve in the frame front varies from the classical four-point touch position (see Chapter 8 for an explanation of four-point touch). This curve in the frame front is often referred to as "face form," because the frame front more closely conforms to the curve of the face.

This curve serves both the cosmetic purpose of improving the frame appearance and the optical purpose of aligning both surfaces of the lenses with the wearer's line of sight.

Allen[1] has shown the correct and incorrect face form relating to the wearer's PD (Figure 5-1). If the wearer's PD equals the "frame PD" (eye size plus bridge size), then no face form is required; the frame front should be straight (Figure 5-2).

If the wearer's PD is less than the eye size plus the bridge size of the frame, then the frame front should be given face form by bending it at the bridge, allowing both cosmetic and optical alignment (Figure 5-3). A perfectly straight alignment of the frame front will tilt the OCs with reference to the line of sight and cause unwanted sphere and cylinder powers (Figure 5-4).

If the wearer's PD is greater than the frame eye size plus the bridge size, then theoretically the bridge should be bent to curve the frame opposite to the normal curve of the face. Although this permits proper optical alignment, it is cosmetically unsatisfactory, and thereby impractical (Table 5-1). Such a frame adjustment should not be done.

Vertical Displacement

Unless otherwise specified, an optical laboratory will make a single vision lens so that the MRP is centered vertically—halfway between the top and bottom of the frame. Low-powered lenses made from traditional materials seldom need an MRP height specified. Optical problems caused by a vertical MRP placement that might need to be above or below the vertical frame center are so minimal with low-powered lenses that few wearers are ever bothered. However, this is not the case when lens powers increase, when different lens materials are used, or when aspheric lens designs are employed. In these instances, vertical MRP placement becomes important.

Optically Correct OC Placement

Consider a lens placed before an eye with the OC of the lens directly in the eye's line of sight (Figure 5-5). As light passes through the OC of the lens, it enters and leaves the lens at right angles to both front and back

TABLE 5-1
Amount of Face Form Required

If	Then
1. PD = Eye size + bridge size	No face form
2. PD < Eye size + bridge size	Positive face form
3. PD> Eye size + bridge size	Negative face form (this is impractical and should not be carried out)

TABLE 5-2
Amount of Pantoscopic Tilt Required*

If	Then
1. Eyes at OC	No pantoscopic tilt
2. Eyes above OC	Pantoscopic tilt required
3. Eyes below OC	Retroscopic tilt required (this, however, is impractical and should not be carried out)

*For each millimeter the eyes are centered above or below the optical centers of the lenses, two degrees of lens tilt are required.

surfaces. The optic axis of the lens and the line of sight of the eye fall in the same place.

Note, however, that a lens with its OC directly in front of the eye should not be tilted. Figure 5-6 shows this incorrectly tilted lens. Tilting the lens when the OC is directly in front of the eye will both induce an unwanted cylinder component and alter the sphere value of the lens. (An optical explanation of this is found in Chapter 18.)

With most frames, the eye is slightly higher than the center of the lens. This is shown in Figure 5-7. The alignment shown in Figure 5-7 is not an optically correct alignment, since the optic axis of the lens does not pass through the center of rotation of the eye. Even though the lens is not tilted, light passing through the center of rotation of the eye also passes through the lens at an angle to both lens surfaces.

Fortunately, lenses are usually worn with the lower lens edge tilted toward the face. This *pantoscopic tilt* is the amount the frame front is tilted with reference to the plane of the face. To avoid the lens aberrations that would otherwise be caused by lens tilt, light following the line of sight through the center rotation of the eye must still pass through the lens OC at right angles. This can be accomplished by lowering the OC of the lens 1 mm for every 2 degrees of pantoscopic lens tilt and is shown in Figure 5-8. (Table 5-2 summarizes the relationship between pantoscopic tilt and OC placement.)

In Figure 5-1, Allen[1] shows several examples of correct and incorrect pantoscopic tilt with respect to vertical

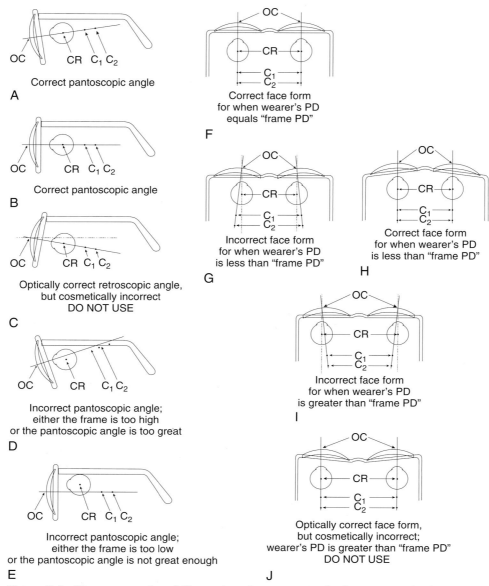

OC   CR C_1 C_2
Correct pantoscopic angle

A

OC   CR C_1 C_2
Correct pantoscopic angle

B

OC   CR C_1 C_2
Optically correct retroscopic angle,
but cosmetically incorrect
DO NOT USE

C

OC   CR C_1 C_2
Incorrect pantoscopic angle;
either the frame is too high
or the pantoscopic angle is too great

D

OC   CR C_1 C_2
Incorrect pantoscopic angle;
either the frame is too low
or the pantoscopic angle is not great enough

E

OC
CR
C_1
C_2
Correct face form
for when wearer's PD
equals "frame PD"

F

OC
CR
C_1
C_2
Incorrect face form
for when wearer's PD
is less than "frame PD"

G

OC
CR
C_1
C_2
Correct face form
for when wearer's PD
is less than "frame PD"

H

OC
CR
C_1
C_2
Incorrect face form
for when wearer's PD
is greater than "frame PD"

I

OC
CR
C_1
C_2
Optically correct face form,
but cosmetically incorrect;
wearer's PD is greater than "frame PD"
DO NOT USE

J

Figure 5-1. Here are a series of illustrations demonstrating both correct and incorrect use of pantoscopic angle and face form, depending upon the placement of the lens optical center. The symbols C_1 and C_2 show the location of the centers of curvature for the first and second lens surfaces. They also indicate the position of the optic axis of the lens. The location of the center of rotation of the eye is denoted by CR and the optical center of the lens by OC. Illustrations **C** and **J** are theoretically correct, but should not be carried out. They may be avoided by using good frame selection procedures. (Modified from Allen MJ: How do you fit spectacles? *Indiana J Optom* 32:2, 1962.)

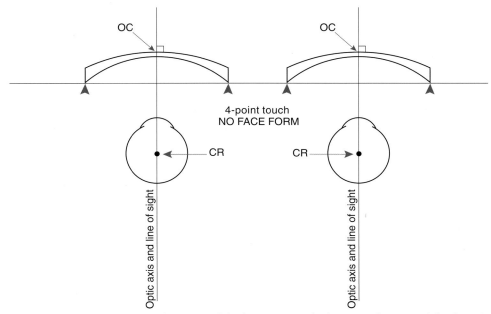

Figure 5-2. When the optical centers of the lenses are at the horizontal center of the frame's lens openings, the geometric center distance ("Frame PD") equals the wearer's interpupillary distance. The lenses should have no face form (a "4-point touch"). When this is the case, light entering along the line of sight strikes at right angles to the front and back surfaces of the lens. This prevents inducing unwanted sphere and cylinder power changes caused by tilting of the optical center.

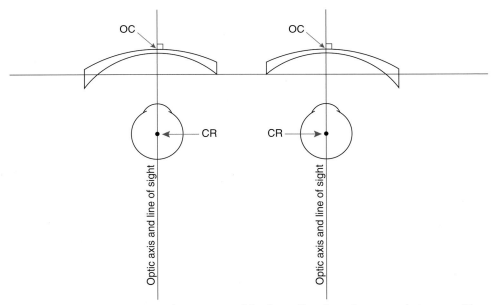

Figure 5-3. To prevent optical error caused by lens tilt, when the wearer's interpupillary distance is less than the frame's geometric center distance ("Frame PD") face form is required. This is because more of the lens blank has been removed nasally than temporally during edging. The object of adding face form to a spectacle lens prescription is to keep the lens surfaces at the optical center perpendicular to the line of sight.

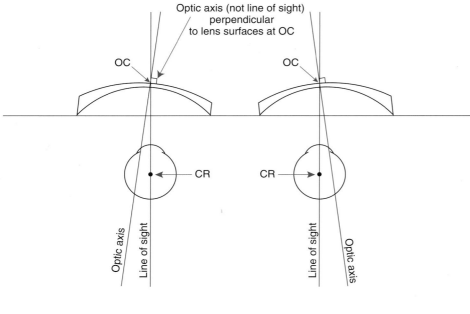

Figure 5-4. In this figure, the glasses are not adjusted to include face form. Because the wearer's interpupillary distance is smaller than the geometric center distance, the line of sight crosses the lens optical centers obliquely. This results in lens tilt, inducing unwanted changes in the sphere and cylinder components of the prescription.

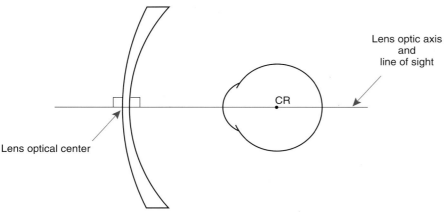

CORRECT

Figure 5-5. A properly adjusted lens allows the line of sight to pass through the optical center of the lens at right angles to the front and back surfaces. If the eye is midway between the top and bottom of the lens, and the optical center is directly in front of the eye, the proper adjustment contains no face form.

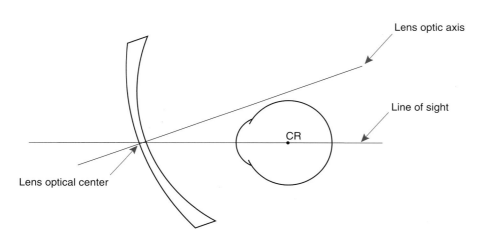

INCORRECT

Figure 5-6. When the optical center is measured for center-pupil height, if the glasses have any pantoscopic tilt, the optic axis of the lens will not pass through the center of rotation of the eye.

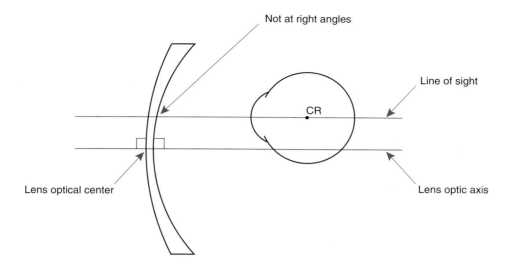

INCORRECT

Figure 5-7. When the eye is above the horizontal midline of the lens, without pantoscopic tilt the optic axis of the lens will not pass through the center of rotation of the eye. This means that the wearer will experience lens aberrations corresponding to the effect of altering lens sphere and cylinder values.

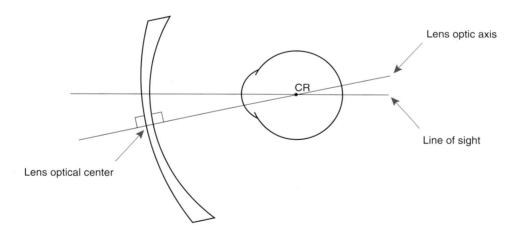

CORRECT

Figure 5-8. A correctly fit pair of glasses will drop the optical center 1 mm for every 2 degrees of pantoscopic tilt. This is also a good fitting situation because the average viewing area is not centered on a point on the lens directly in front of the eye. "The average patient moves his eye through a field of view, which is centered in a slight downward position, since we seldom have occasion to look as far above the horizontal as we do below. Even for viewing tasks other than through the bifocal segment, we look down at the sidewalk, down at store counters, even somewhat downward to drive a car to look at the road directly in front of us.[5]"

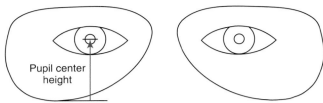

Figure 5-9. To measure pupil center height, mark the location of the pupil on the glazed lens with a short horizontal line or a cross. Pupil center height is the horizontal distance from the lowest level of the inside bevel of the lower eyewire, up to the pupil center.

alignment, and correct and incorrect face form with respect to horizontal alignment.

As a general rule, eyeglasses need to be adjusted so that the lower rims of the frame are closer to the face. This widens the viewing area for the wearer and is more cosmetically appealing. The correct fitting procedure is to first adjust the empty frame for pantoscopic tilt. This angle of tilt in degrees is noted. Next the pupil center height is measured. Afterwards 1 mm is subtracted from the height of the OC for every 2 degrees of pantoscopic tilt. This gives the MRP height.

Summarizing How to Determine MRP Height
MRP height is determined by first measuring pupil center height. Pupil center height is measured with the dispenser's eyes positioned at the same level as the subject's eyes. The subject looks at the bridge of the dispenser's nose. Using a water-based overhead projector pen, the dispenser draws a horizontal line on the glazed lenses through the pupil center for both right and left eyes (Figure 5-9). If there are no glazed lenses in the frame, transparent tape may be used. (The use of transparent tape is described in the section on measuring bifocal heights found later in this chapter.) Next compensate for pantoscopic tilt using the 2-for-1 rule of thumb.

Example **5-1**

A metal frame with adjustable pads and a 40 mm B dimension is selected. The frame and pads are adjusted so that the frame sits on the nose and face as it should after dispensing. The frame front is tilted to the correct pantoscopic angle and is observed to be straight on the face. Neither lens is higher than the other. The frame front has a 10-degree pantoscopic angle. Measure the MRP height and modify this amount to compensate for the pantoscopic tilt.

Solution

In measuring the pupil center height, the distance from the lowest point on the inside bevel of the lower frame eyewire up to the pupil center is measured and found to be 28 mm. If the pantoscopic tilt is 10 degrees, then the height must be lowered by 1 mm for every two degrees of pantoscopic tilt; which in this case is 10/2 or 5 mm. The new MRP height

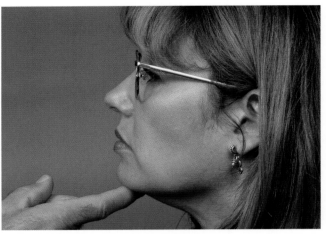

Figure 5-10. If the chin is raised until the frame front is perpendicular to the floor, major reference point height can be measured without compensating for pantoscopic tilt.

is 28 − 5 or 23 mm. (Normally the MRP height would be on the horizontal midline at a height of 20 mm.)

Simultaneously Compensating for Pantoscopic Angle While Determining MRP Height
There is a simple method that makes it possible to compensate for pantoscopic tilt while determining MRP height. The dispenser is positioned at the same level as the subject. With the frame fully adjusted for height, pantoscopic tilt, and straightness, the subject is instructed to look at the bridge of the dispenser's nose. Next the dispenser places a finger under the subject's chin and tilts the subject's head back until the frame front is perpendicular to the floor (Figure 5-10). With the subject's head in this position, a horizontal line is drawn on the glazed lens at the level of the pupil center. The distance from the lowest portion of the inside bevel of the lower eyewire to the horizontal mark on the lens is the MRP height. This height has already been corrected for pantoscopic tilt and does not require any compensation. (This is summarized in Box 5-1.)

MRP Placement for Polycarbonate and Other High Index Materials
It is especially important to measure PDs monocularly and to consider the vertical position of the MRP when using polycarbonate and high index materials. Many of these materials have more chromatic aberration* than crown glass and regular (CR-39) plastic.

Fitting eyewear correctly will help keep many types of aberrations under control (for more on lens aberrations, see Chapter 18). If other aberrations are minimized by good fitting techniques, a small amount of

---

*Chromatic aberration causes objects with high contrast border areas to have rainbowlike color fringes. Chromatic aberration may be visible with high-powered prescriptions made from lens materials with low Abbé values.

BOX 5-1

Steps in Measuring MRP Height

1. Frames are adjusted to fit the wearer, giving attention to nosepads, frame height, pantoscopic tilt and straightness of the frame on the face.
2. Fitter positions himself or herself on the same level as the subject.
3. Subject fixates on bridge of fitter's nose.
4. Fitter tilts wearer's chin back until frame front is perpendicular to the floor.
5. Fitter marks the location of the pupil centers with short horizontal lines on the glazed lens.
6. Fitter measures MRP height as distance from lowest portion of the inside bevel of the lower eyewire to the line on the glazed lens.

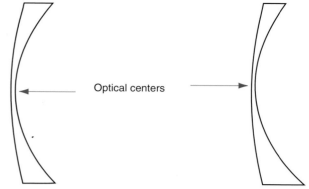

Figure 5-11. Moving the optical center of a high minus lens too far upward will cause the lower edge of the lens to be too thick.

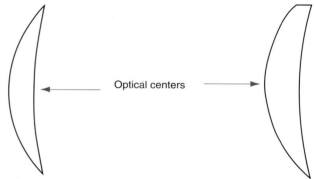

Figure 5-12. These two high plus lenses have the same refractive power. The lens on the left has the optical center half way between the top and the bottom. The lens on the right has the optical center too high for a lens of this power. As a result, the upper edge is excessively thick.

chromatic aberration is less likely to push overall aberration problems into the troublesome area. It should also be noted that the farther from the OC the eye looks, the more evident chromatic aberration may become.

MRP Placement for Aspherics

An aspheric lens typically has a central zone of constant lens surface power, with the power gradually changing toward the periphery of the lens. This means that the central zone must be well positioned both horizontally and vertically. Monocular PD and measured MRP heights are important.

Other Ways of Positioning MRP Height

Some dispensers measure pupil height and do not lower the MRP from this position to compensate for pantoscopic tilt. Although this may help prevent chromatic aberration with distance viewing for polycarbonate and high index lenses, it can cause aberrations because of lens tilt and also result in a thicker lens. Raising the OC of a minus lens makes the top thinner and the bottom thicker (Figure 5-11). Raising the OC of a plus lens makes the top thicker and sometimes increases center thickness (Figure 5-12). Therefore before ordering a high-powered lens with a high OC, it is advisable to consider the resulting edge thickness.

If the dispenser fails to specify an MRP height, the laboratory will center the lens vertically in the frame. For most low-powered crown glass and CR-39 plastic lenses, no problems will be encountered. For polycarbonates, aspherics and high index lenses, the MRP height should be measured.

Notes:

1. It is not advisable to move an MRP height below the horizontal midline (datum line) of the glasses unless the lenses are intended exclusively for near work.
2. When the pantoscopic angle is especially large, it may be advisable to (a) reconsider the frame selected

and choose one that will place the eyes higher in the frame, (b) reduce the pantoscopic tilt, or (c) just not lower the MRP by the full 2-for-1 amount.

Vertex Distance

Vertex distance is the distance from the back surface of the spectacle lens to the apex of the cornea. A 14-mm distance is considered average, although the best fit for spectacles is usually obtained by fitting the frame as close to the eyes as possible without having the lashes rub the lenses.

The depth of the base curve affects the final vertex distance, since each increase of 1 diopter in the depth of the base curve increases the depth of the vertex distance by approximately 0.6 mm. The exact amount of vertex distance increase will depend on the size of the lens. Vertex distance is important when fitting someone with long lashes. Be sure to observe the person from the side with the sample frame. Have the person blink to note the lash clearance. Vertex distance becomes more of a concern in higher powered prescriptions because a change in vertex distance induces a change in both the spherical and cylindrical power of the lenses.

Measuring Vertex Distance With the Distometer

The instrument used to measure vertex distance is the *distometer* (Figure 5-13). The following technique is used to measure vertex distance: With the spectacles in place, the subject is instructed to close the eyes. The flat side of the "scissors" end of the distometer is placed against the closed lid. When the end of the distometer is pressed, the other side of the "scissors" moves out to touch the back surface of the spectacle lens. When the two parts of the distometer touch the lid and lens simultaneously, vertex distance is read from the instrument. The instrument takes average lid thickness into consideration so the reading does not have to be compensated (Figure 5-14).

For more on how prescription powers change with changing vertex distances, see Chapter 14.

MEASURING FOR MULTIFOCAL HEIGHTS

The methods used for segmented multifocals and those used for progressive addition lenses are very similar. The eye reference points are not the same. Progressive lenses

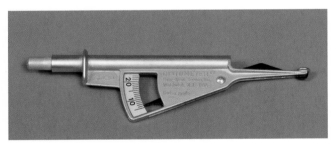

Figure 5-13. A distometer measures the distance from the back surface of the lens to the front surface of the eye.

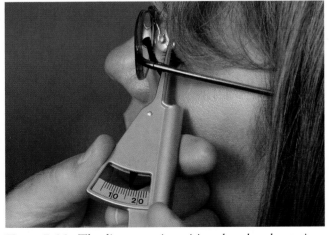

Figure 5-14. The distometer is positioned so that the stationary part of the instrument is against the closed lid. When the probe touches the back surface of the spectacle lenses, the vertex distance may be read from the scale.

use the center of the pupil for reference. Chapter 20 deals specifically with progressive addition lenses. For how to measure for progressive addition lenses, see the section titled "Measuring for and Ordering the Progressive" in Chapter 20.

Measuring for Bifocals

The actual techniques for measuring bifocal height are not any more difficult than measuring the PD. There are, however, a few more considerations that must be taken into account to prevent certain difficulties.

Measurement for segment height should be done using only the actual frame that will be worn, or one of exactly the same size and type. Any variations in size must be precisely compensated for, as previously explained at the beginning of the chapter. The frame must be carefully positioned to sit at the same height at which it will be worn.

Lower Limbus Method

The dispenser positions himself on the same level as the subject and directly in front of him. The subject is instructed to fixate a point straight ahead at eye level—most often, the bridge of the dispenser's nose.

When using the PD rule to measure bifocal height, hold it vertically with the scale extending downward and align the zero point with the lower limbus (Figure 5-15). The bifocal height is indicated by the figure on the scale of the ruler that corresponds to the level of the lowest part of the groove inside the lower eyewire (Box 5-2).

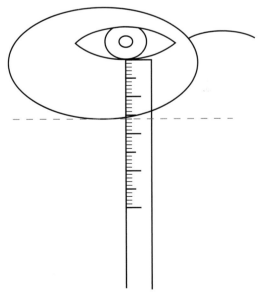

Figure 5-15. Measuring for bifocal height. When using the inside edge of the lower eyewire as reference, an additional amount must be allowed for the depth for the lens bevel in the groove. Although this may vary somewhat, an additional 0.5 mm added to the measure is normally suitable. Alternately, it may be easier to estimate the depth of the groove and measure directly to this estimated location.

The lowest portion of the eyewire must be used, even if it is not precisely under the limbus. Certain frames have a lower eyewire that slants, a problem best illustrated by the aviator frame shape. The distance from the top of the seg to the eyewire immediately below it is notably different from the distance to the lowest part of the eyewire (Figure 5-16).

Lower Lid Margin Method

The lower lid margin is often used as a reference point for measuring bifocal height instead of the lower limbus. The difference is frequently academic because the two are usually in approximately the same position.

BOX 5-2

Steps in Measuring Bifocal Height Using Lower Lid or Limbal Method

1. Fitter positions himself or herself on the same level as the subject.
2. Subject fixates the bridge of the fitter's nose.
3. Holding frame in correct wearing position, the fitter places the PD rule vertically in front of subject's right eye. The zero point is at lower limbus and the ruler scale is positioned downward.
4. For a rimmed frame, the fitter reads the scale at the level of the lowest point where the inside of the groove would be. For a rimless frame, the reference is the level of the lowest point on the demo lens.
5. Repeat for left eye.

Note: If the lenses are being marked for reference instead of using a ruler in front of the face, the glazed lenses are marked at the level of the limbus with a marking pen. When both lenses have been marked, the fitter removes the frames from the subject and measures from the mark down to these reference points.

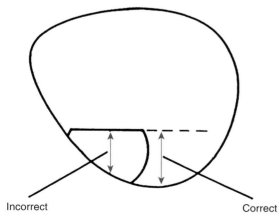

Figure 5-16. The lowest portion of the lens as positioned in the frame must be used in measuring seg height. This is true even if the height at the center of the seg has a different measurement. (*Note:* The segment height is *not* measured using the outside of the frame. The edge of the lens is the reference used.)

The lower lid margin position can vary considerably more than the lower limbus position, however, making the latter a more consistent reference point.

Subjective Determination

Subjective determination is the most accurate means of determining the seg height and of assuring the wearer that the bifocal will be positioned properly. The proper bifocal position for each person, of course, is determined with the occupational and personal characteristics of the individual in mind.

Marking on the Glazed Lens. When the sample frame has glazed lenses, the level of the bifocal can be marked on each lens with a marking pen instead of measuring with the PD ruler. With the dispenser and wearer on the same level and the wearer looking straight ahead, a short horizontal mark is drawn at the proposed level of the bifocal segment line (Figure 5-17). This can be checked before ordering by lengthening the line to simulate the width of the bifocal (Figure 5-18). This way the wearer can be given the opportunity to evaluate the suitability of the proposed height. Ask the wearer to stand and evaluate the position of the line.

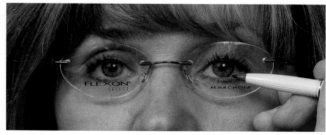

Figure 5-17. Using a marking pen, the proposed level of the bifocal can be drawn on the glazed lens in the new frame. If the wearer will be using old frames, the mark is made on the old lenses.

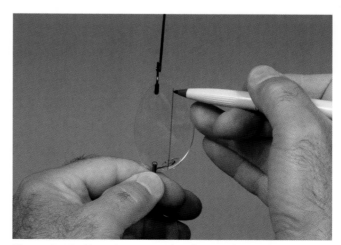

Figure 5-18. Drawing a complete line at the proposed bifocal height will allow the wearer a realistic evaluation of where the segment will be located after the finished lenses are in the frame.

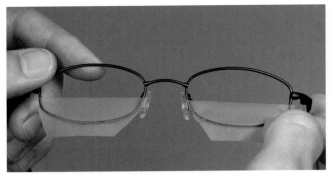

Figure 5-19. To simulate the level of a bifocal segment, a strip of transparent tape is placed across the lower half of each eyewire.

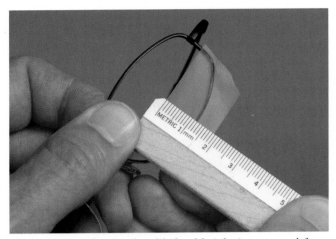

Figure 5-20. The simulated bifocal height is measured from the lowest part of the inside of the lower eyewire.

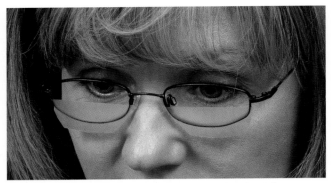

Figure 5-21. Subjectively checking seg height: The wearer should be readily able to locate reading or near point material within the transparent tape area. The same is true when using a frame with glazed lenses that have been marked for height with a lens marking pen.

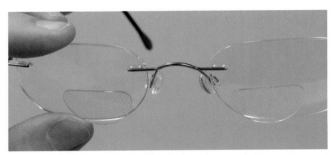

Figure 5-22. Fresnel press-on segments are removable and reusable. They offer a greater degree of reality when asking the wearer to subjectively judge the most appropriate segment height.

Give the wearer something to hold in the reading position. Encourage the wearer to simulate normal working conditions and evaluate whether the line is too high, too low, or just right. If the line is too high or too low, redraw the line and have the wearer reevaluate the new height. When the level is judged as satisfactory, measure the distance from the lowest level of the inside bevel of the lower eyewire up to the drawn bifocal line for each lens.

Using Transparent Tape. The method using transparent tape is slightly more time consuming, but is useful for checking when there are no lenses in the frame. This method also works for checking unequal seg heights. A strip of tape is placed across the lower portion of the empty frame at exactly the level of the proposed segment (Figure 5-19). The proper height is checked in the same way as a regular bifocal (Figure 5-20), and the tape is readjusted if necessary. When the wearer looks into the distance, the taped area should not interfere with vision. When looking up close, the nearpoint material should be seen as if located within the area covered by the tape (Figure 5-21).

Using Fresnel Press-On Segments

By using Fresnel optics, it is possible to produce a uniformly thin, flexible, stick-on lens or prism. Such lenses are normally used to provide high amounts of prism in visual training or to apply prism in certain sections of a lens. However, Fresnel lenses are also available as temporary flat-top bifocal segments. By obtaining a series of Fresnel press-on segments in increasing powers, it is possible to stick the lenses on the wearer's old single vision lenses, or on the glazed lenses in the new frame (Figure 5-22). Having the wearer's prescribed near power in the removable segment will add a dimension of reality that will enable the wearer to judge more accurately the most useful bifocal height for a given work situation.

Measuring For Trifocals

The techniques for measuring trifocals are identical to those for measuring bifocals, except the reference is the top of the trifocal intermediate segment rather than the top of the lower near segment. The trifocal height is the top line (Figure 5-23).

Bifocals enable the wearer to see at two distances clearly: (1) off in the distance through the upper portion of the lens, and (2) at reading distance for the smaller

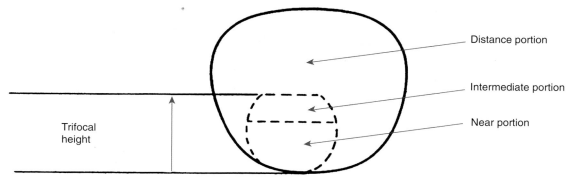

Figure 5-23. No specification for lower seg line is necessary when ordering trifocal lenses. The style of trifocal ordered dictates this position. The top of the intermediate portion is the position measured.

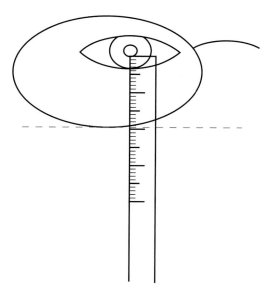

Figure 5-24. Measuring for trifocal height starts as shown. Subtract a full millimeter so that the intermediate seg does not get in the way for distance viewing. If the frame has a groove for the bevel, that must also be considered.

segment area in the lower portion of the lens. When it becomes necessary to see clearly at an intermediate distance (usually an extended arm's length), trifocals are used. Trifocals differ from bifocals only through the addition of an intermediate portion immediately above the near portion, giving the wearer three distances of clear vision instead of two.

Lower Edge of Pupil Method

The lower edge of the pupil method is similar to the lower limbus and lower lid margin methods used for bifocals. For trifocals, however, the lower pupil margin is aligned with the zero mark of the vertically held PD rule. The reading is that point where the scale intersects the level of the inside groove of the lower eyewire (Figure 5-24). Then 1 mm is subtracted to compensate for pupil clearance during fixation of the eye in distance viewing.

Thus if the seg height for a trifocal measures 18 mm from the edge of the pupil, the net seg height ordered would be 17 mm.

Subjective Determination

The subjective technique is again similar to that used for bifocals, with the addition of a test for the third section of the lenses. When an overhead transparency pen and glazed lens are used, the two trifocal lines may be drawn on the lens. The area in between is "colored in" with the pen. Objects viewed through this colored intermediate area will appear tinted.

If the total seg height is lowered, the near portion area will be reduced, and vice versa. For example, assume that a trifocal with a 7-mm intermediate portion is to be fitted 17 mm high in the eyewire. This leaves 10 mm for the near portion of the seg (17 total − 7 intermediate = 10 near). If the top of this intermediate seg is too high, lowering it reduces the reading portion. If the reading portion is increased, the top of the trifocal is raised.

The feasibility of using a trifocal in a given frame can thereby be easily ascertained. If the trifocal seg is deliberately set very low, the resulting small near (reading) portion will probably permit too little reading area; but on the other hand, increasing the reading area may place the trifocal intermediate portion high enough to interfere with distance vision. When no suitable trifocal position in the selected frame is possible, a frame with a greater vertical depth is indicated.

Comparison With Old Lenses

When a person who is currently wearing bifocals is refitted with new bifocals, the segment position may be maintained or changed. If a person is dissatisfied, the complaint will indicate the necessary change in position. If the bifocals were "always in the way," the seg height was too high. If the seg height was too low, the wearer will complain of stiffness of neck caused by constant head-tilting.

Any change that is made, however, should be done via the same techniques described for new multifocal wearers to ensure correct positioning. This is also true for a bifocal wearer changing to trifocals. If the trifocal is merely added to the bifocal height, the tops may intrude into the pupillary area.

Seg Height Factors

If a person is satisfied with the seg height currently worn, but is changing any aspect of the frame, the specifications necessary to achieve the previous seg height may be different. Only with exactly the same frame shape and size will the seg height measurements be identical to the previous order.

One factor that influences the position of the seg is the bridge. The shape and size of the bridge determine the height at which the frame sits on the nose. For example, two frames might both have a vertical dimension of 38, but the bridge on one frame might hold the eyewire higher on the face than a differently shaped bridge on the other frame.

The influence of lens size on segment height is evident in the vertical depth if one frame is a 38 eye size and the other 42. Even if the bridges hold both frames in relatively the same position, as the horizontal size increases, so does the vertical size.

Lens shape influences segment. The seg height might be 15 mm for a narrow frame and 20 mm for a deep frame, yet both frames could place the segment line right at the lower limbus.

When measuring to match the segment height of a new bifocal lens with that of an old bifocal lens, have the person wear his or her old glasses. Note the location of the segment line on the face or in relation to the lower lid. Measure from the lower lid to the seg line: plus if above the lower lid, minus if below it (Figure 5-25, *A*). Place the new frames on the face. Measure the distance from the lower eyewire to the lower lid, then add or subtract the distance from the lower lid to the old seg line (Figure 5-25, *B*).

Other Methods

When a frame lacks glazed lenses, plastic segment-measuring devices are handy and accurate alternatives to the PD-rule method of measuring bifocal height. Such a device may be held in place in one of several ways. One type uses expandable wire springs. Another uses the same principle, but is held in place by three vertical plastic strips: two strips are positioned behind and one strip in front of the upper eyewire. A third design uses double sided tape to hold the device to the frame. In all instances, the scale can be read directly because the clear plastic segment portion is marked in millimeters. Because such devices sit inside the frame bevel, there is no need to compensate for bevel depth. An additional advantage is the fact that they enable comparison of the segment heights of both eyes simultaneously (Figure 5-26). Because frames come with demonstration lenses to

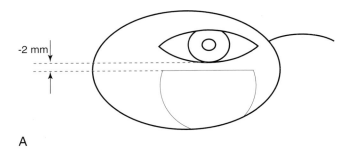

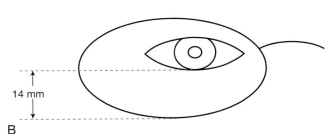

Figure 5-25. Duplicating the old seg height positions for use in the new frame or for a second pair of glasses is done by first measuring from the lower lid, down (or up) to the seg line. The measure will be plus if the old seg line is above the lower lid and minus if it is below it. In the figure, this measurement is –2 mm. Next, with the new frame in place, the distance from the lower lens edge up to the lower lid is measured. In the figure, this measurement is 14 mm. The distance in **(A)** is then added to the distance in **(B)** to determine the seg height for the new or second pair of glasses so that both old and new segment heights match. For the example, this is –2 mm + 14 mm = 12 mm.

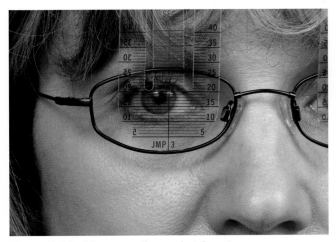

Figure 5-26. Measuring for seg height using a segment measuring device allows for easy comparison of seg heights between left and right eyes.

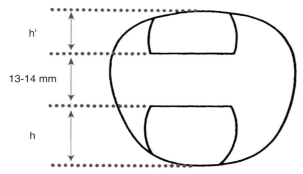

Figure 5-27. The double seg lens. Most double seg lenses have a 13 to 14 mm distance between segs. Measure h′ is therefore dependent upon seg height h and the vertical dimension of the frame chosen.

increase frame stability, these devices are used much less that previously.

Measuring For Double Segs

A double seg lens has near segments in both the lower portion and the upper portion of the lens (Figure 5-27). This upper seg allows the wearer to do near work more comfortably when the working area is above eye level. Double segs are available in several seg shapes.

Measuring for a double seg is done in practically the same manner as for the normal bifocal. The only initial consideration is the lower seg height. This can be measured by any of the methods described previously.

When a double seg lens is ordered, the lower edge of the top segment will automatically be 13 to 14 mm above the lower seg line position. With the frame in place, note the position in the frame where the upper seg will begin. If there will not be a large enough field of view in the upper seg, either a different frame with more area above eye level must be chosen or the lower seg must be placed deeper in the frame to bring down the upper seg. A reasonable minimum area for the upper seg is considered to be 9 mm.[2]

The opposite problem can result if the subject has previously worn the bifocal seg lower than normal. The upper seg will be so low that it will partially obscure distance vision. The lower seg then has to be raised until the upper seg is high enough that it is no longer disturbing the wearer.

When the wearer is unsure of the applicability of double segments to his or her situation, it may be helpful to use a set of Fresnel segments* to demonstrate the application. To do so, subtract 0.50 D from the power of the new bifocal add and select Fresnel segments of this power. Position the Fresnel segments upside down and 14 mm above the wearer's old bifocals.

---

*Fresnel segments were described under the "Subjective Determination" section earlier in this chapter.

Example **5-2**

A new prescription calls for a + 2.00 add. It is possible that the wearer would benefit from an occupational, double-D segment. What power Fresnel seg should be chosen for demonstration purposes?

Solution

Subtract 0.50 D from the +2.00 D add. This reduced +1.50 D add will be the add power of the chosen segment. Find this power in a Fresnel segment. Position the segment upside down so that it adheres to the upper portion of the wearer's old eyeglass lenses, exactly where the upper, occupational segment will be. This demonstration will be realistic if the distance power of the old prescription is not too much different from what the new prescription will be.

Unequal Seg Heights

Both eyes should be measured independently for bifocal or trifocal heights (Figure 5-28). If one eye is higher than the other and the segments are placed at equal heights, the wearer will have a blur area considerably larger than normal; one eye sees the segment line first as the person looks down, then as that eye begins to clear, the other eye sees the line and begins to clear later.

Before prescribing unequal segment heights, be sure to check (using the actual frame to be worn) to be certain that the frame sits straight on the face. A crooked frame obviously will result in unequal segment heights.

When unequal segment heights are used, they should be called to the wearer's attention. Otherwise they will be discovered as an "error."

Transparent Tape or Drawn Line Methods Used Subjectively

To subjectively check the relationship of the two segment heights to one another, have the person look at a given near object and slowly tilt his or her head back until the "line," or top of the tape, first hits the object. Next, alternately occlude the wearer's eyes to determine whether the "line" is at the same point for each eye. If not, move the tape until there is an equalization. Then measure the height of the tape or drawn line from the lower eyewire for each lens (Box 5-3).

Transparent Tape or Drawn Line Methods Used Objectively

To check the segment height relationship objectively using the transparent tape or drawn line methods, have the wearer look at the bridge of the dispenser's nose, as the dispenser tilts the wearer's head back slowly and notes which "segment" reaches the lower pupil edge first. The tape level is readjusted until both "lines" reach the pupils at the same time (Box 5-4).

Segment Height and Vertical Prism

A prism causes the light to deviate from its path to a new direction. A ray of light will be bent toward the base of

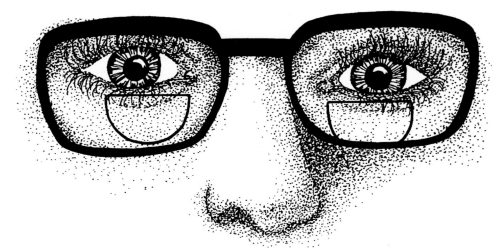

Figure 5-28. A difference in prescribed seg heights is sometimes required so the person's eyes will meet the bifocal line simultaneously on downward gaze.

the prism, causing the image of the object viewed to be displaced in the direction of the apex. This also causes the eye to turn in the direction of the perceived object.

A prism may be necessary in a prescription if there is a slight paralysis of one or more extraocular eye muscles. Without the help of the prism, the person may experience diplopia, or double vision. Even if a person does not have double vision, a prism may be prescribed for ocular comfort. If a tendency for the eyes to turn is present, the person is said to have a phoria condition (i.e., a tendency of the eyes to turn, but with no actual turning manifested) and must exert constant effort to keep both eyes pointing straight ahead. This can lead to fatigue and headaches. A prism can be used to relieve this discomfort. If one eye tends to turn down or up, a vertical prism with the base of the prism up or down is prescribed. If the eyes turn in or out, a horizontal prism with the base of the prism out or in may be prescribed.

When a vertical prism is prescribed, one eye is allowed to turn up slightly more than the other (Figure 5-29). Given equal seg heights, when a person with vertical prism in the prescription is wearing bifocals or trifocals and looks down toward an object in the near field of view, there is a point where one eye crosses the bifocal line before the other. This inequality is not detected in measuring for seg heights if the condition prescribed for is only a phoria.

The inequality of turn can be calculated, however, using the definition of a prism diopter: 1 cm displacement of the image of an object at a distance of 1 m. Assuming 30 mm distance from the back surface of the spectacle lens to the center of rotation of the eye, the difference in the vertical position of the two eyes at the spectacle plane can be calculated. This is the difference in seg height from that which was measured.

According to Figure 5-30, for one prism diopter it can be seen from similar triangles that:

$$\frac{10}{1030} = \frac{x}{30}$$

and so

$$x = 0.29 \text{ mm}$$

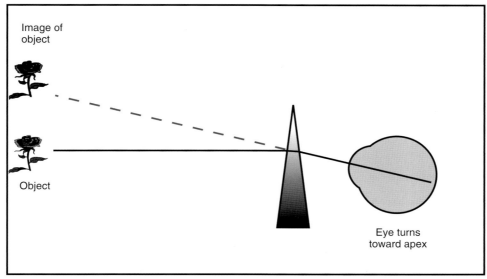

Figure 5-29. A vertical prism causes the eye to turn. This requires an alteration of seg height.

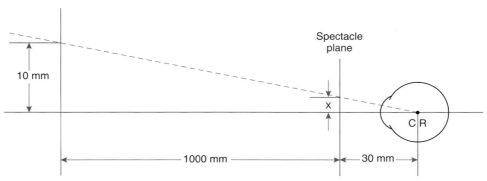

Figure 5-30. Diagram showing required difference in seg heights (X) when one prism diopter of vertical prism is prescribed.

TABLE 5-3 Segment Height Change Indicated in the Presence of Vertical Prism*	
Prism Diopters	**Total Segment Height Difference (mm)**
1	0.3
2	0.6
3	0.9
4	1.2
5	1.5
6	1.8

*When vertical prism is present in a pair of glasses, segment height must be compensated. Each of the prism amounts listed on the left requires a compensated segment height difference as shown on the right.

or approximately 0.3 mm difference for every diopter of vertical prism prescribed.[3]

Therefore, a good rule of thumb for prescribing differences in seg heights is to allow 0.3 mm for every prism diopter, as summarized in Table 5-3.

The seg top is always displaced from its original location in the direction of the apex or point of the prism. (The seg line should be moved in the direction the prism apex points.) If a prescription included three diopters of prism base up before the right eye, then the right seg height should be *lowered* approximately 1 mm from its measured position.

Example **5-3**

A wearer selects a new frame. The dispenser uses the newly selected frame to measure seg height. Both right and left seg heights are measured as 21 mm. If the right lens has 3 Δ of base down prism, what segment heights should be ordered so that the pupils reach the segment lines at the same time once the prism is in place?

Solution

Because the right lens has base down prism, the right eye will turn upward toward the apex of the prism. The amount the eye will turn equals 0.3 mm for each diopter of vertical prism. Therefore the eye turns $0.3 \times 3 = 0.9$ mm, or 1 mm, when rounded. This means that the right segment height must be raised 1 mm. The final seg height should be ordered as:

R: 22 mm.
L: 21 mm.

Example **5-4**

Suppose a wearer has a prescription that reads as follows:

R: $-2.50 - 1.00 \times 180$ 2.5 Δ Base Up
L: $-2.50 - 1.00 \times 180$ 4.5 Δ Base Down
+2.00 add

The selected frame is properly adjusted before seg height measurements are taken. Seg heights are measured using the empty frame. They are found to be:

R: 21
L: 21

How should the seg heights be adjusted to allow for the influence of the prescribed vertical prism once the lenses are in place?

Solution

To solve the problem, first decide which seg height will be raised and which lowered. Because the seg height will be displaced in the direction of the apex (i.e., opposite the base direction), the right seg height will be lowered and the left seg height raised.

To continue solving, next consider how far each seg height must be moved. Remember that each prism diopter yields 0.3 mm of movement. For the right eye, this is 2.5 $\Delta \times 0.3$ = 0.75 mm of movement. For the left eye we find 4.5 $\Delta \times$ 0.3 = 1.35 mm. Therefore, to the nearest millimeter the seg heights will be:

R: 20 mm
L: 22 mm

The same principles that are explained here for segment heights also apply to progressive addition lens fitting cross heights. For more information on how vertical and horizontal prism affects fitting cross heights and monocular PDs, see Chapter 20.

Variations of Seg Height

It is not reasonable to expect every person to be best served with a bifocal segment height that comes to the level of the lower limbus. But because some starting point must be used for seg height determination, the lower lid or limbal margin technique was described. It should be understood that these rules should be used as a basis, or starting point, for professional seg measurement. Other variations influence final seg height placement.

Posture

Perhaps the most obvious influence on segment height is posture. The person who "walks tall" or erect and carries the head back may find that the normally placed segment is constantly interfering with distance vision. This person would benefit from a segment placed at a level lower than usual because tilting the head back moves the segment higher and into the line of sight.

The person with the opposite tendency (i.e., that of carrying himself or herself in a somewhat stooped-over manner) could wear the segment slightly higher than usual.

These extremes in posture should be noted when apparent, although they are not the norm.

Height

A tall person sometimes needs segments set slightly lower than normal because the eyes must turn downward to a greater degree to sight the floor. The bifocal line would be more likely to interfere if placed at the normal level. Shorter persons, however, should not be given higher than normal segs.

Occupational Need

The person who works at a desk all day may need a higher (and wider) segment than the person who works outdoors and who seldom is required to do any close work.

Round Segs

Different types of segs need to be set at different heights because of variance in the distance to the OC of the bifocal segment and in the shape of the seg top. Specifically, round bifocals need to be positioned about 1 mm higher than flat-top bifocals because their upper area is less useful, being limited in extent, and because their OCs fall much farther from the top. The round bifocal is positioned only 1 mm higher because it would be difficult to raise it significantly more without interfering with distance vision.

For example, a round, 22 mm-wide seg has its OC 11 mm from the top. Its widest usable area is also located at that 11-mm-from-the-top distance. If a seg were fitted 14 mm high, the center of the seg and the widest usable area would be 3 mm above the frame's lower rim. If a flat-top seg were used at the same height in the frame as the round seg (i.e., 14 mm high), the OCs would be 9 mm above the lower rim of the frame, as would the widest part of the bifocal.

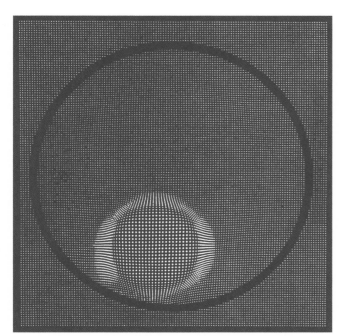

Figure 5-31. A blended bifocal works well for those who desire an invisible near addition, but either do not want or cannot afford a progressive addition lens. (Courtesy of Essilor of America, St. Petersburg, Fla.)

Blended or "Invisible" Bifocals

The so-called *blended bifocal* follows the optical characteristics of the usual round-seg bifocal, except that the demarcation line between the distant portion and the bifocal is obliterated by a polishing process of the lens or lens mold that substitutes a narrow nonoptical transition area for the line of demarcation.

A blended bifocal is not a progressive addition lens. The only resemblance is that in both lens designs the near segment is not obvious. Optically a blended bifocal performs the same as a standard bifocal because only two actual zones of focus exist: one for distance and one for near. Consequently, no aberration or unwanted cylinder is noticeable peripherally.

Distortion is produced around the bifocal segment by the blended area, which varies in width from less than 3 mm to just under 5 mm, depending on the power of the add and the base curve (Figure 5-31). This area serves as the boundary of the bifocal, and permits the lens to be fitted according to the same provisions that affect an ordinary visible bifocal. Both the height of the segment and near PD need to be specified.

Because most blended bifocals are of the round seg type, and because the blend is wider than the usual demarcation line, the bifocal may require either slightly higher placement of the top of the segment or greater depression of the gaze for reading. The manufacturer recommends fitting this bifocal 1 mm higher than is usual for other types of bifocals. The frame used should provide sufficient space in its lower area to contain the bifocal.

The blended area is proportionately less visible in low powers than in higher ones. The tendency for the lens segment to be slightly visible increases with an increase of power in distance or near portions.

High Powered Lenses

Looking away from the center of a high plus lens will cause decreased visual acuity because of lens aberrations. This is especially noticeable in regular, nonaspheric lenses and very strong plus lenses such as are used for aphakic corrections.

For example, a regular nonaspheric +12.00 D lens with a −3.00 D back surface curve will show a power of +11.40 D sphere in combination with a −0.94 D cylinder at a point 25 degrees from the OC. Therefore, it may be seen that the farther from the central area of the lens a person looks, the greater will be the departure from the desired power. Since the power is increasingly affected as a person looks farther from the OC, it is desirable that the reading area of the lens be as close to the distance OC as possible. For these reasons, a straight-top bifocal is more likely to meet this requirement than a round one, and the higher the bifocal is placed in the lens (closer to distance OC), the better the optical requirements can be met.

Children

Bifocals are seldom prescribed for children because of an inability to focus near point material. More often their need for a bifocal stems from a binocular visual problem. Children will normally see clearly through both distance or near portions when viewing near objects. Unless the seg height is properly placed, the child may unconsciously use the distance portion above the seg line for reading or near point work instead of the bifocal portion. To assure that the near addition is being used, the bifocal should be measured and placed so that the seg line *bisects* the pupil. For measuring purposes, the fitter should be on the same level as the child. This ensures that no parallax error occurs. Children adapt quickly and are not bothered by the high seg placement.

The type of bifocal seg commonly used is a wide flat-top style. A wide near area helps to guarantee that the whole near field will be covered by the add, ensuring its prescribed use. (Some practitioners prefer using a progressive add lens for children who need a near addition because the seg is invisible.) If a progressive addition lens is used for children, the fitting cross is placed 4 mm higher than normal (i.e., 4 mm above the pupil center).

Summary

As can be seen, a considerable number of factors can influence the bifocal height. Not all of these have been noted here, but those covered in this section can be summarized as follows.

1. Head back—seg lower; head down—seg higher.
2. Tall persons: seg lower.

3. Adapt the height to the occupational need. Office professions (close work)—seg higher; outdoor occupations (distance vision)—seg lower.
4. Set round segs 1 mm higher.
5. Set seg tops in high plus lenses as high as is practical.

Influence of Vertex Distance on Apparent Seg Height

The apparent height of the segment is dependent on the distance that the lens is from the eye, or the vertex distance.

If a wearer complains that the new bifocals are too high and always in the way, yet from the front the segs look to be exactly the same height in relation to the eyes as the old pair, the lenses are very likely sitting farther from the face than the old ones were.

To illustrate, imagine standing 3 feet away from a window and looking over the window sill at the ground. Approaching the window, more of the ground can be seen, even though the actual height of the sill has not changed. The same is true of the dividing line of bifocals. If the bifocals are farther from the face, they interfere with vision just as if they were placed higher.

The solution is to decrease the vertex distance by changing the adjustment of the pad arms on metal or combination frames (see the section on nose pad adjustments in Chapter 9) or to increase the pantoscopic angle of the frame, tilting the lower edge of the frame toward the face (Figure 5-32). The pantoscopic angle can be increased on almost any type of frame and provides a workable solution because the bifocal section is apparently lowered when it is moved closer to the face.

Because of the relationship between apparent seg height and vertex distance, one seg will appear higher to the wearer than the other if one lens is closer to the face than the other. This possibility should always be investigated if the wearer complains of unequal seg heights (Box 5-5).

Prism-Compensated Segs

When a person has anisometropia (a large difference in power between the left and right eyes), unequal prism is induced when looking through any area of the lenses except the center.

An individual who does not require bifocals is able to avoid the prism by turning the head and keeping the lines of sight of both eyes close to the optical centers of the spectacles. When reading, the chin is dropped to keep the OCs lined up with the material. The amount the eyes turn inward from these points is usually small enough to elicit only a low amount of prism. The prism base is horizontal and is easily compensated.

If the wearer attempts to read by lowering the eyes rather than the lenses, the eyes will move away from the OCs and additionally induce definite amounts of vertical prism. This may be clinically significant. Some

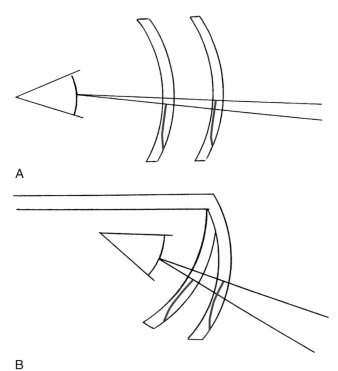

A

B

Figure 5-32. A, Decreasing the vertex distance of a lens from the wearer's point of view will cause a reduction in the apparent height of the seg. **B,** Increasing the pantoscopic angle of a frame also reduces the apparent seg height for the wearer.

BOX 5-5

Seg Adjustments Listed in Order to Be Tried

Segs Seem High	Segs Seem Low
1. Increase pantoscopic tilt.	1. Narrow pads.
2. Decrease vertex distance.	2. Bend pads down by adjusting pad arms.
3. Spread pads.	3. Increase vertex distance.
4. Move pads up by adjusting pad arms.	4. Reduce pantoscopic tilt.
5. Stretch bridge (plastic frame).	5. Shrink bridge (plastic frame).

---

individuals with anisometropia, however, learn to compensate for this.

When an anisometrope is forced to use bifocals or trifocals, the prismatic consequences of the prescription can no longer be avoided because the reading segments must be placed away from the OCs of the distance correction. To predict if this will be a problem, ask the wearer to read through the old (nonbifocal) glasses. If the wearer drops the head to read, he or she is looking through the OCs and may need help in the form of slab-off prism to counteract the unequal prismatic effects. If, however, he or she drops the eyes to read and looks through the bottom of the lenses, the wearer is accustomed to reading through this portion of the glasses and will probably not need any prismatic compensation in the seg (see also Chapter 21).

COMPENSATING FOR AN INCORRECTLY SIZED SAMPLE FRAME

At the very beginning of the chapter, the importance of a properly positioned frame was emphasized. Before measuring for lens placement, the frame must be positioned on the face where it will be worn, otherwise the measurements will be wrong. So with metal frames, the nosepads are positioned for proper height. And as stated earlier, with plastic frames, if the bridge of the sample frame is too small, the frame will sit too high; if it is too large, it will sit too low. But what should be done if the sample frame is not the same size as the frame that will be worn? Unless allowances for frame size differences are made, the lens measurements will be wrong.

If the eye size is too large or too small, the depth of a given frame style will vary uniformly from one size to the next, according to the "boxing" concept of lens size. If the eye size is incorrect, the segment height ordered will need to be changed to allow for the difference in lens depth. Since the usual difference in vertical dimension from one given eye size to the next is 2 mm, the change required in either the optical center (OC) or seg position from the bottom of the eyewire is 1 mm.

Obviously the chance of error is much greater when using a sample with a correct eye size but an incorrect bridge size because compensation for eye size is relatively simple.

When the Eye Size Is Incorrect

Suppose a person needs, for example, a 52□20, but the closest available sample is 50□20. The bifocal is measured using the 50□20, and the height is determined to be 15 mm. If the lenses are ground for the larger frame, a 15-mm bifocal height will place the seg line too low. The question is how much higher must it now be placed?

To determine the answer, consider that a given frame may use the same pattern for all eye sizes. When the eye size is increased by 2 mm across the A dimension, there is effectively 1 mm of lens material being added to the outside edge in every direction (Figure 5-33). This means that the distance from the geometric center to the lower bevel will be increased by 1 mm. At the same time, the distance from the *desired* seg top position to the lower eyewire also increases 1 mm. Therefore, if a 50□20 frame requires that the seg line be 15 mm high, a 52□20 will mandate a 16 mm high seg to maintain the location of the upper line at the desired level. By the same reasoning, a sample frame having an eye size 2 mm too large will measure 1 mm higher than actually required.

Rule of thumb: For an improper eye size, the seg height is corrected by one half the difference between sample frame eye size and desired frame eye size.

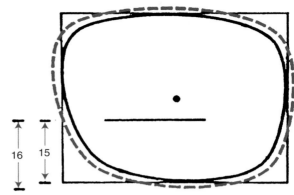

Figure 5-33. The actual sample frame eye size is represented by the solid line. The desired eye size to be ordered is represented by the dotted line and is 2 mm larger. Hence the seg height to be ordered will be 1 mm greater.

As with any rule of thumb, exceptions do occur. They are:

1. If the bridge of the frame is constructed proportionally higher (or lower) in the frame as the eye size changes, the variations will not be constant. (To check this, for an individual frame style, the distance from the bridge crest to a line running tangent to the upper rims is measured. The difference in these measured values between eye sizes should be half the difference between the two eye sizes, as in the rule of thumb.)
2. Because of the wearer's nose-cheek formation, if it appears that a larger eye size will cause the inner, lower eyewire sections of the larger frame size to rest on a different anatomic part of the face, a larger eye size may rest higher on the face than might be expected. Appropriate care should therefore be taken.

If the Correct Bridge Size Is Unavailable

Now consider the case where the correct eye size is available, but the bridge is one size too small. It is still not possible to measure directly using the frame as it sits "normally" when placed directly on the face. When the bridge size is too small, the whole frame will sit too high on the face. Any uncompensated direct measure will result in a seg that is much too low. The right bridge size will allow the frame to be at its correct lower position. Unfortunately, there is no conversion factor possible using a sample frame with the wrong bridge size. Instead the fitter must move the frame down the nose until properly positioned, then hold it in place while measuring for seg height. (This presumes that the fitter is able to accurately estimate where the correct size will place the frame.)

The Alternatives

Of the two situations presented, the more predictably accurate involves an incorrect eye size combined with a correct bridge size. If the fitter has a choice between using either (1) an incorrect eye size and correct bridge size, or (2) a correct eye size and incorrect bridge size, then the first instance should be chosen.

INSTRUCTING THE NEW BIFOCAL WEARER

New multifocal lenses represent a completely foreign experience for the first-time wearer. Some of the resultant problems may be prevented by direct advice ahead of time.

Because of the magnification produced by plus lenses, the wearer can expect objects seen through bifocals to appear magnified, creating the impression that these objects are closer because they appear larger. Curbs look higher than they really are, and staircases become real hazards when observed through the bifocal add. Distance judgment returns to normal after a period of adaptation despite the magnification, and the height of stairs, curbs, and so forth, are properly judged.

The new bifocal wearer will experience differences from well-established habits, and the necessary adjustments to compensate for the differences should be explained to him or her. For example, before wearing bifocals:

1. The floor could be seen by keeping the head erect and dropping the eyes into the lower portion of the lenses.
2. A book could be read by holding the eyes at the center of the lenses and dropping the chin and head.

To correctly use bifocals:

1. The floor is seen by holding the eyes at the center of the lenses and dropping the chin and head.
2. A book must be read by holding the head erect and dropping the eyes into the lower portion of the lenses.

These differences may be contradictory to the wearer's well-established habits. A period of adaptation is required, and the wearer can more easily master the new responses required if he or she understands them ahead of time.

DETERMINING LENS BLANK SIZE

A *lens blank* is a lens before it has been edged to fit into the frame. It may be either finished or semifinished. A *finished* lens blank has the correct powers called for in the prescription and needs only to be edged. A *semifinished* lens blank has only one side of the lens finished, usually the front side; the back side needs to be ground and polished to the correct power.

The dispenser is concerned with lens blank size for several reasons. For single vision lenses, the question is especially pertinent if lenses are to be edged in-house. The lens blank size determines if an in-house edging lab will be able to edge the prescription from finished lenses that are in stock or if the prescription will have to be sent out for surfacing. For multifocal lenses, the question is, given the seg height and PD requested, can the lenses be made for the frame selected?

MBS for Single-Vision Lenses

The PD *measurement* in essence determines the position of the OCs of the lenses and helps decide the total size of the finished lens blank required for the designated frame. It will be recalled from Chapter 2 that the effective diameter (ED) of the spectacle lens is found by taking the distance from the geometric center of the lens to the edge point of the lens farthest from the geometric center and doubling it (see Figure 2-2). If a person's eyes are not at the geometric centers of the frame, the centers of the lenses must be displaced or decentered so they are vertically aligned with the centers of the wearer's pupils.

For example, if the OC of the lens falls at the geometric or boxing center of the frame's lens shape, then a lens blank with a diameter equal to the frame shape's ED is large enough to fill the frame's lens opening. But if the lens must be decentered, then as a general rule 2 mm must be added to the ED of the lens blank for every 1 mm the lens is decentered.*

Using a Formula to Find MBS for Finished Single-Vision Lenses

Minimum blank size (MBS) for finished, single vision lenses can be summarized as a simple formula. The formula is:

$$MBS = ED + 2(\text{decentration per lens}) + 2$$

where *MBS* is the minimum blank size and *ED* is the effective diameter of the frame shape. The decentration per lens is the difference between the frame GCD (the A plus the DBL) and the wearer's PD, all divided by 2. Expressed as a formula, this is

$$\text{Decentration per lens} = \frac{(A + DBL) - PD}{2}$$

Twice the decentration per lens equals total decentration.

In other words,

$$\text{total decentration} = (A + DBL) - PD.$$

This means that the formula for minimum blank size could also be written as

$$MBS = ED + \text{total decentration} + 2\,\text{mm}$$

---

* This rule holds true only when the longest radius from the geometric center of the lens opening is opposite in position (nasal or temporal) to the decentration direction. In other words, if the longest radius of the lens opening is temporal and the lenses are decentered inward (nasally), the rule holds true, as it does if the longest radius is nasal and the lenses are decentered outward (temporally).

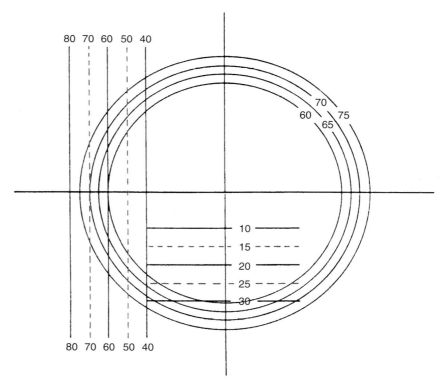

Figure 5-34. Single-vision minimum blank size chart. The blank size chart shown is used as follows: (*1*) Place the frame front face down on the chart with the right lens opening over the simulated lens circles. (*2*) Center the frame bridge over the correct binocular distance PD as indicated by the scale on the left. (*3*) Ensure vertical centration. This is done by positioning the lowest point on the inside groove of the lower eyewire on the lower chart scale. The correct level is one half the B dimension of the frame. (If a vertical positioning for the optical center of the lens is specified, use this height instead.) (*4*) Note which diameter lens circle will just enclose the lens opening of the frame including the eyewire groove. This is the minimum blank size required for a nonprismatic, single vision lens. (Reprinted with permission from Brooks CW: *Essentials of ophthalmic lens finishing*, St. Louis, 2003, Butterworth-Heinemann.)

The last factor in the MBS formula is "+ 2 mm." These additional 2 mm add a slight amount of extra lens material to allow for possible defects on the edge of the lens. Here is an example of how to figure out the MBS for finished single vision lenses.

Example **5-5**

What would the MBS be for a finished, single-vision lens that is to be placed in a frame having the following dimensions?

$$A = 52 \text{ mm}$$
$$DBL = 18 \text{ mm}$$
$$ED = 57 \text{ mm}$$

The wearer's PD is 62 mm.

Solution

First find total decentration.

$$\text{Total decentration} = (A + DBL) - PD$$

In this case,

$$\text{total decentration} = (52 + 18) - 62$$
$$= 8 \text{ mm}$$

Now that the total decentration is known, MBS is determined by

$$MBS = ED + \text{total decentration} + 2 \text{ mm}$$
$$= 57 + 8 + 2$$
$$= 67$$

Therefore if the prescription has no prescribed prism, the smallest finished lens blank that could be used has a diameter of 67 mm.

Determining MBS for Finished, Single-Vision Lenses Using a Drawing

It is possible to use the newly selected frame in combination with a scale drawing to determine the minimum, finished single-vision lens size necessary. This drawing is shown to scale in Figure 5-34. Follow the directions given with the figure legend.

Determining MBS for Multifocal Lenses Using a Drawing

For multifocal lenses, the location of the segment in the frame determines whether or not the semifinished lens blank will be large enough. If the bifocal or trifocal segment is too high, there may be an air space between the bottom of the edged lens and the frame's lower eyewire. It is always an embarrassment to the dispenser when the surfacing lab calls to say that the lens will not cut out for the chosen frame. This can sometimes mean that the wearer must be asked to return to select a new frame. Therefore it is best to try and avoid problems in questionable cases by verifying lens blank size ahead of time. This may be done using actual-size drawings or charts. An example of a chart is shown as Figure 5-35.

All charts basically mimic the semifinished lens. The frame is placed on the scale drawing of the lenses and moved vertically and horizontally to position the lens segment as it will appear in the frame. If the frame's lens

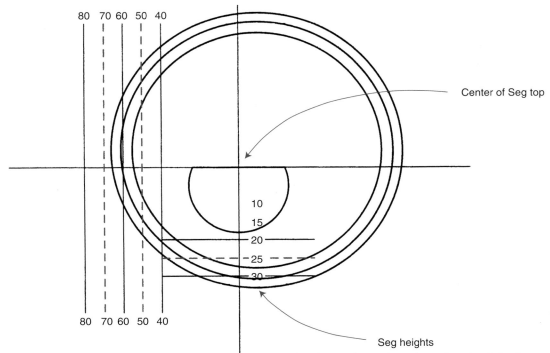

Center of Seg top

Seg heights

Figure 5-35. To use a multifocal minimum blank size chart, place the right side of the frame face down over the chart. Move the frame left or right until the near interpupillary distance line corresponding to the ordered near interpupillary distance is directly in the center of the frame bridge. Move the frame up or down until the correct seg height corresponds to the lowest part of the inside bevel of the lower eyewire. The smallest circle that completely encloses the lens shape is the smallest blank possible for this manufacturer. Because manufacturers' lens blanks will vary, blank size charts for multifocal lenses are not interchangeable.

BOX 5-6

How to Use Scale Lens Drawings to Determine Minimum Blank Size for Multifocal Lenses

1. Place the frame face down on the drawing.
2. Move the frame up or down until the inside bevel of the lower eyewire is over the line corresponding to the correct seg height.
3. Move the frame left or right until the center of the bridge is over the line corresponding to the near PD.
4. Note whether the lens blank completely encircles the frame's lens opening.
5. If encirclement is complete, the blank is large enough. If it is not, the blank is too small.

---

opening is completely covered by the drawn lens, the real lens blank will be large enough (Box 5-6).

If the Multifocal Lens Will Not Cut Out

Sometimes a lens will not cut out because the seg ordered is especially high or unusually low. If a lens will not cut out for this reason, it is possible to move the frame up or down until the drawn lens covers the frame's lens opening, thus determining how much the segment height will need to be decreased or increased so the lens will cut out. This modified height may be read directly from the drawing. Now the dispenser must make a judgment. Can the seg height be modified, or should a different frame or new multifocal lens style be chosen? Often a small change in seg height will allow the chosen frame to be used.

Sometimes a lens will not cut out because the wearer's near PD is too small to permit enough lens decentration. This may be a warning that the frame selected is too large for the wearer. Moving the frame left or right on the minimum blank size chart will show what the near PD must be so that the lens will cut out. (In some cases, it may be permissible to modify the near PD if the bifocal segment is wide enough. For more on this subject, see Brooks: *Essentials for Ophthalmic Lens Finishing.*[4])

REFERENCES

1. Allen MJ: How do you fit spectacles? Indiana J Optom, 32:2, 1962.

2. Dowaliby M: Practical aspects of ophthalmic dispensing. Chicago, 1972, The Professional Press, Inc.
3. Riley HD, Hitchcock JR: Segment height adjustment and vertical prism, Optom Weekly, 66:889-902, 1975.
4. Brooks CW: Essentials of ophthalmic lens finishing, ed 2, St Louis, 2003, Butterworth-Heinemann.
5. American Optical Corporation: Lens information kit; optical cosmetic and mechanical properties of ophthalmic lenses, Southbridge, Mass, 1968.

Proficiency Test

(Answers can be found in the back of the book.)

1. True or false? When measuring for multifocal heights, the place on the eyewire directly below the pupil is used as a zero point.

2. The OC and the MRP are at exactly the same point on the lens except:
   a. when there is a measured MRP height.
   b. when there is prescribed cylinder present in the prescription.
   c. when there is prescribed prism present in the prescription.
   d. when a bifocal segment has a raise instead of a drop.
   e. the OC and the MRP are never at exactly the same point on a lens.

3. When the wearer's PD is less than the A plus the DBL measurements of the frame, then:
   a. positive face form is required.
   b. negative face form is required.
   c. no face form is required.
   d. pantoscopic tilt is required.
   e. retroscopic tilt is required.

4. You have a very small, fashion oval lens shape. The eye size is only 30 mm. The bridge size is 22 mm. The lens powers are −3.50 D spheres. The wearer's PD is 62 mm. In practice, how would you adjust the frame for face form?
   a. a very slight amount of face form
   b. no face form
   c. a very slight amount of antiface or negative face form
   d. a moderate amount of antiface or negative face form

5. True or false? Tilting the wearer's chin back until the plane of the frame front is perpendicular to the floor, and then marking the pupil height is a short cut measuring method for placing the MRP of the lens at the appropriate fitting height.

6. For every 2 degrees of pantoscopic tilt, the OC should be:
   a. raised 0.5 mm above the pupil center.
   b. raised 1 mm above the pupil center.
   c. lowered 0.5 mm below the pupil center.
   d. lowered 1 mm below the pupil center.
   e. There is no relationship between pantoscopic tilt and the vertical placement of the OC.

7. Here is a theoretical question. There are two frames. Both are for the same wearer. In fact, both are the same frame style and size exactly. However, one will be worn with no pantoscopic tilt. The other will have a lot of pantoscopic tilt. Which one should have the highest MRP when the lenses are ordered?
   a. The one with no pantoscopic tilt.
   b. The one with lots of pantoscopic tilt.
   c. There should be no difference in ordered MRP height at all.

8. You measure an MRP height to be 26 mm. The B dimension of the frame is 44 mm and the pantoscopic tilt of the frame is 12 degrees. How high should you order the MRP? (Watch out! This question may not be as straightforward as it appears.)
   a. 26 mm
   b. 24 mm
   c. 22 mm
   d. 20 mm
   e. 18 mm

9. A distometer is used to:
   a. measure the distance between lenses and the frame eye size.
   b. measure the power of a spectacle lens.
   c. measure the PD.
   d. measure the vertex distance.
   e. measure the segment height.

10. The left lens is closer to the face than the right lens. Therefore:
   a. the left seg will seem higher to the wearer than the right.
   b. the right seg will seem higher to the wearer than the left.
   c. there will be no effect on the apparent subjective height of the segs.

11. Which of the following is *not* a legitimate use of a Fresnel press-on segment?
   a. As an aide for determining segment height.
   b. As a temporary bifocal addition.
   c. As a means of changing the distance power of the wearer's existing glasses until such time as their new glasses arrive.
   d. To demonstrate how a double segment lens would work for occupational purposes.

12. For every one diopter increase in base curve, what happens to the vertex distance?
   a. It increases by approximately 0.6 mm.
   b. It decreases by approximately 0.6 mm.
   c. It increases by approximately 1 mm.
   d. It decreases by approximately 1 mm.

13. The wearer's Rx comes back from the lab, but their lashes brush the backs of the lenses with each blink. They do not want to go to a different frame. You cannot alter the bridge. You have done everything you can by adjusting tilt and face form. You still need 1 more millimeter of vertex distance to clear the lashes. You decide to reorder lenses with new base curves. How should you change the base curves?
   a. Increase the base curve by 1 D.
   b. Increase the base curve by 2 D.
   c. Increase the base curve by 3 D.
   d. Decrease the base curve by 1 D.
   e. You cannot solve the problem this way. Change frames.

14. In measuring for a trifocal, we find the distance from the inside bevel of the lower eyewire to the lower edge of the pupil to be 22 mm. What trifocal height should be ordered?
   a. 22.5 mm
   b. 23.5 mm
   c. 24 mm
   d. 20 mm
   e. 21 mm

15. You are measuring a trifocal height for a nylon cord frame in the dispensary. The frame comes with display lenses. To determine trifocal height, you begin by measuring the distance to the bottom of the pupil. This distance measures 21 mm. What seg height would you order?

   a. 22 mm
   b. 21.5 mm
   c. 21 mm
   d. 20.5 mm
   e. 20 mm

16. How should round segment heights be ordered compared with flat-top segment heights?
   a. Round segment heights should be ordered 1 mm lower than flat-top segment heights.
   b. Round segment heights should be ordered 2 mm lower than flat-top segment heights.
   c. Round segment heights should be ordered 1 mm higher than flat-top segment heights.
   d. Round segment heights should be ordered 2 mm higher than flat-top segment heights.
   e. Segment shape has no influence upon segment height.

17. An individual wears 6 Δ of prism base-down before the left eye for a phoria condition. An empty frame is used to measure for bifocal height. What alteration to the measured bifocal height must be made for the left eye?
   a. The left bifocal height must be raised 1 mm above its measured value.
   b. The left bifocal height must be raised 2 mm above its measured value.
   c. The left bifocal height must be lowered 1 mm below its measured value.
   d. The left bifocal height must be lowered 2 mm below its measured value.
   e. The left bifocal height should be left exactly as measured.

18. An individual wears 3 Δ base-up before the right eye and 3 Δ of prism base-down before the left eye to alleviate a phoria problem. If an empty frame is used in measuring for bifocal height, what alteration in those measured values must be made?
   a. Raise the right bifocal 0.5 mm and lower the left bifocal 0.5 mm from their measured values.
   b. Raise the right bifocal 1 mm and lower the left bifocal 1 mm from their measured values.
   c. Lower the right bifocal 0.5 mm and raise the left bifocal 0.5 mm from their measured values.
   d. Lower the right bifocal 1 mm and raise the left bifocal 1 mm from their measured values.

19. A new bifocal wearer must:
   a. keep the head erect and drop the eyes to see the floor.
   b. drop the eyes to read a book.
   c. drop the chin and head to engage in near work.

20. An individual selects a frame with the following dimensions:
    A = 48
    B = 44
    DBL = 20
    The wearer's PD is 62 and the seg height is measured at 21 mm.
    The seg style chosen is a double-D occupational. How much vertical near viewing area will there be at the top of the lens once the lenses are edged and inserted in the frame? (There are two answers below that could be considered as correct, depending upon the brand of lens chosen. You need only select one of the two.)
    a. 5 mm
    b. 6 mm
    c. 7 mm
    d. 8 mm
    e. 9 mm
    f. 10 mm
    g. 11 mm
    h. 12 mm
    i. 13 mm
    j. 14 mm
    k. 15 mm
    l. 16 mm

21. How should bifocal height be positioned for a child?
    a. At the lower limbus
    b. Between the lower limbus and the lower edge of the pupil
    c. 1 mm below the lower edge of the pupil
    d. At the lower edge of the pupil
    e. At the center of the pupil
    f. 4 mm above the center of the pupil

22. You are measuring a child for bifocal height. Here are some measurements: From the inside bevel of the lower eyewire to the lower limbus is 15 mm. From the inside bevel of the lower eyewire to the bottom of the pupil is 19 mm. From the inside bevel of the lower eyewire to the center of the pupil is 21 mm. How high would you order the bifocal?
    a. 15 mm
    b. 18 mm
    c. 19 mm
    d. 21 mm
    e. 25 mm

23. The seg position for the new Rx in a newer-style frame should duplicate the seg position in the old pair of glasses. The old seg height was 14 mm. However, the bifocal line is 2 mm below the lower limbus. For the new frame, the distance from the lowest part of the inside bevel of the lower eyewire up to the level of the limbus is 17 mm. What

bifocal height would you order for the new pair so that the new pair matched?
    a. 14 mm
    b. 15 mm
    c. 16 mm
    d. 17 mm

24. True or false? To lower the apparent height of a bifocal segment from the wearer's perspective, it is possible to increase the pantoscopic angle.

25. A person chooses a frame with an A dimension of 50 mm and a DBL of 20 mm. There is no frame of this size available. The frame must be ordered. It is still necessary to measure for progressive addition fitting cross height. Only a 48□20 frame is in stock. The fitting cross height measured with this frame is 21 mm. What fitting cross height should be ordered?
    a. 19 mm
    b. 20 mm
    c. 21 mm
    d. 22 mm
    e. 23 mm

26. A frame with an eye size of 48 mm and a bridge size of 20 mm is necessary. The only frame available is one with a 50 mm eye size and a 20 mm bridge size. You determine that for a 50 mm eye size frame you would need a bifocal height of 17 mm. What would you order for the 48 mm eye size frame so that the bifocal line will come out at the right place?
    a. 16 mm
    b. 16.5 mm
    c. 17 mm
    d. 17.5 mm
    e. 18 mm

27. A semifinished lens blank:
    a. has both front and back surfaces already ground to the correct curves and power, but has not yet been edged.
    b. has been made to the correct thickness, but does not have the correct surface powers on the front or the back surfaces.
    c. has the front surface at the correct curve, but the back surface is not yet ground to the needed curvature to produce the required lens power.

28. A frame has the dimensions of 49□19 with an ED of 52 mm. The patient's PD is 68 mm. What is the minimum lens blank size required?
    a. 50 mm
    b. 52 mm
    c. 54 mm
    d. 63 mm
    e. 71 mm

29. What is the smallest lens blank size possible for a 50 mm round eye size frame if the lens must be decentered 3 mm per lens?
   a. 50 mm
   b. 52 mm
   c. 54 mm
   d. 56 mm
   e. 58 mm

30. What is the ED of the frame in Question 29?
   a. 48 mm
   b. 50 mm
   c. 52 mm
   d. 56 mm
   e. 63 mm

31. True or false? Lens blank size charts that are made for multifocal lenses are basically a drawing of the semifinished lens that is to be used for the prescription.

32. True or false? If a lens will not work in a certain frame because the lens blank is too small, the seg height or near PD should never be modified so that the frame and multifocal lens style can still be used.

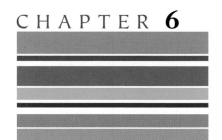

CHAPTER 6

Ordering and Verification

This chapter is basically a guide to procedures followed when ordering and verifying prescriptions from an optical laboratory. Using uniform terminology and a checklist approach assures a minimum of errors, which in turn improves the quality of service to the spectacle wearer.

ORDERING

When ordering a prescription, use the manufacturer's or supplier's own printed form or enter it online if possible. This will prevent many errors or omissions in processing. Online ordering can help prevent errors because the program will often keep the order from being sent until all necessary information is present.

With paper forms, it is very important to print the necessary information. Poor or illegible handwriting usually results in errors.

General Procedures for Forms

Use a separate form for each job ordered, since the form itself may travel with the materials during laboratory processing.

When ordering less than a total frame and both lenses, specify this clearly on the order form. For printed forms, write this in fairly large letters or check the appropriate places on the form.

Do not include superfluous data or information on any forms if such data are not necessary or applicable to the order. For example, do not supply eye size and bridge size if only a temple is being ordered.

Lens Information

When writing the prescription in paragraph form, such as in a letter, always write the data referring to the right lens first, followed by the data for the left lens. For example, "Mr. Hensley was issued a prescription of OD: –3.00 D sphere, OS: –2.75, –1.50 × 175." When written on a blank prescription pad, such a prescription would be written with the left lens value directly below that of the right lens. This would appear as follows:

OD: –3.00 D sph
OS: –2.75 –1.50 × 175

("OD" is, in this instance, the abbreviation for "right eye" from the Latin words *oculus dexter*, whereas "OS" is the abbreviation for the Latin words *oculus sinister*, or left eye.) Always use at least three figures for the sphere and cylinder components. If the dioptric unit is less than 1.00 D, use a prefatory zero before the decimal point, as for example, +0.75 D. Carry figures two places after the decimal point, as for example, +2.00 D (not +2 D) or –1.50 D (not –1.5 D). State the axis as *x*, but do not put a degree sign after the numbers representing the cylinder axis because it may be mistakenly read as an extra zero. For example, 10 degrees may be misread as 100 when written out with the degree sign in longhand as 10°. Many also use 3 numbers for the axis. Therefore it is normal to see a 5 degree axis written as 005.

Check the base curve of the wearer's old lenses, particularly when only one lens is being replaced. (For information on how to measure base curve, see Chapter 13.)

Frame Information

Be sure to specify the style of temple desired if more than one style is available. Print the name of the frame and include the name of the manufacturer (Figure 6-1).

REORDERING FROM EXISTING SPECTACLES

Sometimes it is necessary to use a person's existing spectacle lenses as the basis for ordering another pair of glasses. This can occur in an emergency situation if the person has cracked or broken a lens and the lenses are still in the frame. It may also happen that an individual has a pair of glasses and wants a second pair, but no longer has the written prescription.

Obtaining Lens Information for Existing Spectacles

Although it is possible to read the prescription directly from the current eyeglasses, it is best to contact the prescriber or previous dispenser to verify what was ordered—not just what was received. For example, when taking a prescription from an existing pair of glasses, one may misread a cylinder axis as 170, when the lens is really axis 168. Yet the original order could have called for axis

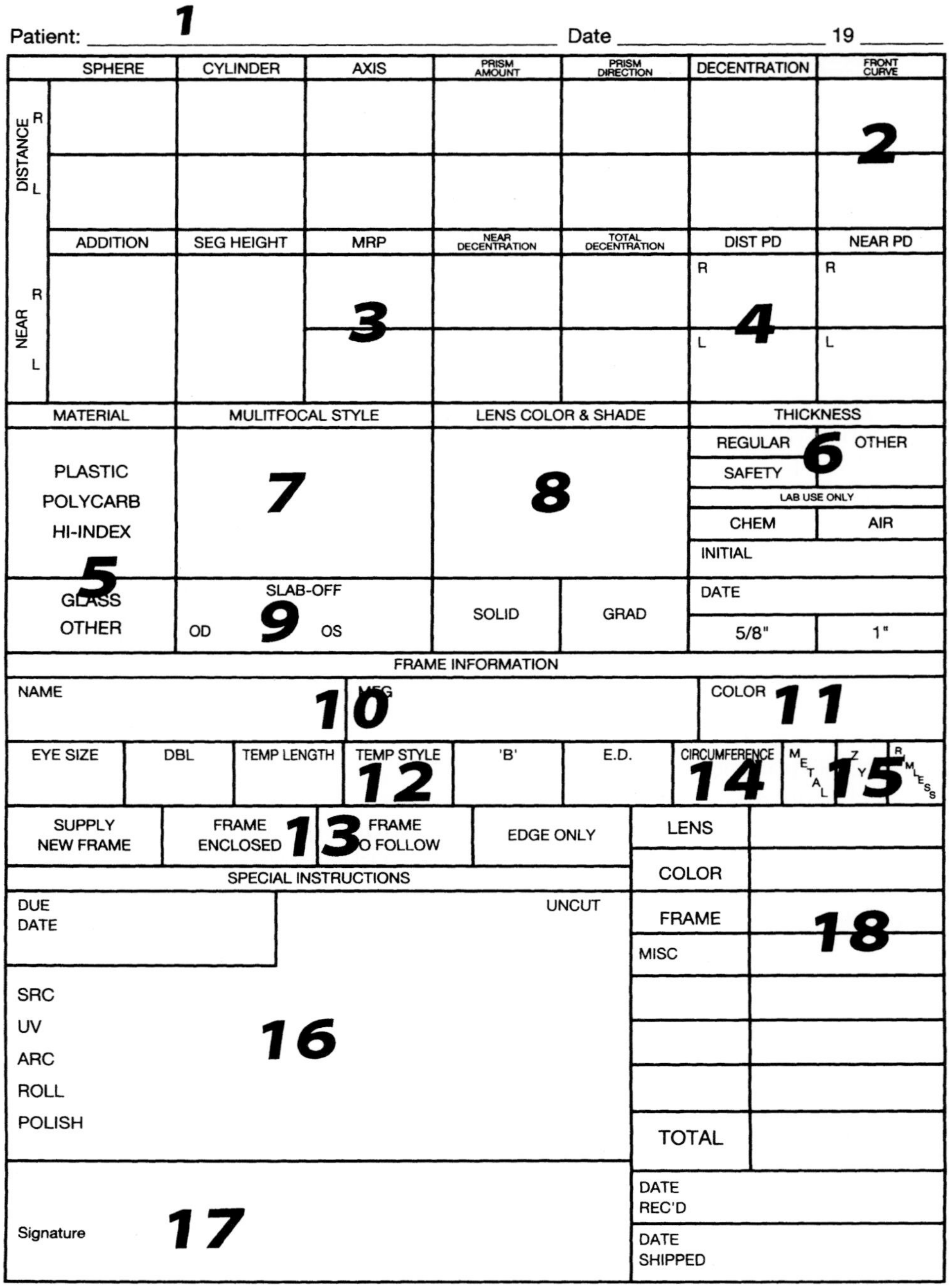

Patient: _____ Date _____ 19 _____

	SPHERE	CYLINDER	AXIS	PRISM AMOUNT	PRISM DIRECTION	DECENTRATION	FRONT CURVE
DISTANCE R							**2**
DISTANCE L							

	ADDITION	SEG HEIGHT	MRP	NEAR DECENTRATION	TOTAL DECENTRATION	DIST PD	NEAR PD
NEAR R			**3**			R	R
NEAR L						L **4**	L

MATERIAL	MULITFOCAL STYLE	LENS COLOR & SHADE	THICKNESS	
PLASTIC	**7**	**8**	REGULAR	OTHER **6**
POLYCARB			SAFETY	
HI-INDEX			LAB USE ONLY	
5			CHEM	AIR
			INITIAL	
GLASS	SLAB-OFF	SOLID	GRAD	DATE
OTHER	OD **9** OS			5/8" 1"

FRAME INFORMATION

NAME	MFG **10**	COLOR **11**

EYE SIZE	DBL	TEMP LENGTH	TEMP STYLE **12**	'B'	E.D.	CIRCUMFERENCE **14**	METAL ZYL RIMLESS **15**

SUPPLY NEW FRAME	FRAME ENCLOSED **13**	FRAME TO FOLLOW	EDGE ONLY	LENS
				COLOR

SPECIAL INSTRUCTIONS

DUE DATE	UNCUT	FRAME **18**
		MISC
SRC		
UV		
ARC **16**		
ROLL		
POLISH		TOTAL
Signature **17**		DATE REC'D
		DATE SHIPPED

◀ **Figure 6-1.** Example order form. Order forms vary considerably from laboratory to laboratory. It is crucial that an order form be completely and correctly filled out. Errors in completing the order form can result in glasses being improperly made, necessitating a costly remake. At the very least, an incomplete order form could delay the order or require that the wearer return so that the missing information can be supplied. Instructions for completing each general area of the form are given below. Areas left blank are self-explanatory.

(1) Some recommend that the wearer's last name be written here in all capital letters, be underlined, and be listed before the first name. This is followed by a comma and the first name printed in small letters.

(2) List only if ordering special base curves. Otherwise leave blank.

(3) List the MRP height *only* if it is other than at half the B dimension. Otherwise this is left blank. Often this is where fitting cross height is listed for progressive addition lenses.

(4) Do not give both binocular and monocular PDs. Use either one or the other, but not both. If you use a binocular PD, write it once, right on the line between left and right boxes.

(5) You must indicate a lens material.

(6) Normally you do not specify a thickness for the lens. Be sure to indicate if the lens is a regular thickness or is for safety eyewear, however. If the frame is a Z87 safety frame, circle "safety" and the lenses will be properly marked to conform to Z87 requirements.

(7) Indicate multifocal type and seg size, or progressive lens brand when appropriate.

(8) Indicate as specifically as possible what color lens you want. Indicate the desired transmission or shade. If the lenses have no tint, write either "clear" or "white." Circle either "solid" for a uniform tint, or "grad" for a gradient tint.

(9) If slab-off is being ordered, indicate the prism amount of the slab-off.

(10) The frame name may be anything from "Harry" to "T849." The name alone is not enough; the manufacturer must be listed as well. It is not uncommon for more than one manufacturer to use the same name or number.

(11) Color may be a number.

(12) Examples: skull, cable, riding bow, library.

(13) Circle one on this row. "Frame to Follow" means the frame is not with the order. It is to be sent later.

(14) If the order is for "lenses only" (edge only), one way to ensure a more accurate fit is to remove the lens from the frame and measure the circumference of the lens with a circumference gauge. This will allow for better duplication of the lens size. However, a digital frame tracer works best.

(15) Indicate whether the frame is metal, plastic, or rimless. This is especially important when the frame is not present. Be even more specific as to lens material if possible.

(16) "Special Instructions" is for calling attention to anything unusual about the prescription. "SRC" means scratch resistant coating; "UV" means add ultraviolet protection (plastic lenses only); "ARC" means antireflection coating (plastic or glass); "roll" means to roll the edges of the lens to make the lens look thinner; "polish" means to polish the edges.

(17) Signature of the person or the name of the office that is ordering the prescription.

(18) This section is for laboratory pricing.

165. So an axis 170 lens is ordered. But what if the new lens comes in as axis 172? The dispenser will likely accept the lens because it is only two degrees off and within ANSI standards. What the dispenser does not realize is that the axis of the lens is really off by 7 degrees, compared with the original prescription.

Take New Facial Measurements

Even when duplicating an old pair of glasses, it is still important to take new facial measurements. Retake the wearer's PD. You may still wish to use the distance between the OCs found in the old glasses, but you need to know the wearer's measured PD. Large differences may indicate the presence of prescribed prism.

If the lenses are either bifocal or trifocal lenses, note where the segment line falls in reference to the lower limbus. This is important if the new segments are to match the old ones. If the lenses are progressive addition lenses, find the location of the fitting cross on the old lenses to verify that it falls in the center of the pupil (see Chapter 20, Progressive Addition Lenses).

When the Wearer's PD Does Not Match the Distance Between Optical Centers

If the wearer's PD that has just been measured does not match the distance between the OCs in the glasses that are being worn, the dispenser's best options are to:

1. Find out where the prescription originated and call to verify the prescription. Specifically ask if the prescription contains prescribed prism. This is always the correct first option, even when the prescription can be easily read from the existing glasses because an error still may have occurred.

2. If the wearer has no idea where the prescription originated and does not want to have a new eye examination, use the PD found in the existing glasses.* You cannot be sure this is not part of the

---

*The exception to this generalized rule would be for lenses with very low powers in the horizontal meridian. If the optical center of a very low powered lens is off, there is very little horizontal prismatic effect produced. This possibility will become more obvious once the reader is familiar with ANSI Z80 Standards for PD and horizontal prism. For low-powered lenses, the distance between optical centers can miss the wearer's ordered PD by a relatively large amount and still produce only a negligible horizontal prismatic effect. When this occurs, the glasses are still considered to be within tolerance.

For example: A lens pair has a power of −0.50 D sphere in both eyes. The wearer's PD is 60. However, the measured distance between lens centers in the old glasses is 64 mm. This means that the resulting prismatic effect will only be 0.20 prism diopters. Unwanted horizontal prism of this amount is well within ANSI standards of acceptability. And it is also highly unlikely that the original prescription included prescribed prism of an amount less than even one quarter diopter.

To summarize, familiarity with ANSI standards for PD-horizontal prism will make it easier to discern when differences such as these are due to allowable tolerances and when there is a truly prescribed prism present in the prescription.

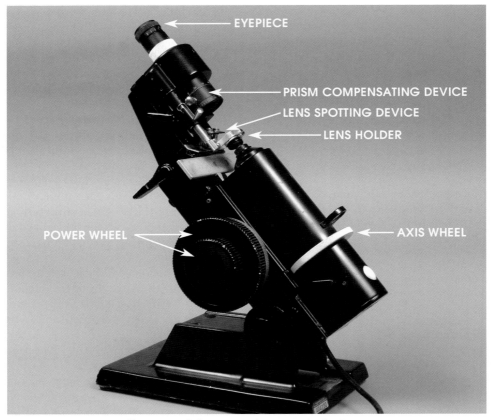

Figure 6-2. A manually-operated lensmeter has certain basic parts common to most instruments.

original prescription and thus should duplicate what is being worn. (Besides, changing an existing prismatic effect may present adaptation problems for the wearer.) You should be certain that the reason for ordering a PD other than the wearer's measured PD is well documented in the record.

Obtaining Prescription Information for Single-Vision Lenses

The heart of the lens prescription is the sphere, cylinder, and axis. These measures of lens power are found using a *lensmeter* (Figure 6-2). Most lensmeters use line targets, but others have targets consisting of a circle of dots. There are lensmeters with internally viewed targets and those with targets projected on a screen. Lensmeters may also work manually or automatically. The most commonly used lensmeters are manual and use a crossed-line target.

How to Find Single-Vision Lens Powers Using a Crossed-Line-Target Lensmeter

When using a lensmeter, begin by focusing the eyepiece to assure an accurate reading. When looking through the eyepiece, imagine sitting on top of a tall building and looking at the street below. This will help relax your accommodation and keep your eye from changing focus,

which can contribute to inaccuracies. First, rotate the eyepiece so that it moves toward the operator's eye—away from the rest of the instrument. Then looking at the *crosshairs and concentric circles* (not the crossed-line, illuminated target), slowly turn the eyepiece back toward the rest of the instrument until the crosshairs and concentric circles *first* come into sharp focus. If you turn too far and pass the first clear focus, again rotate the eyepiece away from the instrument; then slowly rotate it back toward the instrument to the first best focus.

The focusing procedure is only done once and need not be repeated for each pair of spectacles being measured. However, this eyepiece focal adjustment will be different for each individual. When more than one person uses the instrument, the procedure must be repeated for each individual. (Time may be saved by having each person who uses the instrument mark the edge of the eyepiece for their own "zero point.")

Reading Sphere and Minus Cylinder Axis Powers. When reading a spectacle lens prescription, which lens should be verified first? Here is how to decide.

- It is proper to begin with the strongest lens first. For this purpose the strongest lens is defined as the lens with the strongest power in the 90-degree meridian.
- If the lenses have similar powers and there is also prescribed vertical prism in the prescription, then

begin with the lens with the most prescribed vertical prism.

- If it is not evident which lens is stronger and there is no prescribed vertical prism, begin with the right lens.

Place the glasses in the lensmeter so that the back side of the lens is against the lensmeter aperture.

There are two ways to read or write a prescription. One is to read the cylinder in the prescription as a minus cylinder. The other is to read the prescription so that the cylinder is given as a plus power. We will first consider the prescription as being a *minus cylinder form* prescription.

To read a prescription in minus cylinder form, begin by turning the *power wheel* in the high plus direction. Now slowly turn the wheel back in the minus direction. If the prescription is a sphere, with no cylinder component, the illuminated target will clear all at once as shown in Figure 6-3. In older instruments, the target may consist of a single line, which represents the sphere, crossed by three widely spaced lines, which represent the cylinder. A more common configuration consists of three closely spaced lines for the sphere, crossed by three widely spaced lines representing the cylinder.

If the prescription contains a cylinder component, the sphere and cylinder lines will not focus simultaneously. Thus after the power wheel has been turned to the high plus, slowly turn the power wheel in the minus direction. This will cause either the sphere or the cylinder lines to begin to clear. *The sphere lines need to be cleared first.* If the narrower sphere lines begin to focus first, but do not fully clear, the *axis wheel* should be turned until the

sphere lines do clear (Figure 6-4). (It may be necessary to alternately adjust both the power wheel and the axis wheel until the sphere power lines do clear.) If the cylinder lines begin to clear first, the axis wheel should be rotated 90 degrees, causing the sphere and cylinder lines to transfer places. The sphere lines will then be clearer than the cylinder lines. When the sphere lines appear

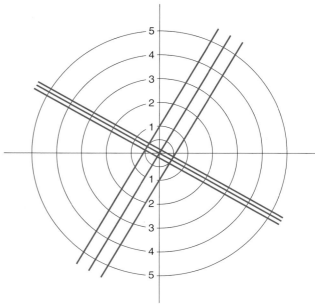

Figure 6-3. When the illuminated target shows both sphere and cylinder lines that are both clear at the same time, the lens is a sphere.

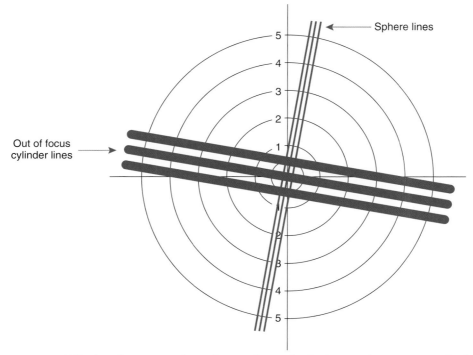

Figure 6-4. Whether the operator is reading a spherocylinder lens in plus or minus cylinder form, the sphere lines must come into focus before the cylinder lines.

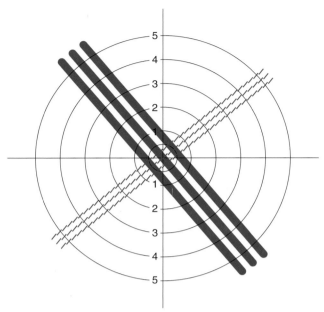

Figure 6-5. If the sphere line will not focus and appears to be diagonally broken, the axis of the cylinder is off. Turn the axis wheel until the sphere lines sharpen. When the sphere lines sharpen, the axis is being read correctly.

clear and unbroken, the value indicated on the power wheel is recorded as the spherical power of the prescription. Note the value seen on the axis wheel, and record this value as the cylinder axis.

Example **6-1**

A lens has an unknown power. Find the sphere power of the lens and the axis of the cylinder when the prescription is to be written in minus cylinder form.

Solution

The power wheel is turned into the high plus, then back into the minus direction. The target does not begin to clear until the power wheel is well into the minus. When it does begin to clear, the three cylinder lines are clearing first instead of the sphere lines. The axis wheel reads approximately 45 degrees. To make the sphere and cylinder lines change places, the axis wheel is rotated approximately 90 degrees. Now the axis is at about 135 degrees, but the sphere lines are still not quite clear. Rather, they appear to be diagonally broken (Figure 6-5).

Lines which appear broken and run diagonally to their intended course indicate that the target lines are not in the proper axis position. The axis wheel is rocked back and forth while the power wheel is "fine-tuned" until the lines are restored to continuity. (A final reading with the power wheel is done by moving the wheel from the minus to the plus direction,[1] then stopping when the lines are first clear.) In this example, the sphere lines become clear when the power wheel reads −4.00 D and the axis wheel reads 135 degrees. These first two parts of the prescription are written as shown in Figure 6-6, *A*.

	Sphere	Cylinder	Axis
R:	−4.00		135
L:			

A

	Sphere	Cylinder	Axis
R:	−4.00	−0.75	135
L:			

B

Figure 6-6. A, When recording the power of a prescription while reading a lensmeter, the first two components to read are the sphere and cylinder axes. They may be recorded immediately. **B,** After the sphere wheel is turned to find the power in the second meridian, the difference between the first and second sphere wheel readings is recorded as the cylinder power.

Finding the Cylinder Power. To find the cylinder power, continue turning the power wheel farther in the minus direction. The sphere lines will blur and the three wide cylinder lines will come into focus (Figure 6-7). When the three cylinder lines are in focus, note the new power wheel reading. The difference between the sphere reading and this new reading is the power of the cylinder. This cylinder value is recorded as a negative number.

Example **6-1** *continued*

In the example given earlier, we had found a sphere power of −4.00 D and a cylinder axis of 135. Find the power of the minus cylinder.

Solution continued

Now we continue by turning the power wheel farther in the minus direction. The sphere line blurs, and the cylinder lines begin to come into focus. When the power wheel reaches −4.75 D, the cylinder lines are clear. The power of the cylinder is the difference between the first and second power wheel readings. The difference between −4.00 D and −4.75 D is 0.75 D. Because the procedure is for a minus cylinder lens, the cylinder power is recorded as −0.75. This is shown in Figure 6-6, *B*. (See Box 6-1 for a summary of this procedure.)

Reading a Lens in Plus Cylinder Form. Some prescriptions are written with the cylinder as a plus value instead of a minus value. When written this way, the prescription is said to be in *plus cylinder form*. To read a prescription in plus cylinder form, lensmeter measuring procedures are basically the same as when reading in minus cylinder form, with one exception. When finding the sphere power, turn the lensmeter power wheel first in the high *minus* direction, instead of the high plus

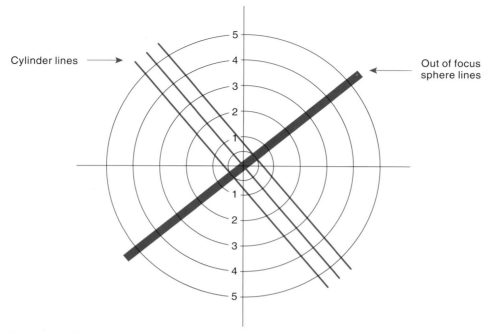

Cylinder lines →

← Out of focus
sphere lines

Figure 6-7. Once the cylinder lines are clear, cylinder power can be figured. Cylinder power is the difference between the current power wheel reading and the reading noted earlier when the sphere lines were clear.

BOX 6-1

How to Find Spherocylinder Lens Power Using a Standard, Crossed-Line-Target Lensmeter

1. Focus the eyepiece.
2. Turn the power wheel into the plus until the illuminated target blurs out.
3. Turn the power wheel slowly in the minus direction until the sphere lines clear.
4. Adjust the axis wheel for optimum sphere line clarity.
5. Record sphere power and cylinder axis.
6. Turn the power wheel farther in the minus direction until the cylinder lines clear.
7. Take the difference between the two power wheel readings and record as a minus cylinder.

---

direction. When the target is blurred out and the power wheel is in high minus numbers, slowly turn the wheel back in the plus direction. If the prescription is a sphere, the illuminated target clears all at once. If the prescription contains a cylinder component, however, the sphere lines must come into focus first. Turn the axis wheel to achieve this. Sphere and cylinder axis may be recorded. (Note that the cylinder axis will be 90 degrees away from what it was when the lens was recorded in minus cylinder form. The sphere value will also be different.)

Next, turn the power wheel further in the plus direction until the three cylinder lines are clear. The difference between the sphere power reading and this new reading is the cylinder power. The cylinder power is

recorded as plus. (Note that the numerical value of the cylinder is the same, whether recorded as plus or minus cylinder power, only the sign is different.)

For more on how to transpose from the plus to minus cylinder form of prescription writing, see the Toric Transposition section in Chapter 12.

Find and Spot the Optical Center of the Lens. After finding the sphere, cylinder, and axis, locate the optical center (OC) of the lens by centering the illuminated target at the intersection of the cross hairs in the eyepiece reticle. This is done by moving the glasses left or right on the instrument table, and moving the instrument table up or down. (In practice, this is done at the same time as sphere, cylinder, and axis values are being found.) Once centered, the lens is spotted using the lensmeter spotting mechanism.

If the cylinder power is high, the sphere and cylinder lines cannot be seen simultaneously. This makes centering of the lens difficult. To center the lens, move it until the sphere line crosses the center of the reticle cross hairs. Then focus the cylinder lines and recenter the lens so that the middle cylinder line crosses the center of the cross hairs. Then repeat the process, going back and forth between sphere and cylinder lines until both are centered without moving the lens.

After the first lens is spotted, move the second lens in front of the lensmeter aperture and determine sphere, cylinder, and axis values for the second lens. Locate the OC of the second lens by centering the target on the reticle horizontally. Do not try to center the lens vertically. Do not move the instrument table up or down.

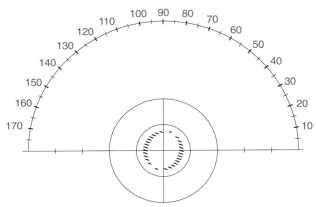

Figure 6-8. When reading a spherocylinder lens with a corona-style lensmeter target, the dots will elongate clearly in one direction. The first clear elongation denotes the sphere power.

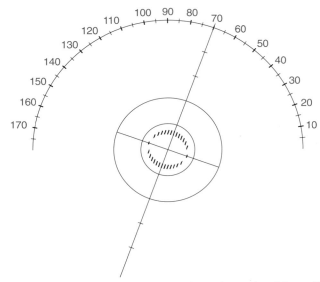

Figure 6-9. With a spherocylinder lens, the circle of dots will elongate a second time. Turn the eyepiece crosshair so that it parallels the direction of elongation. This is the cylinder axis. Here the cylinder axis reads 70 degrees.

If the target is not centered vertically, record the amount of resulting vertical prism seen in the instrument. (How prism is recorded will be explained in more detail later.) Spot the lens once. Now move the instrument table up or down until the target is centered vertically. Spot the lens a second time. The second spotting shows the OC height. It will also be used later on to tell if the prescription is within standards for unwanted vertical prism. The first spotting is used to measure the horizontal distance between left and right OCs.

If there is no prescribed prism in the prescription, this horizontal distance between OCs should equal the wearer's PD. In practice, there is a certain amount of allowable tolerance for error. Tolerances will be covered later in the chapter in the section on lens verification.

The heights of the OCs are measured as the vertical distance from the lowest portion of the lens bevels, up to the level of the spotted OC. When there is no prescribed prism present, the OC and MRP are one-and-the-same. When this is the case, measuring OC height is the same thing as measuring MRP height.

How to Find Single-Vision Lens Powers Using a Corona-Target Lensmeter

Some lensmeters use a circle-of-dots target instead of a crossed-line target to measure lenses. To find the power of single-vision lenses with a circle-of-dots (corona) type of instrument, begin by focusing the eyepiece. This is done in the same manner as previously described for the crossed-line lensmeter.

To find the sphere power, turn the power wheel into the high plus direction until the circle of dots disappears. Slowly turn the wheel back toward the minus direction. If the whole circle of dots clears simultaneously, the lens is a sphere. Sphere power is read directly from the power wheel.

If the dots elongate into clear lines as shown in Figure 6-8, the lens has a cylinder component and the reading

---

BOX 6-2

How to Find Spherocylinder Lens Power Using a Corona-Target Lensmeter

1. Focus the eyepiece.
2. Turn the power wheel into the plus until the illuminated target blurs out.
3. Turn the power wheel slowly in the minus direction until the dots in the target elongate into clear lines.
4. Record the sphere power.
5. Turn the power wheel farther in the minus direction until the dots in the target elongate into clear lines in the other direction (90-degrees away).
6. Turn the measuring hairline until it parallels the direction of elongation.
7. Record the cylinder as the minus difference between the two power wheel readings, and the axis as the degrees indicated by the measuring hairline.

---

just found is the sphere component of this spherocylinder lens. To find the cylinder, turn the power wheel further into the minus direction. The elongated "dots" will blur and re-elongate at right angles to their original direction. When they are once again clear, note the power reading. The difference between the sphere power and this second power wheel reading is the cylinder power.

To find the cylinder axis, use the rotating hairline and degree scale found in the eyepiece. Rotate the hairline until it parallels the direction of elongation of the circle of dots. Note where the hairline falls on the degree scale. This is the axis of the cylinder (Figure 6-9). (For a summary of this procedure, see Box 6-2.)

Obtaining Prescription Information for Multifocal Lenses

Distance powers for multifocal lenses are measured in the same way that powers for single vision lenses are measured. A multifocal differs from a single vision lens because it has additional plus power for viewing at near. This near addition is plus power that is added to the power of the distance prescription.

To measure the distance power of multifocal lenses, place the glasses in the lensmeter in exactly the same way as would be done for single vision lenses (Figure 6-10). The distance power is measured in the manner previously described for single vision lenses.

To measure the add (near addition) power, turn the glasses around backward in the lensmeter so that the front of the lenses are against the lensmeter aperture. Now remeasure the distance power. When measured this way, the power is called *front vertex power.* When measured in the normal way, from the back, the power measured is called *back vertex power.* For higher lens

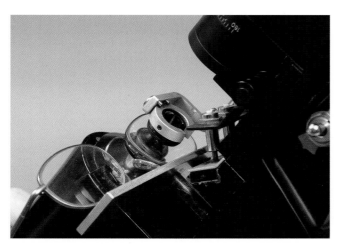

Figure 6-10. To measure the power of single vision lenses or the distance power of segmented multifocals, the glasses are placed in the lensmeter as shown. This measures the prescription in the correct manner. The power being measured is known as the back vertex power.

powers, it is not unusual to find a difference between front and back vertex powers.

It will be noted that the lensmeter-measured cylinder axis for the front vertex power is the mirror image of the axis for the back vertex power. In other words, a lens having a 30-degree back-vertex-power axis will manifest an axis of 150 degrees when turned around.

When remeasuring the distance power as front vertex power, do not measure the lens at the OC. Instead measure the distance front vertex power at a location above the OC. That point should be as far above the OC and inward as the point where the add power will be measured is below the OC and inward (Figures 6-11 and 6-12). This technique ensures that any power variations caused by lens aberrations or lens thicknesses will be the same in distance and near power measurements.

Next measure the power of the lens through the near segment (Figure 6-13). (For a summary of measuring near add power, see Box 6-3). The difference between distance and near power readings is the power of the near addition. When the lens is a spherocylinder lens, the near addition is the difference between the distance sphere and the near sphere power components.

Example **6-2**

A lens has a distance front vertex power that reads +3.87 −1.00 × 020. The front vertex power through the near addition reads +5.87 −1.00 × 020. What is the add power?

Solution

The add power is +2.00, because +5.87 − (+3.87) = +2.00. The sphere power through the add is 2.00 D higher than the sphere power through the distance portion.

Sometimes when lens powers are high, it is difficult to see both sphere and cylinder lines through the add at the same time. It may only be possible to see the cylinder lines through the near segment. This happens because of the prismatic effect that is manifested off the center of the lens. Yet it is still feasible to find the near addition power. Simply take the difference between the distance power wheel reading and the near power wheel reading using the cylinder lines. In this example, the cylinder lines in the distance are clear at +2.87 D. At near the cylinder lines will be clear at +4.87 D. The

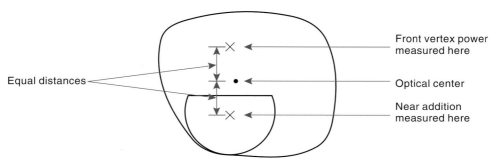

Equal distances

Front vertex power measured here

Optical center

Near addition measured here

Figure 6-11. When measuring the add power of a lens, first turn the lens around. Remeasure the distance power at a point above the optical center. This point should be as far above the distance optical center as the near verification point is below the optical center.

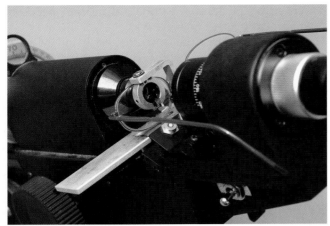

Figure 6-12. To measure multifocal lens power, the glasses must be turned around backward in the lensmeter and distance power measured again, this time as front vertex power. Note that the power is measured as far above the optical center of the lens as the near verification point in the multifocal segment is below the distance optical center of the lens.

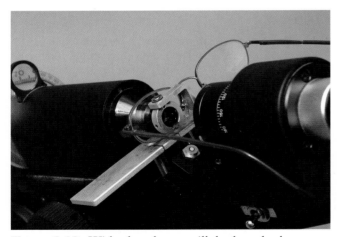

Figure 6-13. With the glasses still backward, the power through the multifocal segment is measured. This difference between distance and near powers is the power of the near addition.

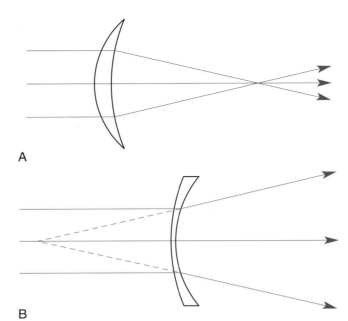

A

B

Figure 6-14. A distance lens is meant to meet the needs of a farsighted eye using a plus lens **(A)** or a nearsighted eye with a minus lens **(B)**. This is done by taking parallel light from a distant object and bringing it to focus at the far point of the ametropic eye.* A lensmeter is made to optically position the illuminated target at that far point. The light from the lensmeter target travels backward through the lens.

difference is still the same +2.00 D add power found using the sphere lines.

If the prismatic effect of the decentered lens causes the entire illuminated target to disappear off the viewing area, it may be necessary to use an auxiliary prism or prism-compensating device to bring it back into view. The use of auxiliary prisms or a prism-compensating device is described later in the chapter.

Why Spectacles Should Be Turned Around to Measure the Add Power

The purpose of a distance lens is to take parallel light and bring it into focus. For a plus lens, this will be a real image (Figure 6-14, *A*), and for minus lenses this will be a virtual image (Figure 6-14, *B*). To measure this type of lens, the illuminated lensmeter target is optically placed at the focal point of the lens. The light from the lensmeter target travels from behind the lens, going through the back of the lens, and out the front. When the light comes out the front of the lens, the rays are parallel and going into the eye piece section of the lensmeter. Thus the distance lens is being measured under the same circumstances as when it is being worn.[2] When being worn, parallel rays enter the lens from the front. (Light paths are reversible.) The focal length is refer-

---

*The ametropic eye has a refractive error and requires a lens prescription for distance vision.

BOX 6-3

How to Measure Multifocal Add Power

1. Turn the glasses around backward in the lensmeter.
2. Measure the sphere value of the front vertex distance power.
3. Measure the sphere value of the front vertex, near power.
4. The difference between the two values is the add power.

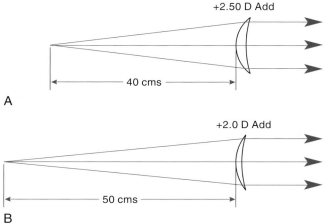

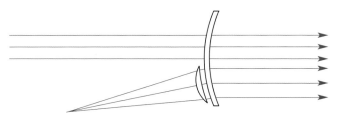

Figure 6-15. The additional plus lens (which becomes the near addition) will change diverging light rays from a near object and make them diverge less. To test for add power accuracy, the reference is in front of the lens, making front vertex power the correct power measurement. Both a +2.50 D add (**A**) and a +2.00 D add (**B**) will cause light diverging from their respective focal points to appear as if coming from optical infinity.

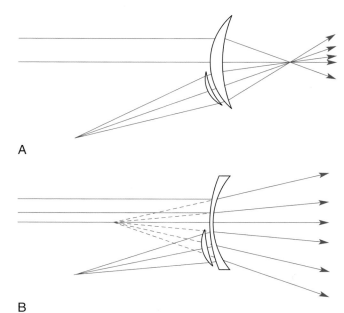

Figure 6-16. When a near object is located at the focal point of the near addition, diverging light is caused to leave the segment as parallel rays. When rays enter parallel, the emmetropic eye* does not have to accommodate in order to see clearly.

---

*An emmetropic eye has no refractive error and does not require any distance prescription.

Figure 6-17. The function of a near addition is to take light from a near object and reduce the divergence of the rays. For both a plus-powered distance lens (**A**) and a minus-powered distance lens (**B**), a near add has the ability to convert diverging light from the near add focal point so that it enters the distance lens parallel.

enced as the distance from the back side of the lens. Therefore the power being measured is called the back vertex power.

Whereas a distance lens is designed to take incoming parallel rays of light and bring them to a focus, a reading addition must take diverging rays of light coming from a near object and change them so they appear to be coming from farther away. In Figure 6-15 diverging light from an object at the focal length of the near segment is seen to be changed to parallel rays when going out the back side of the segment. This is easier to understand when shown together with a distance lens of zero power as shown in Figure 6-16. The person wearing this bifocal lens will not have to focus for a near object viewed through the segment of the lens.

From the previous figure, it is evident how a near (reading) addition is really just a small plus lens which is "added to" the distance lens. To tell if this plus lens segment is focusing the light as intended, we find the focal point by turning the lens around in the lensmeter. This allows the illuminated target to be optically placed at the focal point and referenced from the front surface of the lens. We are now measuring front vertex power.

Combining both distance and near lenses together when the distance lens has plus or minus power gives the situation shown in Figure 6-17. The near addition takes light from a near object and refracts the rays so that optically the rays from the near object resemble light rays coming from a more distant object. Now the distance lens is able to bring the light to a focus to meet the refractive demands of the near or farsighted presbyope.

Measuring the Near Addition When Lens Powers Are Low

It should be noted that when distance and add powers are both low, there will be little difference between add powers found using front and back vertex powers. For this reason, many use the easier method of measuring adds with back vertex powers instead of turning the glasses around. As soon as distance or near powers increase, however, multifocal adds measured with back vertex powers will give wrong results.

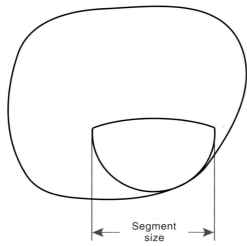

Figure 6-18. The width of a bifocal or trifocal segment is measured at the widest part of the segment.

Identifying Multifocal Segment Style and Size

When ordering a replacement pair or second pair of glasses from an existing pair, it is important to identify the multifocal type. Multifocals are identified by segment style. The most commonly used visible segment styles are flat-top (sometimes called "D" segs), curve-top, and round segs. (For a more complete listing of visible multifocal styles, see Chapter 19, Segmented Multifocal Lenses. For progressive addition lenses, see Chapter 20, Progressive Addition Lenses.)

Measuring Segment Size

Once segment style is identified, segment size must be found. Segment size is measured across the widest portion of the segment—*not* the top of the segment (Figures 6-18 and 6-19). Trifocal sizes are identified by two numbers. The first number is the vertical size of the trifocal section in millimeters. The second number is the widest horizontal measure of the multifocal segment.

Measuring Segment Height

To measure and duplicate the segment height of an existing prescription, first the old segment height for the existing prescription is measured. If the frame will remain the same, so will the old segment height. If a different style frame is to be used, then the location of the old segment line as it appears on the wearer must be duplicated.

For record keeping purposes, the segment height of the existing prescription must be measured. Segment height is the vertical distance from the lowest part of the lens bevel to the top of the bifocal or trifocal segment line. (This has been previously explained in Chapter 5 [pp. 70-71] and was illustrated in Figure 5-16.)

The wearer should be asked if he or she is satisfied with the segment height of the old glasses. If so, the dispenser follows the procedures explained in Chapter 5

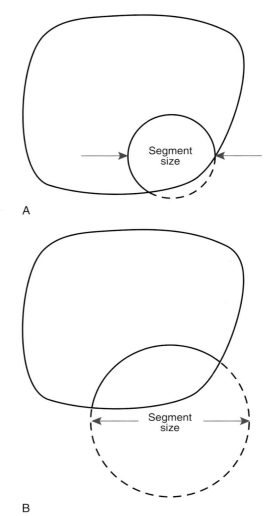

Figure 6-19. The width of a round segment is determined by its diameter. This remains true, even if most of the segment has been edged away, making a physical measurement impossible. In such cases, the size of the segment is determined by estimating the location of segment borders.

[pp. 73-74] for duplicating an old segment height in a new pair of glasses.

If the wearer is not satisfied, or if the dispenser judges the old height to be inappropriate, a new segment height should be determined. How this is done is also explained in Chapter 5 beginning on p. 70.

Identifying Base Curve

The front curve of a multifocal lens is called the base curve. If an individual has more than one pair of glasses of the same power, it is advisable to use the same base curve for both pair of glasses. This is more critical for multifocal lenses than for finished single vision lenses because multifocal base curves change in bigger steps. Changing the base curve may affect the way objects appear to the wearer. Straight lines may seem curved, objects may seem larger or smaller than they actually

TABLE 6-1
Lens Material Possibilities Based on Minus Lens Center Thickness*

If Minus Lens Center Thickness Is:	Possible Material or Function Is:
<1.0 mm	Foreign-origin glass lenses[†]
=1.0 mm or between 1.0 and 2.0 mm	Polycarbonate, Trivex, and some high index plastics
≈1.5 mm	If glass, the lens may be made from certain Corning materials, such as "Thin & Dark" or "Corning Clear 16" glass
	If plastic, some high index plastics
1.9-2.2 mm	CR-39 plastic
≈2.2 mm	Glass
>3.0 mm	"Basic Impact" safety lenses[‡] made from any material

*Warning: It is not possible to identify lens material on the basis of lens thickness!
[†]Glass lenses purchased outside the United States do not have the same impact resistance requirements and may be exceptionally thin.
[†]It is important to note that a thick lens is not a safety lens unless it has been marked on the surface as a safety lens with the manufacturer's identifying mark.

are, and the ground looks to be closer or farther away. Wearers usually adapt to normal base curve changes when lens powers change. But when base curves change and lens powers do not, switching back and forth between two pair of glasses is harder.

Base curves are measured using a lens clock* (lens measure). (For an explanation of how to use a lens clock to measure the base curve of a lens, see the section in Chapter 13 called Finding the Refractive Power of a Lens Surface Using a Lens Measure.)

Identifying Lens Material

It is important that an attempt to identify the lens material in the existing prescription be made. It is simple enough to tell the difference between glass and plastic. Lightly tapping the lens with a metallic object, such as a ring, will result in a characteristically different sound and feel.

Plastic materials are not as easy to differentiate one from another. When a polycarbonate lens is dropped on a surface with its backside down, some compare the sound to that of a poker chip. But a lens already in a frame will not be removed just to perform this procedure!

Polycarbonate and higher index plastics are often made thinner than regular plastic lenses of equal powers. Lens center thickness is measured with lens calipers. Center thickness can be used to help determine the type of material from which the lens is made. Minus lenses have their thinnest point at the optical center. Table 6-1 has some "center thickness clues" for determining what type of material was used to make minus lenses of certain thicknesses. Center thickness is measured at the location

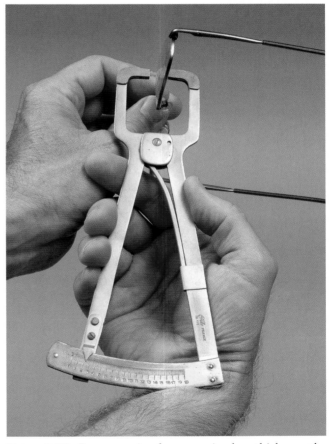

Figure 6-20. In preparation for measuring lens thickness, the optical center of the lens is spotted using the lensmeter. Then the center thickness of the lens may be measured with a pair of calipers as shown in this photo.

of the lens OC as shown in Figure 6-20. But the bottom line is this. *Whenever new glasses are made, the wearer must be advised of the safety factors related to the different available lens materials.*

Suppose a dispenser uses regular CR-39 material to replace a pair of glasses that had been made in a safer

---

*For aspheric and progressive lens surfaces, a lens clock is not a reliable method for finding base curves. Another method must be employed, such as measuring the back non-aspheric curve, lens thickness and back vertex power, then, knowing the index of refraction, calculate the base curve. (ANSI Z80-2005 Standards, pp 24-25)

material, such as polycarbonate. Without active wearer involvement and documentation in the record, this decision could spell disaster. And since people do not always remember what material they have been wearing, their answer cannot be depended upon. In short, *the dispenser should treat the choice of lens materials as if the individual was getting glasses for the first time.*

Identifying Lens Tint

The lens tint of the old pair of glasses should be identified and recorded. (For information on tint types, see Chapter 22). Tints should be considered afresh each time new glasses are ordered. It should not be assumed that the wearer wants the same tint (or lack of tint) as he or she had before.

What to Keep in Mind When Ordering One Lens Instead of Two

Occasionally, it becomes necessary to order one lens instead of two. This occurs when only one lens power changes from the previous examination or when one lens is damaged or broken.

When a single vision lens is being replaced, the major reference point (MRP) height of the remaining lens in the prescription should be measured. The MRP height of the new lens should match that of the remaining partner lens.

When only one lens is replaced in multifocal lenses, the lens should be ordered so that the two segment heights match. This is true unless there is a measured seg height difference between the wearer's left and right eyes.

It is also important that the MRP height of the lens that is *not* being replaced be measured. This is because many optical laboratories do not place the MRP on the 180-degree midline for multifocals with a segment that is set high in the frame. This means that in order for the new lens to match the old lens, *both* MRP and seg heights should be specified. This is true even if MRP height was never specified in the original order (Figure 6-21).

In some countries a lens manufacturer may place the major reference point on their bifocal lenses at a standard distance above the segment line, regardless of segment height. With increasing globalization, this may occur in some lenses sold in the U.S. With this in mind, ANSI Z80.1-2005 Prescription Recommendations defines the term *Distance Reference Point* or *DRP*. (DRP is commonly used with progressive addition lenses, but is not often used for segmented multifocals.) The Distance Reference Point is defined as "That point on a lens as specified by the manufacturer at which the distance sphere power, cylinder power and axis shall be measured."* Therefore if a certain lens manufacturer always places the MRP

---

*ANSI Z80.1-2005 American National Standard for Ophthalmic-Prescription Ophthalmic Lenses-Recommendations, Optical Laboratories Association, Fairfax, VA, 2006, p 8.

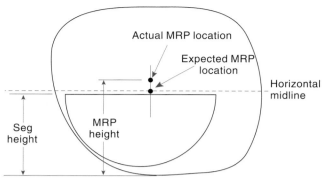

Figure 6-21. When a laboratory receives no specific instructions for MRP height, the MRP is normally placed at midlevel (on the horizontal midline). However, when the seg height is specified at a level that approaches or goes above this horizontal midline, many laboratories place the MRP 3 mm above the seg line. Therefore, when replacing only one lens of a multifocal prescription, the dispenser should either send the old glasses to the laboratory, or tell the laboratory the segment height *and* the MRP height for the new lens. This way the new lens will match the old lens. Failure to specify MRP height when ordering one lens only may result in unwanted vertical prism in the finished pair of glasses.

5 mm above the bifocal segment, then for this manufacturer the distance power would be measured at that point.

ORDERING LENSES ONLY

Ordering "Lenses Only" Using a Remote Frame Tracer

Sometimes a wearer wants new lenses for an old frame, but does not have a spare pair of glasses. When the order cannot immediately be done in-house and the wearer must keep the frame, the order to the laboratory is for "lenses only." The danger in ordering "lenses only" and just specifying frame name and size is that the lens can easily be too large or too small. The error is only evident when the wearer returns, and the dispenser attempts to insert the off-sized lens pair into the old frame. In this situation the method of choice is to remove the lenses from the frame and use a remote frame shape tracer that is connected to the computer in the optical laboratory. With a frame tracer, a stylus can trace the inside bevel of the eyewire. Both shape and size are electronically sent directly to the laboratory (Figure 6-22). In the laboratory this frame information is downloaded into the laboratory computer. The lenses are cut exactly to the traced shape and size. Assuming that the frame did not distort during tracing, after the lenses are returned from the lab, the new lenses should fit into the old frame.

Ordering "Lenses Only" by C-Size

Sometimes there is not a frame tracer available. Without a tracer, it is still possible for the wearer to keep the

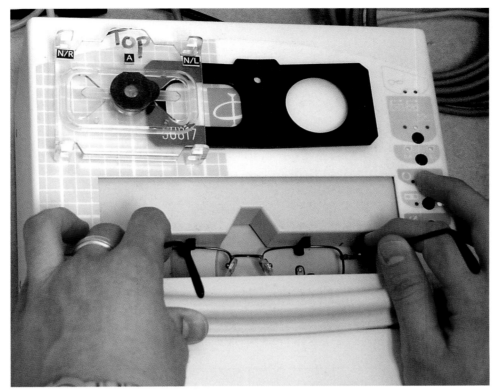

Figure 6-22. A frame tracer uses a stylus to trace the inside bevel of the frame, recording the shape. This shape is then sent to the optical laboratory and downloaded into their lens edger so that the lenses may be edged to exactly fit the measured frame.

frames and still order the lenses. When the shape of the frame is well known, the laboratory may have a factory pattern or an electronically stored shape on hand. However, there may be a variation in size. Simply ordering the size stamped on the frame may not be good enough. In this case, the lens may be removed and a circumference gauge (Figure 6-23) used to find the *C-size** or circumference of the lens (Figure 6-24). When lens circumference is known, lens size can be reproduced with more accuracy.

Ordering "Lenses Only" for a Frame of an Unknown Shape

If the frame name or lens shape is unknown, or if the pattern is not readily available at the laboratory, then it will be necessary to trace the lens and measure for C-size. The procedures for shape tracing and C-size measurements are:

1. Using the lensmeter, spot the distance OCs and the 180-degree line.
2. Remove the right lens from the frame without disturbing the three lensmeter dots (this may

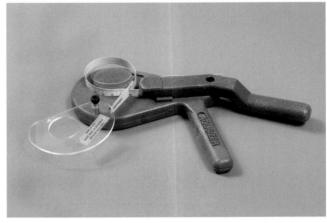

Figure 6-23. A circumference gauge is used to find the circumference of an edged lens.

require spotting over them with a non–water-soluble marking pen; non–water-soluble marks can be removed later using a solvent.)
3. Use a form, such as the one shown in Figure 6-25, and keeping the 180-degree line horizontal, center the lens as if making a pattern (Figure 6-26). In practice one of these forms may not be available. If not, draw an "x" and "y" axis on graph paper and

---

*C-size should not be confused with the C dimension of the lens. The C dimension is used in the boxing system for measuring lenses and frames, and is the width of the lens along the horizontal midline.

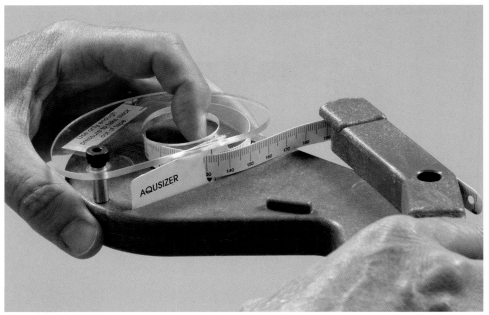

Figure 6-24. To measure the circumference of a lens, place the lens in the gauge front-side-up. Close the tape around the lens and read the circumference directly from the tape.

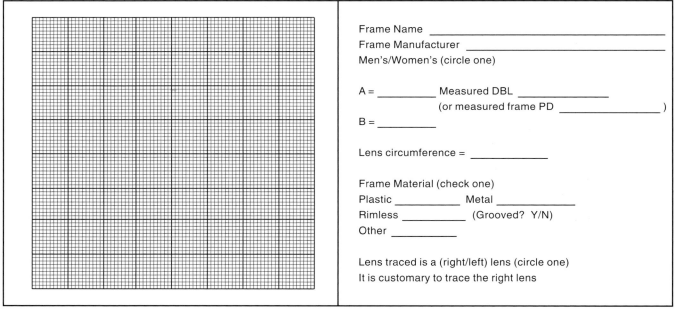

Frame Name _____

Frame Manufacturer _____

Men's/Women's (circle one)

A = _____ Measured DBL _____

(or measured frame PD _____)

B = _____

Lens circumference = _____

Frame Material (check one)

Plastic _____ Metal _____

Rimless _____ (Grooved? Y/N)

Other _____

Lens traced is a (right/left) lens (circle one)

It is customary to trace the right lens

Figure 6-25. Here is an example of one type of form that may be used to trace a lens of unknown shape for a "lenses only" order.

record the necessary information. Graph paper will work just as well.*

4. Trace the lens onto the graph paper, using a sharp pencil. Keep the pencil perpendicular to the paper the whole time the lens is being traced.

5. Measure the actual lens A and B dimensions (not the dimensions of the lens tracing) and record these dimensions. An easy, more accurate alternative* to a simple ruler is to use a Box-O-Graph to measure the lens (Figure 6-27). The tracing is only used for shape, not dimensions.

---

*It is even possible to draw a horizontal line on a blank sheet of paper, then place the lens on the paper with the three dots on the drawn line. Draw around the lens and record all the necessary measurements.

*An even more accurate method uses the same principle as the Box-o-Graph, but features a digital readout. This alternative, sometimes used by optical laboratories, is the Digi-sizer by Precision Tool Technologies. (http://www.precisiontooltech.com)

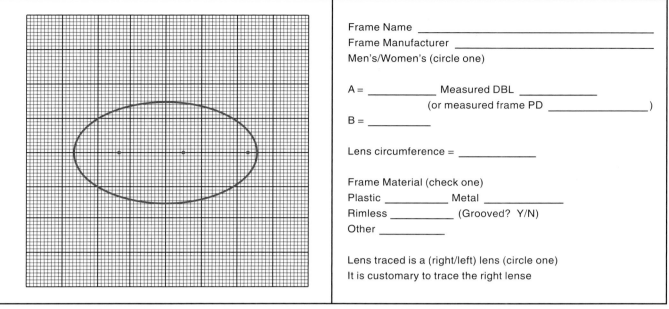

Frame Name _____

Frame Manufacturer _____

Men's/Women's (circle one)

A = _____ Measured DBL _____

(or measured frame PD _____)

B = _____

Lens circumference = _____

Frame Material (check one)

Plastic _____ Metal _____

Rimless _____ (Grooved? Y/N)

Other _____

Lens traced is a (right/left) lens (circle one)

It is customary to trace the right lense

Figure 6-26. Center the lens so that it is exactly in the middle of the grid both horizontally and vertically. The three lensmeter dots must be exactly horizontal but do not have to be exactly on the line; nor does the center lensmeter dot need to be at the origin of the *x* and *y* axes.

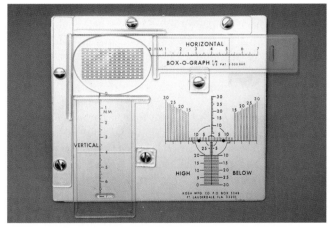

Figure 6-27. For a lens or pattern to be measured correctly using a Box-o-Graph, it must be placed on the surface of the Box-o-Graph in the same orientation as it has in the glasses. Therefore it is helpful to put three lensmeter dots on the lens first so that the 180-degree line is known. If spotted, the three dots on the lens should all fall parallel to the horizontal lines on the device. Both horizontal and vertical Box-o-Graph bars are pushed securely against the lens, and the A and B dimensions read from the scale.

6. Measure the DBL of the frame. Do not rely on the bridge size marked on the frame.
7. Using a circumference gauge, measure the circumference of the lens and record.
8. Record whether the lens is for a plastic, metal, nylon cord, or other type of frame.

9. Indicate whether the lens is a right or a left lens. (It is preferable to use the right lens.) Mark "N" for nasal on the nasal side of the tracing.
10. Replace the lens in the frame and clean up the lenses.

VERIFICATION

Always use the original examination or prescription form rather than the actual order form to verify a prescription received from the laboratory. This will reveal any errors made when filling out the order form as well as any errors made by the laboratory.

Verifying Lens Powers and Determining Error Tolerances

Lens power is verified using the lensmeter, and in the United States tolerances for ophthalmic lens prescriptions are set by the *American National Standards Institute*. The American National Standards Institute, abbreviated *ANSI*, is a nongovernmental agency made up of representative segments of industry. The specific standard for prescription lenses is identified by the number Z80.1 and is titled "American National Standard for Ophthalmics—Prescription Ophthalmic Lenses—Recommendations." The main points of this standard are summarized in Appendix A in the back of the book.

Each aspect of a spectacle lens prescription has a small range of tolerance within which that particular variable of the eyeglass prescription can fall and still be considered acceptable. It must be recognized that it is a difficult task to fabricate a prescription that meets ANSI standards in all variables.

Tolerance for Error in "Sphere" Power and Cylinder Axis

The technique for using a lensmeter to measure a lens of unknown power was explained earlier in this chapter. Verifying a lens of known power with the lensmeter is much the same.

After focusing the eyepiece, the lens with the strongest power in the 90 degree meridian is placed in the lensmeter. If the lenses have similar powers and there is also prescribed prism in the prescription, then choose the lens with the most vertical prism and start with that lens.*

The power wheel of the lensmeter is preset for the expected sphere power, and the axis wheel is preset for the expected axis. If either of these two values is incorrect, the lensmeter's illuminated target will blur.

With the sphere power and axis preset, center the lensmeter target on the reticle. If the mires are unclear, focus the power wheel or axis wheel and note what the sphere power and cylinder axis reads compared with what was ordered.

The question is, how far away from the expected value can the sphere power of the prescription be and still be considered acceptable? According to older ANSI standards, for most lenses, the allowable error tolerance was ±0.12 D and for higher powers, the allowable error tolerance increased. Now the power standard is not based on the sphere power, but on the meridian of highest absolute power. To know if this power is off, we may need to finish reading the full spherocylinder prescription before we can tell if the power is acceptable. So before deciding on power acceptability, we will write our sphere finding down and go on to the cylinder.

Cylinder axis error tolerances vary, depending on the strength of the cylinder power. For small 0.25 D cylinders, the axis can deviate up to 14 degrees either way. If the cylinder power is equal to 1.75 D or greater, however, the tolerance drops to ±2 degrees. An easy way to visualize axis tolerances is to think of a cross with the 0.25 D cylinder on the bottom and 1.75 D on the top. This is shown in Figure 6-28.

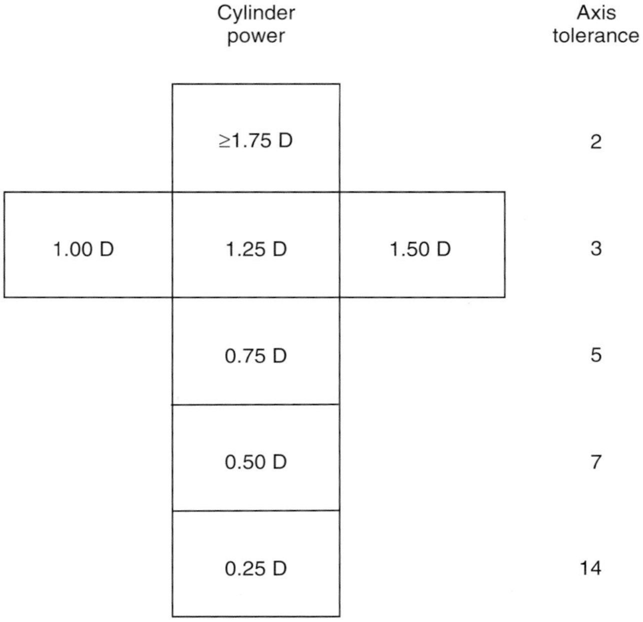

Cylinder Power Verification and Error Tolerance

Cylinder power verification is done by finding the difference between the sphere power reading (where the narrowly spaced sphere lines focus) and the power wheel reading where the three broadly spaced cylinder lines focus. The ANSI standard cylinder power tolerances vary depending on the strength of the cylinder. For cylinder with a power of 2.00 D or less, this tolerance is

---

*Z80.1-2005, American National Standard for Ophthalmics—Prescription Ophthalmic Lenses—Recommendations, Optical Laboratories Association, Fairfax, VA, 2006, p 21.

Figure 6-28. Drawing an "Axis Tolerance Cross" is a simple way to remember the cylinder axis tolerances for each cylinder power.

±0.13 D. For cylinders from 2.25 D through 4.50 D, tolerance is ±0.15 D. Above these powers the tolerance is 4% of the cylinder power. When using a standard lensmeter, this means the cylinder power tolerance is close to 1/8th diopter. These tolerances are slightly greater for progressive addition lenses. Exact tolerances are listed in Appendix A.

Meridian of Highest Absolute Power Error Tolerance

As stated earlier, the power standards for prescription eyewear have changed from looking at sphere power to looking at the power of the lens in the meridian of highest absolute power. So what does that mean? Basically, power standards are stricter for low powers. Up to ±6.50 D, the tolerance is ±0.13 D. For powers above 6.50, the standard is ±2% of the power. (Slightly more error is allowed for progressive addition lenses.)

So what about power standards for a prescription written in minus cylinder form that has a power of −6.00 −4.00 × 180? The sphere power is −6.00 D. This would give the appearance of requiring a standard of ±0.13 D. But what if this lens were written in plus cylinder form? In this case, the lens would be written as −10.00 +4.00 × 090. So is the sphere power for this prescription −6.00 D or −10.00 D? The answer to this question makes a big difference when applying standards that are stricter for low powers and less strict for high powers. For this reason, the power tolerance is no longer based on sphere power, but on the meridian of highest absolute power.

So how can the meridian of highest absolute power be found and verified? The meridian of highest absolute power can be found and verified in two ways.

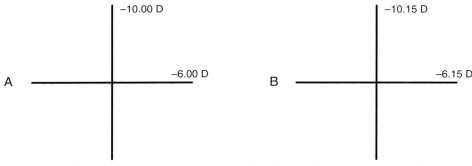

Figure 6-29. To help in reasoning through and understanding lens power verification, put the lens power that was ordered on a power cross. The ordered power in the text example is shown in **(A)**. After the completed eyeglasses have been returned from the lab, place those lens powers on a power cross. The text example for the completed pair is shown in **(B)**.

BOX 6-4

How to Write the Prescription So That the Sphere Power *Is* the Meridian of Highest Absolute Power

If the sphere power is:	And the cylinder power is:	Then do this:
Minus sphere	Minus cylinder	Convert the prescription to plus cylinder form
Minus sphere	Plus cylinder	Leave the prescription in plus cylinder form
		[Exception: If the cyl power is more than twice as strong as the sphere power, then convert the prescription to minus cylinder form.]
Plus sphere	Plus cylinder	Convert the prescription to minus cylinder form.
Plus sphere	Minus cylinder	Leave the prescription in minus cylinder form.
		[Exception: If the cyl power is more than twice as strong as the sphere power, then convert the prescription to plus cylinder form.]

To convert between plus and minus cylinder forms of prescription writing:
Add the sphere and cylinder powers. This is the new sphere power.
Change the sign of the cylinder from plus to minus or from minus to plus. This is the new cylinder value.
Add or subtract 90 from the cylinder axis. This is the new cylinder axis.

The first method is to put the ordered lens powers on a power cross. In our example, the power cross would appear as shown in Figure 6-29, *A*. The two meridians show −6.00 D and −10.00 D. The meridian of highest absolute power is the one with the −10.00 D power. Next we read the power of the lens. Suppose the lens verifies as −6.15 −4.00 × 180. Initially this looks like the lens power fails the standard because the power standard for a −6.00 D power is ±0.13 D. But if we place this on a power cross (Figure 6-29, *B*), we have −6.15 in one meridian and −10.15 in the other meridian. The power standard for a −6.00 D power is ±0.13 D, but for a −10.00 D power the standard is 2% of the lens power, or ±0.20 D. So looking at it this way, the lens would pass.

The second method for finding and verifying the meridian of highest absolute power is to rewrite the prescription so that the meridian of highest absolute power is the sphere. Then we can verify it as sphere power, cylinder power, and cylinder axis in the same manner we are accustomed to reading lenses. Box 6-4 shows how to write the prescription so that it always has

the meridian of highest absolute power as the sphere power. So for our example, we convert the prescription to plus cylinder form, which is −10.00 +4.00 × 090. We read the lens in plus cylinder form and find −10.15 +4.00 × 090. We see that sphere power, cylinder power, and cylinder axis are all in tolerance.

For more on this subject, be sure to read and look at the examples in Appendix A in the back of the book.

Checking for Unwanted Vertical Prism
There are two methods for checking for unwanted vertical prism. The first is the more traditional method. It does not use the refractive power of the lens as part of the decision-making process. The second method uses a cut-off power to help in making the decision, simplifying the process some.

The Traditional Method for Vertical Prism Tolerances. After the sphere, cylinder, and axis for the first lens have been verified, spot the lens and slide the spectacles across the lensmeter table to measure the second lens. Remember the lens with the highest power

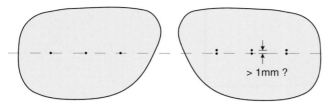

Figure 6-30. This lens has been spotted twice: once at the actual optical center and once where the optical center should be located. Does the vertical difference between the place where the optical center should be and the place where it is really located exceed 1 mm? If it does and the amount read on the lensmeter is also above 0.33Δ, then the lens pair will be out of tolerance for vertical prism.

in the 90-degree meridian is the first to be verified. When the second lens power has been verified, spot the OC of this second lens.

In the event that the second lens will not center, but shows the illuminated target above or below the intersection of the eyepiece crosshairs, the lens is showing unwanted vertical prism. Prism amount is indicated by the numbered concentric circles on the reticle mires (or screen in some lensmeters.) With the illuminated target centered exactly above or below the middle of the crosshairs, read the amount of vertical prism present. If the amount is 0.33Δ or less, the prescription is within ANSI tolerances for vertical prism. If it is greater than 0.33Δ, the dispenser must double-check to be sure that the lens pair has too much vertical prism.

To make this additional check, be certain the lens is centered horizontally, even though the target is off vertically. When it is horizontally centered, spot the lens. Next move the lensmeter table up or down until the target centers vertically. Spot the lens a second time. Remove the spectacles from the lensmeter, and measure the vertical distance between these two spots. This is shown in Figure 6-30. If the vertical difference between these two dots is greater than 1 mm, the lens pair is out of tolerance for vertical prism.

It should be noted that *both* criteria must fail for the lens pair to fail. If the amount of vertical prism exceeds 0.33Δ, but the vertical difference is less than 1 mm, the lens pair passes. If the vertical difference is greater than 1 mm, but the amount of vertical prism is less than 0.33Δ, the lens pair passes. The lens pair only fails when the vertical prism is greater than 0.33Δ *and* the vertical difference exceeds 1 mm.

A Power-Based Method for Vertical Prism Tolerances. ANSI Z80 standards now show a power-based method for determining whether or not unwanted vertical prism is within acceptable standards. The same basic procedure is followed as was explained in the preceding section and the end result is exactly the same as the method just explained above. Here is how it works.

If the power in the vertical meridian of the lens is low (from zero to plus or minus 3.375 D), then the only thing

to worry about is whether or not the amount of unwanted vertical prism is above 1/3 prism diopter. If it is above this amount, the prescription is not within allowable tolerances.

If the power in the vertical meridian of the lens is high (above plus or minus 3.375 D), the amount of vertical prism is not an issue. The only thing to be concerned with is how far the optical centers are away from each other vertically. If they are more than 1 mm apart, then the prescription is out of tolerance. These criteria are summarized in Table 6-2.

Here is the specific procedure for carrying out the power-based method of checking for unwanted vertical prism.

1. Verify the sphere, cylinder, and axis for the first lens.
2. Spot the lens and slide the spectacles across the lensmeter table. Verify and spot the OC of this second lens.
3. If the second lens will not center, move the lens sideways until the illuminated target centered exactly above or below the middle of the crosshairs. Read the amount of vertical prism present and spot the lens.
   a. If the prism amount is 0.33Δ or less, the prescription is within ANSI tolerances for vertical prism.
   b. If the prism amount is greater than 0.33Δ and the power in the vertical meridian is 3.25 D or less, the prescription fails.
4. If the prism amount is greater than 0.33Δ and the power in the vertical meridian is 3.50 D or more, the lens pair may still pass. To find out, continue on with the following steps.
5. Move the lensmeter table up or down until the target centers vertically. Spot the lens a second time.
6. Remove the spectacles from the lensmeter, and measure the vertical distance between these two spots as was shown in Figure 6-30.
   a. If the vertical difference between these two dots is 1 mm or less, the prescription passes.
   b. If the vertical distance between these two spots is greater than 1 mm, the prescription fails.

TABLE 6-2
Allowable Unwanted Vertical Prism Based on Lens Power

If the Power in the Vertical Meridian is	The Allowable Imbalance Tolerance is
±3.25 D or less	0.33 Δ or less of vertical prism
±3.50 D or more	1.0 mm or less of vertical difference in MRP locations

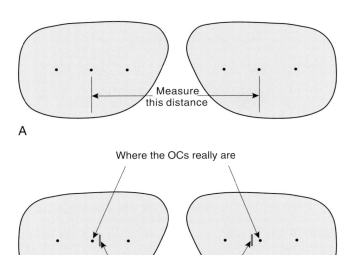

A

Where the OCs really are

PRP locations (where the OCs should be located)

B

Figure 6-31. A, Measure the horizontal distance between the two center lensmeter dots (the locations of the lens optical centers). **B,** Now compare this distance to the distance between the Prism Reference Points. The PRPs are where the ordered distance PD locations should be found. If the difference is less than 2.5 mm, horizontal prism is within tolerance. If the difference is greater than 2.5 mm *and* the lens pair shows greater than 0.67Δ of horizontal prism, the prescription is out of tolerance. When there is prescribed prism in the prescription, the PRP location is where the prescribed prism should be correct (i.e., still at the distance PD.)

Checking for Unwanted Horizontal Prism

By now the spectacle lens pair has both lenses spotted. To check for unwanted horizontal prism, measure the horizontal distance between the center lensmeter dots on the two lenses as shown in Figure 6-31, *A*. Compare this distance to the PD that was ordered. If the difference between the ordered PD and the measured PD is 2.5 mm or less, the prescription passes. If the difference is greater than 2.5 mm, the prescription might fail. We will not know this, however, until we check for horizontal prism tolerance limits.

There are two methods to check for horizontal prism tolerance limits. The first method is easier to understand, but harder to do. The second is harder to understand initially, but is finally easier to do. The second method is the one recommended by ANSI.

Method 1: Spotting the Location Where the Optical Centers Should Have Been. The first method requires spotting the *prism reference point* or *PRP* location. The prism reference point is where the OCs should have been. This is done by measuring from the center of the bridge. Find the right PRP using the right monocular PD (or one half the binocular PD). It is measured from the center of the bridge. Mark this PRP location

on the lens by dotting or drawing a vertical line using a lens marking pen. Do the same for the left PRP using the monocular (or half binocular) PD (see Figure 6-31, B).

Next, center this new PRP mark on the right lens in front of the lensmeter stop. Read and note the amount of unwanted horizontal prism from the lensmeter. Do the same for the left eye. Add both left and right horizontal prism amounts together. If these two amounts are two thirds of a prism diopter or greater, the prescription is out of tolerance. If they are less than two thirds of a diopter, the prescription is within horizontal prism tolerance.

Method 2: Determining if the Wearer's PD is Within the Two-Thirds Diopter Limit. To check for the location of horizontal prism tolerance limits, put the spectacles back in the lensmeter and do the following:

1. For the first lens, place the center lensmeter dot in front of the lensmeter stop. (The stop is that part of the lensmeter against which the back surface of the lens rests.)
2. Note where the wearer's PD *should* be. (This location is called the PRP or prism reference point.)
3. Move the spectacles so that the PRP (the point where the wearer's PD should be) moves toward the lensmeter stop. Watch the illuminated target as the glasses are moved. The prismatic effect seen will increase as the glasses are moved. Keep moving the glasses in this same direction until 0.33Δ results.
4. Spot the lens.
5. Repeat this procedure for the second lens.
6. Measure the distance between the two new lensmeter dots on the two lenses. If the distance between the two new dots equals or passes the wearer's PD, the prescription passes. If this distance does not reach the wearer's PD, the prescription fails.

A Power-Based Method for Horizontal Prism Tolerances. As with the vertical prism tolerances, there is a power-based method for determining whether or not unwanted horizontal prism was within acceptable standards. Again, the end results are exactly the same as in the previously explained methods for determining horizontal prism. This is the procedure.

If the power in the horizontal meridian of the lens is low (from zero to plus or minus 2.75 D), then the only thing to worry about is whether or not the amount of unwanted horizontal prism is above ²/₃ prism diopter. If it is above 0.67 Δ, the prescription is not within allowable tolerances.

If the power in the horizontal meridian of the lens is high (above plus or minus 2.75 D), the only thing to be concerned with is how far the optical centers are away from each other horizontally (i.e., how far the PD is off). If the OCs are more than 2.5 mm away from the wearer's PD, then the prescription is out of tolerance. These criteria are summarized in Table 6-3.

Location of the optical center.
This is the location of lensmeter stop before the frame
and lenses are moved.
(As frame and lenses are moved to the left,
the lensmeter stop does not move.)

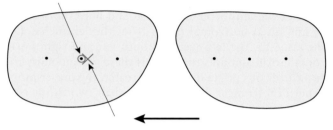

This is where the PRP should be.
Move frame and lenses to the left
until 1/3 Δ results.
(The PRP is the expected location of the wearer's PD.)

Figure 6-32. To check for horizontal prism tolerances, move the spectacles so that the lensmeter stop travels toward the Prism Reference Points. The PRPs are at the intended location of the wearer's PD. Keep moving the spectacles until 0.33Δ results.

TABLE 6-3
Allowable Unwanted Horizontal Prism Based on Lens Power

If the Power in the Horizontal Meridian is	The Allowable Imbalance Tolerance is
From 0.00 D to plus or minus 2.75 D	0.67 prism diopters
Above plus or minus 2.75 D	2.5 mm total

Example **6-3**

Suppose a prescription has a distance power of −0.75 D for both right and left lenses. The wearer's distance PD is 58 mm. We want to verify the prescription for horizontal prism. When the lens OCs are spotted, the distance between them is 63 mm. Is the prescription out of tolerance for horizontal prism?

Solution

Because the optical centers for this prescription are 63 mm apart when they should be 58 mm, the spectacles clearly exceed the 2.5 mm tolerance criterion for horizontal prism. The 2.5 mm criterion would only allow the OC distance to vary from 55.5 mm to 60.5 mm. But this alone does not indicate that the prescription fails ANSI standards. The lens pair has not yet been checked for 0.67Δ horizontal prism tolerance. (Since the power of the prescription is less than 2.75 D, the amount of prism is critical.) To check for horizontal prism tolerance, place the right lens in the lensmeter with the OC at the lensmeter stop as shown in Figure 6-32. Set the lensmeter for the correct sphere power and cylinder axis and be certain that the target is clear.

Because the wearer's PD is smaller than the distance between the OCs and this is a right lens, the glasses are

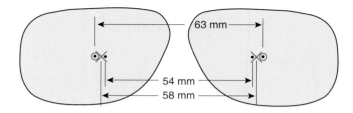

⊙ Lensmeter dots indicating location of lens optical centers
• Lensmeter dots indicating location where of 1/3Δ of horizontal prism is read
✕ PRP locations (The place where the optical centers should be so they will match the location of the wearer's actual PD.)

Figure 6-33. In this case, the distance between the optical centers measures 63 mm, but the wearer's actual PD is 58 mm. However, because we can move the glasses all the way in to 54 mm before a 0.33Δ–per lens reading occurs, the prescription passes. (A −0.75 D sphere prescription could have the optical center separation vary anywhere from 49 to 67 mm and still not fail ANSI Standards for horizontal prism. The lower the refractive power, the farther the optical centers can be off without reaching a total of 0.67 Δ for the pair.)

moved to the left. Look into the lensmeter, move the glasses to the left, and watch the amount of horizontal prism increase. Stop and spot the lens when the prismatic effect reads 0.33Δ.

Repeat this for the left lens. This time move the glasses to the right until the prismatic effect reaches 0.33Δ. Spot the lens. The glasses now look like those shown in Figure 6-33.

Next measure the distance between the new lensmeter dots. This distance proves to be 54 mm. Because this distance overshoots the wearer's PD, the prescription passes, even though it failed the 2.5 mm criterion. (For a summary of horizontal and vertical prism standards, see Appendix A.)

Verifying For Prescribed Prism

A lens that has prescribed prism included as part of the prescription is not centered the same in a lensmeter as a prescription without prism. The prismatic prescription is not centered correctly if the illuminated lensmeter target is at the intersection of the crosshairs. Centering of a prismatic prescription is correct when the illuminated target is located at the point that matches the prescribed prism. When this happens, the lens may be dotted for verification.

Example **6-4**

A right lens prescription reads:

$$+3.00 - 1.25 \times 135, 2.00 \, \Delta \text{ Base Out}$$

How must the lens be centered before it is spotted?

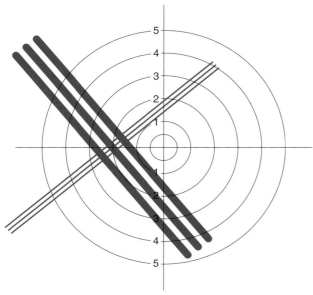

Figure 6-34. In this example, the illuminated target indicates 2Δ of Base Out prism, assuming the lens is a right lens. (If the lens being measured were a left lens, the prism would be 2Δ Base In.)

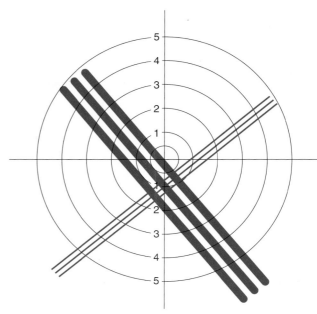

Figure 6-35. This prismatic effect reads 1Δ Base Down whether the lens is a left or a right lens.

Solution

To verify this prescription, the lens must be placed in the lensmeter and moved until the illuminated target is located 2Δ units to the left (temporal) of the crosshair origin (Figure 6-34). (Target center location always corresponds to prism base direction. This is true whether the lens is plus or minus in power.)

Example **6-5**

Another right lens prescription reads

$$+3.00 - 1.25 \times 135, 1.00 \; \Delta \; \text{Base Down}$$

How must the target be centered for this lens before it is spotted?

Solution

Everything except prism is identical to the previous prescription. Therefore in this case, the only difference is that the illuminated target is moved until it is located directly below the cross hair origin, 1 Δ unit down, as shown in Figure 6-35.

Example **6-6**

Suppose a right lens prescription with the same refractive power as in the previous two prescriptions calls for horizontal *and* vertical prism. Prism values ordered were 1Δ Base Down and 2Δ Base Out. How must the illuminated target be positioned for accuracy in verification?

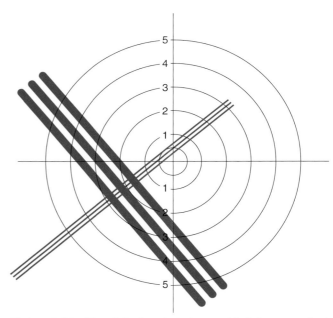

Figure 6-36. If a right lens is being verified for prescribed prism of 2Δ Base Out and 1Δ Base Down, it must be positioned as shown before the lens can be spotted.

Solution

When both horizontal and vertical prism is called for, the illuminated target must be moved both horizontally and vertically. The correct positioning is shown in Figure 6-36.

Verifying High Amounts of Prism

When verifying high amounts of prism with the lensmeter, it is not uncommon for the prism to displace the center of the illuminated target off the lensmeter viewing

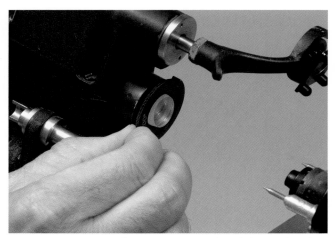

Figure 6-37. An auxiliary prism is used to help verify a lens with a large amount of prism in the prescription. The prism base of the auxiliary prism is placed opposite the prism base direction found in the prescription.

screen. This will leave only sphere or cylinder lines in view, but not both. When this happens, the prism amount is read using one of two methods, depending on the type of lensmeter. One method uses a loose, compensating prism. The other requires a prism compensating device.

Using Loose Auxiliary Prisms to Measure Large Prismatic Effects. Some lensmeters, such as the B&L Reichert, come with prism lenses that are placed in a special lens-holding cell in the instrument. The prism lens is oriented with its base direction opposite to the spectacle lens' prism base direction so that the illuminated target center will be returned to the screen. The sequence of steps for finding prism is as follows:

1. An attempt to read a prescription with a high amount of prism is made, but the lensmeter's illuminated target center is displaced off the viewing screen. Once this has happened, look at the prescription and estimate prism base direction. Estimating is done by observing lens thickness differences. The thickest edge of the lens indicates prism base direction.
2. Measure or look up the wearer's PD. Dot the location of where the MRP should be for right and left lenses according to the wearer's PD. (This procedure was explained in an earlier section of the chapter called "Method 1: Spotting the Location Where the Optical Centers Should Have Been.")
3. Estimate the amount of prism that will be necessary and put the auxiliary prism in the cell of the lensmeter so that its base direction is opposite to the base direction of the prism in the spectacle lens (Figure 6-37). Keep the auxiliary base direction of the prism either totally horizontal or totally vertical.
4. Set the lensmeter cylinder axis at 180 degrees and the sphere power on zero. Look into the lensmeter

and slightly rotate the auxiliary prism until the center line of the illuminated lensmeter target crosses the middle of the crosshairs. This will ensure that the prism base direction is exactly zero or 180 (Base In or Base Out) with no vertical component.* If a large amount of vertical prism is being measured, this will ensure that the base direction is 90 or 270 (Base Up or Base Down), with no horizontal component.

5. Next, place the spectacle lenses in the lensmeter and center the MRP of the lens over the lensmeter stop. If the target does not appear, increase the amount of prism by choosing the next higher auxiliary prism. (Each time a different auxiliary prism is placed in the cell, the alignment process described in the previous step must be repeated.)
6. When the illuminated target is visible on the screen, note the prismatic amount seen in the lensmeter. To figure the total amount of prism, reverse the base direction of the auxiliary prism and add it to the prism amount shown in the lensmeter. In other words if the prism on the screen shows 1Δ Base Out and the auxiliary prism is 6Δ Base In, change 6Δ Base In to 6Δ Base Out and add it to 1Δ Base Out. The amount of prism present in the lens is 7Δ Base Out.

Example **6-7**

A lens cannot be read in the lensmeter without the help of compensating prism. A 5Δ Base In auxiliary prism allows the target to be seen. The illuminated target shows up at a point on the screen that measures as 4Δ Base Out and 1Δ Base Up. How much prism is there in the lens?

Solution

The 5Δ auxiliary prism is oriented with its base opposite that of the prism in the lens. To figure the amount of prism present in the lens, change 5Δ Base In to 5Δ Base Out. Now add the 5Δ Base Out that was neutralized by the auxiliary prism to the 4Δ Base Out and 1Δ Base Up that was viewed on the screen. This makes the total amount of prism 9Δ Base Out and 1Δ Base Up.

Using a Prism Compensating Device to Measure Large Amounts of Prism. Some lensmeters, such as the Marco and Burton lensmeters, come with a prism compensating device† (Figure 6-38). To find prism amount and prism axis direction using a prism compensating device, begin by placing the Prism Reference Point over the lens stop. The *Prism Reference Point* or *PRP* is "That point on a lens as specified by the manufacturer at which

---

*Contributed by Dr. Sarah Huseman.
†A prism compensating device is based on the Risley prism principle. A Risley prism consists of two rotating prisms that work together to vary prism power. Prism power will be zero when the bases of the 2 prisms are oriented in opposite directions. Prism power will be at a maximum when the bases are both in the same direction.

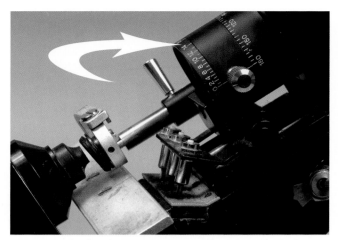

Figure 6-38. A prism compensating device, such as the one shown here, allows a highly prismatic lens to be verified. For lensmeters with prism compensating devices, the lensmeter must always be checked to ensure that the compensating device is zeroed. Otherwise the lensmeter appears to be detecting prism in a lens when there is none.

the prism value of the finished lens is to be measured."* The PRP will correspond to the location of the wearer's monocular PD or to one half the wearer's binocular PD for a given pair of glasses. This is where the MRP of the lens should be.

Turn the power wheel to the sphere power of the prescription and the axis wheel to the correct cylinder axis. Next, move the illuminated target using the prism compensating device so that the larger prismatic component (either horizontal or vertical) may be read.

(Compensating prism power is increased or decreased by turning the knob on the compensating device. Base direction of the compensating prism is changed by physically moving the knob so that it rotates around the axis of the lensmeter.)

Again using the prism compensating device, move the illuminated target onto either the horizontal or vertical crosshair on the measuring reticle. This is done by using just horizontal or just vertical prism. In other words, leave the base direction of the prism compensating device at either 90 or 180. (Remember, the base direction for the lens may be estimated ahead of time just by looking at the thickness differences between temporal and nasal lens edges or by the thickness differences between top and bottom edges.) Read the larger prismatic component that has been neutralized from the prism compensating device. Read the smaller prismatic component directly from the reticle. (See Box 6-5 for a summary of these steps.)

---

*ANSI Z80.1-2005 American National Standard for Ophthalmic-Prescription Ophthalmic Lenses-Recommendations, Optical Laboratories Association, Fairfax, VA, 2006, p 9.

BOX 6-5

Using a Prism Compensating Device to Read Large Amounts of Prism

1. Dot the location of the wearer's eye on the lenses from monocular PD measurements.
2. Place the point of reference over the lens stop. (Use the center pin on the lensmeter's dotting mechanism to be certain that the marked reference point is exactly centered.)
3. Turn the power wheel to the sphere power of the prescription and the axis wheel to the correct cylinder axis.
4. Estimate which prism component is larger, horizontal or vertical. (To do this, look at the thickness differences between temporal and nasal lens edges, and between top and bottom edges, and find the thickest edge.)
5. Physically move the knob on the prism compensating device to position the prism base direction to 180 if horizontal prism is larger, to 90 if vertical prism is larger.
6. Move the internal illuminated target onto either the horizontal or vertical crosshair on the internal measuring reticle. (Turning the knob on the prism compensating device will accomplish this by increasing or decreasing prism amount.)
7. Read the larger prism component from the external prism compensating device.
8. Read the smaller prismatic component from the reticle scale inside the instrument.

Using an Autolensmeter to Verify Lenses

An autolensmeter offers the advantage of requiring less operator expertise than that required for manual types. It also provides a permanent record of the reading when equipped with a printer.

Autolensmeters come in varying degrees of sophistication. The basic sequence for use involves the following:

1. Select lens form and accuracy.
   The operator indicates whether the lens is to be read in plus or minus cylinder form. The level of accuracy is also indicated, since many instruments will read lens power to the nearest quarter diopter, eighth diopter, or even hundredth of a diopter.
2. Position the first lens.
   The lens is positioned by moving it until centered. Instead of viewing a conventional crossed-line or a corona target, the image may consist of a cross that appears on a small screen (Figure 6-39, *A*). As the lens is moved, this cross can be made to approach a large central cross. When the small cross reaches the center of the large cross, the smaller one may become bolder as with the Humphrey Instruments Lens Analyzer (Figure 6-39, *B*).

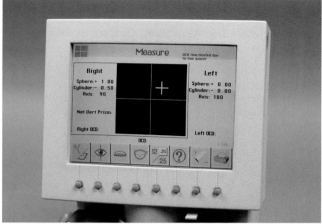

A

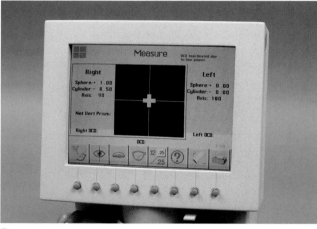

B

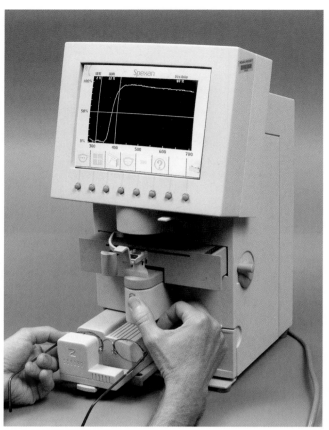

Figure 6-40. Some models of the Humphrey Lens Analyzer autolensmeter will allow the transmission of a lens to be measured. The readout is in the form of a transmission curve.

Figure 6-39. To center a lens with the Humphrey Lens Analyzer model LA 360, the lens is placed in the lensmeter. This may cause the viewing screen to appear as shown in **(A)**, with the small white cross off center. The lens is moved until the small movable cross is centered with the large stationary cross **(B)**.

Some instruments like the Lens Analyzer shown allow the instrument to be operated with or without centering the lens. In one mode, the spectacle lens is positioned with the location of the known PD in front of the instrument's reading stop. The instrument reads both power and prismatic effect at that point. This mode is used when monocular PDs are known.

The second mode allows a reading to be taken at any position on the lens. Once the second lens reading is taken, the instrument uses power and prismatic effect to calculate OC locations, giving the "PD" of the glasses.

3. Spot the lens.
The lens may be spotted with the customary three lensmeter dots if it has been centered as initially described in step 2 above.

4. Position and spot the second lens.
The next step for a single-vision lens pair is to position and spot the second lens. Some autolensmeters have an intermediate step for multifocals whereby the add is measured before the second lens.

5. Print out the results.
Using an Autolensmeter to Verify Transmission. The usual method for finding the transmission of a lens is to use a light transmission meter. (A photo of such a meter may be found in Chapter 22, Figure 22-3.) Yet it is also possible to find the transmission of a lens with the Humphrey Lens Analyzer. The transmission is given as a transmission curve. (Figure 6-40.)

Verifying Lens Segments and Surfaces
Verification of the Multifocal Segment
To verify the size and location of the multifocal segment, check the following:
1. Check segment height.
2. Check flat-top bifocals for tilt by placing a ruler across the seg tops.
3. Measure seg width with a ruler at the widest part of the seg.

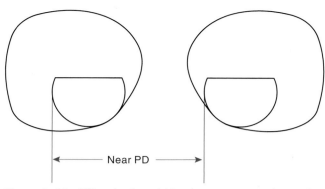

Figure 6-41. When both multifocal segments are identical, it is easier to measure near PD from the left side of one segment to the left side of the other than from center to center.

4. To verify the near PD ordered, measure the distance from the left side of one seg to the left side of the other (Figure 6-41). A lens pair should be within 2.5 mm of the ordered amount to be within standards.

Checking Lens Surface Curves, Size, and Tint
Using a lens clock, check the base curve and look for the presence of warpage. Warpage is revealed by two different surface powers (indicating cylinder power) found on both front and back surfaces instead of on just one surface.

Check the lens size, particularly in a "lenses only" order. Be sure the tint corresponds with that ordered.

Checking for Small Surface and Media Defects
Check for internal media defects, such as bubbles and striae in the lens material. A *stria* is a streak seen in a lens caused by a difference in the refractive index in the material. When seen, a stria occurs in a glass lens. The streak causes a distortion in the object viewed and is not a physical streak like a mark on or in the lens. Also inspect the surface for scratches, pits, or areas of grayness.

The surface is also inspected for waves. A *wave* is a defect in lens surface curvature, which causes a slight, irregular variation in the surface power. It is created during the lens surfacing process and can occur with any type of lens material. Check for waves by holding the lens about 12 inches from the eye and viewing either a grid or some object having a straight edge. Move the lens slowly back and forth. The straight edge should appear smooth. It should maintain its smoothness and become increasingly curved as the straight edge approaches the edge of the lens.

If there is a localized distortion present (Figure 6-42), mark the area and view it through the lensmeter. If the area distorts the lensmeter target, the defect makes the lens unacceptable. However, if the defect is outside of the 30-mm circle that is centered on the MRP, or if the defect is within 6 mm of the lens edge, the lens may be considered acceptable. In fact, the same applies to any small isolated material or surface defects and not just

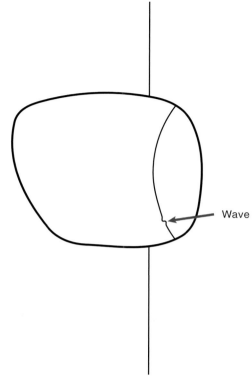

Figure 6-42. To inspect for a wave in the surface of a lens, view a grid or straightedge through the lens, moving the lens slowly so that the image of the line traverses the surface slowly. An irregularity in the otherwise smooth image shows the presence of a wave.

waves. If small, isolated defects are outside of the 30-mm circle or within 6 mm of the lens edge, they are acceptable.

Verification of Frames and Quality of Mounting
First check the quality of the mounting (the lens insertion). The security of the lenses will be revealed by the presence or absence of an air space between lens and frame. Note if the bevel is even, or if chips or other defects are present at the edges.

Check to be sure that the frame concurs exactly with all ordered specifications: (1) style and color, (2) eye size and DBL, and (3) length of temple. Be sure to inspect for possible frame damage, such as scratched or marred surfaces, or rolled eyewires.

Overall Verification
Check the extent of frame alignment (see Chapter 8). In many instances, frames will not be properly aligned but can be adjusted to standard alignment in the office. In some cases this may not be possible because the frame is distorted or stretched too greatly, or because the lens has been twisted because of an error in the position of the cylinder axis.

Errors that are adjustable in the office are probably best corrected by the dispenser. Much time is saved if the prescription does not have to be returned to the laboratory. Errors that cannot be salvaged by the dispenser, however, should *not* be passed on to the recipient. This violates basic ethical principles, and it will eventually result in general dissatisfaction with the dispenser. It may also cause the laboratory to denote the dispenser as careless or unsuspecting. The dispenser who insists on correct and careful work from a laboratory generally receives it.

REFERENCES

1. ANSI Z80.1-1999 American National Standard for Ophthalmics: Prescription ophthalmic lenses—recommendations, Merrifield, Va, 2000, Optical Laboratories Association.
2. How bifocal adds should be measured, Ophthalmic Lens Data Series, Bausch & Lomb, undated.

Proficiency Test

(Answers can be found in the back of the book.)

What is wrong with each of the following (Questions 1-4):

1. OS: −4.25 −0.75 × 010
   OD: −4.50 sphere

2. +4.5 −1.0 × 017

3. +0.50 −1.75 × 12°

4. +2.00 −.75 × 033

5. True or False? Always use the actual order form to verify a prescription received from the laboratory.

6. An individual with badly scratched lenses wants a new pair of glasses. You read the existing prescription from the old glasses to make the new pair. You also measure the wearer's PD. The distance between the OCs in the existing spectacles is found to be significantly different from the wearer's PD. Which of the following reasons for this are possible?
   a. There may be cylinder present in the prescription.
   b. There was an error in making the original glasses.
   c. There is prescribed prism in the original prescription.
   d. Both lenses in the prescription are simply spheres.

7. A wearer breaks her glasses. It is still possible to measure the lens power and distance between OCs in the broken glasses. The prescription is fairly high and there is a large difference between the wearer's measured PD and the distance between OCs found in the broken glasses. The wearer cannot identify the prescriber or place where the prescription originated or the glasses were made. In this case, the glasses should be made with:
   a. The new lens centers set at the wearer's measured PD.
   b. The new lens centers set at the same distance as the old lens centers were set.

8. In using a lensmeter, it is possible to find the power in either plus cylinder or minus cylinder form. Assume you are to find lens power in *minus* cylinder form. The correct procedure is listed below. Fill in the blanks with the correct missing words so that the procedure is correct for minus cylinder form. Also list the numbers you would find if the prescription you were reading had a power of +2.00 −4.00 × 015.
   a. Turn the power wheel into the high _____ numbers.
   b. Slowly advance the power wheel in the _____ direction.
   c. Rotate the axis wheel to cause the _____ lines to come into focus first.
   d. When in focus, record the _____ and _____ values.
      (When reading this particular lens, the numerical values are equal to _____ and _____.)
   e. Move the power wheel a second time, still in the _____ direction, until the _____ lines come into clear focus.
      (This numerical reading is_____.)
   f. The difference between first and second power readings is the cylinder and is recorded as a _____ value.

9. A conventional crossed-line-target lensmeter is being used to find the power of a lens. To measure the prescription in plus cylinder form, begin by turning the power wheel:
   a. In the high plus direction.
   b. In the high minus direction.
   c. In either direction.

10. **A.** A lensmeter is used to measure a lens. The single line is clear at −3.00 D, and the axis wheel reads **20**. With the axis wheel still at 20, the triple lines are clear at −2.50 D. Is this lens being read in plus or minus cylinder form?
    a. Plus cylinder form
    b. Minus cylinder form
    B. What is the power of this lens when written in minus cylinder form?

11. True or False? The proper way to measure near addition power is by turning the glasses around in the lensmeter so that the temples are pointing toward you, then measuring distance and near powers, taking the difference between the two as the near addition power.

12. When a lens is measured in the normal manner, with the back side of the lens against the lensmeter stop, the power being measured is called:
    a. The equivalent power
    b. The effective power
    c. The front vertex power
    d. The back vertex power

13. A lens has a front vertex power in the distance portion that reads +4.87 − 1.25 × 165. The front vertex power through the near addition reads +6.62 − 1.25 × 165. What is the add power?

14. It is necessary to order one lens only for a frame that cannot be sent to the laboratory. The frame is a common frame, and the laboratory has a pattern for it. Leaving off what piece of information when ordering could result in a lens that is unacceptable optically?
    a. The "frame difference" measurement
    b. The height of the lens OC
    c. The ED of the frame
    d. The circumference of the existing lens

15. True or False? When using a pencil or pen to physically trace around a lens to make a drawing for a "lenses only" order, it is also necessary to draw the axis of the cylinder on the lens tracing.

16. True or False? When ordering "lenses only" for a frame of unknown name, suppose a hand drawn lens tracing is made. The tracing is only used for shape, not dimensions.

17. A Box-o-Graph may be used to measure:
    a. The C dimension of a lens.
    b. The circumference of a lens.
    c. The ED of a lens.
    d. The A dimension of a lens.

18. True or False? These all mean the same thing: (1) lens C-size, (2) the C dimension of a lens, and (3) lens circumference.

19. True or False? When making new lenses from an old prescription, the same lens material that was used in the old prescription should always be used in the new lenses.

20. As the power of the cylinder component of a prescription increases, the American National Standards Institute tolerances for how far the cylinder axis can be off mean that:
    a. High cylinder powers require the axis to be more exact.
    b. High cylinder powers allow the axis to be less exact.
    c. High cylinder powers require the same amount of exactness as low cylinder powers.

21. When verifying lens powers for a pair of glasses, always:
    a. Start with the right lens.
    b. Start with the left lens.
    c. Start with the lens with the highest power in the 180-degree meridian.
    d. Start with the lens with the highest power in the 90-degree meridian.
    e. Start with the lens with the highest power in the axis meridian.

22. The American National Standards Institute recommends the following tolerances for acceptable limits of unwanted horizontal prism in a lens pair:
    a. If the PD is more than 2.5 mm off *and* horizontal prism exceeds 0.67Δ, the prescription is outside of acceptable limits.
    b. If the PD is more than 2.5 mm off *and* horizontal prism exceeds 0.33Δ, the prescription is outside of acceptable limits.
    c. If the PD is more than 2.5 mm off *or* horizontal prism exceeds 0.67Δ, the prescription is outside of acceptable limits.
    d. If the PD is more than 2.5 mm off *or* horizontal prism exceeds 0.33Δ, the prescription is outside of acceptable limits.

The American National Standards Institute recommendation for vertical prism or MRP placement for lenses in a frame is (Questions 23 to 25):

23. a. 0.12Δ
b. 0.33Δ
c. 0.50Δ
d. 0.67Δ
e. 1.00Δ

or

24. _____mm difference between left and right MRP heights when no prism is ordered.
a. 0.5 mm
b. 1.0 mm
c. 1.5 mm
d. 2.0 mm
e. 2.5 mm

25. and the prescription is acceptable:
a. if both aspects pass.
b. if either one or the other aspect passes.

26. The American National Standards Institute recommendation for segment height in a mounted or unmounted lens pair is _____.
a. ±0.5 mm.
b. ±1.0 mm.
c. ±1.5 mm.
d. ±2.0 mm.
e. ±2.5 mm.

27. The American National Standards Institute recommendation for near PD tolerance for a mounted lens pair is:
a. ±0.5 mm.
b. ±1.0 mm.
c. ±1.5 mm.
d. ±2.0 mm.
e. ±2.5 mm.

For the following questions indicate whether the prescription is within tolerance according to the Z80.1 Recommendations for Prescription Ophthalmic Lenses. The prescription calls for the following:

$$R: -1.00 - 2.75 \times 175$$
$$L: -0.25 - 0.75 \times 004$$
$$add = +2.25$$
$$PD = 65/62$$
$$seg\ height = 21$$

However, when the prescription comes back from the laboratory, you find the variables to be as follows:

$$R: -1.37 - 2.65 \times 178$$
$$L: -0.25 - 0.70 \times 008$$
$$add = +2.25$$
$$PD = 69/64$$
$$seg\ height = 21.5$$
$$vertical\ prism\ shows\ 0.25\Delta\ Base\ Down\ OS$$
$$horizontal\ prism\ shows\ 0.10\Delta\ Base\ In$$

Tell whether or not the parameter listed is within the standards specified by the American National Standards Institute (Questions 28-37).

28. Right lens meridian of highest absolute power
a. Yes
b. No

29. Left lens meridian of highest absolute power
a. Yes
b. No

30. Right lens cylinder power
a. Yes
b. No

31. Left lens cylinder power
a. Yes
b. No

32. Right lens cylinder axis
a. Yes
b. No

33. Left lens cylinder axis
a. Yes
b. No

34. Far PD/horizontal prism
a. Yes
b. No

35. Near PD
a. Yes
b. No

36. Seg height
a. Yes
b. No

37. Unwanted vertical prism
a. Yes
b. No

38. In trying to measure a lens, it is found that the prism amount present in the prescription is so high that the illuminated target is off of the lensmeter screen. Using the prism compensating device, the illuminated target is moved onto either the horizontal or vertical crosshair on the measuring reticle. This is done by using either only horizontal or only vertical prism.
  a. The larger prismatic component is read from the prism compensating device. The smaller prismatic component is read directly from the reticle.
  b. The smaller prismatic component is read from the prism compensating device. The larger prismatic component is read directly from the reticle.
  c. It makes no difference which prism element is read from the prism compensating device or reticle.

39. Lens warpage is revealed by:
  a. Cylinder found on the front surface.
  b. Cylinder found on the back surface.
  c. No cylinder found on either surface.
  d. Both a and b
  e. None of the above reveals lens warpage.

40. To check for strain in a lens, what instrument is used?
  a. Ophthalmoscope
  b. Retinoscope
  c. Colmascope
  d. Lensmeter
  e. c or d may be used

41. Which error is of no consequence in verifying correctness of frames and lenses?
  a. air space between lens and frame
  b. chips in the lens edge between bevel and lens surface
  c. distortion (unevenness) in lens edge between bevel and lens surface
  d. lens strain in a glass lens near the eyewire in a metal frame
  e. All of the above are of consequence.

42. What is the meridian of highest absolute power for this prescription: $-1.50 -2.75 \times 180$?
  a. -1.50 D
  b. -2.75 D
  c. -4.25 D
  d. -1.25 D
  e. None of the above are correct responses.

43. Write each of these prescriptions so that the meridian of highest absolute power is the sphere power.
  a. $+3.00 -2.00 \times 180$
  b. $-3.00 -2.00 \times 180$
  c. $+3.00 +2.00 \times 180$
  d. $-3.00 +2.00 \times 180$

CHAPTER **7**

Lens Insertion

Inserting a lens into a frame so that the end result is both neat and professional in appearance requires a skill only developed by considerable practice. Numerous techniques are available, and any are acceptable if the end product meets the expressed standards. This chapter presents the steps involved in lens insertion, some of the methods used, and also some of the difficulties that must be avoided.

AN OVERVIEW OF INSERTING LENSES INTO PLASTIC FRAMES

The steps involved in inserting a lens are standard for most plastic frames. The major variant is whether or not heat is used in the process—and if heat is to be used, how much heat is required. When no heat is used, the lenses are "snapped" into place. This is called *cold snapping*.

Adaptations of these basic procedures of lens insertion for special materials are explained later in the chapter. Table 7-1 gives an overview of lens insertion for different frame materials.

Lens Insertion Into Normal Plastic (Cellulose Acetate) Frames

Here are the procedures used to insert a lens into a plastic frame. Although specific for cellulose acetate frame material, there is little difference in technique for other frames.

Heating the Frame
Lenses should be inserted into the frame without bumping the temples. When the endpieces of the frame are hot, if the temples are bumped, the hinge may loosen or become misaligned. Because most plastic frames have *hidden hinges*, which do not go all the way through the plastic, a loose temple is very difficult to repair.

Begin heating the frame by noting the curvature of the lens meniscus compared with the curve of the eyewire (Figure 7-1). Since the lens usually curves more than the eyewire, it is advisable to preshape the upper and lower sections of the eyewire to conform to the meniscus of the lens edge. This makes lens insertion somewhat easier. Before heating the frame, it is advisable to do a "dry run." Hold the lens frame in exactly the position you intend to use when actually putting the lens in the frame.

You must be able to return the frame to this position immediately after it has been heated. Frames cool rapidly and lose pliability quickly, and the few moments salvaged by this preparation may be vital.

Hold the lens with one hand and the frame with the other, in exactly the same manner as they will be held when beginning lens insertion. It is much better to hold the frame by the frame front and not the temples. Holding the frame by the temples vastly increases the possibility of loosening a hinge. Heat only the portion of the frame that is actually going to be manipulated. In the case of lens insertion, this is just one half of the frame front (Figure 7-2, *A*).

Some frame warmers blow hot air onto the frame from both sides of a frame, others only blow air from one direction. When using an air blower that blows from one direction only, be sure to heat both the front and back or top and bottom of the frame front alternately to prevent overheating any one portion.

When using a salt pan, first stir the salt to equalize the temperature, then push some of the salt into a mound in one portion of the pan. Place the section of the frame to be heated just beneath the surface of the salt mound, leaving that portion not to be heated out of the salt and as parallel to the surface of the salt as possible (Figure 7-2, *B*). Move the frame continually and very slowly while under the salt to avoid marking the soft plastic with salt granules. Do not permit the frame to become so heated that it sags or distorts. If salt sticks to a dry frame, additional talcum powder should be added to the salt. (The only two components of the "salt bath" are salt and ordinary talcum powder. Salt conveys heat well, while talcum powder prevents salt from lumping and sticking to the frame.) CAUTION: Because many frame materials are sensitive to excessive heat and coated lenses can be damaged by the high heat of salt pans, it is much safer to use a hot air blower, rather than hot salt. An expensive anti-reflection (AR) coating can easily be ruined by using hot salt to heat the frame.

Inserting the Lens
As stated earlier, begin by noting the curvature of the lens meniscus compared with the curve of the eyewire as was shown in Figure 7-1. Heat the frame and preshape the upper and lower sections of the eyewire to conform

TABLE 7-1
Comparing Lens Insertion By Frame Material

	Amount of Heat	Heating Methods	Edged Lens Size	To Shrink Material	Notes
Cellulose Acetate	Use minimal heat till pliable.	Hot air best. Hot salt or beads acceptable.	On size or up to 0.5 mm above frame size.	Plunge in ice water. Will shrink if previously stretched.	Cellulose acetate is the standard material used for most plastic frames.
Cellulose Propionate	Cold snap the lenses in place if possible. If not possible, use minimal heat.	When necessary use a low heat setting (40° C/105° F) on an air warmer. Avoid using hot salt.	On size.		May help to heat a little at a time to avoid overheating.
Nylon	Use hot water.	Hot water preferred for penetration. Hot air used if hot water not available.	≈ 0.2 mm larger than frame size.	Material does not shrink.	To retain adjusted shape, hold frame in the desired shape until cool. (Running cold water will speed cooling.)
Carbon Fiber	None to minimal. Preferred insertion method: cold snap.	When heat used, hot air at low temperature.	On size to just slightly larger in some cases.	Material does not shrink.	Types of carbon fiber material will vary. So will heat and insertion techniques.
Polyamide	No heat. Cold snap lenses in place.	Hot air for temples only.	Exactly on size.	Material shrinks slightly when heated.	After insertion, loose lenses may be tightened by heating the frame slightly.
Polycarbonate	None.	Cold snap.	On size.	Material does not shrink.	Material does not adjust.
Optyl	High heat. Heat till material bends under its own weight.	Hot air, high temperature.	≈ 0.6 to 1.0 mm oversize.	Material will not shrink, but instead expands with heat. Gradually returns to size as temperature cools.	Material returns to original shape when reheated. Quick cooling stops shrinking process and results in loose lenses.

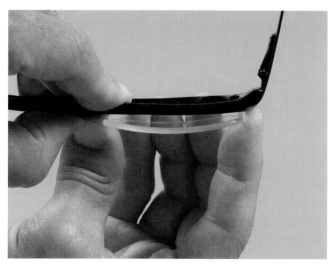

Figure 7-1. The top edge of the frame is compared with the top edge of the lens. If the frame is first curved to conform to the lens, the end result will often be more cosmetically acceptable.

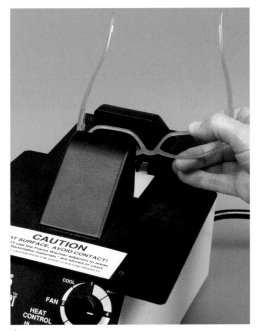

A

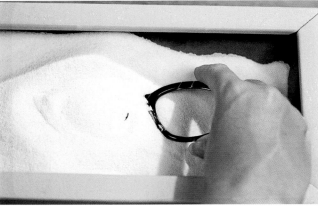

B

Figure 7-2. A, Heat only that portion of the frame that is going to be manipulated. Here a hot air frame warmer is being used to heat the frame. Hot air is the safer method of heating a frame compared with hot salt. **B,** If hot salt is to be used, the frame should be moved slowly under the surface of the salt to help heat it uniformly. Moving the frame also causes it to heat faster, since heat is continually leaving the salt immediately adjacent to the frame and entering the plastic. (Remember: With newer plastic frame materials and many lens treatments, it is not safe to use a salt pan.)

to the meniscus of the lens edge as shown in Figure 7-3.

Method 1—Insert the temporal (outer) edge of the lens into the corresponding portion (outer edge) of the frame (Figure 7-4, *A*). With the thumbs on the surface of the lens and the fingers on the nasal (inner) edge of the frame eyewire, snap the lens into the frame from the nasal (inner) side by applying pressure with both the thumbs and fingers (Figure 7-4, *B*).

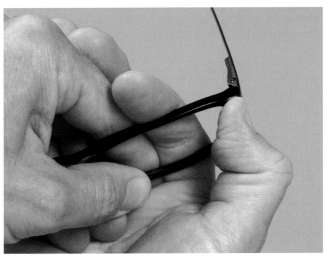

Figure 7-3. To make the frame rim fit the lens better, pre-shape the rims to conform to the meniscus curve of the lens.

Method 2—Insert the upper outer (temporal) edge of the lens into the frame groove (Figure 7-5, *A*), push the upper inner (nasal) edge into the eyewire so that the whole upper edge of the lens is in the frame (Figure 7-5, *B*), push the lower temporal edge in (Figure 7-5, *C*) and conclude by snapping the lower nasal corner in (Figure 7-5, *D*). (See Table 7-2 for a review of these methods.)

Most frame construction makes it easier to insert lenses from the front. Lenses should definitely be inserted into safety frames from the front so they will not be as likely to come out of the frame when struck from the front.

If the frame cools too much before the lens is fully inserted, by whatever method, it is advisable to totally remove the lens before reheating the frame. A heated lens is difficult to handle; also, a frame without lenses heats more uniformly and will stretch more evenly as the lens is inserted.

When pulling the eyewire using any of the methods, the pulling action must be *straight* and caution must be taken not to "*roll*" the eyewire. This rolling results in the front of the eyewire covering less lens than the back, or vice versa, as if the groove were turned at an angle (Figure 7-6). A rolled eyewire holds the lens less securely and disturbs the finished appearance of the spectacles. It also may cause some visual disturbance if the lens bevel is revealed and refracts light.

If during the insertion procedure, the eyewire appears to become rolled, it is helpful to change the direction of insertion (back to front, or vice versa) so that the stress put on one portion of the eyewire is equaled by stress on the other, reversing the direction of the roll.

After inserting the lenses into a conventional plastic frame (made of cellulose acetate) and checking for adjustment, it may be helpful to plunge the frame and lenses into ice water to "set" them. This procedure shrinks the

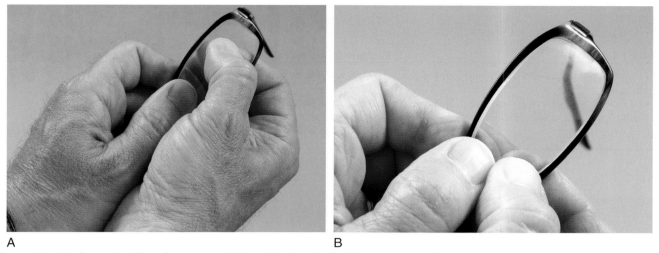

A B

Figure 7-4. Method 1. **A,** Place the temporal edge of the lens in the frame groove. (The first moments of lens insertion are crucial in proper alignment of the lens bevel with the frame groove and must be done quickly.) **B,** The lens should snap in place fairly easily. If extreme force must be used in attempting to snap the lens in place, the process is better carried out using method 2.

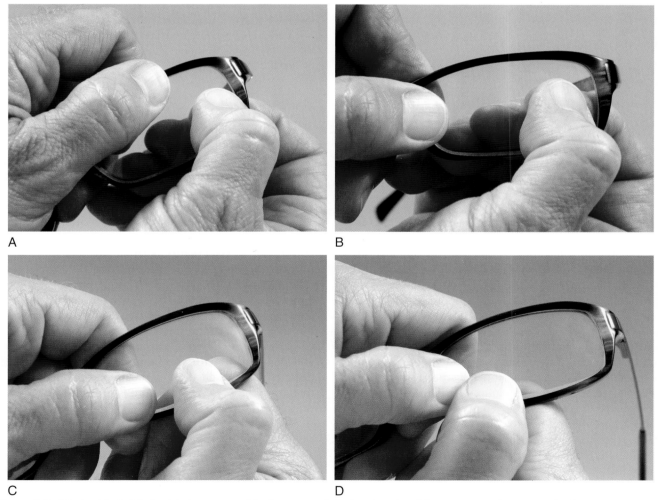

A B

C D

Figure 7-5. Method 2. **A,** Method 2 also starts with alignment of the lens bevel and frame groove, beginning in the upper temporal corner. **B,** When the upper and lower rims of the eyewire have been preshaped to the lens configuration, lens insertion into the entire upper half of the frame may be completed well before the frame cools. **C,** When the upper part of the lens is in the frame, start temporally and begin pulling the lower eyewire around the lens. **D,** Conclude the insertion process by snapping the bevel of the lower nasal part of the lens into the groove.

TABLE 7-2
Procedures for Inserting Lenses Into Plastic Frames

Method 1	Method 2
1. Heat and curve frame top to match lens top	1. Heat and curve frame top to match lens top
2. Heat eyewire	2. Heat eyewire
3. Place outer part of lens in outer part of frame	3. Place upper outer edge of lens in frame
4. Push inner edge of lens in with thumbs	4. Place upper inner edge of lens in frame (top of lens is now in frame)
	5. Pull lower eyewire around lens beginning temporally and ending nasally

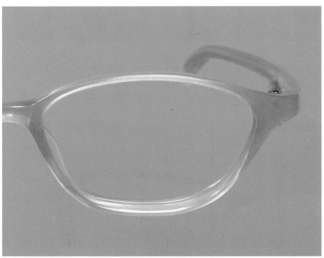

Figure 7-6. This insertion attempt caused the lower eyewire to be rolled forward.

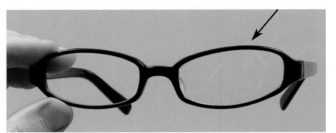

Figure 7-7. After putting the first lens in the frame, lens orientation for the inserted lens should be compared with the empty eyewire. This frame shows too much temporal upsweep.

frame and may help to prevent loose lenses later. Be sure, however, to check the insertion and all adjustment points before "setting" the lenses. A notable exception for using this treatment is the Optyl frame that shrinks as it slowly cools. Plunging such a frame in cold water stops the shrinking process and can result in loose lenses.

Adapting for a Lens That is Too Small

If new lenses have been ordered for an old frame, they may be too small if the frame has been stretched around its old lenses. In these cases, it may be possible to shrink a regular plastic frame to reduce the circumference of the eyewire to accept the new lenses firmly.

First heat the frame front thoroughly until it is quite pliable, then immediately immerse it in very cold water—as cold as possible. Allow the frame to rest in the cold water until it is completely cold to the touch.

If the frame is still too large, repeat the process two or three times. If the frame is still too large after the third treatment, the technique probably will not succeed.

This process can also be used on new frames, although they rarely respond more than slightly.

Checks After Lens Insertion

After inserting lenses, check to be sure the lens is entirely in the groove of the eyewire. Be sure the eyewire is flat or uniformly rounded on the outside; if it is slanted, the eyewire has been rolled. A roll can be corrected by heating that portion of the eyewire involved and either twisting it with the fingers or pressing the frame against a flat surface with a counter-rolling motion. If uncorrectable by this method, it is best to remove the lens and correct the lower eyewire without the lens in it. Then reinsert the lens properly after heating the frame.

Compare the eyewire containing the lens with the empty eyewire adjacent to it. Be sure the lens fits squarely all around and has not been twisted. Note whether or not the eyewire containing the lens is still parallel to the empty eyewire. Observe the upper rim near the bridge and compare it with the empty side. If the plastic is humped or stretched in comparison, the lens is not matching the eyewire shape and is probably altering the initial frame shape (Figure 7-7).

When both lenses have been inserted, an empty sample frame of the same shape may be used to assess the inserted pair. This may be necessary, especially for an untrained eye, because the lensmeter will not reveal a twist of the lens in all cases, such as when the lenses are spherical, or if the bridge or endpiece is askew.

Lens-twisting pliers (Figure 7-8) are used to correct a rotated lens. First, heat the frame and inspect the lens and pliers to be sure that all surfaces are free of salt. Hold the frame in one hand with the upper eyewire toward

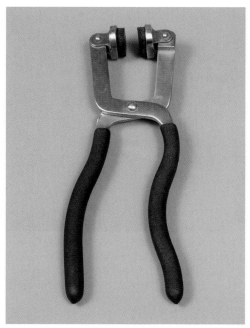

Figure 7-8. Many different types of *lens twisting* pliers are available. There are two important variations in these pliers. 1. One is the "throat depth" of the pliers. The farther the pads are from the central joint of the pliers, the less likelihood there is of inadvertently marking the frame in twisting. 2. The second variation is the vertical dimension of the pads that grip the lens surfaces. Some pads will be too large vertically for frames with narrow vertical depths to the lens.

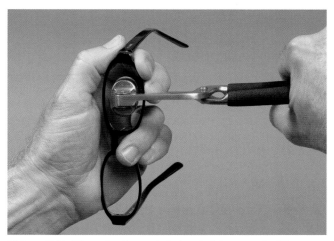

Figure 7-9. Here the frame is being held correctly. However, carelessness in holding the frame results not only in a rotation of the lens, but also in a twisting of the frame bridge.

the palm. When working on the lenses, the forefinger, second finger, and thumb should grasp the area around the endpiece while the third and little finger brace the bridge area (Figure 7-9). Using the pliers to hold the lens, rotate the frame so that the upper eyewire always remains towards the palm when shifting from one lens to the other. The difference then is that for one lens the

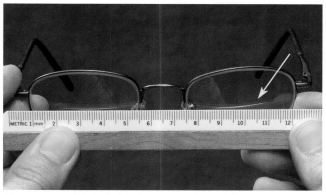

Figure 7-10. If the bifocal is a straight top, both bifocal lines will run parallel to the straight edge. Here there is an error present and the left lens is obviously twisted. It should be mentioned though that parallel bifocal lines do not guarantee that the lenses are not twisted in the frame. The frame front should still be examined for temporal upsweep or nasal humping.

hinges face away from the palm whereas for the other, they face towards the palm.

The pliers should grasp the lens close enough to the lower eyewire to prevent contact between the eyewire and the metal of the pliers. If the pliers press against the hot eyewire, they will invariably dent it.

The same lens adjustment can be made using the fingers of the free hand instead of the pliers to grasp the lens. This adjustment must be performed immediately after lens insertion and before the frame has cooled.

Checking a Bifocal or Progressive Addition Lens

With *straight-top bifocals*, the position of the lenses can easily be checked using a straight edge. This is placed horizontally across the front surface of the lenses at the level of, and parallel to, the straight tops of the bifocal segments.

If both lenses are correctly inserted, both segment tops will run adjacent or parallel to the straight edge. If one or both lenses are improperly inserted, the segment top of one lens will appear at an angle to the straight edge when the straight edge is parallel to the segment top of the other lens (Figure 7-10).

If the segment tops of the lenses are parallel but one lens still appears poorly positioned by the criteria previously mentioned (comparing the frame with lenses versus an empty frame), then the lens blank has been edged in a rotated position. The error cannot be corrected by adjustment; it requires the manufacture of a new lens.

By holding the lenses back to back, it is possible to determine before insertion if either bifocal lens has been edged in a rotated position. The bifocal portions should overlap exactly if equal seg height and decentration were ordered (Figure 7-11). This is true for any type of multifocal lens.

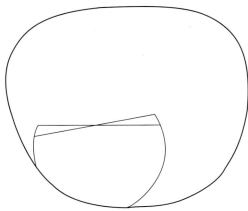

Figure 7-11. When two lenses are held back to back, any error in lens rotation becomes immediately evident. The same technique may be used to check a "lenses only" order when one bifocal seg has been ordered a different height from the other. Their differences will be obvious and measurable.

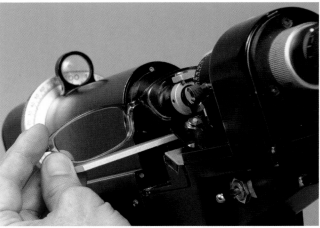

Figure 7-12. Ordinarily, during verification, glasses are positioned to rest flat on the lensmeter table. To aid in determining which way a rotated lens should be turned for lens realignment, it is helpful to set the instrument at the desired axis and rotate the glasses.

These same helps may be used with progressive addition lenses that still have lens markings in place. There are two circles or other marks that denote the 180-degree line. These may be used to check for lens straightness just like the tops of bifocals were.

Judgment of *round-seg bifocals* depends a good deal on noting whether the lenses look like they are straight in the frame and not rotated. (Again, compare the frame with lenses versus an empty frame.) A good reference point for observation is the point where the nasal edge of the seg meets the eyewire. If both bifocals were ordered with equal seg height and decentration, the inner edges of the segs should meet the eyewires at symmetrical points. If one point appears higher up the eyewire nasally than the other, use the lens-twisting pliers to correct it, provided this adjustment does not place the cylindrical correction off axis. If the axis is disturbed, the lens has been erroneously cut off pattern.

To be certain that *single-vision cylindrical lenses* are in the frame straight, preset the lensmeter at the correct sphere power and set the axis reading at the axis called for in the prescription. If the lines in the lensmeter appear to be "off axis," the lens has been inserted in a rotated or twisted position. Raise one side of the glasses, then the other, from the lensmeter table until the lines in the lensmeter appear straight and unbroken (Figure 7-12).

Note the angle at which the frame is sitting, keeping in mind that the rotated lens has now been turned to the proper axis position. (In essence, the frame needs to be twisted around the lens until it sits flat on the lensmeter table again.) To bring the lens to its proper position, dot the lens with the lensmeter marking mechanism. Then heat the eyewire and twist the lens around until these three dots are horizontal in the frame. The lens is then

at its proper axis, which should also result in a symmetrical-looking frame.

If there is nasal humping or a temporal upsweep present for one lens but not the other, the lens has slipped in the edging process or was improperly positioned at the time of the original edging. The only alternative is a new lens.

After the lenses are straight in the frame, adjust the frame into standard alignment.

Removing a Lens

To remove a lens, heat the frame front and place the thumbs on the back side of the lens in the lower, nasal area (Figure 7-13). Brace the front of the eyewire with the fingers. A towel may be placed around the lens to prevent burning of the fingers. (Lenses that were inserted with a "cold snap" method will also be removed cold.) Push the lens in one direction by pressing with the thumbs and bracing or pulling the eyewire in an opposite direction with the fingers.

Insertion Into a Cellulose Propionate Frame

Cellulose propionate material is very similar to cellulose acetate. However, it is more heat sensitive. It may even be advisable to cold snap the lenses in place. When using heat, the frame warmer should be set for a low temperature (40° C/105° F). The closer the edged lens size is to the frame size, the less heat will be necessary. For that reason, it may be helpful to edge the lenses "on size." Because it is not always possible to tell a cellulose acetate frame from a regular plastic frame, and because a number of other frame materials are also sensitive to heat, it is generally advisable to heed the following:[1]

- Use the lowest amount of heat necessary to accomplish the task.

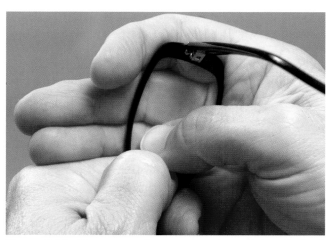

Figure 7-13. To remove a lens, pressure is applied to the back of the lens at the lower nasal portion.

- Heat the frame until it is pliable; not until it actually softens.
- Never leave a frame unattended in a frame warmer.

Insertion Into a Nylon Frame

Insertion of lenses into a nylon frame must be done following the manufacturer's directions to prevent problems.

Because nylon frames do not stretch as much as ordinary plastic frames, the lenses must be edged closer to the frame size than usual. Care must be taken to avoid cutting the lenses too small; this hazard is a common tendency, encouraged by the difficulty of stretching the nylon about the lens. Lenses cut too small will fit loosely after insertion because of the depth of the bevel.

Nylon frames cannot be heated uniformly enough by the usual methods to permit the stretching necessary for lens insertion. The hot air and salt pan methods tend to heat the outer layers of the nylon excessively and leave the deeper portions too cool to stretch. Hot water penetrates the nylon better and permits the eyewires to stretch properly to accept the lenses.

To adjust a nylon frame, the best method is to heat the plastic, bend it as desired, and then hold the frame in the new conformation as it cools. If the frame is released before it is cool, it tends to resume its initial configuration. Holding the frame to the adjusted configuration while running cold water over it may help.

Insertion Into a Carbon Fiber Frame

There are many different carbon frames on the market. The actual material will vary, depending on the manufacturer. This means that the properties of the material will vary some as well. The recommendations of the individual frame manufacturers should be followed.

Great care must be taken if carbon fiber material is heated. Carbon fiber material does not lend itself to adjustment. Although carbon fiber will become some-what pliable with heat, the recommended method of lens insertion for carbon fiber fronts without eyewire screws is to "cold snap" the lenses in place.

Cold snap lens insertion is just what its name implies. The lenses are cut to fit the size of the frame exactly. The frame front is not heated. Instead, the lenses are inserted without heat. They are pushed into the frame in the same manner as they would be for a normal plastic frame. Pressing on the lens "snaps" the lenses into the "cold" frame.

Because of the reputed tendency of a standard CR-39 plastic lens to shrink very slightly over time, some labs use a small amount of heat to insert the lens. The lens may then be ground slightly larger. If heating carbon fiber material, it is much better to use hot air instead of salt or glass beads. A hot air warmer should be on low temperature and the frame heated for 10 to 20 seconds. Be advised, however, that "heat can soften the frame finish, making it easy to scrape the coated surface with the sharp edges of the lens. This can result in a frame that is chipped or flaked, exposing the dull base material.[2]"

Many carbon fiber frame fronts come with an eyewire screw like that found in regular metal frame fronts. The screw opens and closes the eyewire to accept the lens. Lens insertion is done as if the frame were a metal frame (see *Lens Insertion into a Metal Frame* later in this chapter).

Insertion Into a Polyamide Frame

Most of the guidelines for working with carbon-fiber frames also apply to polyamide frames. The nylon-based polyamide material is thin, light, and resists adjustment. The lenses should be sized exactly and cold snapped into place. Oversized lenses simply will not go in, since the material will not stretch. One of the unique features of this material is its tendency to shrink slightly when heated in excess of 230° F.[3] Therefore heating a polyamide frame to insert a correctly sized lens will cause problems. A correctly sized lens would then be too large for the frame. On the other hand, this tendency to shrink somewhat can be an advantage if a lens is a bit too small. After the lens has been cold snapped into place, the lens fit can be tightened by heating the lens and frame together. The polyamide shrinks, and the eyewire contracts around the lens. Do not plunge the frame into cold water.

For polyamide frames, it is best to use a hot air type of frame warmer even when adjusting the temples.

Insertion Into a Polycarbonate Frame

Polycarbonate material is used for certain sports eyewear frame fronts. Polycarbonate does not adjust. Because polycarbonate does not become pliable when heated, lenses must be "cold snapped" into place. Lenses should be cut close to the actual frame size, since polycarbonate neither stretches or shrinks.

Insertion Into a Kevlar Frame

Kevlar is also a nylon-based material. It neither stretches nor shrinks with heat, but does exhibit a degree of pliability. This pliability allows for a more conventional lens insertion. In other words, the lenses do not have to be cold snapped into place. Yet the lenses still need to be cut exactly to size or insertion will prove troublesome.

Insertion Into an Optyl Frame

Optyl, first developed in 1968 by Wilhelm Anger Co. of Traun, Austria, is a material that belongs to the group of epoxy resins. Optyl frames are cast molded rather than cut. They are also 20% to 30% lighter than the more conventional frame materials.[4]

Optyl frames can be identified by trade name and by the characteristic clear colors in which the material is made. Originally, there was always an absence of a metal reinforcement through the temples. They were clear Optyl material and an identifying characteristic. However, Optyl frames also come with temples having traditional metal core reinforcements that have a different composition. Unlike the first type of Optyl temples, these are adjusted with little or no heat.

Because Optyl will not shrink, it is better to cut the lenses slightly oversize. A margin of 0.6 to 1.0 mm too large is customary.

Frames made from the original Optyl material do not begin to soften until the heating temperature reaches 80° C; they can safely be heated to a level of 200° C without bubbling or distorting. Should the frame become distorted, it will go back to its original molded shape on being heated. This can be an advantage when the frame is distorted during lens insertion, but it can also be a disadvantage during frame adjustment, because heating the frame may cause it to lose its adjustment and go back to its original molded form.

To allow lens insertion, the frame should be heated until pliable enough to bend of its own weight: usually about 30 to 60 seconds. The lenses are not so much pushed into the eyewires as placed in them. If the eyewires are not properly surrounding the lenses, the frame should be reheated; the eyewires will adapt to the lenses as the frame attempts to resume its original molded shape.

The lenses must never be forced into a frame that has not been heated to pliability, nor should the frame be plunged into cold water to try to shrink the plastic about the lenses. Optyl expands with heat and returns to size through slow cooling. Plunging the frame into cold water stops the shrinking process and has the exact opposite effect of that desired.

If a glass lens is off axis or inserted in a rotated position, it should be rotated into its proper position only after the frame has been reheated, never while cold. If the lens is plastic, however, it should be removed and reinserted. If plastic lenses are not removed but only rotated, they will be loose after the frame and lenses cool.

Frames made of the original Optyl material do not bend while cold. Attempts to adjust them without heating almost always result in breakage. Since the material bends only when heated, properly adjusted Optyl frames tend to stay in adjustment until again heated.

To adjust the frame, heat only the portion of the frame requiring bending. Since this may be difficult to do for limited areas, such as a portion of the temple about the ear, use a heating unit that can direct heat to a limited area, such as a forced-air unit with a cone attachment that directs the flow of heat. Hold the frame so that the portions adjacent to the area being heated are protected from the heat and do not lose their adjustment.

LENS INSERTION INTO A METAL FRAME

Lenses to be inserted into a metal frame must be edged to the exact size. Therefore, it is more likely that the order will be correct if the laboratory has the wearer's actual frame. In certain instances, however, it will be necessary to order "lenses only." When ordering "lenses only" for a metal frame, then the dispensary must trace the lenses using a remote frame tracer and send the digitized shape to the lab electronically.

If there is not a frame tracer in the dispensary, the laboratory must have the pattern for the frame in question. If there is any doubt about whether the laboratory has the pattern, they should be asked before the order is sent. Without an exact pattern, the frame will have to accompany the order. Once it is determined that the laboratory has the pattern, the chances of getting a good fit for a "lenses only" order are increased by measuring the circumference of the existing lenses. (This is explained in detail in Chapter 6.)

To put a lens in a metal frame, begin by comparing the meniscus curves of the top and bottom of the lens to the corresponding curves of the upper and lower frame eyewires. If they do not match, the lens bevel will not seat squarely in the eyewire groove. Although in most cases these curves will match closely enough to allow a good lens fit, it will occasionally be necessary to use *eyewire forming pliers* (Figure 7-14) to reshape the frame eyewire. Eyewire forming pliers have curved nylon jaws. To increase the meniscus curve, position the pliers along the eyewire, as shown in Figure 7-15, and squeeze lightly. It may be necessary to continue to reposition the pliers stepwise along the upper and possibly lower eyewire until the new curve is evenly formed. (If the eyewire has *too much* curve, the eyewire forming pliers may be reversed to take some of the curve out of the eyewire.)

The best policy is to remove the eyewire screw, put the lens in the rim, and replace the screw. Simply loosen-

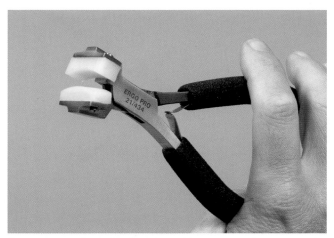

Figure 7-14. Eyewire forming pliers are used to cause the frame eyewire to conform to the meniscus curve of the lens bevel.

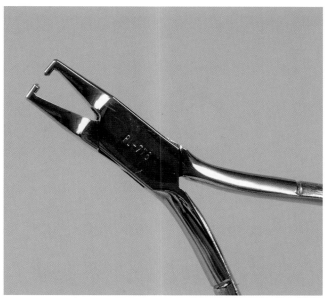

Figure 7-16. Eyewire closure pliers are made to fit into the top and bottom of the eyewire barrel.

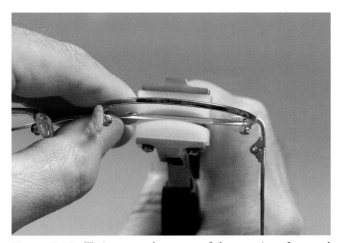

Figure 7-15. To increase the curve of the eyewire of a metal frame, position the eyewire forming pliers as shown in the photo and gently squeeze, repositioning the pliers as necessary.

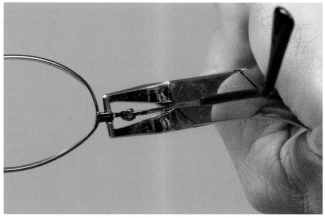

Figure 7-17. By using eyewire closure pliers to squeeze the eyewire around the lens, it is possible to see how well the lens will fit without having to replace the screw. Such pliers are especially handy in the edging laboratory.

ing the screw until it is possible to place the lens in the eyewire may cause the lens to chip during insertion. It is helpful to use *eyewire closure pliers* (Figure 7-16) to aid in seating the lens in the eyewire groove. With closure pliers it is also possible to tell if the lens will be of the correct size (Figure 7-17).

If the lens is too large, some dispensers will attempt to reduce the size of the lens with a hand edger to make it fit. Before attempting this, the dispenser should remember these points:

1. Evenly reducing the size of a lens is difficult. Uneven size reduction will produce gaps between the lens and the frame.
2. Only nonglass lenses should be hand edged. Heat-treated glass lenses may break during hand edging,

and hand edging will destroy the effect of the lens hardening process. Hand edging chemically hardened glass lenses should be followed by rehardening, as impact resistance is reduced by hand edging.

Once the lens is seated in the eyewire, the eyewire screw is tightened. Forcibly tightening the eyewire screw so that it places excessive stress on the lens may cause a glass lens to chip along the edge if struck or may cause a plastic lens to warp. Excessive edge strain may be checked for by using a colmascope, which is a set of crossed polarizing filters.

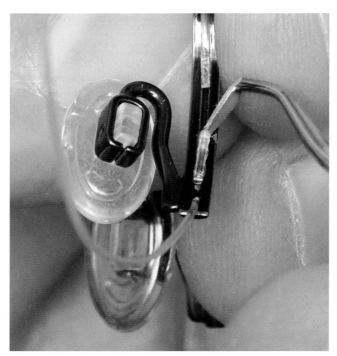

Figure 7-18. When it is difficult to remove a nylon cord from the frame channel of a nylon cord frame, a dental pick makes the job easier.

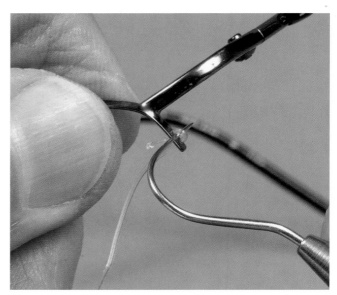

Figure 7-19. When removing an old cord from a nylon cord mounting, a dental pick can catch the tight loop to get the cord out of the holes.

LENS INSERTION INTO A NYLON CORD FRAME

An alternative to the traditional method of beveling a lens and inserting it into a grooved frame is the nylon cord frame. A *nylon cord frame* requires that the lens be made flat on the edge. A small groove is cut into the edge, usually all the way around the lens. A thin nylon string, attached to the frame, is slipped into the grooved lens to secure it in the frame. A nylon cord frame is also referred to by a number of names, including *nylon supra*, a *string mount*, *rimlon*, *Nylor*, and *suspension mounting*.

Mounting a new grooved lens in a nylon cord frame or replacing an old or broken cord on an existing frame requires similar procedures. Once the technique for replacing an old or broken cord is mastered, mounting a new lens in a new frame can be easily done. Therefore, *the first procedure outlined is that of replacing an old or broken cord. We are assuming that at least part of the cord is missing, so we will have to resize the cord to match the lens.*

Replacing a Nylon Cord of Unknown Length

1. *First remove the old cord.* Sometimes it is difficult to remove the end of the cord from the frame groove because it has been wedged securely into the groove. If this is the case, a dental pick can be handy for pulling the end of the cord out of the frame groove (Figure 7-18).
2. *Pull out the old cord.* Next catch the loop with the dental pick (Figure 7-19) and pull out the cord.

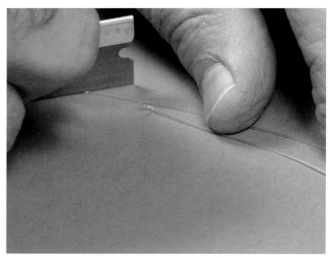

Figure 7-20. Cutting the nylon cord at an angle makes it easier to thread through the holes in the frame and allows it to seat smoothly in the groove under the lens. Here the length of the new cord is being estimated from the old cord that broke off near the point of attachment.

3. *Cut the new cord at an angle.* Since the old cord is missing and the length unknown, start with a very long section of cord. Remember, whenever cutting the nylon cord, always cut the cord at an angle. Both ends of the cord should be cut at an angle to make threading easier and so that the cord seats nicely in the frame. Using a single-edged razor blade is best (Figure 7-20).
4. *Thread the cord into one side.* The cord will need to be attached to the mounting at two locations. Each

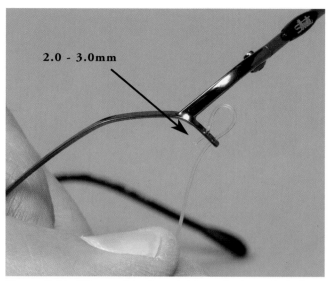

Figure 7-21. The cord is threaded into the lower hole from the inside and back into the upper hole.

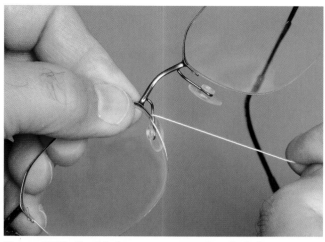

Figure 7-22. In this instance, we need to find the necessary cord length when the cord, or a good portion of the cord is missing. When replacing a nylon cord of unknown length, the cord is pulled snug around the lens, but not stretched.

point of attachment consists of two small holes. Some prefer to start with the nasal point of attachment, others the temporal. For illustration purposes, we will start temporally.

Starting with the temporal point of attachment, thread one end of the nylon line into the *lower* hole from the *lens* side. Then thread the same end into the upper hole, leaving a length of 2.0 to 3.0 mm (Figure 7-21).

5. *Size the cord to the lens.* Slip the other end of the cord through the lower hole at the nasal point of attachment. Do not thread it through the upper hole. Remember, the cord is first threaded from the lens side. With the end of the nylon cord still loose, slip the lens into the upper part of the frame. Thread the cord around the lens and pull the cord snug (Figure 7-22). Do not forcibly pull the cord so that it stretches.

6. *Remove the lens without "losing your place."* Hold the excess end of the cord with the thumb, so that it does not slide out, and remove the lens. (Since the cord was not pulled tight, it should be possible to remove the lens without losing the point of reference for length on the cord.)

7. *Take up the slack in the cord.* Because the cord was not pulled tight around the lens, it is necessary to pull the cord 1.5 to 2.0 mm *farther* through the lower hole so that the lens will be tight enough.

8. *Thread the excess cord through the remaining hole.* Thread the excess cord through the upper nasal hole while maintaining the new position of the cord in the lower hole.

9. *Clip off the excess cord.* Clip the excess cord, leaving 2.0 to 3.0 mm inside the eyewire. (If the cord is clipped at an angle it may lay down in the groove

more smoothly. Nail clippers work as well as regular cutting nippers.)

10. *Press the end of the cord into the frame groove.* First press the cord into the frame groove with the thumb (Figure 7-23, *A*). To get it all the way into the groove, it is helpful to next use a pair of half-padded nylon jaw pliers to push the loose end of the cord down into the groove (Figure 7-23, *B*). (Failure to tuck the cord into the groove will cause the lens to chip or flake because of the pressure of the cord between the edge of the lens and the edge of the eyewire.) Do this both nasally and temporally.

11. *Secure the lens in the upper half of the frame.* The lens is inserted into the frame, beginning in the nasal area (Figure 7-24, *A*), followed by the temporal area (Figure 7-24, *B*). The lens should come in *behind* the nylon cord so that the cord rests on the front surface of the lens.

12. *Stretch the cord into the groove around the lens.* To secure the lens in the frame, the cord must be stretched to fit into the lens groove. This is done using a plastic strip. (Some use a fabric ribbon. However, a ribbon will often fray, leaving threads wedged between the lens and the cord. It is extremely difficult to remove these threads.) Start out with the cord on the front side of the lens. Slip the plastic strip between the nylon cord and the lens, folding the strip back and grasping both ends together. Begin temporally and use the strip to pull the cord around the edge of the lens, seating it into the lens groove on the way around (Figure 7-25).

(*Caution*: There are metal hooks made specifically for stringing lenses. The main hazard

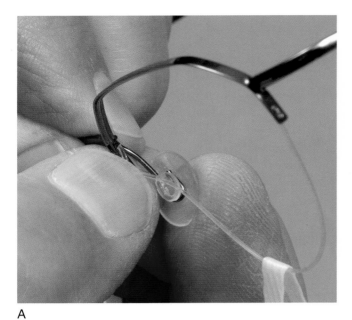

A

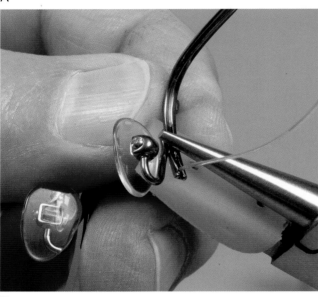

B

Figure 7-23. The cord is cut to the correct length and threaded. Before putting a lens in the frame, the end of the cord is pressed into the groove of the frame. In **(A)** the end of the cord is being pressed into place with the thumb. This may not get the cord all the way in the groove, but will get it started. In **(B)** half-padded pliers are used to press the end of the cord fully into the groove.

of these hooks is the possibility of causing a small flake of the lens to chip out at the groove area. When this occurs, the lens must be replaced.)

13. *Check the cord tension.* Cord tension can be checked in one of at least two ways.
   a. Check the tension at the corner of the lens right after the cord drops into the groove (Figure 7-26), or

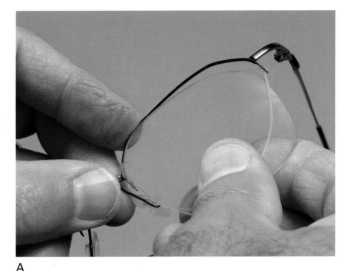

A

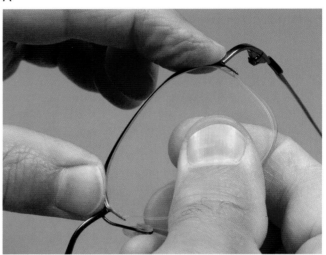

B

Figure 7-24. To put the lens in the frame, begin with the upper nasal corner as shown in **(A)**. Once the upper nasal corner of the lens is in place, the upper edge of the lens can be more easily aligned by moving across the upper rim, as shown in **(B)**.

   b. Check the tension of the cord by sliding the plastic strip toward the bottom of the lens until it is close to the midpoint of the lens cord. Pull fairly hard on the cord with the strip. The strip should pull the cord about 0.5 to 1.0 mm away from the edge of the lens.
14. *Try to rotate the lens.* Once the lens is in place, grasp the lens as shown in Figure 7-27 and attempt to rotate it in the frame. If the lens rotates easily, the cord is not tight enough.

   If the tension is incorrect, the lens should be removed and the length of the cord altered. (It may be necessary to use the dental pick to free the end of the cord from the frame groove. Most often when the fit is wrong, the cord will

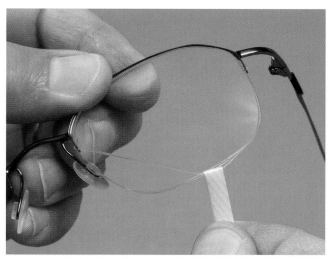

Figure 7-25. The cord must now be pulled around the lens. To slip the nylon cord into the groove in the lens, begin temporally and pull the cord around the lens in a nasal direction. The cord must start out on the front side of the lens.

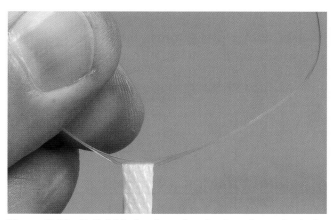

Figure 7-26. Pull fairly hard on the plastic strip to check the tension of the cord. As shown in the figure, the cord should stretch some, but there should be no more than 1.0 mm between the cord and the lens. (Some prefer to check for cord tension at the center of the bottom of the lens.)

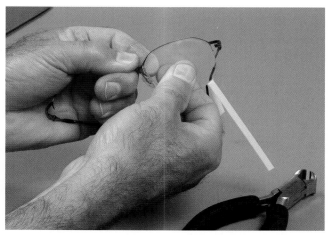

Figure 7-27. Once the lens is in, grasp the lens between thumb and fingers and try to rotate the lens. If the lens rotates easily, the cord is not tight enough.

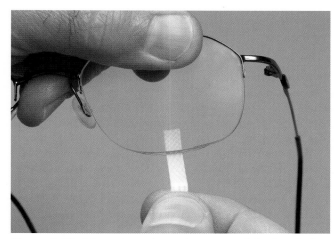

Figure 7-28. Move the strip to the center of the lens before attempting to remove it. If the strip is at or near a corner of a lens when being removed, it may pull the cord out of the groove.

be loose and will have to be shortened. If this is the case, repeat the above steps, beginning with step 8.

15. *Remove the plastic strip.* Once the lens is securely seated, move the plastic strip to the center of the lens edge, release one end of the plastic strip and pull it from between the lens and cord (Figure 7-28). Trying to remove the strip at a corner can pull the cord out of the groove. (For a review of these steps, see Box 7-1.)

Replacing an Old or Broken Nylon Cord

If the nylon cord is old or broken with both parts still intact, the new cord can be cut to match the length of the old cord. The procedure is basically the same as just described for replacing a missing cord, except that we can line up the new cord with the old cord and cut it to match. Remember to cut both ends of the new cord at an angle. If the old cord is in two pieces, line up the longest piece of the old cord and allow extra for the estimated length of the short piece of the broken cord. Cut the new cord to match.

Both temporal and nasal edges are threaded into the frame as described above. Hereafter the remaining steps are the same as previously described.

Cautions for Lenses With Thin Edges

When a lens used for a nylon cord frame has thin edges, the edge may not leave much room for the groove. This means that thin lens material on either side of the groove

BOX 7-1

Procedure for Inserting Lenses Into a Nylon Cord Frame

1. If necessary, remove the old cord.
2. Cut the end of the new cord at an angle.
3. Thread the nylon cord through the lower, temporal hole from the lens side and continue through the upper hole leaving 1.5 to 2.0 mm.
4. Put the lens in and pull the cord snug to size the lens.
5. Hold the excess end of the cord with the thumb and remove the lens.
6. Take up 1.5 to 2.0 mm of slack in the cord.
7. Thread the remaining cord through the upper hole.
8. Cut the cord off 1.5 to 2.0 mm past the hole.
9. Press the excess cord into the frame groove on both sides.
10. Insert the lens in the upper half of the frame.
11. Stretch the cord around the lower half of the lens using the plastic strip.
12. Check cord tension. (Cord should give 0.5 to 1.0 mm.)

may have a tendency to chip, especially during insertion and removal. Plus lenses and thin, high index minus lenses with narrow vertical dimensions may have notably thin areas. Here are some suggestions to avoid chipping thin lens edges:[5]

When putting the nylon cord into the lens, if possible, start with the thinnest part of the lens and finish with the thickest.

To remove a nylon cord, do the reverse; start with the thickest part of the lens edge and end with the thinnest.

Retightening a Loose Nylon Cord Lens

If a lens in an old nylon cord frame is loose or has fallen out, it is prudent to simply replace the cord, as above, rather than retightening the existing cord. Over time an old cord may have lost some of its elasticity. The new cord will have more elasticity, and replacing the old cord avoids the possibility of it breaking later on.

Some dispensers have resorted to removing the lens and heating the old cord. The heat will cause the cord to shrink. When the lens is reinserted, it will be tighter—but only temporarily. Tightening a lens in this manner is not a good practice. The cord will not remain tightened long, and the lens may fall out

unexpectedly, this time to break or become badly scratched.

Nylon Cord Frames With Liners

Some nylon cord frames have liners that fit into the top eyewire channel of the frame. These liners are called *figure 8 liners* because when viewed from the end (in cross section) the liner looks like the number 8. One part of the 8 is smaller than the other.

If it is necessary to replace the figure 8 liner in the top eyewire, take a knife blade, file, or dental pick and dig into the liner, sliding it out either end. Measure the old length of liner and cut a new piece of the same length. To aid in inserting the figure 8 liner back into the top eyewire, make sure the new piece is cut at an angle.

Using the smallest side of the figure 8 first and beginning either nasally or temporally, slide the liner into the top eyewire channel. Feed in the entire piece of liner and center it in the channel. If the liner seems loose, turn it around and use the larger side. Care should be taken not to block any of the four holes used to hold the nylon cord in place.

Frames With Metal "Cords" for Rims

Some frames are made with very thin metal rims. When lenses for these frames are edged with flat edges and then grooved, the rim of the frame slips into the groove in the same manner as a nylon cord would. Because the metal rims are thicker than a nylon cord, the groove must be made wider than it would for nylon cord frames.

CLEANING FRAMES AND LENSES

In the past, the simplest method of cleaning frames and lenses was to immerse them in a mild detergent solution, rub with the fingers or a soft cloth, and dry with a soft, lint-free cloth. Difficult-to-remove lens spots were taken care of using acetone, with care being taken to avoid getting any acetone on the plastic frame. Now, however, the situation is not so straightforward.

Using some detergents as the last cleaning agent for antireflection-coated lenses is incorrect because some detergents contain additives. Use no detergent that contains citrus (which leaves a residue), and none having creams or abrasive material. Acetone should not be used on polycarbonate lenses.

Tables 7-3 and 7-4 summarize the cleaning agents that should be used or avoided for different frame and lens materials.

TABLE 7-3
Cleaning Of Frames

Frame Material	Use	Avoid
Cellulose acetate Propionate Polyamide	Mild detergent* Ultrasonic unit with ultrasonic cleaning solution	Acetone or acetone replacers Alcohol†
Nylon Carbon-fiber Optyl	Mild detergent Alcohol will work for stubborn spots Ultrasonic unit with ultrasonic cleaning solution	Acetone or acetone replacers
Polycarbonate	Mild detergent Alcohol Ultrasonic unit with ultrasonic cleaning solution	Solvents such as acetone
Metal	Mild detergent Alcohol Ultrasonic unit with ultrasonic cleaning solution	Acetone or acetone replacers (which may remove painted trim)

*A mild detergent is one that has no citrus (which leaves a residue), and no creams or abrasive material. A clear detergent, such as clear Joy, works well.
†Propionate material is sensitive to alcohol. Because it is difficult to tell the difference between cellulose acetate and propionate frames, it is safer to avoid alcohol.

TABLE 7-4
Cleaning of Lenses

Lens Material	Use	Avoid
Glass and CR-39 plastic	Mild detergent, alcohol, acetone, or acetone replacer such as "Solves It"*	Abrasives
Polycarbonate and High Index Plastic	Mild detergent or alcohol	Acetone
AR Coated Lenses	AR Coating Lens Cleaner (It is possible to use a mild detergent first, then an AR lens cleaner.)	Detergents with citrus, creams, or abrasive material Acetone Ultrasonic cleaning units

*Available from SeeGreen, Los Angeles, Calif.

REFERENCES

1. Hilco TempMaster Frame Warmer Instructions, Plainville, Mass, Hilco.
2. Bruneni J: Heating carbon frames, Optical Dispensing News, no 33, 2003.
3. Ophthalmic frame: plastic materials guidelines: Bell Optical Laboratories, Dayton, Ohio, undated.
4. How to work with Optyl: Norwood, NJ, 1976, Optyl Corp.
5. Tibbs R: Cord counsel, Optical Dispensing Newsletter, Oct 24, 2000.

Proficiency Test

(Answers can be found in the back of the book.)

1. True or false? When inserting a lens, if success is not achieved on the first try, heat the frame and the partially inserted lens together, then push the partially inserted lens the rest of the way into the bevel.

2. True or false? The lower eyewire of the frame is rolled forward (i.e., front side slanted down) when the lens is inserted. After several attempts to straighten it and reinsert the lens, the forward-rolled eyewire still remains a problem. One solution is to straighten the eyewire and try inserting the lens from the back.

3. If salt from a salt pan sticks to the frame, what may be done to alleviate the problem?
   a. Use newer salt.
   b. Have the heating element checked.
   c. Add talcum powder to the salt.
   d. Use a better product line of frames.
   e. Wash the frames ahead of time.

4. A pair of edged multifocal lenses are held back to back. Their segments overlap exactly. Which of the following statements should **not** be made? (There may be more than one correct response.)
   a. The cylinder axes are correct.
   b. There will be no unwanted vertical prism in the prescription.
   c. Neither of the lenses was edged in a twisted position.
   d. The segment heights are equal.
   e. The total segment insets are equal.

5. The best way to heat nylon frames is by using:
   a. salt.
   b. glass beads.
   c. hot forced air.
   d. hot water.
   e. sand.

6. What type of frame may be heated until it bends under its own weight?
   a. cellulose acetate and propionate frames
   b. Optyl frames
   c. nylon frames
   d. polyamide frames
   e. none of the above

7. What frame material(s) shrink(s) when plunged into cold water?
   a. polyamide
   b. cellulose acetate
   c. Optyl
   d. carbon fiber
   e. propionate

8. What frame material(s) may shrink slightly when heated?
   a. polyamide
   b. cellulose acetate
   c. Optyl
   d. carbon fiber
   e. propionate

9. Which frame materials do best by "cold snapping" the lenses into place?
   a. polyamide
   b. Optyl
   c. carbon fiber
   d. polycarbonate
   e. Kevlar

10. Types of frame materials that do not adjust very well are:
    a. polyamide
    b. Optyl
    c. carbon fiber
    d. polycarbonate
    e. cellulose acetate

11. True or false? Polycarbonate frames neither stretch nor shrink when heated.

12. A pair of frames is labeled "Optyl." The temples have metal reinforcing running the length of the temples. These temples:
    a. require a considerable amount of heat before being adjusted.
    b. do not require very much heat before being adjusted.

13. How much should an edged lens for an Optyl frame usually deviate from the marked frame size?
    a. 0.2 to 0.4 mm smaller than marked
    b. exactly as marked
    c. 0.2 to 0.6 mm larger than marked
    d. 0.6 to 1.0 mm larger than marked
    e. 1.0 to 1.4 mm larger than marked

14. To remove the lenses after a cellulose acetate frame is heated, it is easiest to push a lens out by placing the thumbs on the:
    a. front side of the lens temporally, pushing the lens with the thumbs while pulling the eyewire with the fingers.
    b. front side of the lens inferior nasally, pushing the lens with the thumbs while pulling the eyewire with the fingers.
    c. back side of the lens centrally, pushing the lens with the thumbs while pulling the eyewire with the finger.
    d. back side of the lens superior temporally, pushing the lens with the thumbs while pulling the eyewire with the fingers.
    e. back side of the lens inferior nasally, pushing the lens with the thumbs while pulling the eyewire with the fingers.

15. Eyewire closure pliers are used:
    a. to press a stubborn lens into an eyewire that is otherwise too small for the lens.
    b. to form the eyewire of a metal frame to the meniscus curve of the lens.
    c. to close the eyewire of a metal frame around the lens to allow for lens size evaluation.
    d. to grasp the eyewire of the frame while tightening the eyewire screw.

16. True or false? Hand edging a chemically treated glass lens without retreating it is acceptable. It is not necessary to chemically treat the lens again like it is necessary to reheat treat a heat-treated glass lens after hand edging.

17. When restringing a nylon cord mounting, the ends of the cord are threaded through two holes in the nasal and two holes in the temporal side of the frame. Which hole is threaded first?
    a. The cord is always threaded through the upper hole first.
    b. The cord is always threaded through the lower hole first.
    c. It does not matter which hole is threaded first.

18. We are inserting a grooved lens in a nylon cord frame. The nylon cord is the correct length and in the mounting. Now the upper part of the lens is pressed into the upper eyewire of the frame. When this is being done, where should the cord be?
    a. On the front surface of the lens.
    b. In back of the lens.
    c. Cord position does not matter.

19. To get the end of a nylon cord out of the groove mounting when it is stuck in the groove, the best thing to use is:
    a. your fingernail.
    b. finger nail clippers.
    c. a tooth pick.
    d. a dental pick.

20. For a nylon cord frame, the tension of the cord is checked before removing the plastic strip used to slip the cord into the lens groove. The strip is positioned toward the bottom of the lens until it is close to the midpoint of the lens cord. The cord is pulled fairly hard with the strip. The strip:
    a. should pull the cord about 0.5 to 1.0 mm away from the edge of the lens.
    b. should pull the cord about 1.5 to 2.0 mm away from the edge of the lens.
    c. should pull the cord about 2.5 to 3.0 mm away from the edge of the lens.
    d. should not pull the cord away from the edge of the lens at all.

21. True or false? When the cord of a nylon cord frame has lost its elasticity, remove the lens and heat the cord. This will shrink the cord, retightening the lens. The lens will remain tight almost as long as it did after first being inserted.

22. When the lens is completely inserted into the frame bevel, yet the lower edge appears to be sticking out slightly, what is the problem most likely to be?

23. What type of lens will not give evidence of being twisted or rotated in the frame when being checked in a lensmeter?

24. A pair of glasses is being verified. One lens is obviously in a rotated position, yet the axis of the cylinder for this lens is correct when read on the lensmeter. What might be the cause?

25. If a cellulose acetate frame has been stretched by a previous lens that was ground too large (making the new lenses too small for the frame), what is the best way to remedy the problem?

26. What is the easiest way to check for a rotated lens after lens insertion when the lenses are flat top multifocals?

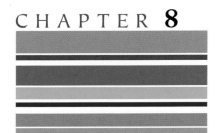

CHAPTER **8**

Standard Alignment

A dispenser must be able to bring a frame into proper alignment before he or she can make a pair of glasses fit properly. Actual manipulative procedures required in fitting are first studied and mastered while learning to "true" the frame. This chapter both teaches proper standard alignment and prepares the groundwork for frame fitting.

STANDARD ALIGNMENT OR "TRUING" OF FRAMES

A frame received from an optical laboratory is theoretically supposed to have been *trued* (i.e., brought into standard alignment). A frame in standard alignment has been adjusted to certain impersonal standards that are independent of the type of face to which it is to be fitted. Standard alignment is intended to ensure that adjustments required to fit the wearer are responsive to the wearer's physical characteristics and not to irregularities in the frame itself that may be produced while the frame is fashioned in the laboratory.

Since, in actual fact, some frames may not have received this adjustment in the laboratory, it is essential that it be performed by the dispenser before attempting to adjust the spectacles for the individual wearer. The best time to preadjust is when the prescription is being verified.

"Truing" spectacles is a good starting point for adjusting them, especially spectacles that have been worn for a long time without recent adjustment. The same would apply to spectacles brought in by someone other than the wearer, or spectacles that have been stepped on, run over, or damaged in some other way. These frames must be brought back into standard alignment before additional adjustments can be attempted.

A general rule for standard alignment is to begin with the bridge, then work with the endpieces, and handle the temples last. Obviously, changes made in one part of a frame may influence the alignment in another part. Bending the bridge, for example, may change the relationship of the temples. Handling the bridge first, and the other parts in order, helps to eliminate having to go back and realign parts.

Adjustable plastic frames must almost always be heated to be aligned. Metal frames and parts do not require heating, except for metal parts that are covered with plastic.

This chapter is divided into sections on bringing plastic frames, metal frames, nosepads, and rimless frames into standard alignment. For instructional purposes, it is easier to consider each of these as separate and distinct types. In practice, however, there are a great variety of frames having characteristics that cross over. Some frames are hybrids of two or more types. This means that, in the end, the dispenser must often use the techniques learned in more than one section on a single frame.

It is advisable to first read the section on plastic frames before jumping to the metal or rimless sections. This is because the first section introduces terminology that is used, but is not as thoroughly explained, in the later sections.

SECTION A
Standard Alignment of Plastic Frames
HEATING THE FRAME

Standard plastic frames* must be heated for any alignment. Standard procedure for adjusting the frame should be followed, beginning with the bridge.

Only that area of the frame requiring adjustment should be heated to avoid the possibility of disturbing an aligned area by mistake. Frames may be heated using forced hot air, or a "salt pan" containing heated table salt, or a pan containing heated small glass beads. The method of choice for heating frames is forced hot air.

Hot Salt or Glass Beads

Even though an explanation of how to use hot salt or glass beads is included, it should be noted that it is not recommended. Forced hot air is preferable because some of the newer frame materials are adversely affected by heating them using a salt pan. In addition, lens coatings may be damaged by the heat and abrasion of hot salt against the surface. Even if the coating appears undamaged after heating using a salt pan, the coating may not

---

*Cellulose acetate and cellulose propionate frames are considered to be standard plastic frames. For more on how various plastic frames respond to heat, see Chapters 1 and 7.

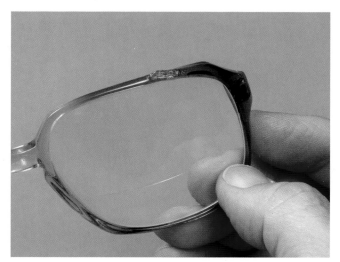

Figure 8-1. An example of a frame that has been overheated, resulting in bubbling of the plastic on the upper rim.

BOX 8-1

Points to Remember in Heating Frames

WITH HOT AIR:
1. Heat only the portion of the frame to be worked on.
2. Rotate the frame in the heat. (This is especially important for warmers having heat coming from one direction only.)
3. Check the type of frame material. Some materials can stand more heat than others.

WITH SALT OR BEADS:
1. Ask yourself, "Should this frame material or these lenses be subjected to salt or beads?" If there is any doubt, use hot air.
2. Always stir the salt (or glass beads) first.
3. Keep the area of the frame being heated parallel to the surface of the salt.
4. Keep the frame moving slowly.
5. Heat only the portion of the frame to be worked on.

---

last as long. If lenses are returned in an unexpectedly short time because of a haziness or crazed* surface when normal care has been exercised by the wearer, the difficulty may have begun right in the dispensary. New dispensers have difficulty identifying frames or lenses that would be damaged with indiscriminate use of a salt pan. Therefore, if a salt pan is being used in the practice, it is safer to require novices to use a forced air warmer.

When using a salt pan, stir the salt to equalize the heat before inserting the frame. A wooden spoon is an excellent tool for this purpose; it does not get hot to the touch and can also be used to push the salt into mounds for heating specific parts.

Insert the frame into the salt just under the surface and as parallel to the surface as possible. The frame may bubble or distort if it is angled so that one portion is too close to the heating element (Figure 8-1). Moving the frame about while in the salt also helps to prevent this problem. If the frame is not moved, even cellulose acetate frames may acquire small indentations in the plastic surface. These small indentations will appear to dull a smooth, highly polished jet black frame. For this reason, some advise against using a salt pan for black frames.

Talcum powder may be mixed with the salt to prevent the salt from sticking to the frame and from lumping. Salt will also stick to a frame that has been cooled in cold water and again placed in the salt while still wet. For this reason, warm-air heating is preferable for a wet frame.

Forced Hot Air

The method of choice for heating frames is forced hot air. When using hot air to heat a frame, move or rotate the frame to prevent overheating of one area and to ensure even heating of the different surfaces, especially

if the hot air warmer only supplies air from one direction. The surface plastic of a frame will bubble if overheated by forced hot air on one side only. This may happen before the frame is hot enough to become pliable.

For a summary on heating frames, see Box 8-1.

THE BRIDGE

Since a number of things may be in error in relation to the bridge, the bridge itself is judged mainly by the effect it has on the plane of the lenses. Readjusting the lenses to their proper planes is accomplished by first heating the bridge area, then grasping the frame by the lens areas and adjusting according to the correction desired.

When using a salt pan to heat the bridge, stir the salt in the pan and form it into a centrally located peak running across the pan. Place the frame in the pan, temples up, and draw the bridge through the peak of the salt mound. Repeat until the bridge is pliable enough to be bent (Figure 8-2).

When using hot air, concentrate the air stream on the bridge. This may be done with a cone attachment placed over the air exit or by partially closing the exit depending on the type of warming unit being used. Move the bridge through the hot air stream until it becomes pliable. Once the bridge is pliable, it can be adjusted as necessary to effect the desired correction.

The bridge can be out of alignment because one lens is pushed up or one lens is pushed back in relation to the other. If one lens is higher than the other, they are said to be out of *horizontal alignment*. If one lens appears to be farther forward or backward than the other, they are said to be out of *vertical alignment*.

---

*Surface crazing is microcracking that looks like dried mud.

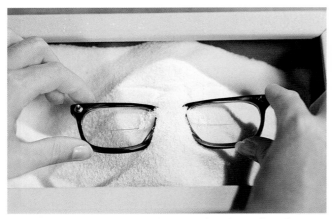

Figure 8-2. To heat the bridge area, first form the salt into a centrally located peak running across the pan, then draw the bridge through the peak of the salt mound.

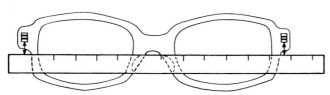

Figure 8-3. Checking for horizontal alignment. This frame shows proper alignment because the distance between ruler and endpiece reference point is equal on both sides.

Horizontal Alignment

It is not easy to check for horizontal alignment of a plastic frame because there are not always clear reference points. To check for horizontal alignment, place a ruler or straight edge across the back of the frame at the top of the pads, if any. If there are no pads, there may be a point where the sculptured shaping of the bridge area ends (this area serves as a nosepad). Both endpieces should be equidistant from the straight edge when it is aligned horizontally (Figure 8-3). A practiced eye may be more helpful than a ruler.

Rotated Lens

There are two common causes for a frame being out of horizontal alignment: a rotated lens and a skewed bridge. A lens rotated in the frame will cause the top of the eyewire to either hump up at the nasal bridge or one endpiece to appear upswept in shape. (See Figure 7-7 in the previous chapter.) To correct the problem, use lens rotating pliers. How this is done is explained in Chapter 7.

Skewed Bridge

When viewed from the front, a skewed bridge will cause one lens to appear higher than the other (Figure 8-4). This problem usually only happens after the glasses have been dispensed and something has happened to them.

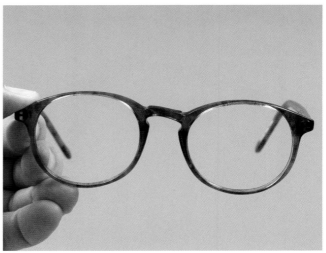

Figure 8-4. An example of a skewed bridge. It will be noted that neither of the lenses shows any twisting. The error is manifested by one lens being higher than the other. (This photo shows the frame from the front. The next photo, correcting the problem, is taken from the back of the frame.)

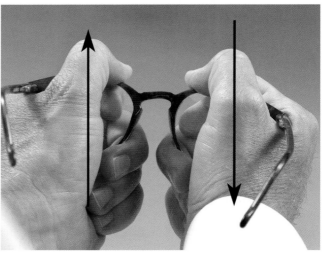

Figure 8-5. To correct for a skewed bridge, heat the bridge and force one side up and the other down. This is the same frame as was shown in the previous figure, but the frame is now facing in the other direction. (Note which way the temples are pointing.)

To correct a skewed bridge, first heat the bridge, then grasp the front with an eyewire in each hand as shown in Figure 8-5. Force the eyewires in opposite directions until the tops of the eyewires are parallel. Of course, the lens must be in the frame for this procedure to succeed. When pressing the lenses in opposite directions, it is important that their frontal planes be kept parallel so that X-ing of the frame is not inadvertently introduced. X-ing will be described in more detail below.

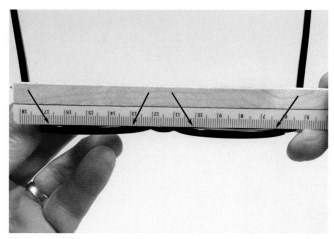

Figure 8-6. Checking for four-point touch. The frame eyewire touches at each place where the ruler crosses the eyewire. This indicates correct alignment when the "frame PD" equals the wearer's interpupillary distance.

Vertical Alignment (Four-Point Touch)

To check for vertical alignment, or *four-point touch*, place a ruler or straight edge so that its edge goes across the inside of the entire front of the spectacles below the nosepad area. Theoretically the frame eyewire should touch at four points on the ruler (i.e., at each place where the ruler crosses the eyewire [Figure 8-6]). However, this ought to only be the case if the frame is small compared with the wearer's head size,* otherwise face form is required.†

Face Form

Face form or *wraparound* is when the frame front is just slightly rounded to the form of the face. Most frames are constructed with at least a degree of face form. This is especially true of large frames and thick metal frames. Frames with face form will not conform to the four-point touch test, but must be symmetrical nonetheless. The temporal sides of the eyewires should touch, and the nasal sides should be equidistant from the ruler (Figure 8-7).

Too much face form would be evident if the two nasal eyewires are a great distance from the ruler. Too little face form is the case if neither temporal eyewire, but only the nasal eyewires, touch (Figure 8-8).

The remedy for either too much or too little face form is to alter the bridge. First warm the bridge until it is pliable, then grasp the frame by the lenses and eyewires with thumbs on the inside and fingers on the outside. Bend the bridge by turning the lenses inward or outward (Figure 8-9).

---

*A strict four-point touch should be used only if A + DBL = wearer's PD.

†For an explanation of why the frame should have face form and how much it should have, see the section on "Face Form" in Chapter 5.

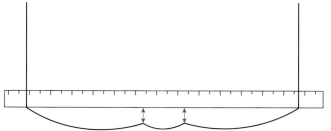

Figure 8-7. For those frames that will not or should not conform to a perfect four-point touch, the nasal sides of the eyewire should be equidistant from the ruler.

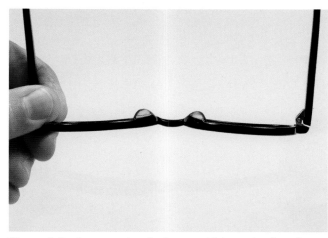

Figure 8-8. An example of a frame with negative face form.

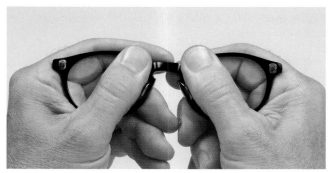

Figure 8-9. As is often the case in dispensing, symmetry is important. To achieve a good bend when changing the face form of a frame, the glasses are grasped symmetrically, immediately adjacent to the bridge.

X-ing

Another type of vertical misalignment may also be discovered while checking for four-point touch. The frame front may be twisted so that the planes of the two lenses are out of coincidence with each other. This is called *X-ing* because the eyewires of the frame front form an X when viewed from the side (Figure 8-10). From below, the frame with X-ing appears as shown in Figure 8-11.

X-ing causes the temples to be out of line with each other. Whenever the temples do not appear parallel, the

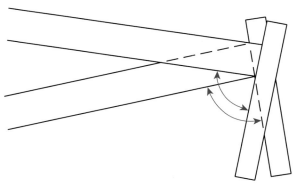

Figure 8-10. X-ing may be identified by the characteristic "X" the eyewires make with one another when viewed from the side.

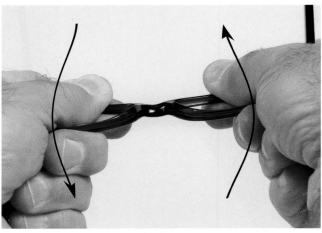

Figure 8-12. In grasping the frame to correct an X-ing error, the wrists move in opposite directions.

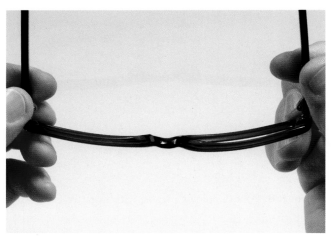

Figure 8-11. This is how a frame with X-ing appears when viewed from below.

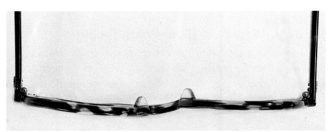

Figure 8-13. Here is an example of lens planes that are variant or out of coplanar alignment. In spite of the improperly bent bridge, the lenses remain parallel to one another.

frame should first be examined for X-ing before other methods of realigning the temples are tried.

X-ing is corrected by grasping the eyewires as shown in Figure 8-12, and rotating the hands in opposing directions until the planes of the lenses are parallel.

Variant Planes

Another form of vertical misalignment is when the lens planes are *variant*, or *out of coplanar alignment*. In this situation, the lens planes are parallel, but one lens is farther forward than the other (Figure 8-13). This error usually becomes apparent when the four-point touch test is used, although it may easily be overlooked otherwise.

To correct a frame with lenses out of coplanar alignment, first heat the bridge and grasp the frame in the manner shown in Figure 8-9, just as would be done in correcting a frame having too much face form. This time, however, push the entire eyewire away from you on one side, and pull it toward you on the other side, all the while keeping both lens planes parallel to each other.

THE TEMPLES

After horizontal and vertical preadjustments have been made to the bridge and eyewires, the third area considered in truing a frame is the temple area. The open temple spread is checked first because the adjustments may affect the endpieces. After this, temple parallelism is considered, followed by alignment of the temple ends. Finally the temple fold angle is corrected.

Open Temple Spread

The *open temple spread*, or *let-back*, is that angle that each open temple forms in relationship to the front of the frame. To afford a true picture of the temple spread initially, the temple shafts must be straight. Before going further, stop and straighten the temple shafts. Any curve to the temple shaft should be eliminated by heating the temple and straightening it with the hands.

It is the normal condition of the temple to be opened out slightly farther than a 90-degree angle; usually 94-95 degrees. Before actually fitting the wearer, it is not always desirable to spread the temples to more than 90 degrees because it may be necessary to bring the temples back in again. This often proves more difficult than was flaring them out originally.

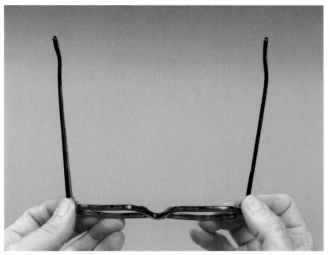

Figure 8-14. The temples on this frame are spread too far for a frame in proper alignment. The spread should be decreased until the temple and the frame front are at a 94- to 95-degree angle to one another.

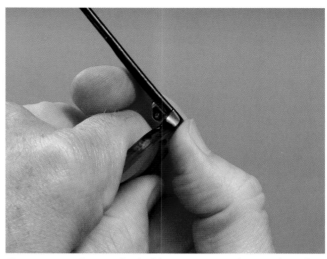

Figure 8-15. One method of decreasing temple spread involves holding the frame by the lens and eyewire while pushing the endpiece back with the thumb.

Temples Spread Too Far

Temples flaring out more than 95 degrees are spread too far for standard alignment (Figure 8-14). There are several methods for correcting this problem, but all involve the same principle: The endpiece must be heated and bent around so that the temple will not be able to open out as far.

With the temple spread to the wide-open position, begin the procedure by heating the desired area. Having the temple fully spread makes it easier to tell when the endpiece has been bent enough. This is because it is possible to see the extent to which the temple is being forced inward. If the frame has a hidden hinge, take care to avoid bumping or knocking the temple because this can loosen it.

The following methods can be used for endpiece adjustment to reduce temple spread:

1. *Using the thumb*—When the endpiece is hot, hold the frame by the eyewire and push on the endpiece with the thumb (Figure 8-15). If there is a metal shield on the frame front, place a cloth between the thumb and the front to prevent burning the skin.
2. *Using a flat surface*—Heat the endpiece and grasp the eyewire and lens with both hands. Use a flat surface, and press the endpiece of the frame down on the surface to force it backward (Figure 8-16, *A* and *B*). The surface must be smooth and free from grit or salt grains. An irregular surface or foreign matter, such as salt grains, will mark the front of the frame when the frame is pressed against the surface.

    Often the corner of the lens may pop out when this method is used. If this happens, turn the frame around and push the corner of the lens with the thumbs while supporting the eyewire from behind

with the fingers. This will pop the lens back into the frame. This may occur several times during the procedure in especially difficult cases and is to be expected.

3. *Bend eyewire and endpiece*—When the endpiece will not bend enough using the above two methods, take the lens out of the frame. With the frame empty, the eyewires and endpiece may be bent backward more easily (Figure 8-17). After reshaping the frame, reinsert the lens.

    Before concluding that the temple has been brought in sufficiently by any of the above methods, however, check between the endpiece and the end of the temple. If a salt pan was used, a few grains of salt can become lodged here and prevent the temple from opening as far as it normally would. The frame appears to be aligned until it is washed off, then the salt dissolves and the temple opens back out.

4. *Bend the butt portion of the temple*—If none of the previous three methods proves successful, this method can be used. It is usually only employed with older frames, and as a last resort because the cosmetic appearance of the frame suffers.

    Heat the temple and grasp the butt end of the temple with half-padded pliers as near the hinge as possible. (Half-padded pliers are shown in Figure 8-18.) Then grasp the temple near the pliers with the free hand and bend the temple inward (Figure 8-19).

5. *Sink the hidden hinge deeper into the frame front*—In cellulose acetate frames with hidden hinges, the temple spread can be reduced by sinking the front hinge slightly deeper into the plastic. This is done by removing the temple and heating the hidden hinge with a soldering iron or a Hot Fingers unit. It does not take very much depth change to

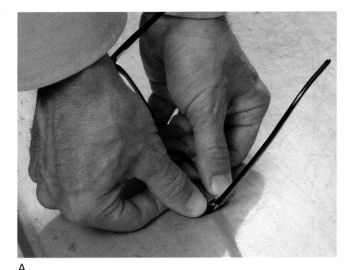

A

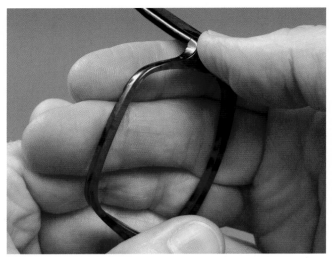

Figure 8-17. Brace both eyewires with the forefinger and press the endpiece with the thumb to decrease the temple spread.

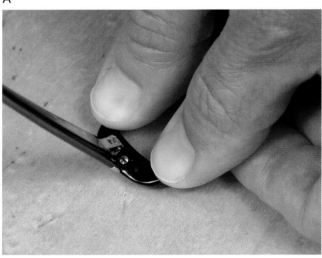

B

Figure 8-16. One of the easiest and most successful methods of reducing temple spread is pressing the endpiece against a flat surface. **A** and **B,** Here are two views of how this is done.

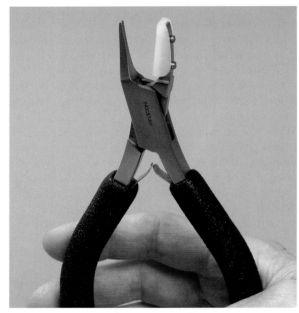

Figure 8-18. Half-padded pliers hold the frame securely. The nylon-padded jaw prevents the frame from being marred by that jaw of the pliers. The unpadded jaw may be flat or rounded.

significantly decrease the temple spread. (For more on how to do this, see the section on Hidden Hinges in Chapter 10.)

Temples Not Spread Enough

Occasionally the temples are not spread enough after the lenses have been inserted and the bridge area straightened. There are at least three things that may be done to correct the problem when this occurs:

1. *The lens may not be completely in the frame at the endpiece.* Check to see if the lens is in place. If not, press the lens back into the groove. This may solve the problem.
2. *The endpiece needs to be bent outward.* Heat the endpiece area and pull the endpiece outward with the fingers while supporting the lens with the

thumbs (Figure 8-20). Never pull on the temple because this will only loosen it and will not get to the root of the problem.

3. *File the butt end of the temple.* When neither of the previous methods work, it may be necessary to file the temple. This may occur when the temples come inward considerably, as when lenses with steep front curves are used. The reason may be the additional curve added to the frame front because the eyewires are shaped to conform to the curved lenses.

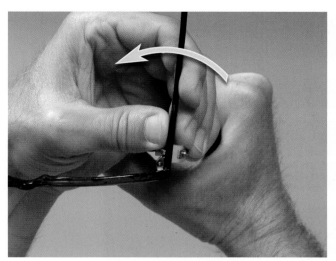

Figure 8-19. If no other method proves successful, it is possible to bring the temples in by grasping the temple butt with half-padded pliers and bending the temple with a free hand.

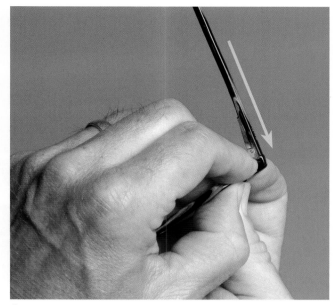

A

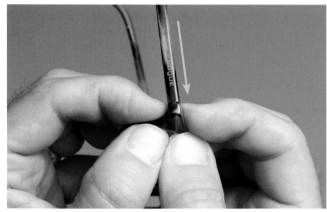

B

Figure 8-20. To spread the temples, heat the endpiece and pull back with the fingers while pressing with the thumbs. (This is shown from two different views in **A** and **B**.) This should cause the angle of temple spread to increase. If, by chance, the lens was not completely in the temporal groove of the frame, it could be a major cause of the temple being insufficiently spread. If the lens is not in the groove, this action should also cause the lens to pop back into place.

To correct this problem, file the end of the temple at the hinge area where it contacts the front of the frame, using a fairly rough file (Figure 8-21). It is extremely important to note that filing for this purpose is done only on the temple—never on the frame front. Individual replacement temples of identical manufacture will often fit at varying angles on the same front. If the front were filed instead of the temple, the result might be an unusually large temple spread if the temples were replaced.

To file the temple, brace the glasses against something solid or hold the frame with the temple folded, with the knuckle of the index finger over the edge of a tabletop for support (Figure 8-22). File the end evenly and uniformly. Periodically, open the temple fully so that its abutment against the endpiece may be observed. Note whether or not the end of the temple is fully touching the endpiece.

One common filing error results in a gap at either the top or bottom of the butt end area of contact with the endpiece (Figure 8-23). A second common error, if the temple is filed too much on the inside, leaves only a small area of contact between the temple and the frame front (Figure 8-24). The first error is particularly undesirable cosmetically. Both errors cause difficulty after a period of wear because the area under concentrated pressure eventually gives way and allows the temple to flare out too far, loosening the glasses.

It is usually not possible to file very far before hitting what appears to be a metal reinforcing piece, which is actually a part of the hinge itself. It does not damage or weaken the frame to file on this piece; in fact, it is unavoidable if much filing is required.

4. *Bend the temple outward.* If none of the above solutions are possible, as a last resort bend the temple outward at a location approximately ¾-inch down the temple from the endpiece. This is usually done using half-padded pliers to hold the butt end of the temple and the other hand to bend to temple outward, similar to the bend that was shown in Figure 8-19.

For a summary of temple spread problems and their solutions, see Table 8-1.

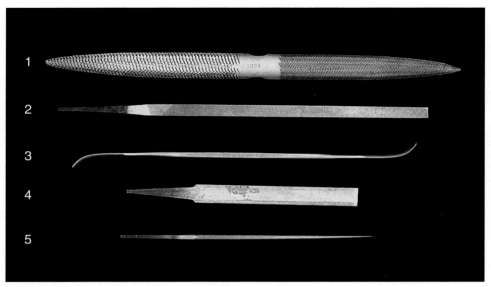

Figure 8-21. Standard files used in dispensing. From top to bottom: *1, Zyl file*—used to file plastic parts of a frame. Although both ends are coarse, one is less coarse than the other for variations in speed of filing. *2, Pillar file*—finer than the zyl file, this file is often used to file metal parts of a frame. *3, Riffler file*—this spoon-shaped file is good for getting at small, hard-to-reach areas. It is used with thumb or finger in the arc of the "spoon." *4, Slotting file*—used for reslotting screws, or making a slot where none previously existed. *5, Rat-tail file*—for classic-type rimless mountings this file was used to reduce lens thickness in an area to allow for proper lens strap grasp. It is also used to smooth the inside of a drilled lens hole.

Temple Parallelism

For frames to be in standard alignment, the temples need to be parallel to one another. One temple should not be angled down more than the other. When looking at the glasses from the side, the angles the temples make with the frame front determine temple parallelism. The angle spoken of here is often called the *pantoscopic angle*. Pantoscopic angle is the angle the frame front deviates from the vertical when the glasses are held with the temples horizontal.*

Viewing the frames from the side, the angle is designated as "pantoscopic" when the lower rims of the frame front are closer to the face than are the upper rims. A proper pantoscopic angle may vary from as little as 4 degrees up to 18 degrees. If the glasses were to be adjusted so that the lower rims are tilted *outward* from the face, the glasses are said to have *"retroscopic"* instead of pantoscopic tilt. Retroscopic tilt is seldom ever appropriate.

In any case, to test whether or not the temples are parallel, position the glasses *upside-down* on a flat surface with the temples open. Then note if both temples sit flat or if one temple is not touching the flat surface. If it is difficult to tell, first touch one temple and then the other to see if the frame wobbles back and forth or if it sits solidly. This procedure is known as the *flat surface touch*

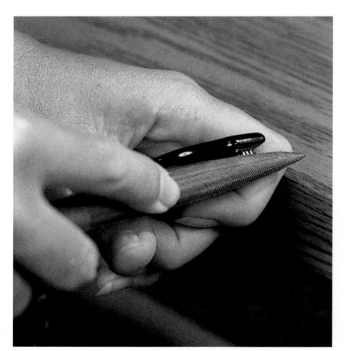

Figure 8-22. Even though a specially designed bench brace is the method of choice, a frame may be successfully held for filing by bracing one knuckle over the edge of a table.

---

*The technically correct definition of the pantoscopic angle refers to the angle formed between the frontal plane of the face and the plane of the frame front when the glasses are being worn.

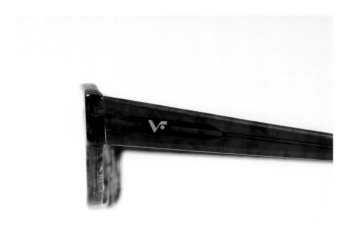

A

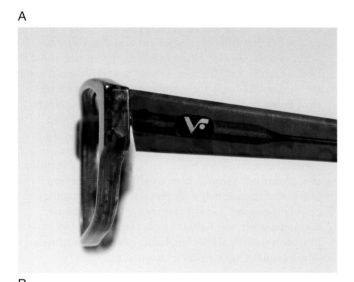

B

Figure 8-23. The frame pictured in **(A)** shows the proper abutment between temple and frame front, whereas the frame in **(B)** is the result of uneven or hurried filings.

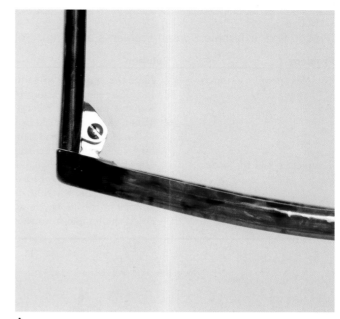

A

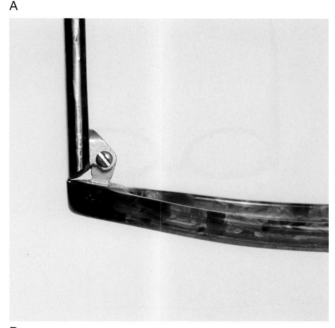

B

Figure 8-24. Viewed from the top, the frame in **(A)** shows how temple and front should abut. The improperly filed temple in **(B)** will not hold alignment. Because so much force is on such a small area, within a short period of time the plastic will be compressed, allowing the temple to open too far.

test (Figure 8-25). If the frame wobbles, it needs correction or it will sit on the face at an angle.

A common mistake is to check for temple parallelism with the glasses placed on the table right side up instead of upside down. If this is done and the bent-down portion of one temple is bent down even the slightest bit more than the other, or if one temple bend is located even the least bit farther forward than the other bend, the flat surface touch test for temple parallelism will not work.

There are five possible sources for incorrect temple parallelism:

1. Incorrect temple parallelism will result if the *endpiece* is not straight. This can happen because:
   a. The lens is not inserted into the frame squarely at the endpiece area. Check this first. It will cause the overall temple angle to be affected. If the lens is only slightly out of the eyewire, heat that area of the frame and press the lens back into the groove. It is usually not necessary to remove and reinsert the lens.
   b. The endpiece is simply angled improperly. If the endpiece was bent upon insertion of the lens, heat the endpiece area. Use the fingers, protected by a lab towel, to bend the endpiece.
2. Another cause of error could be a bend in the *temple shaft* itself (Figure 8-26). This should also be

TABLE 8-1
Plastic Frame Temple Spread Problems and Their Solutions

Problem	Solution
Temples spread too much	1. Heat the endpiece, press it back with the thumb. 2. Heat the endpiece and press it against the table top. 3. Remove the lens and bend the endpiece and the eyewire near the endpiece. Reinsert the lens. 4. When the frame is old or will not respond to the above methods, grasp the temple butt with half-padded pliers and bend the temple as close to the pliers as possible. 5. Sink the hidden hinge deeper into the frame front using a soldering iron or Hot Fingers unit.
Temples spread too little	1. Check to see if the lens is in the temporal groove of the frame. 2. Bend the endpiece forward. 3. File the temple where it abuts with the front. 4. If none of the above are possible, bend the temple outward at a location approximately ¾-inch down the temple from the endpiece.

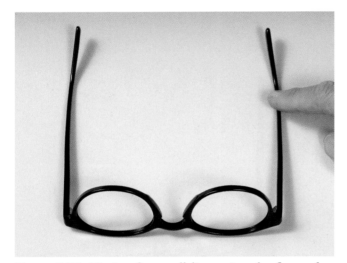

Figure 8-25. Testing for parallelism using the flat surface touch test.

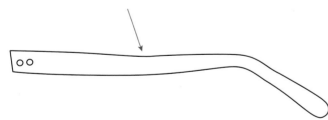

Figure 8-26. A bend in the shaft of one temple may cause the glasses to wobble when placed on a flat surface with the temples open.

checked early on as it can easily occur, but is also easily corrected. This situation is readily solved by heating and straightening the temple shaft.

3. It is even possible for temples to stray from parallel because the bridge of the frame has been twisted. This problem should have been discovered earlier in the alignment process and is called X-ing. It was explained earlier.

4. For frames without hidden hinges, the problem might be that of loosened or broken *hinge rivets*. This should also be ruled out. The rivets are most likely involved if the temple seems wobbly even after the screw has been fully tightened. (For more on this, refer to the section called *Repairing the Hinges* in Chapter 10.) A loose hidden hinge could also cause the same problem. (Again, see Chapter 10.)

5. After the above problems have been ruled out, the *hinges* themselves are likely at fault and may require straightening. Here is how to solve the problem. Close the temple a few degrees from the completely opened position. Grasp the frame front near the endpiece with one hand. Angle the temple by grasping it with the other hand near the butt area and forcing it up or down (Figure 8-27).

Since it is not always possible to change the pantoscopic angle using the hands only and no tools, here is a tool-based method to change the angle:

If the endpiece has enough space, grasp it with half-padded pliers. The padded jaw of the plier should be in the front and the unpadded jaw in the back. The jaw in the back is braced against the hinge rivets in the endpiece to support them. Use a second pair of *angling pliers* (Figure 8-28) to grip the hinge by the top and bottom of the screw. Angle the hinge by twisting the pliers until one temple is level with the other (Figure 8-29). As when making the adjustment without pliers, the temple should be closed very slightly so that the temple butt end is not in contact with the endpiece. If this is not done, the bend is hindered by contact between temple and endpiece.

If there is not enough space to grasp the endpiece, use the angling pliers alone, and hold the frame front with the hands to change the pantoscopic angle.

NOTE: The frame should *not* be heated when any of the pantoscopic angling operations are performed, since softening of the plastic may result in loosening of the rivets. A hidden hinge may accidentally be detached entirely from the front if the frame is heated.

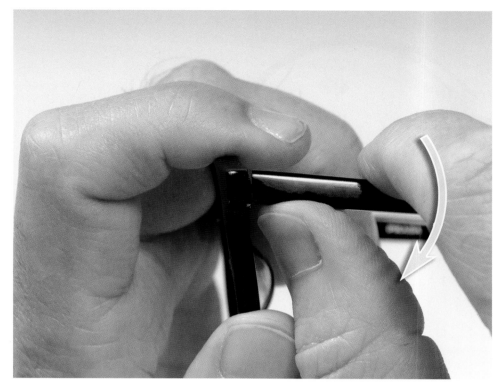

Figure 8-27. This photo shows a commonly used method for changing the pantoscopic angle of the temple. This will not be successful if the temple is fully opened. If it is, there is no space to angle the temple. The butt of the temple must not quite be in contact with the frame front.

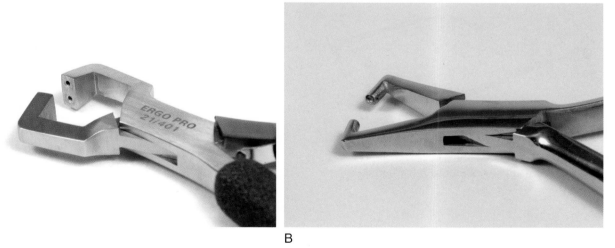

A

B

Figure 8-28. Angling pliers. Traditional angling pliers are shown in **(A)**. Note the indentations on the inside of the jaws used to grip the screw. Since these pliers are a bit bulky and sometimes difficult to get into hard-to-reach areas, a modified, a narrower version is shown in **(B)**.

For a summary of possible sources for unevenness of pantoscopic angles, see Box 8-2.

Aligning the Temple Ends

Proceeding toward the back of the frame, the next area to be aligned is the bent-down portion of the temple: the temple ends. When the temple ends are to be bent down, a good standard alignment demands that both ends of both temples be bent down equally as viewed from the side (Figure 8-30).

Both temple ends should also be bent inward very slightly (Figure 8-31) because the average head has this

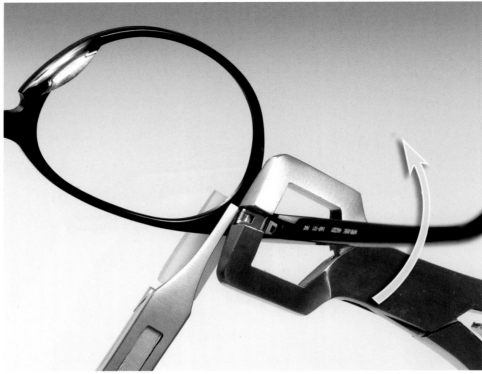

Figure 8-29. This technique for changing the pantoscopic angle is excellent, but cannot always be carried out because of endpiece design. With wrap around endpieces, the endpiece can be grasped at another location.

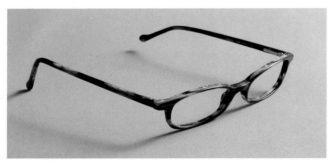

Figure 8-30. In this photo, the temple ends are not bent down equally. Standard alignment requires that both be bent to the same angle.

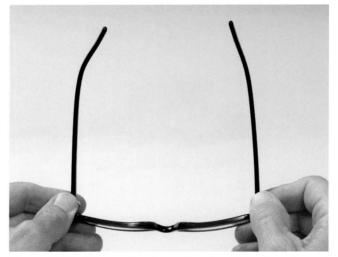

Figure 8-31. The ends of temples should be bent inward slightly to conform to the average head shape. The inward bend should be symmetrical, not like the example shown where the left earpiece is bent farther inward than the right.

BOX 8-2

Possible Problems If Pantoscopic Angles Are Uneven (The Frame Fails the Four-Point Touch Test)

1. The lens is not fully in the temporal frame groove.
2. There is a bend in the endpiece.
3. The temple is bent along the shaft.
4. The frame has a twisted bridge (X-ing).
5. For frames with hinge rivets, a rivet is loose or broken.
6. The hinge is bent, or needs to be bent.

---

conformation. If heating is done with a salt pan, it is important that the ends of the temples be held in the pan parallel to the surface (Figure 8-32, *A*) and not perpendicular (Figure 8-32, *B*). If the temple end is inserted into the salt, the tip is usually overheated.

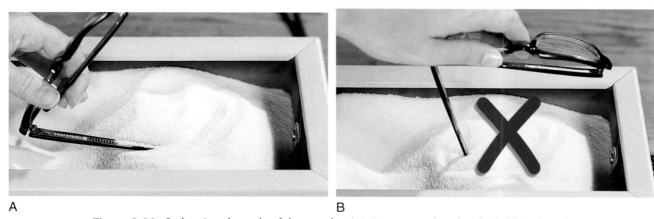

A   B

Figure 8-32. In heating the ends of the temples, it is important that they be held in the salt parallel to the surface, as shown in **(A)**. Sticking the temple end perpendicularly into a salt pan as shown in **(B)** often results in overheating the tip and should be avoided.

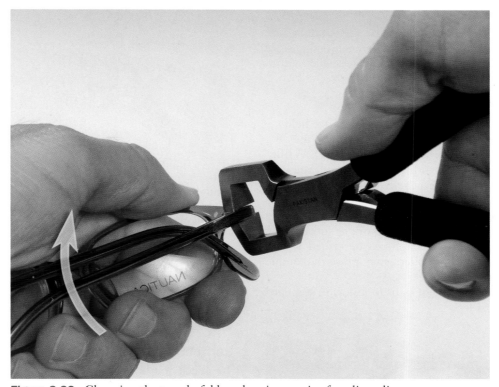

Figure 8-33. Changing the temple-fold angle using a pair of angling pliers.

Temple-Fold Angle

The final alignment step is to fold the temples to the closed position and observe the angle formed as the temples cross. The temples should fold so that they are parallel to one another or form slight angles from parallel. These angles should be symmetrical and should cross each other exactly in the center of the frame, in line with the center of the bridge. Proper adjustment to this configuration permits the spectacle to easily fit into a standard case for glasses.

There are two common methods of changing the temple-fold angle:

1. In the first method, the frame front is held with one hand. Angling pliers grasp the top and bottom of the hinge screw and are used to do the actual bending (Figure 8-33). Since the hinge being bent is metal, it is not necessary to heat the frame.
2. The second method of angling the temple fold uses *finger-piece pliers.* These pliers have jaws that are parallel and have space between the jaws when fully closed (Figure 8-34). They are also referred to as *Fits-U* pliers. These pliers were originally designed for adjusting the old finger-piece mountings, but are also excellent for adjusting the temple-fold

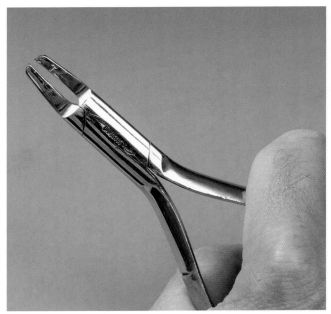

Figure 8-34. Finger-piece pliers were originally designed for adjusting the old finger-piece mountings. These pliers are an excellent tool for adjusting the temple-fold angle.

angle. With the temple folded, the pliers are held parallel to the endpiece hinge screw, so that the hinge is grasped on both sides (Figure 8-35). While the frame front is held with the other hand, the hinge is angled until it reaches the proper position (Figure 8-36).

Changing the temple-fold angle by simply bending the temple with the hands does not work as successfully as using pliers as in the techniques described above. Using hands alone, without pliers, may cause the temple to split at the hinge.

For an overall summary of steps to follow in standard alignment, see Box 8-3.

SECTION B
Standard Alignment of Metal Frames

Metal frames are aligned according to the same principles as plastic frames and, when in standard alignment, should meet approximately the same standards as well. The primary difference lies in the methods of manipulation used to bring the frame into alignment and the presence of adjustable nosepads.

Metal frames require heating only in those places where plastic coats the metal. All other bends are done "cold."

Pliers are used for the majority of adjustments. Since the pressure of metal jaws may mar or disfigure the finished surface of the frames, it is essential to use padded pliers or to cushion at least one jaw of nonpadded pliers by attaching friction or adhesive tape to it.

The order of procedure for aligning metal frames is the same as that used for plastic frames, beginning with the bridge.

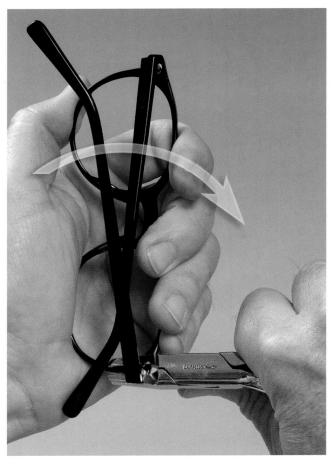

Figure 8-35. With the temple folded, finger-piece pliers are held parallel to the endpiece hinge screw so that the hinge is grasped on both sides.

THE BRIDGE

As with plastic frames, the planes of the lenses are observed to determine bridge alignment as it relates to the overall vertical and horizontal alignment.

Horizontal Alignment

To check for horizontal alignment of a metal frame, place a ruler or straight edge across the front of the frame at the point of attachment of the pad arms. In most frames, the endpieces will be considerably higher than the level of the pad arms, making the horizontal alignment judgment difficult. The endpieces should be equidistant from the ruler.

Rotated Lens

For metal frames, like plastic, there are two common causes for a frame being out of horizontal alignment. The first is a rotated lens, a condition characterized by a nasal or temporal upsweep in one lens causing the tops of the lenses to be out of parallel. To correct for a rotated lens in a metal frame, loosen the eyewire screw and turn the lens until it aligns correctly with its partner; then retighten the screw.

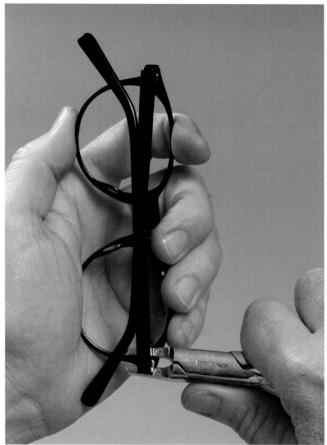

Figure 8-36. While the frame is held with the other hand, the hinge is angled until it reaches the proper position as shown.

BOX 8-3

Steps in Standard Alignment or Truing of Frames

Step 1. Horizontal alignment
 a. Check for a rotated lens.
 b. Check for a skewed bridge.

Step 2. Four-point touch (vertical alignment)
 a. Check for X-ing.
 b. Check for variant planes (or lenses out of coplanar alignment).

Step 3. Open temple alignment
 a. Check the temples for straightness of shaft.
 b. Check for angles of the temples when fully opened for symmetry.

Step 4. Temple parallelism (flat surface touch test)
 a. Check for bent endpiece.
 b. Check for loose or broken rivets or loose hidden hinge.
 c. Check for bend in the temple shaft.
 d. If none of the above is at fault, the hinge is to be bent.

Step 5. Alignment of the bent-down portion of the temple
 a. Check for equality of downward bend.
 b. Check for equality of inward bend.

Step 6. Temple-fold angle
 a. Check for central crossing of the temple shafts when folded.
 b. Check for a fold that permits the insertion of the spectacles into a standard case.

Skewed Bridge

The second cause of horizontal misalignment is a skewed bridge, in which case both lenses are oriented identically but one lens is somewhat higher than the other. Correcting a metal frame with a skewed bridge can be difficult, depending on the bridge design.

To correct bridge skewing with only the hands, grasp the front as was done for a plastic frame, with one eyewire in each hand as was shown in Figure 8-5. Force the eyewires in opposite directions until they are level. Much care must be exercised with this procedure because it is carried out with the lenses in place, making the danger of chipping a lens high.

Horizontal skew cannot always be corrected using pliers because of bridge construction. Metal frames of a bridge construction similar to the rimless variety may be altered as described in the section on rimless and semirimless mountings.

Vertical Alignment (Four-Point Touch)

As when performing the four-point touch test with plastic frames, a ruler or straight edge is necessary to determine whether or not the frame is in alignment. Metal frame construction is so varied, however, that establishing a four-point touch when straddling the inner parts of the frame eyewires is more often impossible than possible. The test is used to analyze the symmetry of the frame front.

Face Form

Metal frames are usually designed with face form, especially in the larger eye sizes. Some very stout metal frames are not intended to meet the literal requirements of the four-point touch test and cannot be adjusted to do so. When checking vertical alignment, there are two questions to keep in mind:

1. Does the frame have a four-point touch or a face-form curve?
2. If the frame has face form, are the two nasal eyewires equidistant from the ruler or is one farther from it than the other?

Either pliers or hands may be used to change the degree of face form in a metal frame. If using pliers, use two pairs to grip the bridge near each eyewire. Rotate the pliers in opposite directions to each other to either increase or decrease the bridge curvature (Figure 8-37). The jaws of both pairs of pliers should be padded to prevent marking the frame.

Frames with reinforcing bars at the bridge do not lend themselves readily to the application of pliers. Most metal bridges may be altered by grasping the lenses and eyewires between the thumbs and forefingers and carefully bending the bridge (Figure 8-38). Undue stress at the lens/eyewire area must be avoided because at this

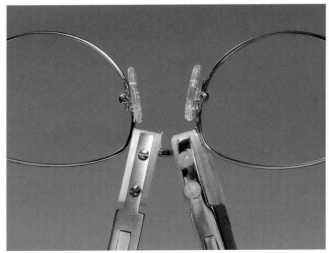

Figure 8-37. These double-padded pliers are rotated in opposite directions to either increase the bridge curvature (add face form) or decrease it. Pliers' jaws coming in contact with metal, especially the outer side of a metal frame, should be padded to avoid marring the finish.

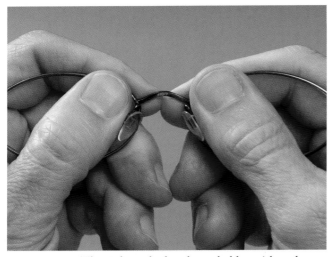

Figure 8-38. This is how the hands are held to either change the face form of a metal frame or to remove X-ing. Care must be taken because undue stress at the lens/eyewire area may result in chipping of the lens edge.

point stress may result in flaking (chipping the edge) of the lens.

X-ing

The misalignment known as X-ing is exactly the same in metal frames as in plastic and can be discovered by the same means. With metal frames, X-ing may be corrected by grasping the lenses and eyewires between the thumbs and fingers as in changing the face form, but apply the pressure in a rotary or twisting manner to align the lenses. As noted, care must be exerted to prevent stress at the lens/frame edge.

It may be possible to correct X-ing with two pairs of pliers. Using double-padded pliers, grasp the bridge in a manner similar to that shown in the previous Figure

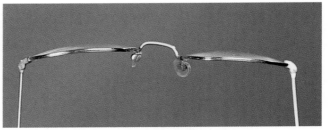

Figure 8-39. When lenses are out of coplanar alignment in a metal frame, the correct procedure for realignment is considerably harder than that with zyl frames.

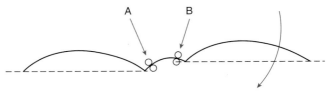

Figure 8-40. In beginning the correction of lenses out of coplanar alignment, the pliers holding the bridge portion nearest the wearer's face (pliers A) are used to hold the frame, while pliers B serve as the bending pliers.

8-37. Pull on one plier while pushing on the other to make the lenses parallel. Using pliers may reduce stress otherwise placed on the eyewires.

Variant Planes

When the misalignment is that of the two lenses being in different lateral positions, yet still parallel to each other (Figure 8-39), the frame can be corrected in one of two ways.

A metal frame with the problem of lenses out of coplanar alignment can often be handled in the same manner as was done for a plastic frame, but without heating it. The frame is bent with the hands by grasping the lenses and eyewires with the thumbs and fingers and forcing the frame into alignment as was seen in Figure 8-9.

If the first method will not work, the second method for variant plane correction uses two pair of pliers and involves two procedures. First, grasp the bridge with two pliers, each a short distance from either eyewire. The pliers holding the bridge portion nearest the wearer's face (pliers *A*) are used to hold the frame, whereas the pliers gripping the bridge portion farthest from the face (pliers *B*) serve as the bending pliers (Figure 8-40). Bend the bridge as if increasing the face form, until the nasal side of the bridge (which had been forward) is on the same plane as that of the other side of the bridge. The lenses will now appear to be angled in relation to each other (Figure 8-41).

Now using pliers *B*, which previously did the bending, as a holding pliers, move pliers *A* to that portion of the bridge between the eyewire and pliers *B* (Figure 8-42). Bend the bridge outward at this point with pliers *A* until the lenses are parallel (Figure 8-43).

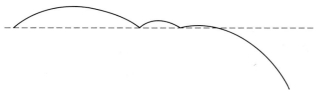

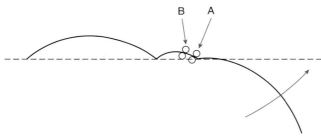

Figure 8-41. The bridge is bent as if the face form were to be increased until the nasal side of the bridge, which had been forward, is on the same plane as that of the other side of the bridge. The lenses now appear angled in relation to each other.

Figure 8-42. Now pliers B that previously did the bending are used as holding pliers. The other pliers (pliers A) are moved to that portion of the bridge between the eyewire and pliers B. The bridge is bent upward at this point by pliers A until the lenses are parallel.

Figure 8-43. The final stage in correcting for lenses out of coplanar alignment returns the metal frame to a proper four-point touch configuration.

THE TEMPLES

As with plastic frames, the temples are used to gauge how the next area is adjusted, starting with the open temple spread. Adjustments often affect the endpieces. After open temple spread, temple parallelism is again checked, temple ends are aligned, and lastly the temple fold is adjusted.

Open Temple Spread

The temple should be at the same angle to the front as it was for a plastic frame; that is 94 to 95 degrees. Also as in the case of plastic frames, it is not usually desirable to spread the temples to more than 90 degrees before fitting them to the wearer.

Temples Spread Too Far (Decreasing the Temple Spread)

If the temples are spread too far apart, there are several ways to bring them back into alignment. Here are a few selected methods.

First method: Use a pair of half-padded pliers as bending pliers. Half-padded pliers have a small metal jaw on one side and a nylon-padded jaw on the other. Grip the outside of the endpiece (Figure 8-44). Hold the front firmly near the endpiece with the free hand. (When

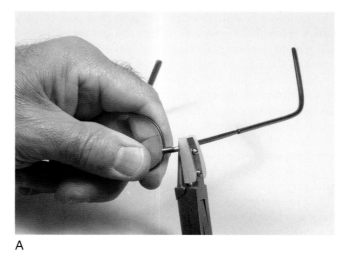

A

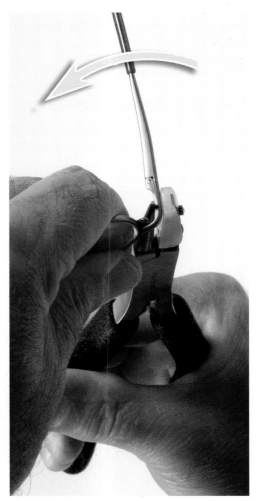

B

Figure 8-44. If the temples are spread too far apart, a pair of half-padded pliers may serve as bending pliers and grip the outside of the endpiece. **A,** Side view. **B,** Top view.

the endpiece is wide enough, use a second pair of thin pliers to hold the endpiece where it joins the eyewire.) Rotate the bending pliers around until the temple has reached the desired temple-spread angle.

Second method: Close the temple and grip the hinge from below with the thin pliers. (Since no visible external frame areas are being gripped, it is not essential that the pliers be padded.) Rotate the pliers, bending the endpiece area inward (Figure 8-45). Because of the risk of chipping the lens, whenever there is sufficient space available, use a second pair of pliers to grip the frame near the lens so that the eyewire area is not stressed (Figure 8-46).

Third method: The endpiece can be bent using another method that does not involve pliers, but only a smooth flat surface. With both hands, hold the frame by the lens and eyewire just adjacent to the endpiece. (The closer to the endpiece the frame is held, the less danger there is of breaking a lens.) Hold the frame front perpendicular to the table surface, and push the endpiece against the surface until there is enough bend to hold the temple at its proper spread angle (Figure 8-47).

Temples Not Spread Enough (Increasing the Temple Spread)

When the temple spread is too small, it can be increased by using the reverse of the first two methods described above for decreasing the temple spread.

First method: This is exactly the reverse of method one above. Grasp the outside section of the endpiece with padded pliers. (This was shown in Figure 8-44.) Bend the endpiece outward to the proper spread while supporting the front at its junction with the endpiece.

Second method: Use the reverse of the second method listed above. Close the temple, grasp the hinge, and bend the endpiece outward. As noted before, certain kinds of frames allow enough space at the endpiece to permit a second pair of pliers next to the eyewire as holding pliers. This takes any possible strain off the eyewire, reducing the possibility of chipping a lens.

For a summary of temple spread problem solutions, see Box 8-4.

BOX 8-4

Alternative Methods of Increasing or Decreasing the Temple Spread on Metal Frames

1. a. Grasp the endpiece with the hand (or when possible, use thin half-padded pliers as holding pliers).
   b. Use thin-padded or half-padded pliers as bending pliers and grasp the endpiece near the hinge. Bend the endpiece in or out.
2. Close the temple, grip the hinge barrels, and bend the endpiece either inward or outward.
3. Push the outside of the endpiece against a flat surface to bend the endpiece inward.

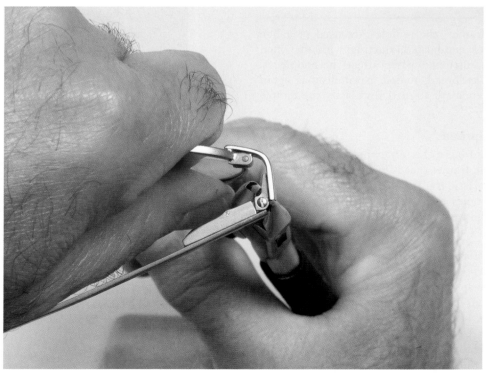

Figure 8-45. Use the hand to grasp the frame front firmly at the endpiece. Decrease temple spread with the pliers. If there is risk of chipping the lens, remove the lens first.

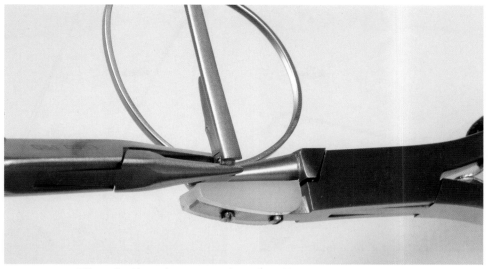

Figure 8-46. The risk of lens chipping can be reduced by using holding pliers while reducing temple spread.

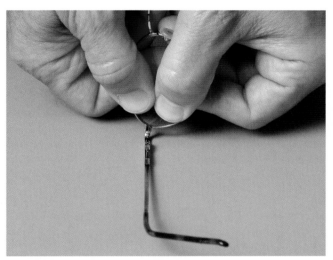

Figure 8-47. To decrease temple spread, the frame front may be held perpendicular to a flat surface and the endpiece pushed against it.

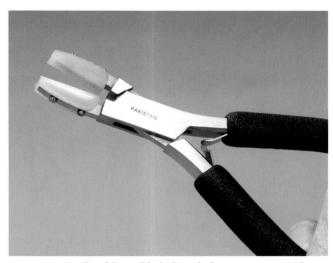

Figure 8-48. Double-padded pliers help to prevent marks on the frame during frame adjustment.

Temple Parallelism (Changing the Pantoscopic Angle)

Temple parallelism refers to the relative pantoscopic angles as viewed from the side. Testing proper temple parallelism is done in exactly the same manner for metal frames as for plastic.

Place the glasses upside down on a flat surface and note if one or both temples touch the surface (flat surface touch test). If the frame wobbles, the pantoscopic angle must be adjusted.

The normal pantoscopic angle varies anywhere from 4 degrees to 18 degrees. By keeping this in mind, it is relatively easy to decide which temple to bend up or down. If the difference between the two angles is extreme, it may be necessary to bend one temple up and one down to make the angle equal on both sides.

There are several ways to change the pantoscopic angle of a metal frame:

1. *Hands only.* The simplest way is to grasp the eyewire and lens close to the endpiece on the same side of the frame as the temple that needs to be angled and bend the temple up or down by hand. The frame will bend at the endpiece or at the hinge.

   Though not desirable, it is sometimes necessary to close the temple a few degrees to allow the hinge to bend. One disadvantage to this method is that it may leave a V-shaped gap at the point where the temple butt and endpiece join. This should be avoided.

2. *Two padded pliers.* Using a pair of bracing pliers with one metal and one nylon jaw (half-padded pliers), hold the endpiece on the front of the frame if there is room, or just anterior to the hinge if there is not. The second pliers, used for bending, should be double-padded pliers (Figure 8-48) to grasp the

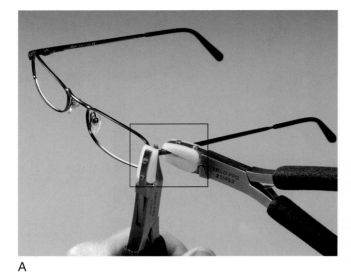

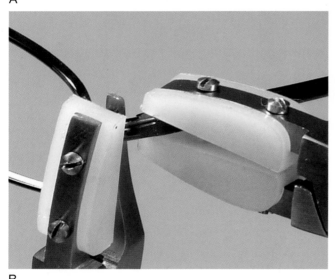

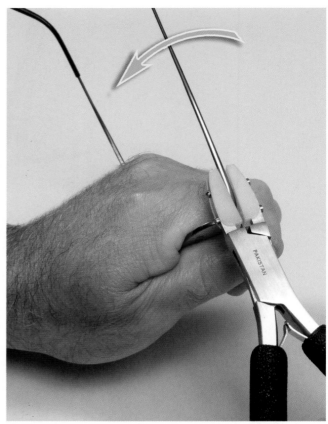

Figure 8-50. When the endpiece is too small, the pantoscopic angle can be changed without holding pliers. If the frame does not have enough flexibility, the lens may be removed first.

B

Figure 8-49. To change the pantoscopic angle, hold the end-piece, grasp the top and bottom of the hinge area, and reangle the temple.

temple close to or directly on the hinge. It may be prudent to remove the lens if the frame is stiff or there appears to be a possibility of chipping the lens. Grasp the frame as shown in Figure 8-49, and reangle it up or down.

3. *One hand and one double padded pliers.* It may be possible to do the bend as described in the previous method without a pair of bracing pliers. This may be done by grasping the endpiece and temple from the front with the double-padded pliers parallel to the temple as shown in Figure 8-50.

4. *One hand on frame front and angling pliers.* Another method of changing the temple-angle is to bend the endpiece with angling pliers. Grip the hinge by the screw head and tip of the screw with the angling pliers (Figure 8-51, *A* and *B*). Holding the frame front firmly, rotate the angling pliers until the desired angle

is reached. The front may be held by the hand near the endpiece, or the endpiece may be secured with pliers to better ensure against chipping the lens.

5. *Gripping the eyewire screw.* When one method does not seem to work, or helps but does not fully accomplish the task, there must be other ways to do the same thing. With some frames it is possible to change the pantoscopic angle by grasping the eyewire screw and angling the temple as shown in Figure 8-52. Only frames constructed in certain ways will allow for this. And this should not be used as the first attempt to change the pantoscopic angle, either.

6. *Angling pliers and one hand on temple.* Angling pliers may be used to change the pantoscopic angle without affecting the endpieces. This may be useful if the endpieces appear to be even. Grip the hinge with angling pliers in the customary manner. This time, however, do not rotate the pliers; instead use them as holding pliers. With the other hand, bend the temple shaft down (Figure 8-53). The pantoscopic angle correction is produced by a change in the hinge angle instead of by a change in the endpiece angle.

For a summary on changing the pantoscopic angle with metal frames, see Box 8-5.

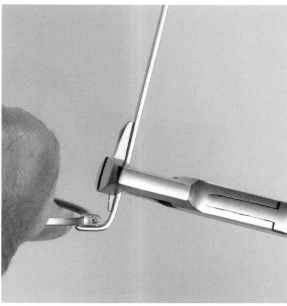

A   B

Figure 8-51. The pantoscopic angle of the temple angle may be changed by gripping the top and bottom of the temple screw with angling pliers and bending the temple upward or downward. This is shown from a side view in **(A)** and from a top view in **(B)**.

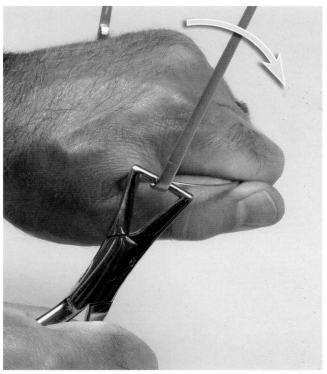

Figure 8-52. Here the pantoscopic angle is changed by grasping the eyewire screw instead of the hinge. Notice that thin angling pliers are used because the standard angling pliers may be too bulky to get into this small area.

BOX 8-5

Alternative Methods of Changing the Pantoscopic Tilt on Metal Frames

1. a. Grasp frame front close to hinge.
   b. Bend temple down by hand.
2. a. Hold the endpiece with half-padded pliers (see Figure 8-48).
   b. Grasp temple on top and bottom of hinge with double-padded pliers.
   c. Bend up or down.
3. a. Hold frame front with hand (see Figure 8-50).
   b. Grasp temple on top and bottom of hinge with double-padded pliers.
   c. Bend up or down.
4. a. Hold front near endpiece with hand (see Figure 8-51).
   b. Grip hinge with angling pliers.
   c. Bend with pliers.
5. a. Hold front near endpiece with hand.
   b. Grasp eyewire screw with angling pliers (see Figure 8-52).
   c. Bend with pliers.
6. a. Hold hinge steady with angling pliers (see Figure 8-53).
   b. Grasp temple with hand and bend down.

Aligning the Temple Ends

The endpiece, or bent-down portion of metal frame temples are aligned in the same manner as that used for plastic frames. Several precautions must be taken, however, to keep from damaging the frame during the adjustment process.

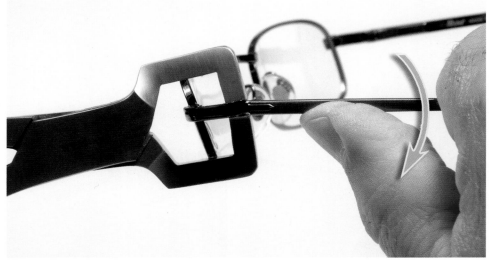

Figure 8-53. The temple angle may be changed by bending the hinge instead of the endpiece itself. This can be done using angling pliers to hold the hinge while the temple shaft is bent down with the other hand.

The conventional skull temple on a metal frame usually has a plastic covering over the end of the temple. This affords a more comfortable fit. Because of the plastic, it is usually necessary to apply some degree of heat to this part of the frame before it can be manipulated to effect adjustments. Different types of temples require varying amounts of heat.

Temples with a clear plastic covering heat very quickly and should be heated only slightly (just slightly warmer than body temperature). The plastic can easily be bubbled by overheating or distorted by being bent while too pliable. New frames bend quite satisfactorily at low or no temperature. The plastic in old frames, however, is usually too brittle to bend without more extensive heating.

Other frames have a fairly heavy piece of metal running through the temple ends. These frames exhibit more resistance to bending because of the thickness of the metal. A common error is to assume that this resistance is due to insufficient heating. The result is overheating and distortion of the plastic when it is bent. To prevent this error, heat the entire plastic portion slightly, but concentrate the heat on the portion that must absorb the bend. Quite a bit of force may be necessary even when the heating is done correctly.

Temple-Fold Angle

The procedure for changing the temple-fold angle in a metal frame varies according to the type of endpiece being used. Two common methods are presented here. One uses double-padded pliers and the other uses half-padded pliers.

In the first method, hold the frame front firmly in one hand and grip the top and bottom of the hinge area with double-padded pliers similar to the manner pictured in Figure 8-54, *A*. Rotate the pliers in the direction neces-

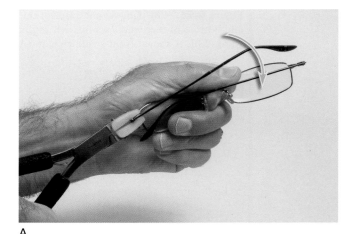

A

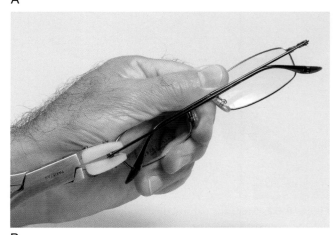

B

Figure 8-54. To change the temple-fold angle on commonly used types of metal frames, hold the frame front in the hand firmly, temples closed. Grip the top and bottom of the hinge area with double-padded pliers as shown in **(A)** and bend the temple so that it returns to and maintains its correct parallel alignment as seen in **(B)**.

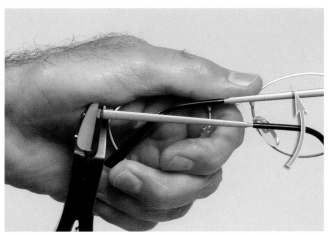

Figure 8-55. The temple fold angle may be changed using half-padded pliers on the endpiece and bending the folded temple to parallel.

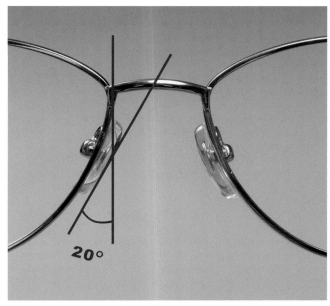

Figure 8-56. In standard alignment of nosepads, the angle most clearly seen when viewing from the front is termed the *frontal angle.*

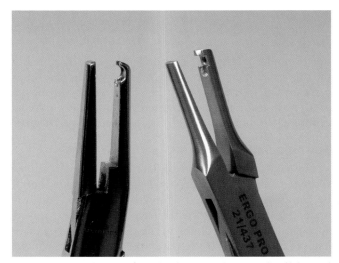

Figure 8-57. The type of pad-adjusting pliers used will depend on the type of pad on the frame.

sary to line up the temples in their correct parallel alignment (Figure 8-54, *B*).

In the second method, the frame front is held by hand in the same manner as method one. With temples closed, the endpiece is gripped with the half-padded pliers as shown in Figure 8-55. The temple is turned until parallel.

SECTION C
Standard Alignment of Nosepads

As with the frame front and the temples, there is a specific standard alignment for nosepads that should be used during the preliminary adjustment of the frame. Obviously, final adjustment of the pads will vary extensively with the individual shape and flare of the nose of the intended wearer. However, pads adjusted to a proper standard initially facilitate individual adjustment later.

There are three basic angles that are used for reference when aligning nosepads. These are the frontal, splay, and vertical angles. To be in standard alignment, these angles must fall within certain limits and be the same for both right and left nosepads.

FRONTAL ANGLE (VIEWED FROM THE FRONT)

The *frontal angle* of the nosepads refers to the vertical position of the pads in relation to each other when viewed from the front. The tops of the pads should be closer together than the bottoms, angling in toward each other approximately 20 degrees from a true vertical (Figure 8-56).

Most pads can be "rocked" about a swivel joint. The pads should be slanted for the frontal angle by the same amount. This is most easily done using pad-adjusting pliers to grip the pad as a whole. Pad adjusting pliers are made in a variety of ways, depending upon the construc-

tion of the nosepads for which they are intended (Figure 8-57). The frame front is held securely in one hand and the pad angled by turning the pliers to the angle desired (Figure 8-58).

When evaluating one of the pads, the play exhibited by that pad should be equal on each side of the desired position for the correct frontal angle. In other words, a pad should not have to be rocked to one extreme in order to match the frontal angle of the other pad.

If one pad has a lot more play in the *amount* of rock it shows, the amount of play may be reduced on some pad types by tightening the looser pad with pliers. The way this might be done depends upon how the pad is made.

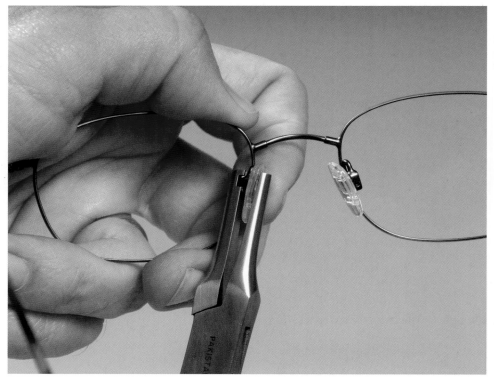

Figure 8-58. The correct method for using pad-adjusting pliers.

For example, it may be done on some pads by pressing on the attachment point with one jaw while the other rests on the face of the pad. For pads which slip into a small box on the pad arm, tighten the amount of rock by crimping the box into which the back of the pad snaps.

Pad Spacing

While viewing the frontal angle, observe the amount of space between the eyewires and pads. Both pads should be equidistant from their respective eyewires. An estimated ideal position is for the face of the pads to appear approximately 1 mm closer to the nose than the eyewire itself (Figure 8-59). If the pads are spread too far apart, the rim of the frame could possibly rest directly on the nose. Both pads should also be equal distances from their respective eyewires; otherwise, the frame will not center properly on the face. Proper correction procedures for these errors are described in detail in Chapter 9 when discussing changing the distance between pads.

Pad Height

A third point of observation is whether or not both pads occupy the same horizontal plane (again, see Figure 8-59). If one pad appears higher than the other, the pad arm may be bent upward. It is essential that both pads be in identical rocking positions because if one is erect and one is slanted, their heights may appear dissimilar. Again, specifics of adjustment technique are described fully in Chapter 9 in the sections that review changing the height of pads.

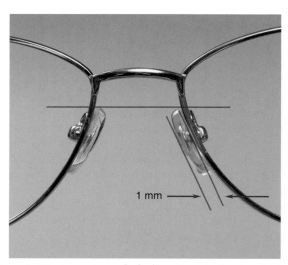

Figure 8-59. An estimated ideal position is that in which the faces of the pads appear approximately 1 mm closer to the nose than the eyewire itself. Both pads should also be at the same height, as shown by the horizontal red line.

SPLAY ANGLE

Remembering that the nose is wider at the base than at the bridge and that the face of the pads should rest fully on the nose, it is apparent that the back edges of the pads should be farther apart than the front edges. This difference then between the back and front edges of each pad, viewed from the top or the bottom, is the *splay angle*.

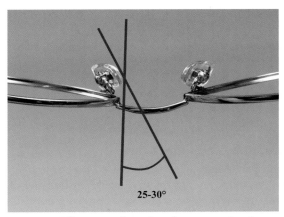

Figure 8-60. The second angle of concern in the proper alignment of nosepads may be seen by viewing the frame from above. This angle is referred to as the *splay angle*.

For initial alignment, a splay angle of 25 to 30 degrees is satisfactory (Figure 8-60) and may be achieved through the use of the pad-adjusting pliers.

VERTICAL ANGLE (VIEWED FROM THE SIDE)

The angle most often neglected in the standard alignment of nosepads is the *vertical angle*. This angle is especially important in ensuring proper weight distribution under the pad. Ideally the longitudinal (top to bottom) axis of the pad face is in contact with the nose surface in the direction of gravity. In other words, the longitudinal axes of the pads should be vertical on the face. (If the nosepads are round instead of elongated, there is no vertical angle.)

Since most spectacles are worn with a certain amount of pantoscopic tilt, the pads will need to be inclined so that the bottoms are slightly closer to the frame front than the tops. Then when the glasses are positioned on the nose with their proper pantoscopic angle, the pads will be approximately vertical (Figure 8-61). For the initial alignment, a vertical alignment angle of approximately 15 degrees is acceptable. This may be achieved in one of three ways:

1. *Using pad-adjusting pliers.* Grasp the pad on its surface with the pliers as was shown in Figure 8-58 and rotate. (In some instances it may be necessary to grip the pad from the top instead of the bottom to adjust the vertical angle.)
2. *Thin-nosed pliers on the pad arm.* For adjusting the vertical angle, because there may not be room to do this adjustment with pad adjusting pliers, thin-nosed pliers are used. The pad arm is grasped directly behind the pad from above or below.
3. *Grasping the box behind the pad arm.* Some nosepads are attached to the pad arms with a small box. It is possible to reangle some pads by grasping the box behind the pad. This is shown in Figure 8-62.

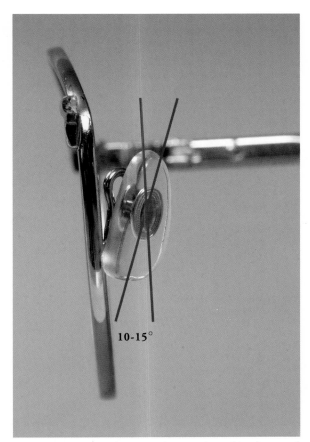

Figure 8-61. The angle most often neglected in the standard alignment of nosepads is the *vertical angle*. This angle is especially important in ensuring proper weight distribution under the pad. When the glasses are worn, the frame front will not be straight up and down, but will be angled. The long axis of the pad will be straight up and down.

Pads Must Have Equal Distances From the Frame Front

While viewing from the side to check for the proper vertical angle, also note the distance of each pad from the front of the frame. Both pads should extend back an equal distance. The pads should be equal not only in height and inclination, but also regarding this distance. If these three details are precise, one pad will practically hide the other when the pair is observed directly from the side. To correct for an error of this nature, use the techniques described in Chapter 9 in the sections on changing the height and vertex distance of pads.

A Humorous Way to Remember the Three Pad Angles*

Here is a clever way to remember which pad angle is which and how they move:

1. Put your thumbs under your arms and flap your arms like a chicken. This movement corresponds to the frontal angle.

---

*Contributed by Dr. Michelle Chen.

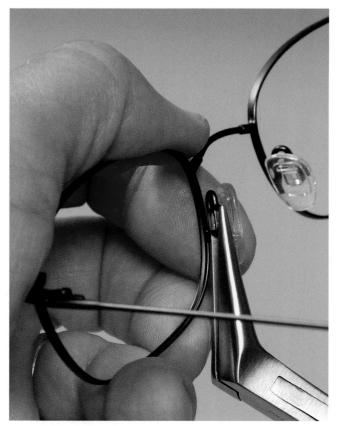

Figure 8-62. If one of the pad angles is out of adjustment, it is possible to correct the angle by grasping the box behind the pad with the pliers and adjusting the angle. Some silicone pads have a tendency to split or tear with stress. This technique avoids the pressure that would be applied to the pad were the pad face to be grasped.

2. Hold your hand straight up in front of you and rotate your wrist in the typical "Miss America" wave. This mimics the splay angle.
3. Imagine being the person on the tarmac at the airport using two orange flashlights to direct an airplane taxiing toward you. To get the plane to move directly toward you, you hold the flashlights straight up and down. Now, bending your elbows, move both flashlights forward and backward. This corresponds to the vertical angle.

SECTION D
Standard Alignment of Rimless Eyewear

RIMLESS CONSTRUCTION AND LENS MATERIALS

In the past, rimless eyewear was the most fragile of eyewear. This made the alignment and adjusting of rimless glasses tedious and risky because it was very easy to chip the lens. This is still the case when older mountings or inappropriate lens materials are used. Rimless are still more difficult to adjust than plastic and metal frames.

Yet when the appropriate tools are used and procedures followed, results and safety are excellent.

Newer mountings use a variety of methods to give extra stability to the mounting. In the past, the lens was held in place with one hole nasally and one hole temporally. Now there may be more than one hole, or a hole and an edge notch used in combination. As a result, these constructions hold their adjustment.

Appropriate Lens Materials

If appropriate lens materials are used for rimless mountings, lens chipping is vastly reduced. At the time of this writing, the best lens materials for rimless mountings are Trivex and polycarbonate. Both hold up extremely well, but Trivex is less likely to develop small stress splits next to the drilled hole. Some labs will only warranty Trivex or Trivex and polycarbonate.

Many high index plastic materials are suitable for rimless, though not performing as well as Trivex and polycarbonate. Though still used some, conventional CR-39 plastic is not a good choice.

Although glass lenses used to be used in rimless mountings years ago, they should not be used now. Chemically tempered glass is physically possible to use with rimless, but inappropriate. Heat-treated glass lenses are impossible. The combination of strain patterns produced by the heat treatment and the induced strain at the mounting points will result in a broken lens in short order.

ALIGNING THE BRIDGE

Whereas the bridge or pad arm origins and the end-pieces serve as the line of reference for frames, the *mounting line* serves as a line of reference for rimless mountings. The mounting line is defined as "the line which passes through the points on the eyewires or straps at which the pad arms are attached.[1]" The end-pieces may be attached on this line, or as may be the case, above or below this line.

Horizontal Alignment

Horizontal skew can be noted by placing a straight edge at the mounting line or parallel to it. If the temples are attached to the lenses on the mounting line, all four points should line up on the straight edge. If the temples are not on the mounting line, the nasal points should be on the straight edge, and the points of attachment of the temples should be equidistant from the straight edge (Figure 8-63).

If the lens is out of horizontal alignment and the frame is new, there is a chance that one lens has been improperly drilled. It may be more likely, however, that the bridge of the frame is bent. Figure 8-64 shows a mounting that is out of horizontal alignment. The problem may be corrected as follows:
1. *Using rimless bracing pliers and double-padded pliers.*
   One of the issues with rimless mountings is

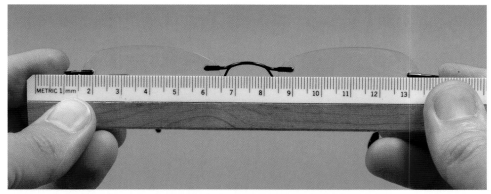

Figure 8-63. Checking the horizontal alignment of a rimless pair of glasses. Here the ruler is placed on the temporal holes. The nasal holes should be equidistant from the ruler.

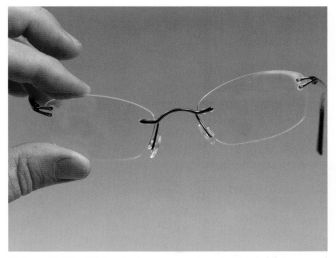

Figure 8-64. This rimless mounting is out of horizontal alignment.

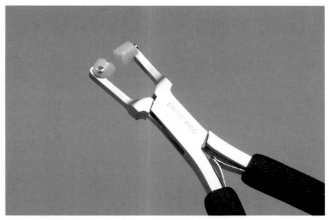

Figure 8-65. Rimless bracing pliers are used to hold rimless eyewear at the point of attachment to the lens. With this particular type of pliers, one jaw is fixed and one jaw pivots. The jaw that pivots (in this figure, the jaw on the left) is to be placed on the front surface to compensate for the lens base curve.

protecting the lens mounting points from stress during the adjustment process. Too much stress on the lens at the mounting point can cause the lens to loosen or fracture. The type of pliers that is designed for reducing stress is referred to as rimless bracing pliers. One example of such pliers is shown in Figure 8-65. The bridge may be realigned by holding a nasal drill point with bracing pliers, grasping the bridge with double-padded pliers, and bending the bridge as shown in Figure 8-66.

2. *Using two pair of double-padded pliers.* A rimless bridge can also be corrected for horizontal misalignment using two pair of double padded pliers as shown in Figure 8-67.

Vertical Alignment (Four-Point Touch)

After the horizontal alignment has been corrected, the next step is checking for a four-point touch. This is done in approximately the same manner as for plastic or metal frames. Place a straight edge on the inner sides of the lenses somewhat below the pads (Figure 8-68, *A*). In

theory the nasal and temporal sides of both lenses should touch the straight edge. Then repeat the test by placing the straight edge somewhat above the pads (Figure 8-68, *B*). The nasal and temporal sides of both lenses should again touch the straight edge. (In practice, because the wearer's PD is usually smaller than the "frame PD", the nasal lens edge may not necessarily touch the straight edge, but must be equidistant from it.)

X-ing

If the nasal and temporal sides of both lenses in *both* upper and lower positions do not touch the straight edge, X-ing of the lenses has occurred. Because of the way rimless lenses are mounted, it would be possible to have a four-point touch exactly in the center of the lenses but still have X-ing. For that reason, the four-point touch test is done at both the top and the bottom of the lenses.

Face Form

While testing for a four-point touch, it may be found that too little or too much face form exists. To increase

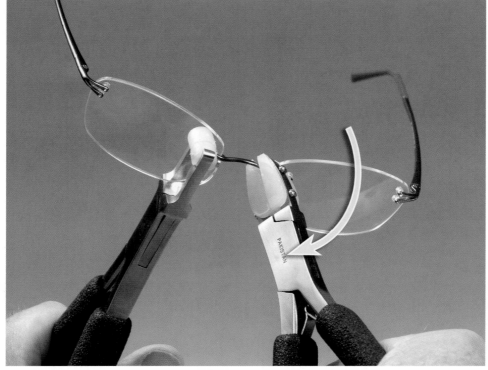

Figure 8-66. Here is one method for adjusting horizontal alignment using a combination of rimless bracing and double-padded pliers. To correct the horizontal misalignment shown in Figure 8-64, hold the nasal point of attachment with the rimless bracing pliers and bend the bridge downward with the double padded pliers.

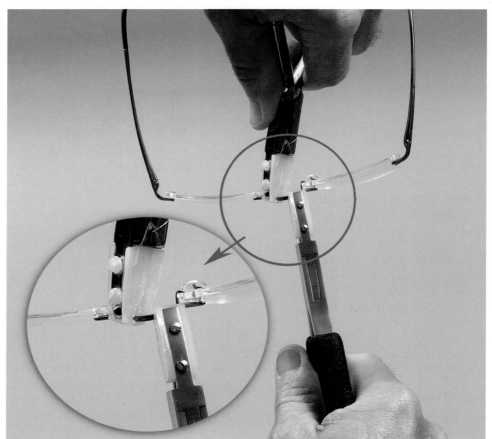

Figure 8-67. Horizontal misalignment may also be corrected by grasping the bridge with two pair of double-padded pliers. This is still the same frame with the same misalignment as was shown in Figure 8-64. Here the frame is viewed from the top. The left pliers hold the bridge, replacing the rimless bracing pliers. The right pliers bend the bridge downward to realign it.

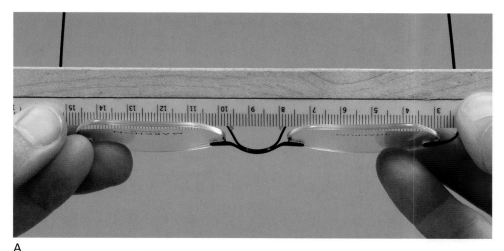

A

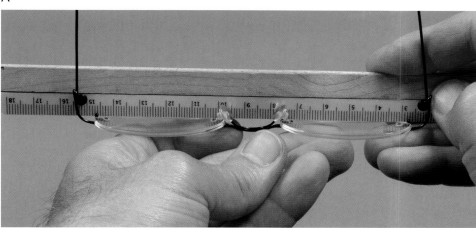

B

Figure 8-68. A, The check for four-point touch on a rimless mounting is begun by placing the straight edge on the inner side of the lenses **below** the pads. **B,** The check for four-point touch on a rimless mounting is completed by placing the straight edge on the inner side of the lenses **above** the pads. By checking both above and below the nosepads, it is easier to tell if the bridge has any propeller-like, X-ing effect.

or decrease face form, grasp the mounting at a nasal point of attachment with rimless bracing pliers and bend the bridge backward or forward using double-padded pliers (Figure 8-69). The bend in the bridge will take place between the two pliers. For maintaining symmetry, it may sometimes be helpful to partially bend the bridge, then switch the rimless bracing pliers to the nasal point of attachment of the other lens and complete the bend.

THE TEMPLES

In the sequence of standard aligning rimless mountings, the temple area is considered next, just as it is with plastic and metal frames.

Open Temple Spread

If the spread of one or both temples is at too great (Figure 8-70) or too small an angle, the error may be

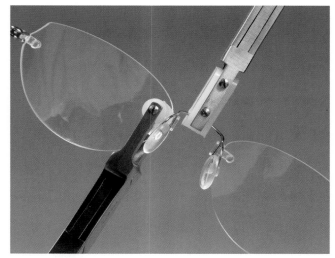

Figure 8-69. To increase or decrease face form, grasp the mounting at a nasal point of attachment with rimless bracing pliers and bend the bridge backward or forward using double-padded pliers.

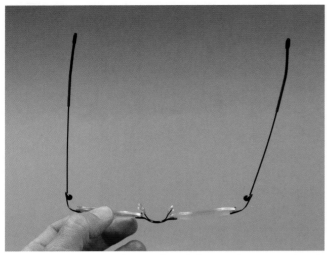

Figure 8-70. The right temple of this rimless mounting is spread too far and must be realigned.

corrected by *bending the endpiece.* To do this, grasp the temporal point of attachment of the lens with rimless bracing pliers. Then grip the endpiece with half-padded pliers from either above (Figure 8-71, *A*) or below (Figure 8-71, *B*). The unpadded jaw of the pliers must be on the inside of the endpiece. If the temple is spread too far, the endpiece is bent inward as is shown in Figure 8-71, *C.*

It is also possible to increase or decrease the temple spread by using tri-angling pliers. Tri-angling pliers* have two round parts to one side of the pliers and a single, rounded section on the other jaw. By positioning and squeezing the pliers as shown in Figure 8-71, *D,* the temple spread may be increased or decreased. (This type of pliers may also be used to adjust other types of frame corners or to reshape a clip-on to match the shape of the frame.) Care must be taken not to mark the frame.

If it is not possible to bend the endpiece, then *bend the temple.* Do this by gripping the butt end of the temple with pliers as close to the hinge as feasible. Then grasping the temple as close to the pliers as possible with the thumb and forefinger of the free hand, bend the temple itself.

Temple Parallelism

Using the flat surface touch test previously described for plastic and metal frames, check the parallelism (relative pantoscopic angles) of the temples. If one temple does not touch, the cause may be a bend in the temple itself, either at the attachment to the frame or just before the curl of the endpiece. This can easily occur with comfort cable temples, as seen in Figure 8-72. Or the bend may also be gradual, extending the length of the shaft. The solution here is to remove the unwanted bend, usually using the hands alone.

---

*Available from Western Optical Supply, Inc. Santa Fe, New Mexico.

If the temple itself is not bent, the fault lies in the angle of the endpiece. Figure 8-73 shows what this error looks like. Here are some commonly used methods for correcting this problem (basically a difference in right and left pantoscopic angles).

Using rimless bracing and double-padded pliers. Open the temple and grasp the lens at the temporal mounting point with the rimless bracing pliers. Using double-padded pliers, grasp the endpiece as shown in Figure 8-74, *A* or *B.* Then rotate the double-padded pliers so that the pantoscopic angle of the temple is increased or decreased, causing the temple to move down or up.

Using rimless bracing and endpiece angling pliers. This method is the same as the one above with one difference. Instead of double-padded pliers, endpiece angling pliers are used to grasp the top and bottom of the temple screw (Figure 8-75). The endpiece angling pliers are rotated, bending the endpiece and moving the temple upward or downward.

Bending the temple by hand. It is possible to hold the lens at the temporal point of attachment and bend the temple up or downward by hand as shown in Figure 8-76. This is probably the least satisfactory method because it is not as easy to control the place where the frame is actually bent. Using two sets of pliers assures that the bend takes place between the locations of the two pliers.

Aligning the Temple Ends

Procedures used to align the bent-down portion of the temple for skull temples on a rimless mounting are the same as outlined for metal frames.

Cable temples are best aligned using the hands alone. Cable temples must be bent much farther than other temples because they tend to spring back to where they were before.

Temple-Fold Angle

The temples, when folded, should meet the same requirements as described for plastic and metal frames. The same general adjustment routine is followed as for plastic and metal frames, except that the point of attachment to the lens must be held with rimless bracing pliers to prevent undo stress on the lenses and their points of attachment.

Fold the temples to a closed position and look at how they cross one another. They should preferably overlap, or at least cross at the center of the frame. Figure 8-77 shows a rimless mounting with uneven temple fold angles.

To correct the temple fold angle, grasp the temporal point of attachment with rimless bracing pliers and the endpiece and butt portion of the closed temple with double-padded pliers. Angle the temple upward or downward with the double-padded pliers as shown in Figure 8-78.

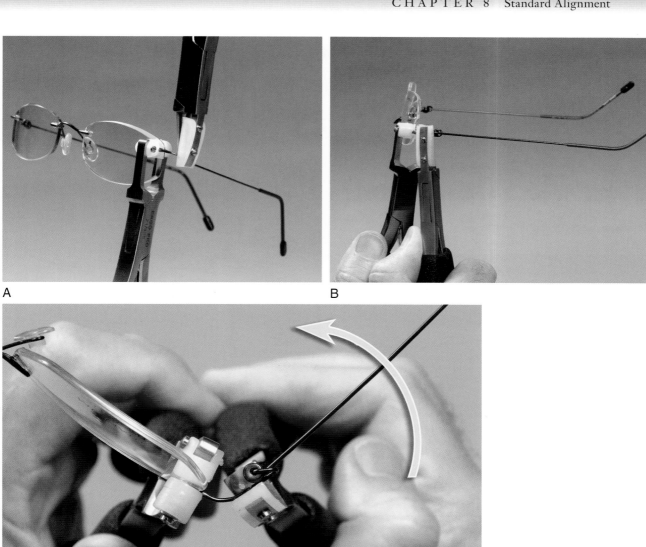

A

B

C

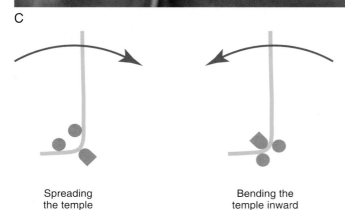

Spreading
the temple

Bending the
temple inward

D

Figure 8-71. **A,** To increase or decrease the temple spread for a rimless mounting, grasp the temporal point of attachment of the lens with rimless bracing pliers. Then grip the endpiece with half-padded pliers from above and bend the endpiece either outward or inward. **B,** Some may prefer to grip the endpiece area from below with both pliers to bend the endpiece in or out. **C,** Hold the frame front steady with rimless bracing pliers (*left*) and rotate the half-padded pliers to bend the endpiece, bringing the temple inward or outward. **D,** Tri-angling pliers may be used to increase or decrease temple spread on certain rimless frames without putting stress on the lenses.

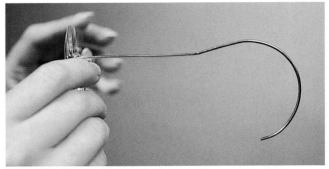

Figure 8-72. An unwanted bend may occur at the position on a cable temple where metal coiling begins.

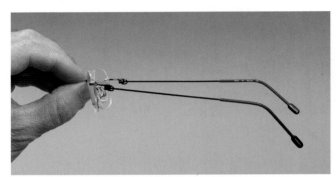

Figure 8-73. The temples of this rimless drill mount are not parallel. The difference in the two pantoscopic angles will cause the frame to fail the flat surface touch test.

OTHER RIMLESS ADJUSTMENTS

Rimless Nosepad Alignment

The nosepads of rimless mountings should meet the same specifications laid down for metal frames. The chief distinction in technique is that the bending of the pad arms should not be attempted unless the base of the pad arm is sufficiently supported to prevent stress on the mounting point and lens.

This support can be given by holding the mounting point with rimless bracing pliers while adjusting the pads with pad adjusting pliers. Sometimes it may be sufficient to support the lens mounting point by holding the mounting point tightly between thumb and forefinger.

A Loose Lens

Any drilled rimless lens may loosen if the lens screw is not tightened down sufficiently.

If the fault lies with the *screw*, it need simply be tightened. The screw may be tightened using a regular screwdriver, but care must to taken not to slip off the screw and scratch the lens. There is a screwdriver with a sleeve around the blade that helps to stabilize the screwdriver and keep it from slipping onto the lens (Figure 8-79). Keep in mind that an overtight screw may crack the lens. This lens screw used for a rimless lens is sometimes

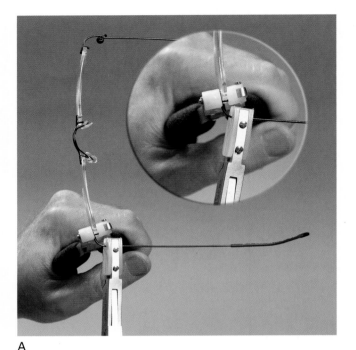

A

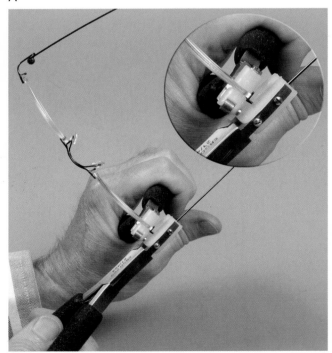

B

Figure 8-74. A, To correct for unequal pantoscopic angles, the dispenser grasps the lens at the temporal mounting point with the rimless bracing pliers and rotates the temple with double-padded pliers. **B,** This method of grasping the endpiece of a rimless mounting is just a variation of that shown in **A.** The temple is still rotated upward or downward.

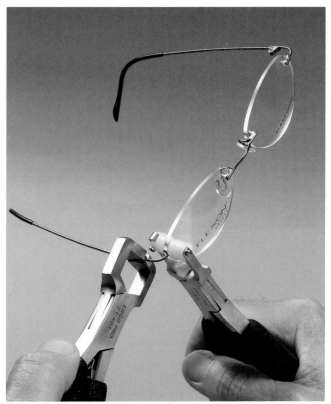

Figure 8-75. A very popular variation on changing the pantoscopic angle uses endpiece angling pliers to angle the temple.

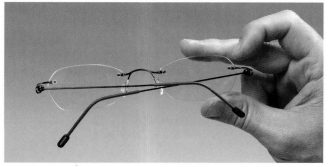

Figure 8-77. A rimless mounting with unequal temple fold angles.

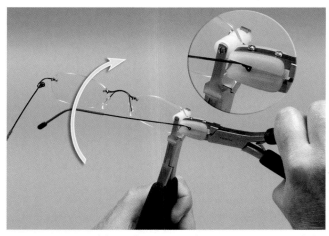

Figure 8-78. Holding the temporal mounting point of the lens, angle the temple with double-padded pliers.

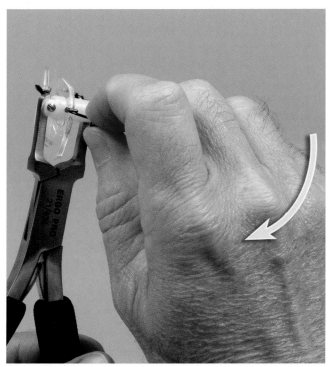

Figure 8-76. A quick alternative for changing the temple's pantoscopic angle uses rimless bracing pliers to hold and makes the bend with the free hand.

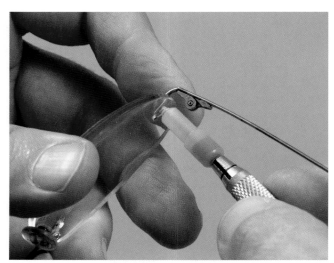

Figure 8-79. A screwdriver made especially for rimless lens screws. The plastic sleeve stabilizes the screwdriver and lessens the risk of slipping off the screw and scratching the lens.

referred to as a "glass screw" because in former days the screw went through glass lens material.

Some find it helpful to protect the surface of the lens by placing several layers of transparent tape over the lens surface so that if the screwdriver slips, it is less likely to damage the lens surface. If the tape leaves a residue, remove it with alcohol.[2]

REFERENCES

1. Cline D, Hofstetter HW, Griffin JR: Dictionary of visual science, ed 4, Radnor, Pa, 1989, Chilton Trade Book Publishing.
2. Carlton J: Fitting tip: Scotch tape to the rescue, Optical Dispensing News, no 139, June 25, 2003.

Proficiency Test

(Answers can be found in the back of the book.)

1. True or false? "Truing" means the same thing as "standard alignment."

2. True or false? It is safer to use hot salt to heat frames than hot air.

3. When the frame front is tested for four-point touch, but only touches on the two temporal eyewires, the frame:
   a. is skewed.
   b. has face form.
   c. is out of coplanar alignment.
   d. has X-ing.
   e. none of the above.

4. A rotated lens can be detected:
   a. when checking horizontal alignment.
   b. when checking vertical alignment.
   c. when checking for four-point touch.
   d. when checking for equality of pantoscopic angle.

5. A situation where the frame front is somewhat twisted, with the planes of the two lenses being out of line with one another, is called:
   a. twisting.
   b. a skewed bridge.
   c. X-ing.
   d. wraparound.
   e. none of the above.

6. An error in standard alignment where, when viewed from the front, one lens appears to be somewhat higher than the other, is called:
   a. X-ing.
   b. propeller effect.
   c. wraparound.
   d. lens out of coplanar alignment.
   e. skewed bridge.

7. When one lens is farther forward than the other, the frame:
   a. has a skewed bridge.
   b. has too much face form.
   c. has X-ing.
   d. is out of coplanar alignment.

8. The temples of a frame do not open far enough. The dispenser standard aligning the frame does not know how wide the wearer's head is. Therefore, when putting the frame in standard alignment, it is not always a good idea to spread the temples to more than how many degrees?
   a. 85 degrees (with reference to the frame front).
   b. 90 degrees (with reference to the frame front).
   c. 95 degrees (with reference to the frame front).
   d. 100 degrees (with reference to the frame front).
   e. The degree spread is not important as long as both temples are spread equally.

9. (Indicate which of the following statements are true and which are false.) To decrease the temple spread for standard plastic frames, one could:
   a. heat the endpiece and press it against a flat surface.
   b. file the frame front.
   c. file the butt end of the temple where it contacts the endpiece.
   d. heat the endpiece and push on it with the thumb.

10. To increase the temple spread for standard plastic frames, one should first try to spread the temple by heating the endpiece and bending it outward. If this and all other measures fail, then it is possible to increase the temple spread by filing. To do this:
    a. file the frame front only.
    b. file the temple only.
    c. file both front and temple evenly.
    d. file temple first and then the front. But file the front only after reaching the metal piece in the temple.

11. When filing temples on a plastic frame, filing the metal piece (a part of the hinge) in the temple:
    a. is permissible.
    b. should be avoided because it decreases the holding power of the temples.
    c. never comes into question because the metal never comes back that far in the temple.
    d. none of the above.

12. (Indicate which of the following are true and which are false.) A frame's inability to meet the flat surface touch test could be caused by:
    a. the lens not being all the way in the groove causing the endpiece not to be straight.
    b. broken or loose hinge rivets.
    c. a bend in the temple shaft.
    d. a bent hinge.

13. When checking for equality of pantoscopic angle in the standard alignment process, it is best to first place the glasses on the table which way? As in A or B?
    a. A, right side up
    b. B, upside down

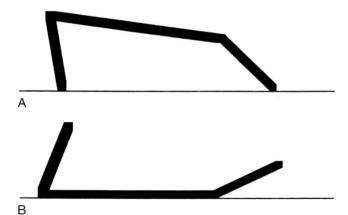

A

B

14. Suppose the bent-down portion of one temple is bent down more than the other. The frames are placed on a table as in figure A above.
    a. When viewed in this way, the left and right pantoscopic angles will appear unequal even if they are not.
    b. When viewed in this way, the left and right pantoscopic angles will appear unequal. This is a sure indication that they really are unequal.

15. One should not use heat in adjusting a conventional plastic frame when:
    a. bending the endpieces.
    b. changing the bridge area.
    c. changing the pantoscopic angle.
    d. bending the temple earpiece.
    e. one should always use heat when adjusting a plastic frame.

16. Of all the tools listed below, which could be a good choice for changing the temple-fold angle of plastic frames?
    a. cutting pliers
    b. a zyl file
    c. half-padded pliers
    d. square-round pliers
    e. finger-piece pliers

17. True or false? The angle that the temple forms, when fully opened, in relationship to the front of the frame is called "let-back."

18. The temples of a plastic frame, when fully opened, do not open wide enough. This problem may be corrected in one of several ways. Which is not a possible solution to this problem?
    a. The lens may not be completely inserted into the frame groove at the location of the endpiece. Heat the frame and insert the lens completely.
    b. Heat and bend the endpiece outward.
    c. File the butt end of the temple.
    d. Heat the butt end of the temple and bend the temple outward.
    e. Use a soldering iron or Hot Fingers unit and heat the hidden hinge so that it will sink deeper into the frame front.

19. "Retroscopic tilt" is manifested:
    a. When the top of the frame front is closer to the wearer's face plane than the bottom of the frame front.
    b. When the bottom of the frame front is closer to the wearer's face plane than the top of the frame front.
    c. When one lens is closer to the wearer's face plane than the other lens.
    d. When one lens is higher on the wearer's face than the other lens.

20. True or false? In standard alignment, the temple fold angle is not correct until both temples are parallel, even if the temples cross in the center of the frame.

21. True or false? When changing temple spread on metal frames, a method that would never work is to push the outside of the endpiece against a flat surface.

22. Identify the angle illustrated.
    a. nasal angle
    b. vertical angle
    c. retroscopic angle
    d. frontal angle
    e. apical angle

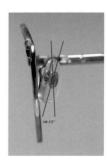

23. Which nosepad angle is best viewed from the top or bottom of the frame?
    a. Frontal
    b. Splay
    c. Vertical

24. Which nosepad angle is most closely related to the pantoscopic angle?
    a. Frontal
    b. Splay
    c. Vertical

25. Which nosepad angle disappears when the nosepads are round instead of elongated?
    a. Frontal
    b. Splay
    c. Vertical
    d. None of the nosepad angles disappear.
    e. With round pads, none of the nosepad angles matter.

26. On an adjustable pad bridge frame, the tops of the two nosepads should normally be closer together than the bottoms of the two nosepads. If this is not the situation, but instead the bottoms of the pads are closer together than the tops, which nosepad angle is off?
    a. Frontal
    b. Splay
    c. Vertical
    d. Cannot tell from the information given

27. In standard alignment, the distance of the face of the pad from the nasal eyewire of the frame is normally how many millimeters?
    a. 0 mm
    b. 1 mm
    c. 2 mm
    d. 2.5 mm
    e. 3 mm

28. Pad adjusting pliers
    a. grip the pad arm behind the pad
    b. grip the face of the pad and the back of the pad

29. When remembering nosepad angles in a humorous way, which pad angle corresponds to the angle mimicked by a chicken flapping its wings?
    a. Frontal
    b. Splay
    c. Vertical

30. Where should a four-point touch be checked on rimless spectacles? (Choose the best, single answer from the choices given.)
    a. below the nosepads on the backs of the lenses
    b. above the nosepads on the backs of the lenses
    c. both above and below the nosepads on the backs of the lenses
    d. at the level of the pad arm attachments on the fronts of the lenses
    e. at the level of the pad arm attachments on the backs of the lenses

31. When checking the four-point touch in a rimless mounting, it is found that the straight edge contacts the four proper points above the nosepads, but below the nosepads the straight edge only touches the left lens and not the right. What error has occurred?
    a. too much face form
    b. too little face form
    c. lenses out of coplanar alignment
    d. horizontal misalignment
    e. X-ing

32. Of the lens materials listed, which material is most likely to break, crack, or develop stress splits at the mounting point when used for rimless drill mountings?
    a. CR-39 plastic
    b. Polycarbonate
    c. Trivex

33. Of the lens materials listed, which material is least likely to break, crack, or develop stress splits at the mounting point when used for rimless drill mountings?
    a. CR-39 plastic
    b. Polycarbonate
    c. Trivex

34. The use of two pairs of pliers at one time is most likely to be of benefit with which type of frames?
    a. Cellulose acetate plastic
    b. Metal frames
    c. Rimless mountings
    d. There is no difference

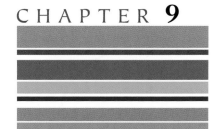

CHAPTER **9**

Adjusting the Frame

The purpose of this chapter is to convey the fundamental principles required for the mastery of an art: fitting the frame properly. If the material covered here is not mastered, many of the other principles learned in other sections of the text will not work because the spectacles may not be worn as intended.

CAUSES OF COMPLAINT

The role of the physical features of a pair of spectacles and how well they are fit to the individual is crucial to satisfaction and the ability of the individual to adapt to the new prescription. Kintner,[1] in his study of the relative role of the physical features serving as factors affecting the wearing comfort of spectacles, concluded that the overwhelming majority of complaints were related to the fit of the frames—a direct result of the frame selection and spectacles adjustment. Many wearers seem more likely to tolerate spectacles in which the prescriptions are slightly awry if the frames fit comfortably. A wearer is not as likely to tolerate spectacles if the frames fit poorly even if the prescription is correct.

The comfort and suitability of the fitting seem to be the most significant criteria for satisfaction.

SECTION A
Overall Frame Adjusting
THE FITTING PROCESS

A new frame should be in standard alignment (refer to Chapter 8) when it is received by the fitter. As discussed previously, however, this is not always the case, so it is wise to check the frames and put them into standard alignment, if necessary, before attempting to adjust them to the wearer's face.

All rules applying to the fitting of new frames for a first dispensing will also apply to the readjustment of frames that have been worn over a period of time and have come out of alignment.

Putting the Frames On

It is preferable to begin the fitting procedure by having the fitter put the frame on the wearer's face for the first time. If the frame requires a good deal of additional adjustment, the fitter should recognize this and remove the frame immediately so that the wearer does not become falsely concerned that the glasses may not be right for him or her.

To place the spectacles on the wearer, hold them by the temples, pulling slightly outward to facilitate slipping the glasses on easily, and guide the ends of the temples just over the ears and down (Figure 9-1). If the temples must be spread a great deal to get them on, use one of the methods outlined in Chapter 8 to adjust the temple spread. This will allow the temples to open wide enough to permit the frame to rest on the nose without pressure against the side of the head.

Triangles of Force

The fitting triangle described by Stimson[2] is composed of the three points where the spectacles contact or put pressure against the head. The apex of the triangle is the contact point on the crest of the nose, and the endpoints of the base of the triangle are the two pressure points just above the roots of the ears, one on each side of the head (Figure 9-2). Since pads are often used for frames, there may actually be two resting points to the apex of the triangle.

Achieving the Proper Temple Spread

The temple-spread angle of the frame should be such that the shafts of the temples exert no pressure, even if touching, on any area of the face or temple before the point of the head at which they should exert pressure—*just above the root of the ears.* This position is usually the widest portion of the head.

Temples Not Spread Enough

If the temples are not spread far enough, there will be too much pressure on both sides of the head, causing the temples to bow out (Figure 9-3). This forces the frame forward until the temples are opposite a narrower part of the head. When the frame slides forward, the pressure that tends to bend them is somewhat relieved (Figure 9-4).

If the glasses are fitted in this manner and the temple spread is never corrected, the glasses will not only tend to slide down, but as they do so, the bent-down portions of the temples will pull against the backs of the ears.

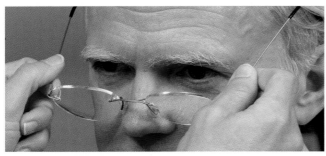

Figure 9-1. The fitter holds the spectacles by the temples, usually spreading them a bit more than they are set for to avoid forcing them on the head.

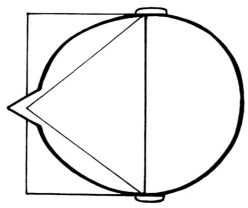

Figure 9-2. The fitting triangle is the connection of only three points upon which "pressure" may be exerted. These are the crest of the nose and the sides of the head just above the roots of the ears. The pressure on the nose is from the weight of the frame.

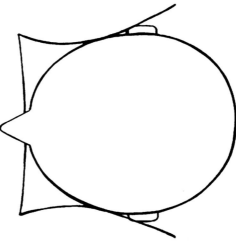

Figure 9-3. Even though the illustration is exaggerated, it can be seen how pressure is exerted on the head and a negative bow in the temples created.

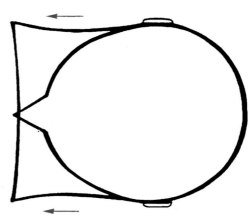

Figure 9-4. In an attempt to return to their original shape, the temples cause the glasses to slip. This creates a situation with the worst characteristics of both tight- and loose-fitting glasses. Not only do the glasses slip forward, but they may also hurt behind the ears.

Then not only do the glasses slip down as if they were loose, but they hurt behind the ears as well. The wearer experiences the disadvantages of both loose and tight glasses at the same time.

The first step in the entire adjustment procedure is to achieve the temple-spread angle that permits the front to rest easily on the nose without being forced forward. This is done by adjusting the endpieces so that the temples do not exert pressure against the sides of the head at any point in front of the ears. The temple shafts may touch the sides of the head, but should not exert pressure. The adjustment should be such that the corner of a sheet of paper may be slipped between the temple shaft and the side of the head. The only place where pressure is allowable is above the root of the ears.

If the head is very round or is wider in front of the ears than above the ears, it may be necessary to bend the temples into an arc that follows this wider portion of the head, but eventually presses the head only at the desired point (i.e., immediately above the root of the ear).

Temples Spread Too Far
If the temple angle is too wide for the patient's head, the glasses will tend to slide down the nose. More often this occurs if the frame has been worn for some time. The specific methods used to reduce the temple-spread angle can be found in Chapter 8.

Equality of Lens Vertex Distance
At this point, it is advisable to check the glasses for equality of vertex distance. This is done by having the wearer tilt his head forward while the dispenser views the glasses from above (Figure 9-5). If the glasses have been properly aligned and the wearer's head is symmetrical, both lenses will be the same distance from the wearer's face. If, however, the temple spread is unequal with one temple angling farther in or out than the other, or if one side of the wearer's head is somewhat wider than

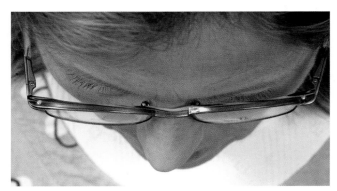

Figure 9-5. The lens in front of the wearer's left eye is closer because one temple is pressing harder on the side of the head than the other.

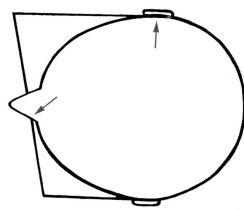

Figure 9-6. If the wearer complains of the frame hurting one side of the nose, unequal temple-spread angles might be suspected.

the other, one lens will be closer to the face than the other.

The necessary correcting procedures for this inequality will be directly indicated by the way the frame positions itself. If, as in Figure 9-5, the wearer's right lens is farther from the face, there is more pressure over the wearer's right ear than the left, forcing the right side out. (The principle is the same as was described in Figure 9-4, except that one temple is under more stress than its partner, forcing that side forward.) The remedy to the problem can be approached two ways.

1. It may be that the right temple is not spread far enough, making this side fit too tight. The solution is to open the temple out farther. This is done in the same manner as for standard alignment.

2. It could also be that the right temple is correctly fitted, but the left temple is too loose. The right only has the *effect* of pushing its side forward because of the lack of counteracting pressure on the left side. Here the solution is to bring this left temple inward, decreasing the spread. Again, the techniques used are the same as those described for standard alignment of the frame.

In practice, often both temples are adjusted somewhat, one being brought in, the other opened out. As stated before, regardless of whether the problem lies with the glasses or the head shape, the solution is the same, and is indicated by the way the frame positions itself. Table 9-1 presents a simple way to remember these adjustments.

If the glasses should be dispensed incorrectly, with one temple not spread sufficiently, after being worn for some time the ear on this same side *and* the opposite side of the wearer's nose will become sore. This results from the clothespinlike effect of the tighter side of the frame pinching the face (Figure 9-6). Therefore if a person complains of the frame hurting one side of the nose, an improper temple-spread angle might be suspected.

It should be noted that in approaching the problem of vertex distance inequality, it is a good idea to first check to see if one of the temples is not straight, but bowed in or out. If the temple is bowed or bent, straighten it first.

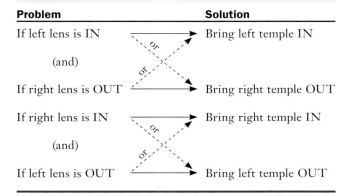

TABLE 9-1		
To Move One Lens Closer to the Face (IN With IN, OUT With OUT)		
Problem		**Solution**
If left lens is IN	⟍ *or* ⟋	Bring left temple IN
(and)	*or*	
If right lens is OUT		Bring right temple OUT
If right lens is IN	⟍ *or* ⟋	Bring right temple IN
(and)	*or*	
If left lens is OUT		Bring left temple OUT

A single bowed temple can cause a vertex distance inequality in the same way as differences in temple-spread angles.

THE FRONT

The adjustment of the frame front takes place after making certain the temple spread angles are right. Here is the two step overview:
- First, the proper pantoscopic angle or tilt of the frame front is set.
- Next the straightness of the frame on the face, when viewed from the front, is adjusted.

It is clear that proper pantoscopic angle and frame straightness should precede any bridge adjustments. This is because changes in the angle of the frame front will directly affect how the nosepads rest on the nose. If the nosepads are adjusted so they sit flat on the nose first, and then the whole frame front is reangled for a new pantoscopic angle, a problem has been created—the pads will no longer be sitting flat on the nose.

Pantoscopic Angles

The usual tilt of the frame front may be anywhere from 4 to 18 degrees from the vertical. It will only approach the upper (18 degree) extreme in the case of exceptionally protruding eyebrows. In evaluating the pantoscopic angle, the lenses or rims of the frames should touch neither the brows nor the cheeks.

(The optical reasons for varying amounts of pantoscopic tilt were described in Chapter 5.)

Straightness of the Frame on the Face

If the frame is crooked on the face, adjustment of the pantoscopic angle at each endpiece will allow the frame to be leveled when viewed from the front.

The first possible cause of a crooked frame is incomplete standard alignment. If the temples are not parallel and fail the flat surface touch test, then the frames cannot be expected to sit straight on the face. However, even if the temples are parallel, there may still be a problem.

Most heads are not symmetrical. One ear is often slightly higher than the other. In such instances, even previously standard-aligned glasses with temples parallel will appear tilted on the face when viewed from the front.

The solution is the same whether the cause is the frame or the face. The pantoscopic tilt* (or more concisely, the angle the temple makes with the frame front) needs to be changed on one or both sides.

If the right side of the frame is too high, the right temple must be angled up. This allows the frame to drop down farther on that side before the temple contacts the top of the ear.

However, it may not be advisable to decrease the pantoscopic angle on the higher side. Sometimes this will cause the frame front to have too little pantoscopic tilt when viewed from the side. If this is the case, the opposite temple may be angled down instead. This increase in the pantoscopic tilt of the opposite side accomplishes the same result because it raises the side that is too low.

Often both raising one temple and lowering the other are required. One bend alone may be insufficient to level the frame. Stated simply, if the right side of the frame front is up, bend the right temple up. Or looking at it from the other side—if the left side is down, bend the left temple down. Table 9-2 shows this in an easy-to-memorize chart.

When the ears are at unequal heights on the head, changing the pantoscopic angle to straighten the glasses

---

*The primary definition of pantoscopic angle that relates to fitting is "the angle that the frame front makes with the frontal plane of the wearer's face when the lower rims are closer to the face than the upper rims" (see Glossary). However, during the standard alignment process, pantoscopic angle usually refers to "that angle by which the frame front deviates from the vertical . . . when the spectacles are held with the temple horizontal."

TABLE 9-2

To Move One Lens Higher on the Face (UP With UP, DOWN With DOWN)

Problem	Solution
If left lens is UP	Bend left temple UP
(and)	*or*
If right lens is DOWN	Bend right temple DOWN
If right lens is UP	Bend right temple UP
(and)	*or*
If left lens is DOWN	Bend left temple DOWN

---

on the face will cause the glasses themselves to lie crooked when placed on a flat surface. If this is not pointed out to the wearer, he or she may think the glasses are in error and be suspicious of the quality of the fitting. Always call this to the wearer's attention.

Reference Points

Although it is helpful to refer to the eyebrows when determining the level of the frame, facial asymmetry can cause one lens to appear higher than the other even when this is not really the case. The frame front should not be aligned solely on the basis of eyebrow height or the position of the eyes in the head because either of these features may be asymmetrical. Instead, overall appearance of both eyes and brows should be used. If due to facial asymmetry the frame conforms better to facial features when fitted slightly higher on one side, then it should be fit that way.

If bifocals are being dispensed and have been correctly measured using a properly adjusted frame for each eye independently, the logical reference point is the relationship between the bifocal line and the lower edge of the pupil. To judge this objectively, tilt the wearer's head back and note whether or not both segment lines intersect the pupils at the same point. (For a more complete description of both objective and subjective techniques, see Chapter 5.) The same may be said for the fitting cross markings of progressive addition lenses. Fitting crosses should be centrally positioned before the pupils.

Other Sources of Error Causing the Frame Front to Appear Crooked

When the glasses are crooked, the following areas should also be checked in determining the source of error.

1. Are the unequally angled temples caused by bent endpieces or just the hinges?
2. Are the temples themselves bent?
3. Is the bridge skewed?
4. Is one ear farther back than the other? (If the temples are the same length, this may cause one

bent-down portion to strike an ear at a different position of the bend than the other, giving the same effect as one ear being higher.)

THE TEMPLES

When all adjustments having to do with the front of the glasses have been done—open temple angle, pantoscopic angle, height, vertex distance, and pad positions on the nose—final attention is paid to the adjustment of the temples.

If the previous front adjustments are satisfactory, the spectacles will stay in proper position on the face *if the head is held erect* even though the temples are not fully adjusted. This is true as long as the first point of contact of the temples is at the sides of the head just above the ears. Note: This is the correct time to adjust the nose-pads. We have not yet covered nosepads. If the frame does have nosepads, they need to be adjusted before the ends of the temples are adjusted. Nosepads are covered in Section B of this chapter.

Lateral pressure—The pressure of the temples against the sides of the head just above the ears is increased, if necessary, by decreasing the temple spread. This can be done by any of the methods described earlier in Chapter 8, such as bending the endpiece areas in.

The correct amount of lateral pressure is such that the patient feels no pressure or, if pressure is felt, no discomfort. The glasses should stay firmly in place even if the head is lowered. This should be true even though the backs of the temples have not as yet been adjusted.

An important point to remember in fitting temples is that the best way the glasses are held in place is with friction, not pressure. Friction is increased when the contact with the side of the head is maximized. With that in mind, adjustment of any type of library or skull temple will work best if the inside of the temple is parallel to the head in three places: 1) along the temple shaft, 2) above the root of the ear (Figure 9-7), and 3) along the slope of the head behind the ear.

This may require rotating the temple about its long axis. To do this, heat and twist the temple.

Earpiece or curl—When the lateral pressure is satisfactorily applied, attention is given to that portion of the temple that lies past the top of the ear. Adjustment varies depending on the type of temple used and will be considered according to temple type.

Fitting Straight-Back and Skull Temples

A straight-back or library temple has no vertical bend behind the ear. As the name implies, it goes straight back. A skull temple is bent down behind the ear.

Many temples can be fit with or without a bend at the ear as a skull or straight-back temple. To begin with, we will consider how to fit a temple without a bend. In doing so, we can consider first the way the temple fits against the side of the head. Later we can add the bend.

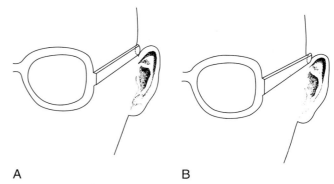

A   B

Figure 9-7. A library or skull temple should be adjusted so that the whole side of the temple is parallel to the slope of the head above the root of the ear. **A,** Proper parallel fit. **B,** Not parallel.

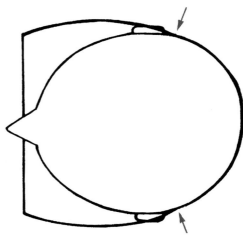

Figure 9-8. A common dispensing error committed by an untrained fitter is that of bowing the temples to achieve a snug fit.

All the principles applying to a straight-back or library temple also apply to the skull temple.

Adjustment of straight-back temples consists of bending inward that portion of the temple that lies just past the top of the ear. This is done in such a way that the inside surface of the temple lies fully against the portion of the head directly behind the top of the ear. The temple must contact the head continuously from the top of the ear back, exerting uniform pressure all along that area.

A common error used to tighten up a frame that slides down the nose is to bend the very last portion of the temple too far inward. The result is that the end of the temple exerts excessive pressure at a single point on the head. This maladjustment usually bows the rest of the temple away from the head (Figure 9-8). At first the wearer is happy because the glasses no longer slide down the nose. But the inward bend of the temple displaces the upper lobe of the ear and eventually digs a painful

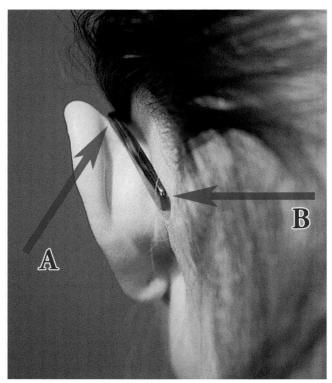

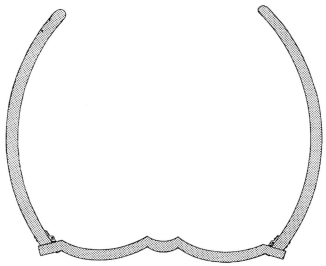

Figure 9-10. Pressure created by bowing the temples is transferred to frame bridge and endpiece areas, causing them to give over a period of time. The illustration shown is a natural outcome of continually increasing temple bowing to maintain a snug fit.

Figure 9-9. The error in the previous figure is shown in this photo of a skull temple. Note how the temple presses both outward on the lobe of the ear (*arrow A*) and inward against the side of the head (*arrow B*).

pit into the side of the head where the tip presses against it (Figure 9-9). This all too common error is seen with both straight-back and skull temples.

When bent inward too far, the excessive pressure of the tips against the head causes the endpieces and the bridge to give, bending out. This in turn eventually releases the lateral pressure that holds the frame up. For the inexperienced fitter unaware of the source of error, the erroneous "remedy" is usually more of the same. This means increasing the temple arc to restore the tip's contact against the side of the head. A vicious circle occurs, resulting in widely bowed temples and an excessively bent frame front (Figure 9-10).

If the structure of the skull is such that there is a dip or hollowed-out convolution in the side of the head, heat the temple and bend it to follow the side of the head as precisely as possible. The objective is to establish as much friction through contact of the surfaces as possible so that a "disc brake" action is introduced. The dispenser may heat and press an indentation into the bent-down portion of a skull temple with both thumbs. Because of this, many call this "adding a thumbprint" to the temple. If this is too difficult to do with the thumbs, eyewire forming pliers can be used as shown in Figure 9-11. (These pliers were pictured earlier and are normally used to shape the eyewire of a metal frame as was seen in Figures 7-14 and 7-15.)

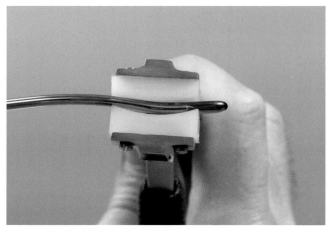

Figure 9-11. The end of this temple is being shaped to conform to a slight hollow in the side of the wearer's head. This dip in the temple is often referred to as a "thumbprint" because it may be pressed into the temple using both thumbs. Here it is being pressed into the temple using eyewire forming pliers.

If the frame front has been properly adjusted, the lateral temple pressure correctly applied, and the friction contact of the temple ends well established, then the spectacles will remain secure without hurting.

Positioning the Temple Bend

The proper position of the bend in the temple lies just *past* the top of the ear. The downward slant of the earpiece should parallel the slope of the back of the root of the ear. If it even touches the root of the ear, it should just barely touch it (Figure 9-12). Above all, the temple

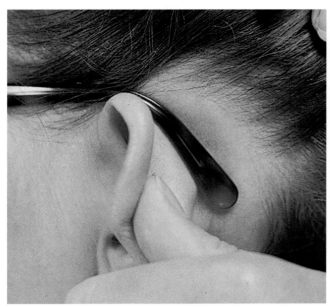

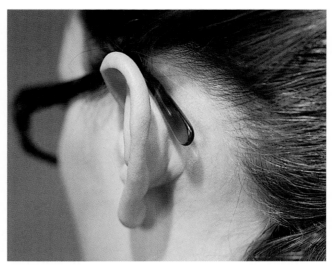

Figure 9-14. Properly positioning the location of the bend is incomplete if the bent-down portion of the temple stands away from the side of the head.

Figure 9-12. A properly positioned temple bend occurs just behind the top of the ear. This allows the bent-down portion of the temple to parallel the upper root of the ear.

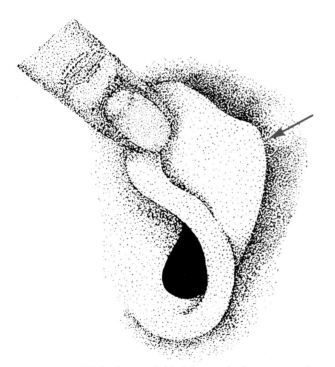

Figure 9-13. With the ear folded forward, the arrow points out the most sensitive portion of the ear. Pressure from the temple on this area should be avoided.

must not press into the crease between ear and head or on the small cord of cartilage that helps in connecting the ear to the head (Figure 9-13).

The earpiece portion of the temple should not be just bent down (Figure 9-14). It must be positioned against the side of the head, usually requiring inward angling.

Shape the descending earpiece portion to match the convolutions of the mastoid process, which is a lump on the side of the head behind the ear. It should exert even pressure throughout its length, just as with the straight-temple types.

Temples Too Long or Too Short
If the temples are too long or too short, the position of the temple bend can be modified. There are, of course, limits as to how far the bend can be moved because too radical a change will result in the earpiece being too long or short. A change of the bend position is more easily and satisfactorily performed for plastic temples than for temples made entirely from metal. Some metal temples may need to be replaced by properly sized temples.

Since temples are manufactured in steps of 5 mm, there is always a possibility that a temple may not fit quite as precisely as desired on a given head. If this is the case, the position of the bend can be changed. The position of the bend also needs to be changed in cases where the correct length is not available or where an error in ordering the correct length has been made. The suggested procedure for changing the position of the bend is as follows:

1. *Note bend position*—The front should be positioned so that the glasses are seated as they will be when worn. Often new glasses or frame samples fit much too loosely, allowing the glasses to slip down on the nose. When this happens, the temple slips forward until stopped by the ear. As a result, the temple bend appears to be properly situated, when in actuality the temples are too long. To avoid this problem, stand with the wearer seated, and grasp the glasses around both endpieces with the left hand. Hold them on the face where they should

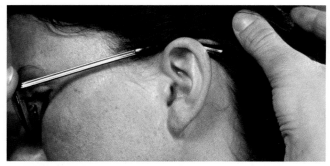

Figure 9-15. The desired location of the temple bend is accurately determined only if the glasses are properly positioned. Error in bend placement is prevented by holding the frame in place.

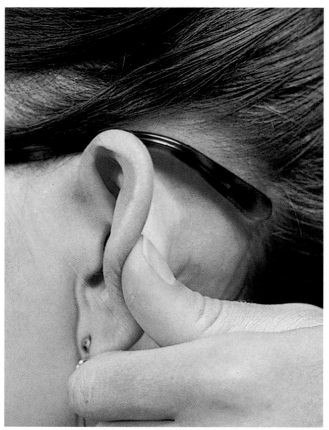

Figure 9-16. If the temple shaft is too long, the bend will occur past the desired position.

actually sit. The right hand is then free to move the hair back or bend the ear forward to inspect for proper fit (Figure 9-15). For the left temple, switch hands and repeat the procedure. It cannot be assumed that both temples will fit the ears correctly just because one does. Faces are not symmetrical; sometimes two separate temple lengths are indicated.

If the shaft is *too long*, the bend will occur beyond the desired position, which is just barely past the top of the ear (Figure 9-16). This permits the spectacles to move forward until the earpiece rests against the cartilage in back of the ear.

It is possible to simply increase the angle of the bend in the temple until the bent-down portion just touches the back of the ear. The fallacy here is that there are only two points of contact—the top of the ear and the back of the ear—resulting in an extremely painful spot behind the ear after continued wearing. Instead the position of the bend in the temple should be moved so that the temple fits correctly.

If the shaft is *too short*, the bend will occur forward of the top of the ear, causing the bent-down portion to rest on the posterior slope of the cartilage. This usually raises the temples up off the ear so that the bend itself is visible along the side of the head and the end of the temple pushes against the back of the ear (Figure 9-17).

2. *Estimate new bend position*—Observe the relationship of the bend to the position it should occupy above the ear and estimate a new position for the bend. Observe each ear separately because the two sides of the head and face may not be symmetrical.

3. *Straighten and bend, or bend and straighten*—Heat both the original bend area and that portion of the shaft where the new bend is desired. Hold the shaft of the temple firmly in one hand and grasp the bent portion with the fingers of the other hand, with the thumb braced on the bend (Figure 9-18). Pull the end up so that the entire temple is straightened.

Move the fingers of the hand holding the temple shaft so that the temple is braced at the new bend point by the thumb and forefinger. Push the protruding end with the thumb of the other hand until it bends over the forefinger of the holding hand to the desired angle (Figure 9-19).

For some, it may be too difficult to add a new temple bend with the hands alone. In this case, there is a pair of pliers that is designed for this use. *Temple bend pliers* may be positioned at the desired location of the temple and the bend added as shown in Figure 9-20.

The desired position of the bend may be more exactly marked with a water-soluble felt-tipped marking pen or a grease pencil to eliminate the guesswork. It may be necessary to reheat the temple before adding the new bend if the resistance to bending is great.

Physically Lengthening and Shortening of Temples

Some metal frames come with bent-down portions that have a metal core, but a plastic outer portion. These types of temples are unique in that they may be shortened or lengthened beyond what would be expected. It is even conceivable to shorten some plastic temples. Both possibilities are explained in Chapter 10.

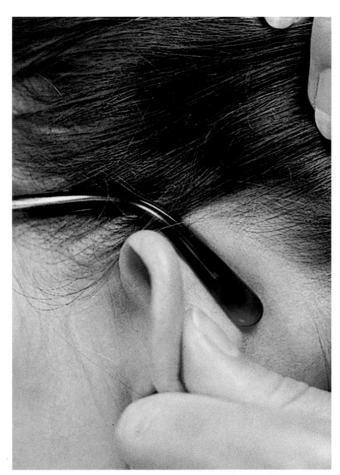

Figure 9-17. If the shaft is too short, the bend will occur too far forward. Note how this raises the temple up off the ear so that the bend itself is visible.

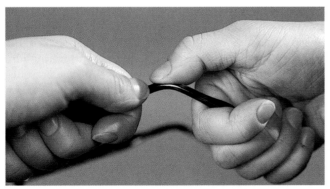

Figure 9-18. Straightening the temple to move the bend to a new location may be done as shown. If the bend is to be moved forward, it may also be done by first placing a new bend at the desired location; then removing the old bend.

Summary of Temple Fitting Criteria

In summary, the temples should meet all of the following criteria:

- The shaft of the temple should not exert pressure on the face or head at any point in front of the position just above the ears. The point just above

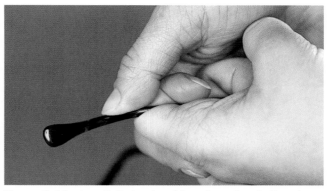

Figure 9-19. A well-fitting bend is a sharp bend. Creating a good, sharp bend may be done by forcing the end of the temple over the knuckle.

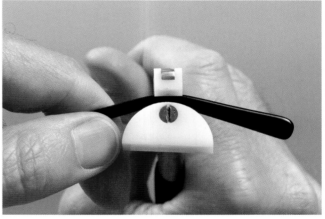

Figure 9-20. A temple bend may be added using temple bend pliers. The temple will still need to be heated, but should not be overheated to avoid marking the plastic.

the ears should receive the lateral pressure of the temples.

- The bend should be just at the point immediately following the top of the root of the ear, so that it does not rest on either the top of the root of the ear or push against the back of the origin of the ear (Figure 9-21).
- The bent-down portion should be angled so that it approximately parallels the posterior descending slope of the root of the ear (crotch of the ear) without either pressing into the crease between the ear and the head or the cord located there.
- The cross section of the shaft, if other than round, should be parallel to the slope of the head and lie with its widest part against the head.
- The bent-down portion (earpiece) should slope with its widest part flat against the side of the head. It should be so shaped and convoluted that it follows the depression behind the ear (the ischium hollow) and the elevation following below it known as the mastoid process. There should be even pressure

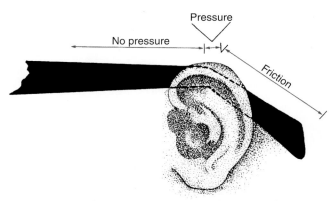

Figure 9-21. The proper location for the temple bend is at the point immediately behind the top of the root of the ear. The only place where pressure is indicated is against the side of the head immediately above the ear. Beyond this point, the hold should be by friction on the order of a disc brake.

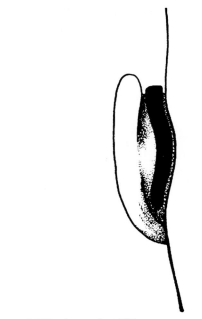

Figure 9-22. A temple will be more comfortable and hold the frame in place better if it parallels the anatomical shape of both head and ear.

throughout the entire area (Figure 9-22). The ends of the temples should not gouge the back of the head or exert greater pressure than the balance of the earpiece.

Optyl Temples

Temples made of Optyl are adjusted to meet the same criteria as temples made of other materials. There are two basic types of Optyl temples. The first is made from the same material as the Optyl frame front and can be identified by the lack of a metal reinforcement running the length of the temple. A special technique is required for this type of temple, since Optyl frames will return

to their original molded form when heated. The second type is called LCM, or light coated metal.

Adjusting Temples Made From Original Optyl Material

Adjusting temples made from the original type Optyl material requires sufficient heat for bending. Attempts to bend an Optyl temple without heat or without sufficient heat will result in a broken temple. Heat only that portion of the frame that requires bending. Hold the rest of the temple so that the adjacent portions not being adjusted are protected from the heat. After heating and bending the temple to the desired position, hold the temple in that position until it cools enough to retain the new shape. (Some frame warmers have a cool air option that can be used to cool down the heated area.) Because heated Optyl material will return to its original shape, failure to hold it in position will allow it to revert somewhat. When making a second bend in a new area of the temple, the first area must be shielded from heat. Otherwise the progress made thus far will be lost.

It is possible to extend the length of an Optyl temple having no metal reinforcing wire by heating the temple so that it is hot enough to allow it to be pulled and stretched. In so doing, it may be possible to use a temple that would otherwise be too short even if the bend were moved as far back as possible.

Adjusting Optyl LCM Temples

The second type of Optyl temple has a plastic of a different composition covering a metal core. It is referred to as an LCM temple and should be marked with the letters "lcm." These LCM temples are extremely malleable and can be adjusted with only a minimum of heat. In contrast to the original Optyl material temple, the LCM temple does not return to its original shape when heated. Remember, to tell the difference between the two temples, look for a lack of a metal reinforcing wire to identify the original material temple, and the presence of the initials "lcm" to identify the light-coated metal temple.

Spring Hinge Temples

Temples with spring-loaded hinges have been much improved. When spring temples were first introduced, they were much more appealing to the wearer than to the dispenser. Because they did not originally have the strength and resiliency of today's designs, it was necessary to fit them so that they were stretched halfway open when fit. In other words, the midpoint of the tension-spread area would fall at the natural position of the temple when placed on the wearer.

Better engineered spring hinges have changed all that. Now the spring hinge temple is fit in exactly the same manner as any other temple. It should fit on the head so that under normal wearing circumstances, the spring hinges are not flexed. The advantage of spring

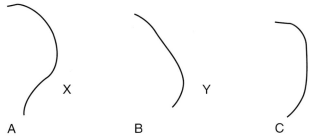

Figure 9-23. The so-called crotch of the ear may follow different contours, three of which are shown. (Redrawn from Stimson RL: Ophthalmic dispensing, ed 2, Springfield, Ill, 1971, Charles C Thomas.)

temples is not that they hug the head any differently than normal, well-fitted temples. They do not. The advantage of a good quality spring hinge is that it allows the frames to retain their adjustment longer.

When people put their glasses on and take them off day after day, there is a certain amount of stress placed on the frames. The temples are forced open beyond the point for which they were adjusted. Eventually, they begin to loose their adjustment. Temples with spring hinges prevent that stress because the spring in the hinge absorbs it.

Frames with spring hinges are less likely to require readjustment or repair when struck with a ball, an elbow, or when knocked from the face. This is because, once again, the spring hinge allows the temple angle to bend outward, then rebound, rather than to bend and stay bent.

Spring temples are adjusted behind the ears exactly as any other temples. The same rules apply to the position of the temple bend as well.

Riding Bow and Cable Temples

Riding bow or cable temples can be used in situations where a skull temple will not hold the spectacles adequately, such as for children or for individuals engaged in rough physical activity. Riding bows are made from plastic; cable temples from coiled metal.

To fit a cable or riding bow temple, the temple should follow around the root of the ear but should not press against the root of the ear at any point before point X at the back of the ear as shown in Figure 9-23, *A*. The cable should lie close to the root of the ear from point X to the end of the temple because it is this contact that holds the spectacles in place. The very last few millimeters of the temple should be turned back away from the ear to keep the end from digging in. Figure 9-24 shows the end of the temple before it has been adjusted. The end of the cable should be bent back and slightly away from the side of the head. This is done with double-padded pliers as shown in Figure 9-25. The completed bend is shown in Figure 9-26.

When the shape of the cable corresponds to the shape of the portion of the ear, which attaches the ear to the

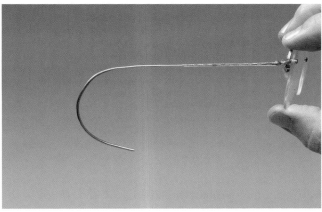

Figure 9-24. Here is what the end of a cable temple looks like before the tip of the temple has been adjusted.

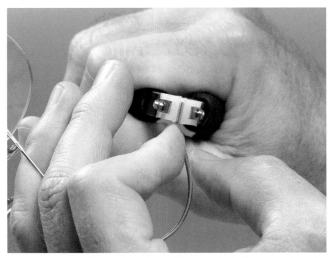

Figure 9-25. The end of the cable temple is bent so that the end will not dig into the crotch of the ear. Hold the temple right next to the double-padded pliers so that the bend will be sharp and well-defined.

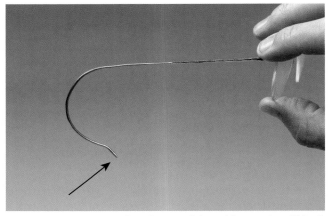

Figure 9-26. Here is what the tip of the cable temple will look like after the bend at the tip is complete.

head, as shown in Figure 9-23, *B*, the cable should pass the point marked Y without pressure before curling to grasp the balance of the ear.

When the ear is shaped as shown in Figure 9-23, *C*, the temple should exert pressure on the ear only during the last 10 or 15 mm of the temple length. This type is difficult to adjust because the temple bend is almost at right angles.

Temple Length
When the necessary cable temple is not on an available sample, the proper length may be estimated by adding 0.75 inch, or approximately 20 mm, to the length of the equivalent, correctly fitting skull temple.

A cable temple of the correct length should stop just short of the lower lobe of the ear (Figure 9-27, *A*). Cable temples that are too short will not have enough length to grip the lower area where it is needed (Figure 9-27, *B*). Cable temples fitted too long have a tendency to dig into the lower earlobe (Figure 9-27, *C*).

Hearing Aids and Fitting Eyewear
For a time, a large number of hearing aids were made to fit in the temples of a person's spectacle frames. With the continued development of smaller hearing aids, combined with rapidly changing eyeglass frame fashions, in-temple hearing aids are now rare.

Most aids fit in or behind the ear, or are a combination of both. In-the-ear aids require no special considerations when fitting and adjusting temples. Hearing aids with a behind-the-ear component work best if the temple style chosen is as thin as possible. One of the very best choices, although not readily available, is the cable temple. The cable hugs the base of the ear and is out of the way of the hearing aid.

Skull temples that are thin enough can sometimes be adjusted to closely match the fit of a cable temple, at least for the upper part of the back of the ear. They must closely follow flush against the side of the head. The thinner the bent-down portion of the temple is, the less will be the interference with the aid.

GENERAL INSTRUCTIONS TO THE WEARER ON FRAME HANDLING

There are many different sets of instructions appropriate for different types of wearing situations. Bifocal wearers will be given different advice on use than progressive addition lens wearers. Those instructions and precautions are addressed in the section of the text that covers each particular topic. As for the handling of eyeglasses in general, here are a few suggestions:
1. To keep eyeglasses in adjustment better, glasses are best taken off using two hands.
2. When removing glasses with the right hand only, grasp the right endpiece, lift the right temple off the ear, and move the glasses to left side of the face so

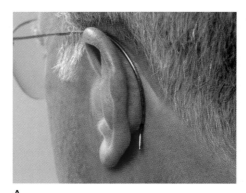

A

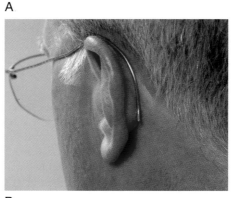

B

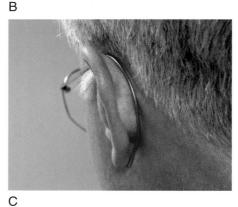

C

Figure 9-27. In judging correct cable temple length, observe where the temple ends as it wraps around the ear. **A,** The correct length cable temple should stop just short of the lower lobe of the ear. **B,** Cable temples that are too short do not have the length to grip the lower portion of the ear where it is most necessary. **C,** Cable temples fit too long have a tendency to dig into the lower ear lobe. If no shorter temples are available, it is possible to clip off the end of the temple with cutting pliers and solder the new end. A small ball of solder at the tip will make a smooth surface and keep the coiled cable from unraveling.

that the left temple comes off the ear easily. Do the opposite for the left hand only.
3. For frames with cable and comfort cable temples, grasp the right endpiece with the right hand and the tip end of the left cable temple with the left hand (Figure 9-28). Pull the left temple off the ear and

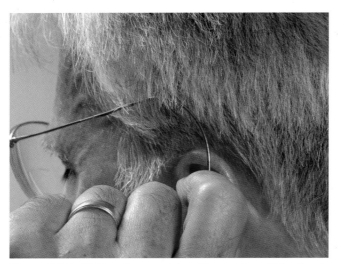

Figure 9-28. Taking frames with cable temples off the face is done by grasping the tip of one temple and pulling it back and around the ear while holding the other temple near the frame front.

swing the glasses to the right so that the right cable temple comes off the ear easily.

4. To lay the glasses down on a table or dresser with the temples open, place the glasses on the surface upside down. When the temples are closed, place the glasses with the folded temples down. Never place the glasses on a surface with the lenses facing down.

5. Do not leave the glasses on the dashboard of a car or where they will be exposed to heat.

6. When not being worn, glasses do best in a case. This is especially true when being carried in a purse or pocket.

7. Rinse the lenses before wiping them with a cloth, unless the cloth is specifically designed for the lenses. Remember that the frames need cleaning too. Washing frames and lenses in a mild detergent, as when doing dishes, is appropriate.

For more on cleaning frames and lenses, see Cleaning Frames and Lenses, Chapter 7, including Tables 7-3 and 7-4.

SECTION B
Fitting Adjustable Nosepads

Adjustable nosepads give tremendous versatility when fitting and adjusting frames. Unfortunately, many are unfamiliar with the basics of how to adjust nosepads correctly and are afraid of making changes. This section presents step-by-step methods for doing just what is needed to correctly position the frame.

Where adjustable pads and pad arms are available, the frame can be altered in height by widening or narrowing the distance between the pads. It should be remembered, however, that increasing or decreasing the distance between pads will not only lower or raise the frame on the face, but also allow the frame to fit closer to or farther from the eyes.

There are primarily two types of adjustable pad arms. The older type is shaped like a question mark; the more common like an upside down U or a gooseneck.

PROPER PAD ANGLES FOR ADJUSTABLE PADS

With any pad adjustment that moves a pad arm, it can be expected that afterwards the face of the pad may no longer sit flat on the nose. The pads must then be realigned to their proper positions so that frontal, splay, and vertical angles are once again correct. These angles were explained in Chapter 8, pages 161-164.

Remember: Adjust the pantoscopic angle (tilt of the frame front) *first* before adjusting the three pad angles. The tilt of the frame front changes how the pads sit on the surface of the nose. Adjusting the pantoscopic angle after aligning the pads means that the pads will have to be aligned all over again a second time.

Achieving the Proper Pad Angles for Adjustable Bridges

The adjustment of rocking pads is most easily performed using pad-adjusting pliers. (See Figure 8-57 in Chapter 8.) These special pad pliers come in a variety of configurations. They should be chosen for the pad attachment type on the frame. Attachment styles change with the times, so the type of pad adjusting pliers that has been in the office for years may no longer be appropriate for the frames being currently used.

Pad adjusting pliers, when chosen properly, have one jaw that holds the base of the pad securely without crushing the pad socket or attachment, and another jaw that cradles the face of the pad. The pad can readily be adjusted for splay, vertical, and frontal angles using these pliers. Snipe-nosed or other flat-jawed pliers can also be used and are intended to be used on the pad support arm. If used on the face of some pads, they may indent or mar the pad face surface.

For pads to be adjusted to rest correctly on the surface of the nose, they should fulfill the following criteria:

1. The pads should rest halfway between the crest of the nose and the inner corner of the eye (Figure 9-29).

2. The long diameter of the pads should be perpendicular to the floor when the head is erect (as also seen in Figure 9-29).

3. The full surface of the pads should rest uniformly on the nose. If either the lower, upper, inner, or outer edge of the pad presses unevenly on the surface of the nose, the nose will show imprint or

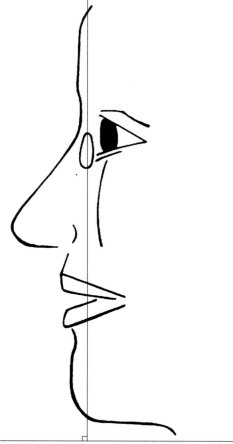

Figure 9-29. The proper resting position for adjustable pads is halfway between the crest of the nose and the inner corner of the eye. The long axis of the pad should be perpendicular to the floor.

cutting marks after wear, or may become too sensitive for continued wear.

To correct these problems, the pad face should be readjusted as listed below:

1. If the lower edge cuts in (as in Figure 9-30), change the frontal angle by moving the bottom of the pads apart.
2. If the top edge cuts in (as in Figure 9-31), change the frontal angle by moving the lower part of the pads closer to each other.
3. If the front edge cuts in (as in Figure 9-32), decrease the splay of the pads.
4. If the back edge cuts (as in Figure 9-33), increase the splay of the pads.
5. If the cutting edges seem oblique, the pad is not vertical. Alter the vertical angle and readjust to correct for one or more of the errors listed above.
6. If the upper part of the pad surface seems to be parallel to the nose, but the lower part cuts in, or vice versa, change to a flexible, silicone pad that will conform more readily to changes in nasal angles.[†]

When Pad Angles Are Correct, But Still Slide Down or Hurt

Sometimes even when the pad angles are correct and the frame is adjusted properly, the glasses still have a tendency to slide. This may occur when the frontal angle of the nose is almost straight up and down. When this happens, replace the nosepads with replacement pads

---

[†]If the wearer does not like the feel of silicone pads, it is possible to heat the stiff plastic pads and bend them to match the curve of the nose surface. This condition may occur where the very upper part of the bridge of the nose is thin and straight, and the nose suddenly flares and splays widely within the dimension of the pad.

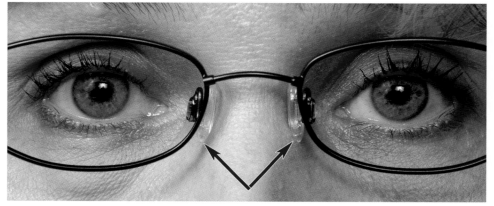

Figure 9-30. Here the lower edges of the pads cut into the nose surface. If the skin on the nose is flaccid, the error is not as visible. It can be detected if the glasses have been worn for a period of time by U-shaped red marks on the nose. The frontal angle is wrong and must be corrected.

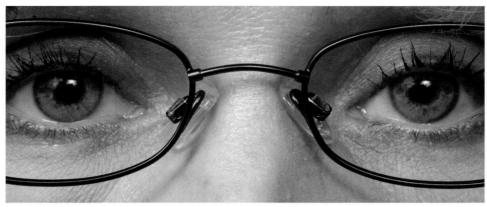

Figure 9-31. If the upper edges of the pads indent, the frontal angle must be more vertically oriented.

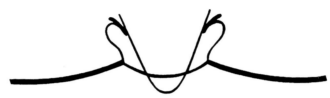

Figure 9-32. This illustration, viewed from the top in cross section, shows a pad splay angle too great for the nose. The splay angle of the pads must be decreased.

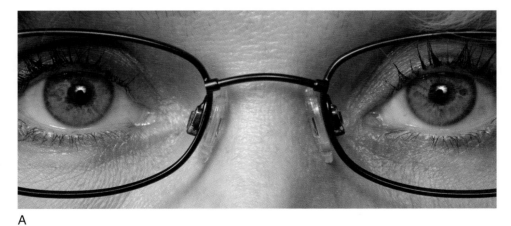

A

B

Figure 9-33. In **A** the splay angle of the pads needs to be increased. The back edges of the pads will cut into the flesh of the nose unless corrected. In **B** the same situation is shown schematically in cross section.

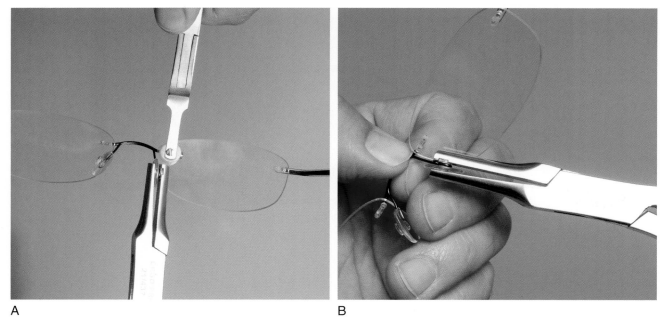

A   B

Figure 9-34. A, Depending upon frame construction, holding the lens with rimless adjusting pliers while adjusting the pad angle may prevent damage to the lens at its point of attachment. For this particular frame this is actually not the best option since the pad arm is attached directly to the bridge. A better option is shown in **B. B,** If the frame is constructed with the pad arm attached more to the bridge, holding the bridge while adjusting the pad may be sufficient.

made from silicone material. This assumes, of course, that the pads are not already of the flexible silicone variety.

Another alternative is to replace the existing pad with a larger pad. This is especially helpful when the pad is causing an irritation to the skin, as often happens in older wearers as the skin loses its elasticity.

A third possibility is to replace both pads with a *strap bridge*. A strap bridge is like two adjustable nosepads that are joined together in straplike fashion. The strap bridge increases the surface area upon which the frame weight rests and is shown in the next chapter as Figure 10-44.

Strap bridges are adjusted like regular nosepads because each side of this flexible bridge has its own pad arm. To get full benefit from the replacement bridge, care should be taken to assure that the upper strap area rests on the crest of the nose and assists in bearing the weight of the frame.

Adjusting Pad Angles for Rimless or Semirimless Mountings

When adjusting the pads of a rimless mounting, certain precautions should be taken to prevent damaging the lens at the point of attachment. A good option is to use rimless adjusting pliers (as were shown in Figure 8-65) to hold the lens at its nasal point of attachment, while adjusting the pad angle with pad adjusting pliers (Figure 9-34, *A*). Some frames may not make this an absolute necessity because the pad arm is attached to the top of the bridge. In this case, or when rimless adjusting pliers are not available, it is possible to hold the bridge of the

frame while adjusting the pad, as in Figure 9-34, *B*. Another option is to hold the lens with the thumb and forefinger at the point of attachment while adjusting the pads (Figure 9-35). Which option may be best may depend upon the construction of the frame.

FRAME HEIGHT AND VERTEX DISTANCE

Achieving the Correct Frame Height

Once the pantoscopic angle has been established satisfactorily, the next step is to place the frame at the correct height. Most judgments for single-vision lenses are based on the position of the frame relative to the brows and orbits (Figure 9-36). It is not difficult to change the vertical height for frames with adjustable pad bridges. For frames with adjustable pad bridges, frame heights can be changed by widening or narrowing the distance between pads.

The primary reasons for widening or narrowing the bridge area are shown in Box 9-1.

Proper Vertex Distance

On occasion it becomes necessary to change the distance between the frame and the face. This is referred to as changing the *vertex distance*, or more specifically, the distance from the front surface of the eye to the back of the spectacle lens. This type of change might be required if, for example, the top of the frame were resting against the brows or the bottom eyewire touching the cheeks and neither error could be corrected by a change of pantoscopic angle. Increasing the vertex distance is also

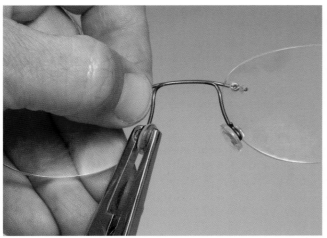

Figure 9-35. If there are no rimless adjusting pliers available, a precaution while adjusting pad angles is to hold the lens tightly between thumb and forefinger at the point of attachment. This helps remove some of the stress from the lens during adjustment. The most appropriate procedure from the three shown in this and the previous two figures will depend upon frame construction. In this figure sequence (Figures 9-34, *A*, 9-34, *B*, and 9-35) the most appropriate procedure for the frame is shown in Figure 9-34, *B*.

BOX 9-1

Reasons for Widening or Narrowing the Frame Bridge Area

WIDENING THE BRIDGE AREA WOULD BE APPROPRIATE IN CASES IN WHICH:
1. The frame is too high on the face.
2. The bifocal or trifocal segments are too high.
3. The progressive addition fitting cross heights are too high.
4. The bridge is too small for the nose.
5. The lenses are too far from the eyes

NARROWING THE BRIDGE AREA WOULD BE APPROPRIATE IN CASES IN WHICH:
1. The frame sits too low on the face.
2. The bifocal or trifocal segments are too low.
3. The progressive addition fitting cross heights are too low.
4. The bridge is too large for the nose.
5. The lashes rub the back surface of the lenses.

often necessary to keep the eyelashes from brushing against the back surface of the lens.

Decreasing the vertex distance, or bringing the frame closer to the face, may be required for purely cosmetic reasons. Decreasing the vertex distance will also provide a wider field of corrected vision. For example, the closer a person stands to a window, the farther to the left and right he or she can see. By the same principle, the closer the frame is to the face the more side area is visible through the lens, with a resulting increase in the overall field of view (Figure 9-37, *A*). Increasing the pantoscopic

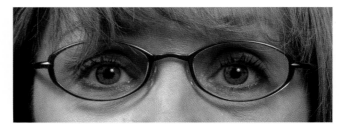

A

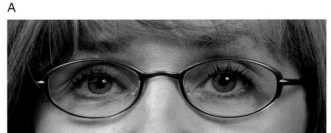

B

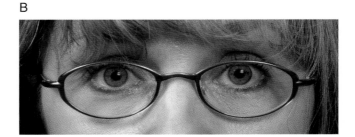

C

Figure 9-36. For conventional eyewear, frame height is based on a combination of eye, eyebrow, and orbit positions. In **A** the frame rides too high. In **B** the height is correct for the frame shown. In **C** the frame is too low. In the past, some large frames have even been designed with upper rims above the brows. As fashion continues to circle around, this could happen in the future. In any case, such frames should still be fitted at a height that conforms to standards discussed in Chapter 4, Frame Selection.

tilt also increases the lower field of view (Figure 9-37, *B*).

For the bifocal wearer, moving the frame closer to the face increases the field of view above the bifocal without the necessity of lowering the segment. (This same effect can be produced by increasing the pantoscopic tilt. See Chapter 5 for specifics.)

When quite strong lenses are involved, precise vertex placement becomes very important. In some instances, small alterations in the vertex distance of the finished spectacles may affect vision profoundly.

ADJUSTING NOSEPADS WITH INVERTED U-SHAPED PAD ARMS

Changing the Distance Between Pads for "Inverted U-Shaped" Pad Arms

The inverted U-shaped pad arm varies in how much it may be adjusted, depending upon how high the U arches. If there is not much length to the pad arm, the extent that it may be adjusted is limited. But if there is "extra"

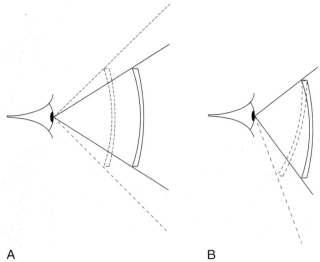

Figure 9-37. When a lens is moved closer to the eye, the field of view increases **(A)**. Pantoscopic tilt also increases the field of view in the lower lens area **(B)**. This is particularly helpful for increasing the near viewing area through bifocals, trifocals, and progressive add lenses.

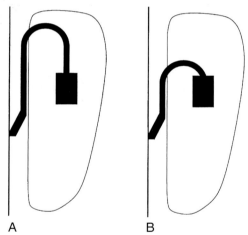

Figure 9-38. The U-shaped pad arm **(A)** has sufficient length to allow frame height and vertex distance changes. The pad arm **(B)** will allow only minimal changes in height and vertex distance, although it may allow some change in the distance between pads.

length to work with, the dispenser will have more latitude in making frame height and vertex distance changes (Figure 9-38).

Most pad adjustments may be done in two movements. The first move makes the change; the second move completes the change and restores the proper pad angle. (This assumes we get it right the first time!)

Widening the Distance Between Pads

When the distance between pads is too small and does not fit the nose, we need to widen the distance between pads. To *widen* the distance between pads, grasp the pad with pad adjusting pliers (Figure 9-39, *A*).

1. First tilt the top of the pliers outward (temporally). *The pivot point is at the point of attachment of the pad arm.* This will cause the top of the U to tilt away from the nose, bending the pad arm at its base (Figure 9-39, *B*). This moves the pad temporally and changes the frontal angle.
2. Next, without removing the pliers from the pad, tilt the bottom of the pliers outward. *Now the pivot point should be the top of the pad arm's inverted U.* This will cause the U to bend at the top, with the center of the pad moving temporally (Figure 9-39, *C*). While the first bend will change the frontal angle of the pad, the second bend will restore it. Figure 9-39, *D* shows the left pad "widened" and the right pad still in the original position.

Narrowing the Distance Between Pads

To *decrease* the distance between pads, the same type of two-step sequence occurs as was described for widening the distance between pads, except that the bends are in a nasal or inward direction instead of outward.

1. For the first bend, the top of the pliers are tilted inward (nasally). *Again the pivot point is at the point of attachment of the pad arm.*
2. For the second bend, follow up by tilting the bottom of the pliers inward, completing the bend, and restoring the frontal angle. *The pivot point is the top of the pad arm's inverted U.*

Moving the Frame Left or Right

(This adjustment uses a combination of the two adjustments that have just been explained: narrowing the distance between pads and widening the distance between pads.)

A frame may sit too left or right on the face as shown in Figure 9-40. There are two possible causes for this problem.

1. The nosepads on the frame are asymmetrical.
2. The wearer's nose is asymmetrical.

When the Nosepads Are Asymmetrical

The first possible cause for a frame sitting too far to the left or right on the wearer's face is that the nosepads on the frame are asymmetrical. If the fault is with the frame, the pads themselves are moved slightly too far to one side or the other, even though they may sit flat on the nose and be comfortable (Figure 9-41). The problem is corrected by moving one pad nasally and the other pad temporally. The procedure for moving one pad nasally is the same as was described for decreasing the distance between pads. The procedure for moving the other pad temporally is the same as was described for increasing the distance between pads.

Adjust both sets of pad arms so that they are mirror images of each other. The left and right pad arms are made to be symmetrical.

When the Wearer's Nose Is Asymmetrical

The second possible cause for a frame being too far left or right is that the person's nose is asymmetrical. This

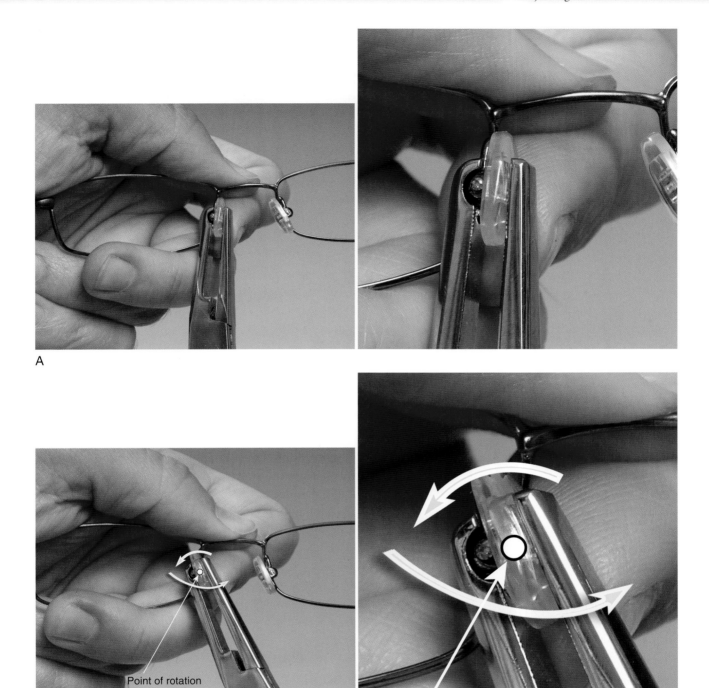

A

B

Point of rotation

Continued

Figure 9-39. To increase the distance between pads for frames having U-shaped pad arms:
- Grasp the pad with pad-adjusting pliers **(A)**.
- Tilt the top of the pliers outward temporally **(B)**. The point of rotation is at the point of attachment of the pad arm. This will decrease the frontal angle.

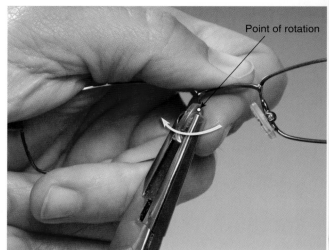

Point of rotation

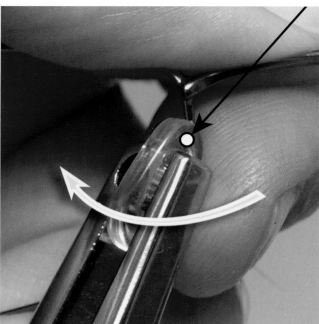

C

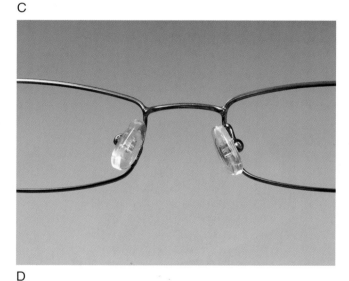

D

Figure 9-39. cont'd
- Next turn the bottom of the pliers temporalward with the pivot point being the top of the pad arm's inverted U **(C)**. This will move the face of the pad temporally and will allow the frontal angle of the pad to be returned to the necessary angle.
- **D,** The pad on the left pad has been "widened" (moved outward).

is quite a common occurrence because many people have had a broken nose at one time or another. If the break was far enough back on the nose it will cause the frame to sit off center, even though the pad arms and pads are symmetrical.

To check for such an error, look at the frame from the straight-ahead position. If the frame is toward the *right side of the wearer's face*, bend the pad arms at their *bases in the direction of the wearer's right lens* and then realign the pad angles. If the frame is toward the *wearer's left*, bend the pad arms toward the *left lens*. The direction of the bend may be remembered logically by keeping in mind that moving the pad arms one way pushes the frame in the opposite direction. It may be remembered by rote by thinking "Frame to the right, move pads to the right.

RIGHT-RIGHT," and "Frame to the left, move pads to the left. LEFT-LEFT.*

---

*Up to this point we have simple consistency for memorization purposes between observed error and proper correction of that error. The consistent relationship between the direction of the error and the direction of correction for that error helps simplify any required memorization.
For equality of vertex distance: One lens in, bend same temple in: IN-IN. One lens out, bend same temple out: OUT-OUT.
For straightness of the frame on the face: One side up, bend same temple up: UP-UP. One side down, bend same temple down: DOWN-DOWN.
For symmetry of the frame on the face: Frame to the right, move pads to the right: RIGHT-RIGHT. Frame to the left, move pads to the left: LEFT-LEFT.

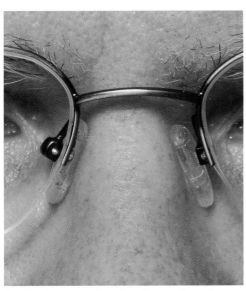

Figure 9-40. An example of a frame that sits too far to the wearer's left. Note that when the pads are shifted to the wearer's right, the frame shifts to the wearer's left.

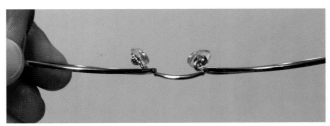

Figure 9-41. In this photo, the pad angles are basically symmetrical, but the pads themselves are moved too far to one side. This defect as shown from above will cause the frame to sit too far to the wearer's left, as was shown in the previous figure.

Changing Frame Height, But Not Vertex Distance

Changing the Height of Pads for Inverted U-Style Pad Arms

Most of the time a frame will be moved higher or lower on the face by narrowing or widening the distance between pads. (This procedure was described earlier.) However, narrowing or widening the distance between pads will also cause the frame to move farther from or closer to the eyes. The distance from the lenses to the eyes is called the vertex distance. To keep the vertex distance the same, the distance between the pads must remain the same. This means that in order to change the height of the frame, the location of the pads relative to the frame front must move up or down.

Moving the frame higher or lower on the face without changing the distance between pads is accomplished for inverted U-style pad arms by changing the location of the bend or loop at the top of the U in the pad arm. Lowering the frame can be accomplished by one of two

methods. The first is easier and requires only two primary bends.

Lowering the Frame: Method 1. To lower the frame on the face without changing the vertex distance, the location of the bend in the pad arm is moved closer to the pad. This is shown in Figure 9-42. The adjustment itself may be made with two bends. These are:

1. Grasp the pad with pad adjusting pliers as seen in Figure 9-43, *A*. While exerting an upward pull on the pad, bend the pad arm until the posterior part of the U is almost perpendicular with the frame front (Figure 9-43, *B*). The pad arm is now shaped more like an "L" than a "U."
2. Bend the pad arm back down, while pushing upward with the pliers (Figure 9-43, *C*).

It may be necessary to repeat these two steps if the pad has not moved up enough. Without an upward pull during step 1 and an upward push in step 2, there will not be any appreciable change in pad height. The finished pad is shown in Figure 9-43, *D*. The other pad is then adjusted to match.

This method will usually work. But if the frame pad will not move enough using this technique, then the more complicated Method 2 technique may be used.

Lowering the Frame: Method 2. Using this method to move the frame lower on the face, the bend in the inverted U must still be moved closer to the pad. The new bend can be placed more easily if the old bend is removed first.

Here are the Method 2 steps for moving the frame lower on the face:

1. Begin by grasping the pad with pad adjusting pliers as shown in Figure 9-44, *A*.
2. Bend the pad up far enough to practically straighten the pad arm (Figure 9-44, *B*).
3. Once the pad arm is straight, use square-round, snipe nose, bent-snipe, or a similar type of thin pliers to grasp the pad arm closer to the pad (Figure 9-44, *C*). How close the pliers are positioned in reference to the pad will depend upon how much higher on the face the frame must be moved.
4. Rotate the pliers until the full U-shaped bend is restored (Figure 9-44, *D*). By comparing the position of this pad to the other one (Figure 9-44, *E*), it can be seen that the newly adjusted pad is noticeably higher.
5. Next equally alter the other pad.

In the end, both pads should still have the same horizontal distance between them. Therefore they will rest on the same position of the nose as before. Because they have been moved higher, the frame will be lower on the face.

Raising the Frame Without Changing the Distance Between Pads

Raising the Frame: Method 1.

To raise the frame on the face without changing the vertex distance, the location of the bend in the pad arm is moved closer to

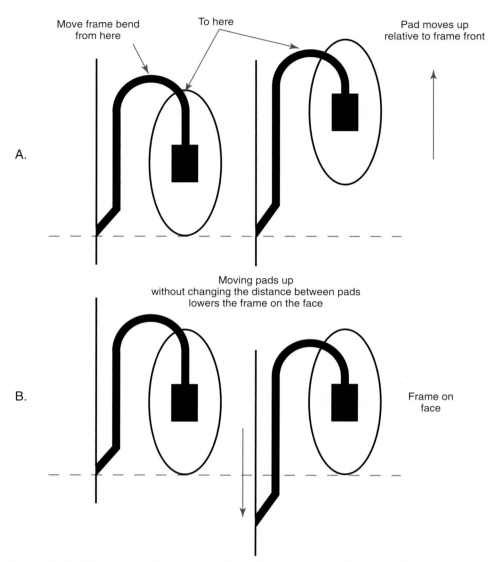

To lower frame height only:
move pads up by changing bend location

Move frame bend
from here

To here

Pad moves up
relative to frame front

A.

Moving pads up
without changing the distance between pads
lowers the frame on the face

B.

Frame on
face

Figure 9-42. To lower the frame on the face without changing the vertex distance, the pads are moved up, but the right and left pads are still the same distance apart. This means that the pads will rest on the nose as they did before. However, this means that the frame, being lower relative to the pads, will also be lower on the wearer's face. **A,** If the bend in the pad arm is moved closer to the pad, the pad moves up. **B,** Because the pad will sit on the nose where it did before, the frame will be lower.

the frame. This method is the reverse of that described in Method 1 for lowering the frame and does not work as easily. Even though it is theoretically feasible to make this adjustment with two bends, it may need to be repeated.
1. Grasp the pad with pad adjusting pliers. While exerting a downward pull on the pad, bend the pad arm until the posterior part of the U is almost perpendicular with the frame front.
2. Still exerting a downward pull on the pad, bring the pad arm back to its correct angle. (Care should be

taken so as not to inadvertently pull the pad away from the frame front.)

Raising the Frame: Method 2. Method 2 for lowering the frame is practically a repeat of Method 2 for raising the frame, with only minor changes. Here is how it is done.
1. Begin by grasping the pad with pad adjusting pliers.
2. Bend the pad up far enough to practically straighten the pad arm.
3. Once the pad arm is straight, use square-round, snipe nose, bent-snipe, or a similar type of thin

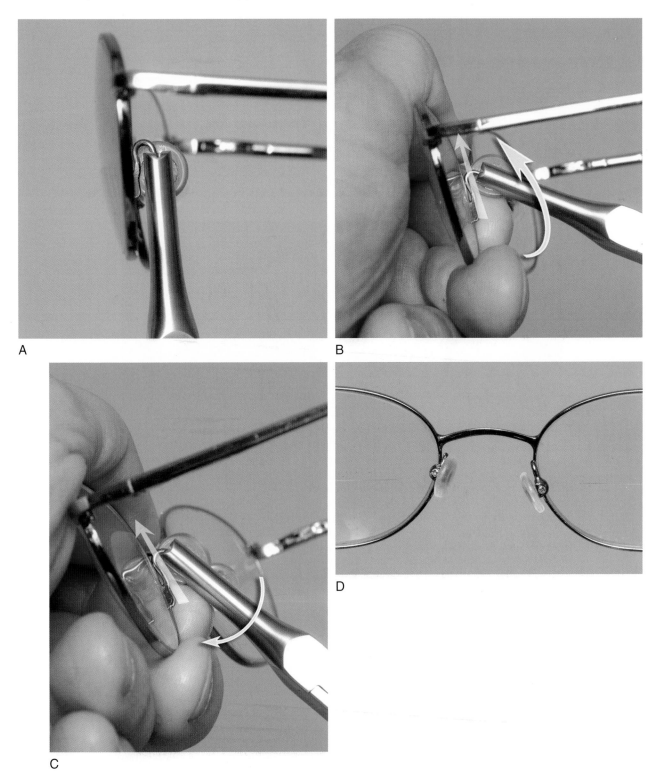

A

B

C

D

Figure 9-43. To raise the pad (lowering the frame on the face), grasp the pad with the pad adjusting pliers **(A)**. The pad may be raised in two moves. First bend the pad horizontally while pulling up **(B)**. Second the pad is returned to its former location. While turning the bottom of the pad back downward, simultaneously push the top of the pad upward as shown in **(C)**. The upward pull **(B)** and upward push **(C)** cause the location of the bend in the U to move closer to the pad. This raises the position of the pad relative to the frame front. **D,** The difference in pad height produced by this adjustment.

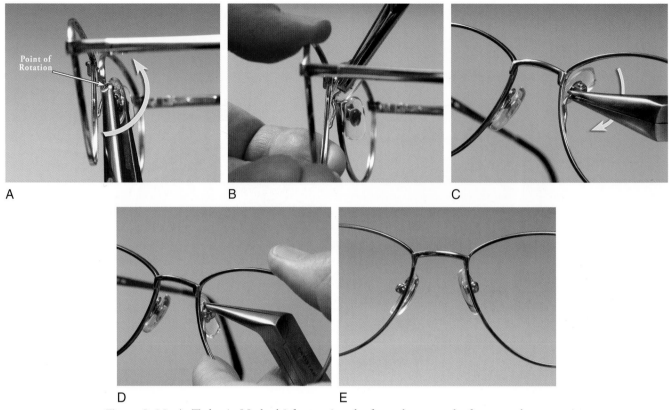

Figure 9-44. **A,** To begin Method 2 for moving the frame lower on the face, start by grasping the pad with pad adjusting pliers. (It is also possible to use thin-nosed pliers and grasp the pad arm instead of the pad.) The point of rotation will be the top of the bend in the pad arm. **B,** The pad arm has just been straightened. By removing the bend, the pad arm can be rebent at a new location. (At this point in the sequence, the pad could either be raised or lowered, depending upon the location of the new bend.) **C,** In this figure, bent snipe-nosed pliers have been moved closer to the pad in preparation for placing the new bend. When the bend occurs, the point of rotation will be where the pliers are grasping the pad arm. **D,** The new bend location is much closer to the pad than it had been. **E,** The bend is now complete and pad height location between left and right pads may be compared. The pad on the right is considerably higher. After the pad on the left is adjusted to match, the frame will be higher on the face by an amount equal to what now shows as the difference in pad heights.

pliers to grasp the pad arm *closer to the point of attachment of the pad arm to the frame front.* How close the pliers are positioned depends upon how much lower on the face the frame must be moved.
4. Rotate the pliers until the full U-shaped bend is restored.
5. Next equally alter the other pad.

Both pads should still have the same horizontal distance between them, will rest on the same position of the nose, and because they have been moved lower, will cause the frame to sit higher on the face. This is illustrated in Figure 9-45.

Changing Vertex Distance, But Not Height

It is possible to change the vertex distance by narrowing or widening the distance between pads. A secondary effect is an increase or decrease in the overall height of the frame. When frame height changes must be avoided, pad bridges should be adjusted another way.

Moderately Increasing the Vertex Distance for Frames With Inverted U-Style Pad Arms

The sequence for moderately increasing the vertex distance can be done with just two bends. This is shown in Figure 9-46. Here is how it is done:
1. The pad is grasped with pad-adjusting pliers and the top of the pad is rotated away from the frame front (Figure 9-46, *A*). The point of rotation is at the point of attachment the pad arm. The pad arm bends at the point of attachment. This changes the vertical angle of the nosepad.
2. The vertical angle can be immediately corrected without repositioning the pliers. The angle is changed by moving the lower part of the pad away from the frame front. The point of rotation is the top of the inverted U. The rotation of the pliers is indicated by the arrow shown in Figure 9-46, *B*. This corrects the vertical angle (Figure 9-46, *C*). The end result is seen in Figure 9-46, *D*.

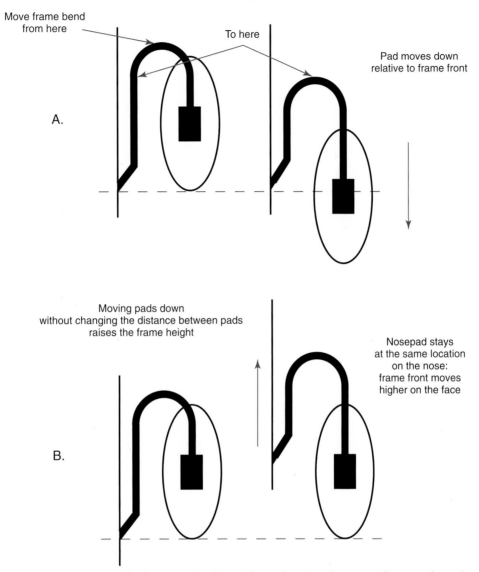

To raise frame height only:
move pads down by changing bend location

Move frame bend
from here

To here

Pad moves down
relative to frame front

A.

Moving pads down
without changing the distance between pads
raises the frame height

Nosepad stays
at the same location
on the nose:
frame front moves
higher on the face

B.

Figure 9-45. To raise the frame on the face without changing the vertex distance, the pads are moved down, but both right and left pads are still the same distance apart and rest on the nose where they did before. But the frame will be higher on the wearer's face. **A,** If the bend in the pad arm is moved closer to the pad arm's point of attachment, the pad moves down. **B,** Because the pad will sit on the nose where it did before, the frame will end up higher.

Significantly Increasing the Vertex Distance for Frames With Inverted U-Style Pad Arms

The idea behind significantly increasing the vertex distance with upside down U-shaped pads is a simple one. Imagine a piece of coat hanger shaped into an upside down U. To increase the distance between the legs of the U, imagine grasping both legs and strenuously pulling them apart. The coat hanger wire is malleable and yields easily. The legs are now farther apart, but the top of the upside down U is longer and flat. Fortunately, this radical adjustment is seldom required.

To significantly increase the vertex distance for a frame having inverted-U style pad arms, we must flatten the top of the pad arm. To begin the process, use square-round pliers and position them at the upper area of the bend in the pad arm. Remove the bend by rotating the pliers as shown in Figure 9-47, *A*. Next, position the pliers closer to the pad arm's point of attachment. Position the round jaw where the inside of the bend will be (Figure 9-47, *B*). Rotate the pliers so that the pad arm turns straight back (Figure 9-47, *C*). The new bend causes the pad arm to have an approximately 90-degree angle. Now slide the pliers closer to the pad

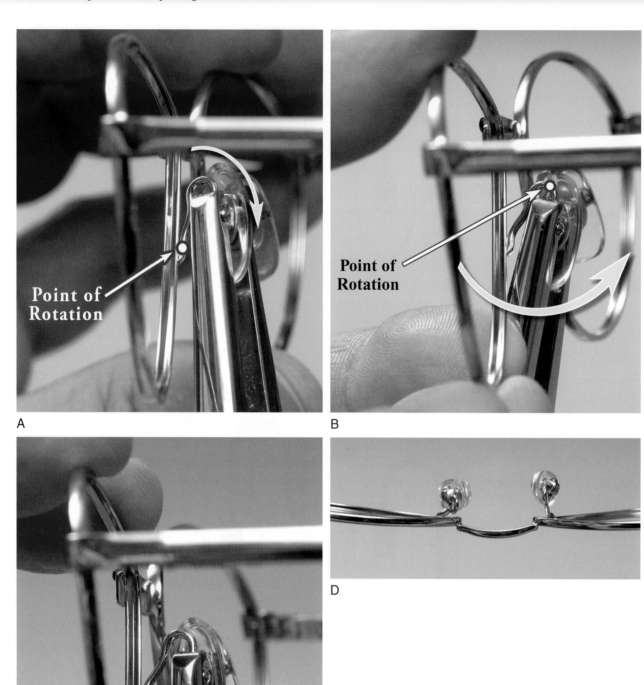

A

B

C

D

Figure 9-46. Here is the sequence for increasing the vertex distance without changing the height of the frame on the face. **A,** The pad is grasped and the top of the pad moved away from the frame. **B,** The bottom of the pad must now be moved away from the frame to complete the adjustment. **C,** The adjustment is complete. **D,** The pads are shown from the top and the difference between left and right pads is evident. Now the pad on the left will be adjusted in an identical manner to match the pad on the right.

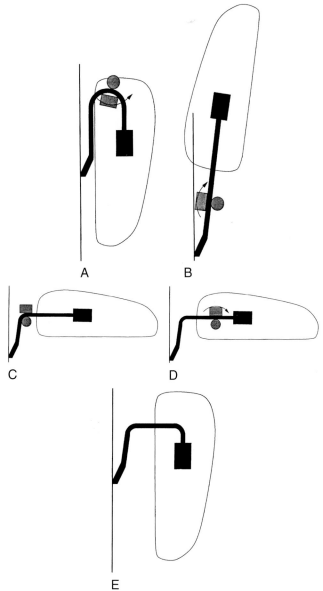

Figure 9-47. **A,** To remove the bend, the pliers are rotated as shown. Here the square-round pliers are shown with the square jaw on the inside so that the point of rotation is the center of the round jaw. (If the bend is too tight to allow this, the round jaw may need to be placed on the inside of the curl.) **B,** To effectively lengthen the pad arm, a new bend will be placed nearer to the point of attachment with the frame. The new bend will not be the only bend. **C,** In accomplishing this bend, the round jaw of the pliers was placed on the inside of the bend. The pad arm has been bent so that the top of the new curl will be flat. **D,** Next the pliers are rotated as shown. **E,** This is the theoretical appearance of a completed vertex distance change. The individual bends will not always look as neatly squared off in practice.

(Figure 9-47, *D*) and place another 90-degree angle in the pad arm. When complete, the pad arm should appear as seen in Figure 9-47, *E*.

Decreasing the Vertex Distance for Frames With Inverted U-Shaped Pad Arms

To decrease the vertex distance, the pads must be positioned closer to the frame front. As with most of the more common pad adjustments, this adjustment may be done with just two bends. The pad is grasped with pad adjusting pliers as in Figure 9-48, *A*. Here is the sequence:

1. Bend the bottom of the pad away from the frame front while pressing the top of the pad in toward the frame front as shown in Figure 9-48, *B*.
2. Next swing the bottom of the pad toward the frame front without allowing the top of the pad to move (Figure 9-48, *C*). If the pliers do not have enough room to swing the lower part of the pad inward, turn them upside down and grasp the pad from above.

The completed work is shown from the top in Figure 9-48, *D* where right and left pad distances can be compared. The pad should still have the same alignment angles as before (frontal, splay, and vertical). It is just farther forward. When both pads are completed, the frame will rest closer to the eyes.

ADJUSTING NOSEPADS WITH QUESTION MARK–STYLE PAD ARMS

Nose pads supported by pad arms that look like a question mark when viewed from the top were the predominant type of pad arm. Now they are definitely a minority. However, they do continue to appear, sometimes as part of a "hybrid" combination of the inverted U and question mark. These types of pad arms are very versatile and in some ways allow easier changes in frame height and vertex distance.

Changing the Distance Between Pads for Question Mark–Style Pad Arms

Regardless of pad or pad arm style, widening the distance between pads will lower the frame and allow it to sit closer to the face. Narrowing the distance between pads will raise the frame and cause it to sit farther from the face.

Widening the Distance Between Pads (Question Mark Style)

When working with question mark style pads, some prefer to use pad adjusting pliers on the face of the pad; others would rather use thin-nosed pliers and grasp the pad arm directly.

Square-round pliers as shown in Figure 9-49. When using square-round pliers, the round jaw will be the pivot point of the pliers (Figure 9-50). It is easier to use

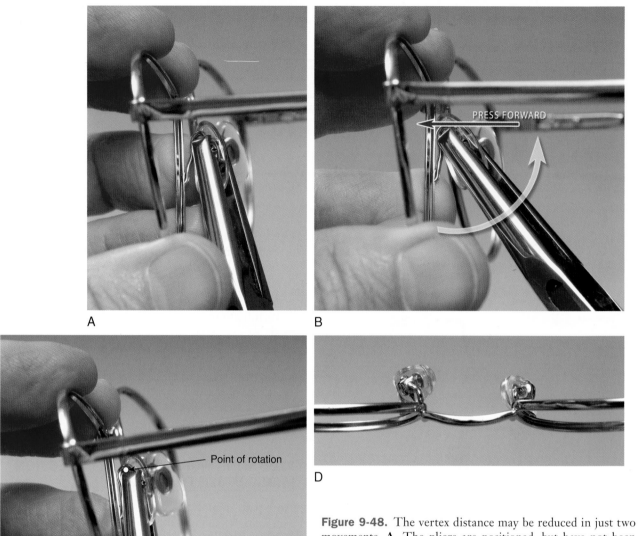

A

B

C

Point of rotation

D

Figure 9-48. The vertex distance may be reduced in just two movements. **A,** The pliers are positioned, but have not been moved yet. **B,** The top of the pad is pressed forward. To get the top of the pad solidly forward, the bottom of the pad is rotated back some. **C,** The bottom of the pad is pressed and/or rotated forward. (If there is not enough room for the pliers from below, grasp the pad from above or use thin pliers to grip the pad arm itself.) **D,** The pad on the right is seen to be closer to the frame front than the pad on the left. When the pad on the left is equally adjusted, the frame will sit closer to the face and eyes.

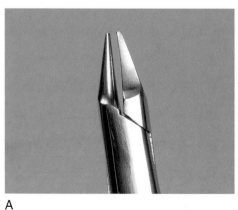

A

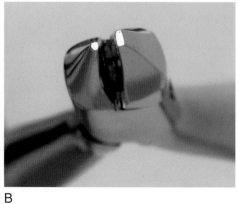

B

Figure 9-49. The square-round (flat-round) pliers are used for pad arm manipulation. **A,** The left side of the jaw is round, the right side is squared off and flat on the inner surface. This is seen more easily from above **(B)**. The design allows the pad arm to be solidly gripped and smoothly bent.

thin-nosed pliers with question mark style pads than with inverted U-shaped pad arms because the pad arm is more easily accessible from the top or the bottom.

Widening the distance between pads can be done in two moves with either type of pliers. The first changes the position of the pad arm, but messes up the splay angle. The second move reangles the splay angle. Here are the two moves for widening the distance between pads using *pad adjusting pliers*:

1. Grasp the pad with pad adjusting pliers and move the pad arm temporally (outward). The bend takes place at the point of attachment of the pad arm and rotates around that point (Figure 9-51, *A*).
2. Correct the splay angle by rotating the pliers with the point of rotation at the center of the pad-arm

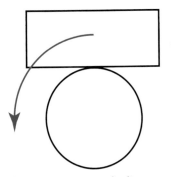

Figure 9-50. To use square-round pliers most effectively, position the pliers so that the round jaw is the pivot point for the bend.

curl (Figure 9-51, *B*). Compare the right and left pads in Figure 9-51, *C*. The pad distance on the left has been widened; the one on the right has not.

Here are the two moves for widening the distance between pads *using square-round pliers*:

1. Grasp the pad arm near the base with square-round pliers held vertically. Bend the pad arm outward. Remember to place the round jaw on the side of the direction the pads are to be moved. Pivot the pliers around the round jaw.
2. Holding the pliers vertically, grasp the pad arm directly in back of the pad and reangle the splay angle.

Narrowing the Distance Between Pads (Question Mark Style)

Narrowing the distance between pads is done the same as widening the distance between pads, except the direction of movement is nasal (inward) instead of temporal (outward). Here are the moves (Figure 9-52):

1. Bend the pad inward.
   a. When using pad adjusting pliers, grasp the pad and bend the pad arm inward so the bend takes place at the point of attachment of the pad arm.
   b. When using square-round pliers, grasp the pad arm near the base with square-round pliers held vertically and bend the pad arm inward. Place the round jaw on the side of the direction the pads are to be moved and pivot the pliers around the round jaw as shown in Figure 9-50.

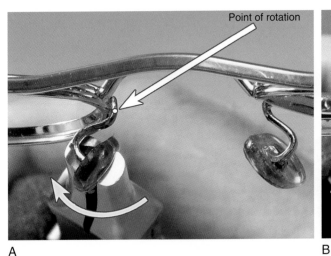

A

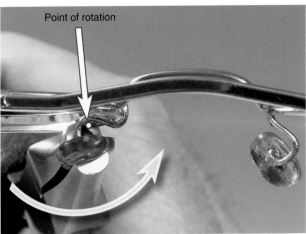

B

Figure 9-51. A, To widen the distance between pads for frames with question mark style pad arms, there are two moves required. This sequence uses pad adjusting pliers. The first move is to grasp the pad with and bend the pad arm outward. The bend takes place at the pad arm's point of attachment. **B,** Here, for the second move in widening the distance between pads, the splay angle is corrected. The pad face is rotated as shown. **C,** The left pad has been moved to the widened position, the right pad has not yet been adjusted. The center line is for reference so that the change in pad distance will be more readily evident.

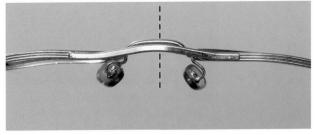

C

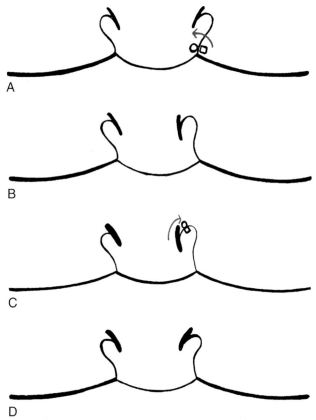

A

B

C

D

Figure 9-52. Summarization of the sequence of steps for narrowing the distance between pads with question mark type pad arms. Only one pad is adjusted for the sake of comparison.

2. Correct the splay angle of the pads.
   a. Use pad-adjusting pliers to correct the splay angle of the pad, or
   b. Use square-round pliers to do the same thing as shown in Figures 9-51, *B* and 9-53.

Moving the Frame Left or Right With Question Mark–Style Pad Arms

(Remember that this adjustment uses a combination of the two adjustments that have just been explained: narrowing the distance between pads and widening the distance between pads.)

When the frame sits too far left or right on the face as was shown in Figure 9-40, remember that there are two possible causes for this problem:
1. The nosepads on the frame are asymmetrical.
2. The wearer's nose is asymmetrical.

To correct the problem, bend one pad arm inward (as in narrowing the distance between pads) and the other outward (as in widening the distance between pads). The entire sequence when using square-round pliers is shown in Figure 9-54.

Changing Frame Height but not Vertex Distance for Question Mark–Style Pad Arms

To change the frame height, but not the distance from the frame to the eyes, the distance between the pads must remain the same, but the pads must be either higher or lower. This will move the frame down or up.

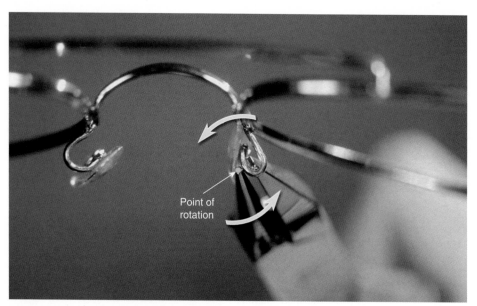

Point of rotation

Figure 9-53. Square-round pliers being used to correct the splay angle of the nosepad and complete the pad narrowing process (*top view*). The point of rotation is at the center of the round jaw of the pliers.

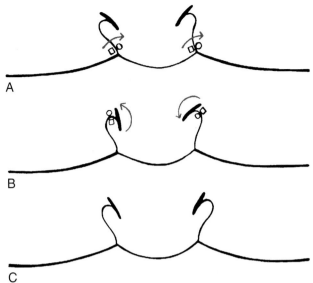

Figure 9-54. **A,** Even though both pad surfaces are correctly angled, both pads are too far to the left. This will cause the frame to be shifted to the right. Bending the pad arms back to their proper position throws the pad angles off **(B)**. These must be reangled as shown in **B** to achieve correct alignment **(C)**.

Suppose we change the question mark style pad arms so they angle downward when leaving the eyewires instead of coming off at right angles. If the pads now rest on the same place on the nose as previously, the lenses will be situated higher on the face in relation to the eyes than previously. The reverse is true if the pad arms are angled up.

Lowering the Frame: Question Mark Pad Arms

To lower the frame, the adjustment is done in two moves. The first bend moves the pad upward; the second corrects the messed-up vertical angle. Here is the procedure:

1. With the pliers held horizontally, grasp the entire pad arm between the pliers' jaws and simply bend the arm upward. (Figure 9-55, *A* shows how the bend is done, and Figure 9-55, *B* shows what the pad looks like after this first step is completed.)

    Correct the vertical angle of the pad. To adjust the angle of the pad, use square-round pliers held vertically. Grasp the pad arm behind the pad halfway into the curl area and return the pad to its original angle (Figure 9-55, *C* and *D*). It may be necessary to grasp the pad arm from above to complete the bend and to fully return the pad to the correct vertical angle.

2. Pad-adjusting pliers can also be used to correct the vertical angle if sufficient room between pad and eyewire is present and if care is taken not to accidentally bend the pad arm back to its original position.

Raising the Frame: Question Mark Pad Arms

To raise the frame, the sequence is the same as for lowering the frame with one exception—the pad arm is bent downward instead of upward. The procedure is:

1. With the pliers held horizontally, grasp the entire pad arm between the pliers' jaws and bend the pad arm downward.

2. Correct the vertical angle of the pad. To adjust the angle of the pad, use square-round pliers held vertically and grasp the pad arm behind the pad.

Increasing the Vertex Distance Only for Frames with Question Mark–Style Pad Arms

Extending the pad arms will increase the vertex distance between the lenses and the eyes. Here is the sequence of adjustments for pad bridges with question mark style pad arms:

1. Open the pad arm curl. Position the square-round pliers so that the square jaw is inside the pad arm curl and the round jaw is outside. Open out the curl of the pad arm by compressing the jaws and rotating the pliers slightly (Figure 9-56, *A*). This adjustment increases the distance from the lens to the pad. When a radical increase in vertex distance is necessary, it is possible to open the pad arm out completely (Figure 9-56, *B*). This is done by squeezing a section of it at a time, gradually moving the positions of the jaws closer to the pad while squeezing with the large part of the pliers near the pliers' throat until the pad arm is absolutely straight.

2. Replace the curl nearer to the pad. Flattening the curl of the pad arm, by whatever method, will turn the pad away from its proper angle so that its surface faces straight back, or nearly so. The pad arm will now require a new curl, which should be placed closer to the pad than it was previously. To put the curl in correctly, hold the square-round pliers vertically and grip the pad arm at the desired position of the curl. Position the round jaw so that it will be on the inside of the new curl (Figure 9-56, *C*). Using the round jaw as a pivotal point, rotate the pliers until the pad reaches its proper position. Figure 9-56, *D* shows an example of how the pad arm should look when finished.

If difficulty is experienced in getting the curl to bend exactly at the desired place, it may be helpful to use a second pair of pliers as holding pliers. With these, the pad arm can be held firmly at a point approximately halfway between the pad and the point of attachment to the frame. This two-pliers technique is extremely useful for antique rimless mountings where bracing is necessary to prevent chipping the lens near the pad arm. It also allows the pad arm to be curled without inadvertently bending it at its base.

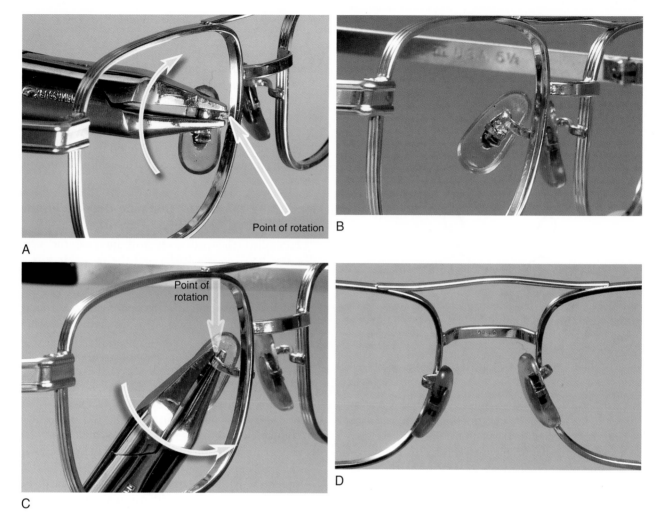

Figure 9-55. A, To raise the pads on frames with question mark pad arms, thin pliers are used to grasp the entire pad arm and bend it upward. This will lower the frame on the face. **B,** After the question mark type pad arm has been bent upward, the pad will be considerably higher, but has an incorrect vertical angle. The pad must be reangled. **C,** Reangling the pad to correct the vertical angle after having raised the question mark style pad arm is done by grasping the curl close to the pad. This can be done with square round (or thin-nosed) pliers as shown here. **D,** Note how much higher the pad on the right is than the pad on the left. When both pads are adjusted, the frame will sit considerably lower than previously.

Decreasing the Vertex Distance Only for Frames with Question Mark–Style Pad Arms

Bringing the pads closer to the lenses will decrease the vertex distance. Here is the two-step sequence used to bring about this change for pad bridges with question mark style pad arms. (See Figure 9-57, *A* to see what the pads look like before starting the adjustment.)

1. Grasp the pad arm at its base with the round jaw toward the temporal side of the frame (Figure 9-57, *B*). Bend the pad arm towards the lens. This will throw the splay angle off (Figure 9-57, *C*).

2. Position the square-round pliers in the curl of the pad arm with the round jaw on the inside of the curl (Figure 9-57, *D*). Tighten the curl by rotating the pliers around the round jaw. This should move the pad closer to the frame, correct the splay angle, and return the pad it to the original distance between pads.

When the adjustment is complete, the reangled pad should duplicate its original angle (Figure 9-57, *E*).

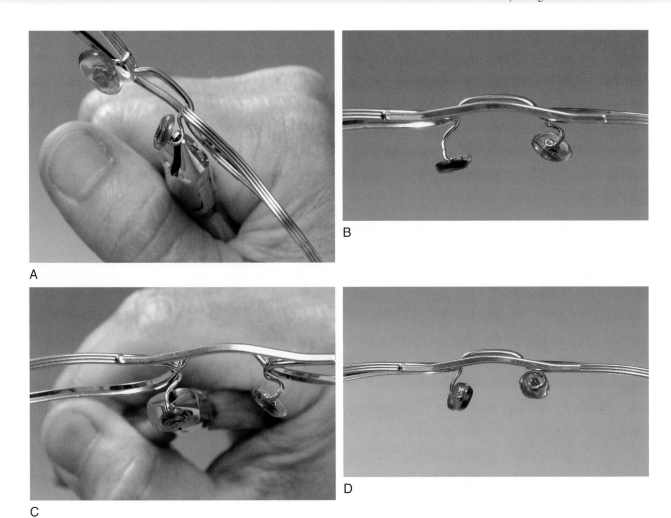

Figure 9-56. **A,** Increasing the vertex distance without changing frame height: To straighten the question mark type pad arm, the curl of the arm is flattened by compressing the jaws and rotating the pliers slightly. Note the location of square and round jaws. Because the curl must open up, the square jaw is on the inside of the curl. (Frame shown from below.) **B,** Here the pad arm curl has been opened up and the pad faces back. (Frame shown from above.) **C,** A new curl is to be placed in the pad arm so that it has a longer effective length. By noting the position of the square-round pliers, it is possible to predict the location of the new curl. (Frame shown from above.) **D,** The pad arm on the left has been lengthened. That on the right is in its normal position. (Frame shown from above.)

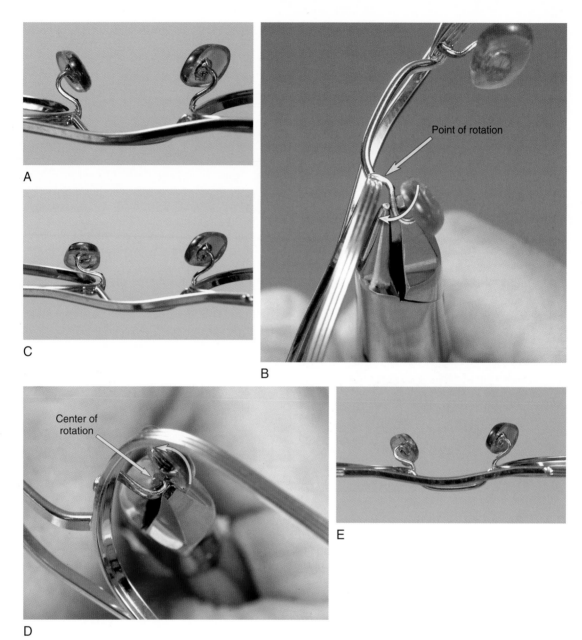

Figure 9-57. A, Here is how the pads and pad arms appear before shortening the effective length of the pad arms. This will decrease the vertex distance from frame to eyes. The pad on the left will be moved. (Frame shown from above.) **B,** To decrease the vertex distance, bend the pad arm temporally. The bend takes place at the point of attachment of the pad arm. (Frame shown from below.) **C,** The pad arm on the left has been bent outward at the base in the first part of decreasing the vertex distance. The splay angle has been thrown off. (Frame shown from above.) **D,** To complete the decrease in vertex distance, tighten the curl of the pad arm. This moves the pad closer to the frame, corrects the splay angle, and returns it to where the distance between pads will be the same as it was before. Note that the square-round pliers grasp the curl with the round jaw on the inside of the curl. (Frame shown front view from below.) **E,** The pad arm on the left has been effectively shortened. The pad arm on the right is positioned normally. After the pad arm on the right has been adjusted, the vertex distance will be considerably less than before. (Frame shown from above.)

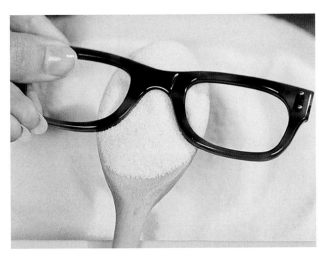

Figure 9-58. Use hot salt scooped up in a wooded spoon to heat fixed pads on a plastic frame in preparation for changing their splay angle. Hot air works equally well or better.

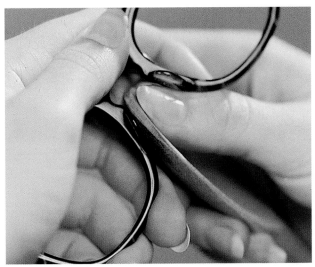

Figure 9-59. Bending the pads back on a plastic frame using the back surface of a wooden spoon. If hot salt is used to heat frames, a wooden spoon is commonly used to stir the salt and makes a handy flat surface to angle the fixed pad back.

SECTION C
"Nonadjustable" Bridge Adjustments

ACHIEVING THE PROPER FITTING ANGLES FOR NONADJUSTABLE PLASTIC BRIDGES

For plastic frames without adjustable pads, checking for correct bridge fit at the time of frame selection is essential. The size must be right and all fitting angles correct. Nonetheless, in certain circumstances it may still be possible to correct a problem after the fact.

Modifying Fixed Pad Bridges

A limited number of plastic frames have a bridge with small, "built-in" pads made from the same material as the frame. They should sit flat on the nose from the beginning and should not have to be adjusted. But suppose a frame bridge without adjustable nosepads, but with these small, fixed pads has the correct width and is parallel to the nose when viewed from the front. The bridge size and frontal angle have been correctly chosen. In spite of this, the splay angle is incorrect, and the attached plastic pads flare in such a manner that their inner edges project into the backward sloping surface of the nose and indent it. This condition will produce both visible and potentially painful signs.

The flare of the pads can be altered by heating the pads and modifying their angle of attachment to the front. To heat the nosepads, use a spoon to scoop up some hot salt from the salt bath and hold it against the pads (Figure 9-58), or direct a concentrated stream of hot air against the pad. To flare the pads outward, use pressure from a smooth flat object, such as a spoon bowl (Figure 9-59).

Modifying Sculptured Bridges

A frame with a "sculptured bridge" has no pad at all. Rather, the bridge area of the frame rests directly on the nose. Frames that have a sculptured bridge rather than pads cannot be altered in angle unless the plastic is filed to a new form. When a coarse file is used, the area should be subsequently smoothed down with fine-grain emery paper. Buffing the area afterward using a rag wheel and buffing rouge will restore a good polish to the frame for cellulose acetate or propionate frames. If no wheel is available, acetone may be applied repeatedly until an acceptable smoothness results. (Newer frame materials may require the application of a polyurethane furniture finish.) It should be kept in mind that filing the bridge as described may cause the frame to sit somewhat lower on the face than previously. When a sculptured bridge does need alteration, it is usually a result of poor frame selection.

FIXED BRIDGE HEIGHT AND VERTEX DISTANCE CHANGES

Properly selected fixed bridge frames should already be at the correct height. If they need to be changed in their height, there are certain limited ways to accomplish it.

In plastic frames and other "nonadjustable" fixed-bridge frames, the height can be affected only by altering the distance between the lenses—either by narrowing or widening the bridge. This adjustment forces the frames to ride on either a wider or narrower part of the nose. Since the nose widens from top to bottom, the frames will be correspondingly either higher or lower than they were before the change in bridge width.

In fixed-bridge frames, even the vertex distance position can usually only be attained by widening or narrowing the bridge. (Again the necessity of altering vertex distance should have been prevented by proper bridge or frame selection during the fitting.)

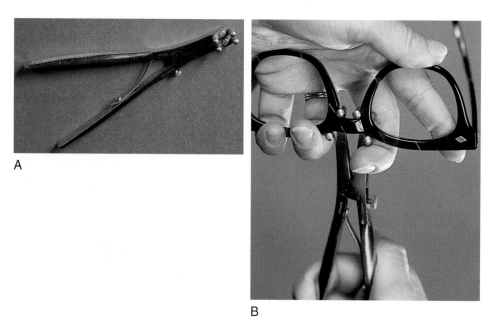

Figure 9-60. A, Bridge-widening pliers. **B,** The procedure for using those pliers. The design of the pliers works better for keyhole bridges than saddle bridges.

If the bridge is widened, it will not only lower the frame but also permit it to sit farther back on the nose, bringing it closer to the eyes. On the other hand, if the bridge is narrowed, it may not only raise the frame, but will cause it to sit forward on the nose, farther from the eyes.

It should be noted that when the physical width of the bridge is widened or narrowed, this will also widen or narrow the distance between the optical centers of the lenses. While this may be tolerable for lower-powered lenses, it may cause problems with unwanted prismatic effect as the power of the lenses increase. Thus, if any adjustments to the physical width of the bridge are being considered, remember:

1. Low-powered lenses may make alterations to the distance between lenses acceptable. "Acceptable" would mean that the change would not cause the lens prescription to go outside of ANSI Z80 Recommendations for Prescription Ophthalmic Lenses.
2. Adjustments to the physical bridge size that will affect the distance between lens centers should be done before the lenses are ordered so that the wearer's PD will be correct when worn.
3. If the above two situations cannot be accomplished, then the adjustment should not be done.

Plastic Frames

Changing the distance between lenses in plastic frames can be accomplished in several different ways. The following methods are those primarily used:

Using Pliers to Change Bridge Size

To use pliers to change the bridge size of a plastic frame, measure the width of the bridge from lens to lens to obtain a starting measurement. Heat the bridge area of the frame. To widen the bridge, place bridge-widening pliers (Figure 9-60, *A*) in the bridge area, and squeeze (Figure 9-60, *B*).

To narrow the bridge, bridge narrowing pliers are sometimes used (Figure 9-61, *A*). Again, place the pliers on the heated bridge area and squeeze (Figure 9-61, *B*).

Note the amount of change by remeasuring until the proper width is achieved, then try the frame on the wearer to verify the alteration. The use of widening or narrowing pliers does not guarantee success. In actual practice, such pliers are successful with only a very limited number of plastic frames.

Using a Dowel Rod to Change Bridge Size

Vertical sections of dowel rods are used for changing bridge size. A $^3/_8$-inch rod is used for narrowing, and a $^5/_8$-inch rod for widening the bridge. To change bridge size using a dowel rod, hold the frame by the eyewires and pull the preheated bridge around the dowel while keeping the lenses parallel (Figure 9-62).

On the narrow dowel rod, this procedure increases the bow of the bridge and moves the lenses closer to one another. On the wide dowel rod, the bridge is stretched, decreasing the bow and separating the lenses farther apart.

Using a Staking Tool to Change Bridge Size

A staking tool is a multiple-use tool used in the repair of frames. It is possible to purchase an accessory for the tool that allows the bridge to be reformed (Figure 9-63). It works in a manner similar to the bridge-reducing pliers. This does not have a very good success record either.

There is no staking set accessory for widening a bridge.

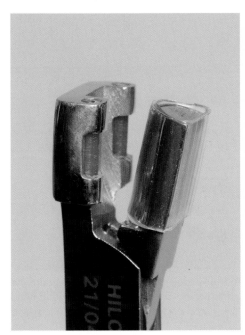

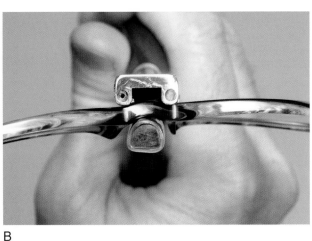

Figure 9-61. A, Bridge-narrowing pliers. **B,** The procedure for using narrowing pliers is shown.

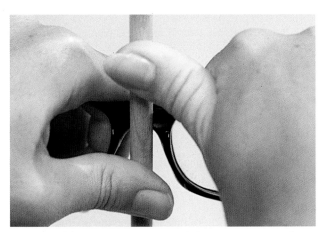

Figure 9-62. The technique used for narrowing a plastic bridge when using a dowel rod.

Using the Hands Alone to Change Bridge Size

Many dispensers prefer to modify the bridge using only the hands. This preference is a personal one and may be due to the possibility of marking the frame or because of either a lack of or dissatisfaction with other tools. To change the bridge size using the hands alone, do the following:

Heat the bridge *only*. Leave the lenses in the frame and try not to heat any other part of the frame.

To widen the bridge, heat the bridge considerably and grasp the frame around each lens. Pull outward. With materials used today, it may only be possible to widen the bridge by ½ millimeter.

To narrow the bridge, heat and reheat the frame. That is, heat the bridge until it is very hot (but not so hot as

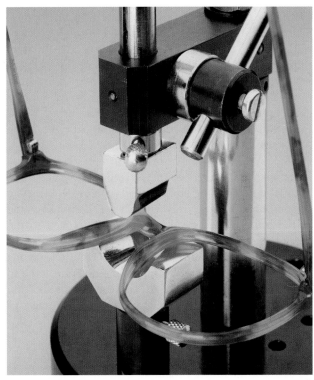

Figure 9-63. A bridge reducing accessory is available for staking sets. The accessory works on the same principle as the bridge-narrowing pliers. (Courtesy Hilco, Plainville, Mass.)

to bubble the plastic) and wait just a bit, then reheat it till very hot again. Repeat this several times. Set the frame down for about 10 to 15 seconds, and then reheat the bridge one last time. Now wait about 8 seconds before pushing the lenses together.

Grasp the frame front by the eyewires, hold the frame against the midsection of the body for stability, and either push the eyewires together or pull them apart, depending on the modification desired.

The reason for heating and reheating the frame in this manner is so that the outer "skin" of the bridge will be cooler than the inside of the bridge. Now when the bridge is compressed, the center will bulge forward without wrinkling the outer surface.[3]

When attempting to widen or narrow the bridge, take care to avoid simply pushing the lower sections together or pulling the bottoms of the eyewires apart (adding unwanted upsweep to the frame). This is especially important when the prescription has a cylinder component because the axis can be shifted. Recheck the cylinder axis after changing the bridge to make sure that such a shift has not occurred. If none of these four methods work very well, there are ways to customize the frame that may do the job.

Changing the Bridge Size by Customizing the Frame
The plastic frame can be customized in one of several ways. These methods are often more successful than those just described above. These customizing methods include:

Adding adjustable pad arms or a unifit bridge. This is done by drilling and press fitting, or by using a Hot Fingers unit. (See "Retrofitting" Plastic Frames with Adjustable Nosepads, Chapter 10.)

Using build-up pads. The bridge on a plastic frame can sometimes be altered to fit an especially narrow or unusual nose by using build-up pads (Figure 9-64). Even silicone stick-on nose pads will cause a slight narrowing of the bridge. Both types of pads are attached to the area of the frame that would normally rest on the nose. For a complete explanation on how acetate or silicone build-up pads may be used to change both frontal and splay angle, and how they are applied, see the section entitled Replacing Nosepads on Plastic Frames in Chapter 10.

RECHECKING THE FRAME FIT

After completing the steps in fitting the frame as given in this chapter and as summarized in Box 9-2, recheck the following before considering the fit final.
1. Are the glasses at the correct height vertically?
2. Is one lens or one multifocal segment higher than the other, or are progressive lens fitting crosses directly in front of the pupils?
3. Is the pantoscopic tilt correct?
4. Are right and left vertex distances equal?

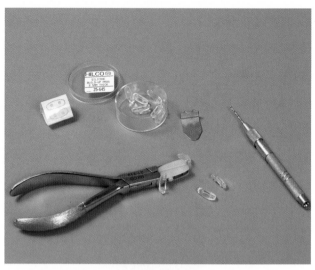

Figure 9-64. Silicone nose pads mounted onto plastic frames with adhesive or with small drilled holes will not only reduce slippage, but also slightly narrow the effective width of the bridge.

BOX 9-2

Steps in Fitting

STEP 1: TEMPLE/ENDPIECE ANGLE
a. Check for proper temple spread angle.
b. Check for equality of lens distances from the eyes, viewing from the top.

STEP 2: PANTOSCOPIC ANGLE
a. Check tilt of lenses from a side view.
b. Check for straightness of the frame on the face from a front view.

STEP 3: NOSEPADS OR BRIDGE AREA
a. Adjust the frame for proper height when necessary.
b. Adjust the frame for proper vertex distance when necessary.
c. Adjust nosepads for maximum surface contact.

STEP 4: TEMPLES
a. Temples are adjusted to exert slight pressure over the tops of the ears.
b. The temple bend is moved to its proper position when necessary.
c. The bent-down portion is contoured to match the side of the head and back of the ear.

After the fitter gains experience, it will be found that many of the steps can be done simultaneously because it will be possible to see and correct more than one thing at a time.

---

5. Is the temple pressure along the side of the skull correct?
6. Is the temple bend positioned correctly relative to the tops of the ears?
7. Does the bent-down portion of the temple angle downward correctly?

BOX 9-3

Summary of Adjustments for Moving the Frame on the Face

TO MOVE FRAME AWAY FROM FACE
1. Narrow adjustable pads (also raises frame)
2. Increase effective length of pad arms
3. Shrink (narrow) bridge of plastic frame (also raises frame)
4. Decrease face form (make front straighter)

TO MOVE FRAME CLOSER TO FACE
1. Spread adjustable pads apart (also lowers frame)
2. Decrease effective length of pad arms
3. Stretch (widen) bridge of plastic frame (also lowers front)
4. Increase face form (make front more curved)

TO MOVE FRAME OFF THE CHEEKS
1. Decrease pantoscopic tilt
2. Raise the frame by narrowing bridge or pads or bending pad arms down
3. Increase vertex distance by narrowing bridge or pads or extending pad arms

TO MOVE FROM OFF THE BROWS
1. Increase pantoscopic tilt
2. Lower the frame by widening bridge or pads or by raising pad position
3. Increase vertex distance by extending pad arms

Note: attempting to move frame forward by narrowing bridge or pads may raise it further.

TO MOVE FRAME HIGHER ON FACE
1. Shrink or narrow the bridge (plastic)
2. Add pads to plastic bridge
3. Narrow distance between adjustable pads
4. Lower vertical position of adjustable pads

TO MOVE FRAME LOWER ON FACE
1. Stretch or widen the bridge (plastic)
2. Spread adjustable pads apart
3. Raise vertical position of adjustable pads

TO MOVE ONE LENS CLOSER TO THE FACE
1. If left lens is IN, bring left temple IN and/or if right lens is OUT, bring right temple OUT
2. If right lens is IN bring right temple IN and/or left lens is OUT, bring left temple OUT

TO MOVE ONE LENS HIGHER ON THE FACE
1. If left lens is UP, bend left temple UP and/or if right lens is DOWN, bend right temple DOWN
2. If right lens is UP, bend right temple UP and/or if left lens is DOWN, bend left temple DOWN

---

8. Do both right and left bent-down portions of the temples follow the contour of the side of the head? (In other words, does the posterior portion of the temple need to be formed to follow the curvature of the side of the head?)

When nosepads are present, recheck these points:

1. Is the distance between pads correct for the wearer?
2. Are the pads sitting on the correct part of the nose for the wearer?
3. Do the frontal angles of the pads correspond to the frontal angles of the wearer's nose?
4. Do the splay angles of the pads correspond to the splay angles of the wearer's nose?
5. Are the longitudinal axes of the pads perpendicular to the floor? (In other words, does the vertical angle of the pad equal the pantoscopic angle of the frame front when the glasses are being worn?)
6. Overall, do the pads sit flat on the surface of the nose?

Test for equality of temple tension on each side by lifting the temples off the ears slightly and pulling the front forward gently. Equality of temple adjustment can also be checked by placing the thumbs on the sides of the temples of the frame and the fingers directly behind the wearer's ears (between the back of the ear and the bent-down portion of the temple). Do this simultane-ously for both ears, using both hands, to obtain an accurate estimate of equality of adjustment.

The wearer should put the glasses on and take them off several times to see if they rest in the proper place. This exercise will reveal if the wearer puts his glasses on in such a way that they rest in some unusual manner, such as with the temples high on the head or in the hair. In such cases, it may be necessary to alter the frame by changing its vertical position, pad angles, or pantoscopic tilt.

The wearer should be made aware of any deliberate irregularities in the glasses, such as unequal seg height or pantoscopic angles.

If attention is not specifically called to these irregularities, the wearer is often mistakenly left with the impression that something is wrong with the glasses.

(For a summary of adjustments on how to move the position of the frame on the face, see Box 9-3.)

REFERENCES

1. Kintner EA: The relative role of physical features of spectacles as factors in wearing comfort. Master's Thesis, Bloomington, Ind, 1970, Indiana University.
2. Stimson RL: Ophthalmic dispensing, ed 2, Springfield, Ill, 1971, Charles C Thomas.
3. Yoho A: Back in plastic, Eyecare Business, March 2003, pp. 44-47.

Proficiency Test

(Answers can be found in the back of the book.)

1. Which of the following may *not* be a cause of one lens being higher than the other?
   a. one earpiece being bent down considerably further than the other
   b. an upward bend in one of the temple shafts
   c. a skewed bridge
   d. one ear higher than the other
   e. nosepads spread too far

2. If the frame is crooked with the right side higher than the left:
   a. bend the right temple down
   b. bend the right temple up

3. If a bifocal wearer complains that the bifocal line is too high and the frame has adjustable nosepads, and if cosmetics will allow:
   a. decrease the distance between pads.
   b. increase the distance between pads.

4. Which is *not* a possible *solution* for the frame sitting too high on the face?
   a. increase the distance between adjustable nosepads
   b. move the vertical position of adjustable nosepads downward
   c. choose a different frame

5. If the eyelashes rub the back surface of the lenses, the fitter should:
   a. spread the temples.
   b. raise the frame.
   c. increase the vertex distance.
   d. spread the nosepads.

6. Which of the following is not a possible cause of *both* lashes touching the lenses?
   a. not enough pantoscopic tilt
   b. base curves that are too flat
   c. adjustable nosepads that are positioned too close to the frame front
   d. adjustable nosepads that are too close together

7. If the top of the frame front touches the eyebrows, what is *not* a possible solution to the problem?
   a. choosing a different frame
   b. moving the adjustable nosepads farther away from the frame front
   c. increasing the pantoscopic angle
   d. All of the above are possible solutions to the problem.

8. One lens is closer to the wearer's face than the other. How could this be corrected?
   a. Increase the temple spread (bend the temple outward) on the side closest to the face.
   b. Increase the pantoscopic tilt on the side closest to the face.
   c. Decrease the temple spread (bend the temple inward) on the side closest to the face.
   d. Tighten the temple tension behind the ear on the side farthest from the face.

9. If the wearer complains that the glasses feel snug, but still slip down the nose, one likely cause is that:
   a. the bridge size is too large.
   b. the bridge size is too small.
   c. too much pressure is being applied by the temple shafts on the sides of the head in front of the ears.
   d. too much pressure is being applied to the sides of the head behind the ears by the very tips of the temples; no pressure is being applied to the sides of the head in front of the ears.

10. True or false? Narrowing the distance between adjustable nosepads causes the frame to sit higher on the face, and somewhat closer to the face.

11. True or false? Strap bridges are a replacement for adjustable nosepads. They help increase the weight-bearing area. Unfortunately, they are not adjustable like the pads they replace.

12. The wearer has a previously broken, crooked nose. The new frame has an adjustable pad bridge. When the glasses are put on the wearer, the frame front sits too far to the wearer's left. (Any references to left or right in the responses below are from the wearer's point of view.) What should be done to correct the problem?
    a. Move both right and left pads to the right.
    b. Move both right and left pads to the left.
    c. Move the right pad to the right and the left pad to the left.
    d. Move the right pad to the left and the left pad to the right.

13. When viewing the wearer from the front, it is discovered that the frame sits too far to the wearer's right. What might be causing this?
   a. Both pads are too far to the wearer's left.
   b. Both pads are too far to the wearer's right.
   c. The wearer's nose is crooked.
   d. Both a and c are possible causes.
   e. Both b and c are possible causes.

14. True or false? The wearer is looking straight ahead. If the dispenser views the glasses from the side and the nosepads are properly adjusted, the long axis of the pads should be perpendicular to the floor.

15. True or false? Most pad adjustments may be done in two movements. The first move makes the change; the second move completes the change and restores the proper pad angle.

16. If *both* nosepads press flat against the side of the nose, yet hurt or cause indentations on the nose, what is a possible cause?
   a. The temple spread is not even.
   b. The pads need to be spread farther apart.
   c. The pads are too small for the weight of the frame.

17. A correctly fitting cable temple should have the tip of the temple located where?
   a. at the lower lobe of the ear
   b. slightly past the lower lobe of the ear
   c. just short of the lower lobe of the ear

18. Which of the following statements about temples with good quality spring hinges is false?
   a. Frames with spring hinges are less likely to require readjustment or repair when struck with a ball, an elbow, or when knocked from the face.
   b. Spring temples are adjusted behind the ears exactly as any other temples would be.
   c. The temple bend location is positioned exactly the same for spring hinge temples as for temples without spring hinges.
   d. Frames with spring hinges should be adjusted so they are tighter than frames with normal, well-fitted temples.

19. True or false? When choosing a frame for individuals with behind-the-ear hearing aids, the best temple design is one that is thin and conforms to the back of the crotch of the ear.

20. True or false? Here is the procedure for taking off a pair of glasses that have cable temples. The wearer should grasp the left endpiece with the left hand and the tip end of the right cable temple with the right hand. The right temple is pulled off the ear and the glasses swung to the left so that the left cable temple comes off the ear easily without causing the glasses to lose their adjustment.

21. The temples on a frame do not open the same amount. One has a greater temple spread than the other. When this is the case, the lens that will be closer to the eye will be the lens:
   a. on the same side as the looser (more widely spread) temple.
   b. on the same side as the tighter (less widely spread) temple.

22. The temples on a frame do not open the same amount. One has a greater temple spread than the other. When this is the case, the side of the nose that could become irritated is:
   a. on the same side as the looser temple.
   b. on the same side as the tighter temple.

23. The temples on a frame do not open the same amount. One has a greater temple spread than the other. When this is the case, the ear that is likely to become irritated will be:
   a. the ear on the opposite side of the tighter temple.
   b. the ear on the same side as the tighter temple.

24. When a wearer's frames are both slipping down the nose and hurting behind the ears, the most probable solution would be to:
   a. move the temple bend farther forward on the temple.
   b. move the temple bend farther back on the temple.
   c. increase the temple spread.
   d. decrease the bridge size.
   e. angle the tips of the temples inward.

25. A wearer comes into the office. His frames are out of adjustment. The left lower rim touches his left cheek and the right side of the frame front is higher than the left side. It also appears that there is just a bit too much pantoscopic angle on the frame. Given the choices below, if you can only make one choice, which choice would be the best?
   a. Bend the left temple upward.
   b. Bend the left temple downward.
   c. Bend the right temple upward.
   d. Bend the right temple downward.
   e. Bend the left temple upward and the right temple downward.

26. Which of the following problems would not be helped or solved by widening the frame bridge?
   a. The frame is too high on the face.
   b. The bridge is too small for the nose.
   c. The lashes rub the back surface of the lenses.
   d. All of the above problems would be helped or solved by widening the frame bridge.

27. When being worn, the only appropriate place for eyeglasses to exert pressure is:
    a. on the sides of the head at the very ends of the temples.
    b. on the sides of the head directly above the ears.
    c. in the crease between the back of the ear and the side of the head.
    d. There should never be any pressure exerted by the frame.

28. True or false? Attempts to conform the temple earpiece to follow the depression in the side of the head behind the ear do not result in sufficient improvement in fit to make fitting efforts worthwhile.

29. Contemporary frames having spring hinge temples should be adjusted so that:
    a. the temple pressure against the sides of the head is considerably less than for frames without spring hinges.
    b. the temple pressure against the sides of the head is slightly less than for frames without spring hinges.
    c. the temple pressure against the sides of the head is the same as for frames without spring hinges.
    d. the temple pressure against the sides of the head is slightly greater than for frames without spring hinges.
    e. the temple pressure against the sides of the head is considerably greater than for frames without spring hinges.

CHAPTER **10**

Frame Repairs and Modifications

An important service that should be provided is frame repair. Most necessary repairs will be minor, although occasionally a major job will be requested. Going hand in hand with repairs are modifications to frames that must be performed to make a frame fit just right. This chapter provides methods and hints for performing these tasks as quickly and efficiently as possible.

SCREW REPLACEMENTS AND REPAIRS

Most major frame repairs require a lot of time. As a result, replacement of broken parts is usually more cost effective. Occasionally, however, a major repair can provide a vital service to a wearer if it enables him to continue wearing a much-needed prescription.

Minor repairs also take time but usually not more than would be expended in aligning a new pair of glasses. Perhaps, more important, is how much these repairs are appreciated.

This chapter begins with the two most common problems: screw repairs and pad replacements, followed by the third most common, temple repairs.

Correctly Using an Optical Screwdriver

When using an optical screwdriver, the screwdriver should *not* be held like a pencil (Figure 10-1). Instead, place the handle end in the palm of the hand, as shown in Figure 10-2, *A*. (Typically the end of the handle is made to rotate, making this technique work more smoothly.) Grasp the screwdriver, as shown in Figure 10-2, *B*. Now brace the frame on the edge of the workbench (Figure 10-3) or on a bench block so that if (or rather *when*) the screwdriver slips, the sharp tip will not go halfway into your finger.

A Note on Screwdriver Types

There are many different types of optical screwdrivers available, from ones with brass shafts and no-roll handles, to others having large, round hardwood handles that fill the palm of the hand. There is also an ergonomic type shown in Figure 10-4 with a handle that can be bent to conform to the hand.

It can be tricky enough just to hold a tiny screw between thumb and forefinger. Getting it screwed into

the hole far enough to get started is even harder. Here are two options to help in this matter.

- There is a "pick-up" screwdriver with spring-loaded retractable jaws for holding small screws until they catch the threads in the barrel.
- Another option is a special screw-holding tool that grips the screw so that it can be more easily pressed into the hole (Figure 10-5).

Check to make sure that the blade of the screwdriver is in good condition. Damaged blades can damage screw heads. And regardless of what screwdriver is used, the blade size needs to match the screw. (Most optical screwdrivers have reversible blades with different widths on each end.)

Another helpful tool is a screw-lift tool. This is used after the screw is loose and ready to be removed. This tool is used to lift the screw from the hole without dropping and losing it (Figure 10-6).

Loose Screws

The constant opening and closing of temples sometimes turns the temple screw and loosens it. Although a loose temple does not necessarily affect the fit or stability of the glasses, most wearers would like to see the problem fixed. If the screw is loose and has not been fully turned, simply tighten it.

Sometimes even after tightening a temple screw, the temple may still be loose and floppy. In this case the temple barrels may need to be realigned. Realignment of temple barrels is discussed later in the Misaligned Hinge Barrels section.

Using a Sealant to Keep Screws Tight

One solution for a screw that continually loosens is to use a screw-locking adhesive sealant on the screw threads to hold it tight. A sealant does not just keep the screw from loosening. It also keeps it from corroding. A corroded screw will lock up over time, making removal difficult. Most optical suppliers carry these products.

Some prefer to use clear nail polish instead of a sealant, painting the head of the screw and the threads to prevent turning. This method is most successful on screws located in a recessed position (Figure 10-7).

217

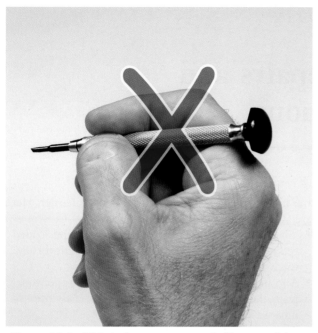

Figure 10-1. This is the wrong way to hold a screwdriver.

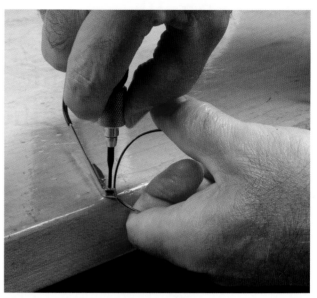

Figure 10-3. Safety first. Always brace the frame against something. Do not hold the frame so that when (not if, but when) the screwdriver slips, it will not penetrate your other hand.

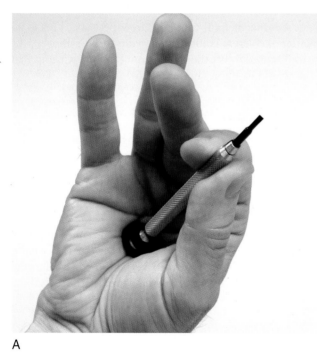

A

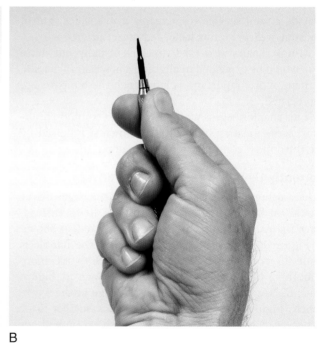

B

Figure 10-2. A, This photo shows how to grasp the optical screwdriver so that the rotating end of the handle is in the palm of the hand. **B,** With the handle end cradled in the center of the palm, grasp the optical screwdriver as shown.

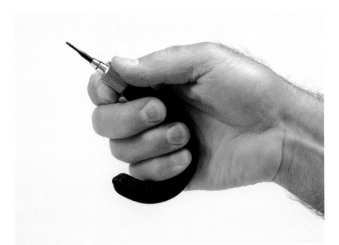

Figure 10-4. There are a large variety of optical screwdrivers available, including this ergonometric one that bends to find the size and shape of the hand.

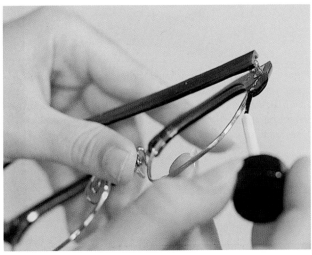

Figure 10-7. Use clear nail polish to seal a tightened screw in place and prevent it from loosening up. This combination frame has an eyewire screw recessed under the top rim.

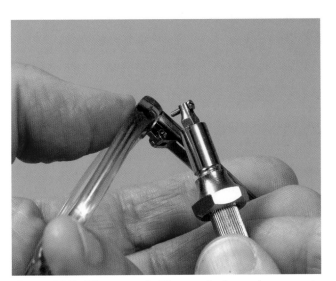

Figure 10-5. The screw-holding tool places the screw in hard-to-reach places where fingers cannot always go.

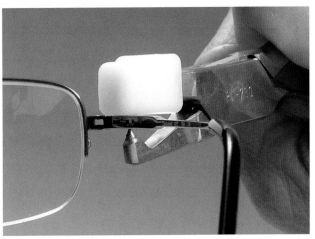

Figure 10-8. Flaring pliers will flare a rivet or screw tip to prevent it from backing out.

Peening Screw Tips to Keep Screws Tight

For temple screws whose tips protrude beyond the barrels, it is possible to put a rivetlike head on the end of the screw. This can be done in one of several ways including:

1. Tapping it firmly with the small end of an optician's hammer to keep the screw from backing out.
2. Using flaring pliers designed to flare out the ends of the screws and rivets (Figure 10-8).
3. Peening down the end using a staking set, such as the one shown later in the chapter in Figure 10-53, but with a concave-end peening tool.

Once the tip of the screw has been flared, it may later be necessary to file the tip to remove the screw.

Using Replacement Self-Locking Screws to Keep Screws Tight

Self-locking replacement screws have an epoxy type of coating on the threads that keeps the screw from backing

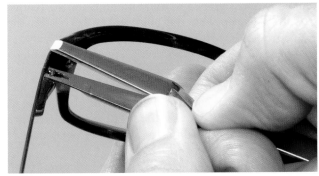

Figure 10-6. The screw-lift tool allows a loosened screw to be removed with less chance of being dropped.

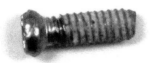

Figure 10-9. This type of self-locking replacement screw has an epoxy type of coating on the threads that keeps the screw from backing out. It is removable and can be used again. As would be expected, each time it is taken out and replaced, it loses some of its adhesive characteristics.

---

out (Figure 10-9). These screws can be removed and used again, as when an eyewire screw must be removed and replaced when changing prescription lenses.

The preceding methods of keeping screws tight are summarized in Box 10-1.

Other Methods Used to Keep Screws Tight

Some frames have built-in systems to keep the screws in place. These frames are designed with a small setscrew in the side of one of the barrels or with a small nut that grasps the tip of the protruding screw.

Optyl frames present a slightly different situation because many times the hinge area is protectively coated with Optyl material. To tighten, loosen, or remove a screw, the hinge area must be heated before the screw can be turned.

Replacement Screws for Spring Hinges

In many spring hinges, the screw holds the spring within the temple in tension. Because of this it is often difficult to line up the barrels on the endpiece with the barrel on the temple when replacing a temple screw. Unless some special tools or specialty screws are used, accomplishing a screw replacement may take more than two hands.

When attempting to insert a screw and turn it into place when the temple barrel is under tension, it is not uncommon to have the screw go in at an angle instead of straight up and down. If the screw is screwed in at an angle, it may cause the threads in the barrel to strip. In an effort to prevent this, Hilco makes a self-aligning spring hinge screw. This stainless steel screw is longer and has a tapered tip. The tip acts as a lead to align the hinge barrels (Figure 10-10). Once the screw is seated, the excess screw that sticks out can be snapped off with regular pliers; cutting pliers are not needed. The broken

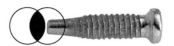

Spring hinge screw

Figure 10-10. The spring hinge screw is tapered at the tip. This allows the screw to more easily slip into the small open area between the nonaligning temple and frame front barrel holes. (Courtesy of Hilco, Plainville, Mass.)

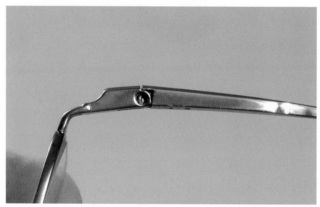

Figure 10-11. This picture shows that when spring hinge temples are placed on the frame front, their barrel holes do not line up. They do not line up because the spring in the temple is not stretched.

end may be peened down with peening pliers or a staking tool for a neater look and more secure hold.

Once the screw is in place, flex the temple outward to see how good the action on the spring temple is. If it opens but will not spring back as it should, loosen the screw slightly. The tension of the tight screw may be holding it open. The use of lubricating oil, such as "3-in-1" may help in keeping the spring working well without sticking.

Spring Hinge Alignment Tools. Because of the difficulty of putting a spring hinge temple back on a frame while inserting the screw in the temple, several types of spring hinge alignment tools have been developed. Here is how to use one such tool.

Figure 10-11 shows how the barrels in the temple and frame front do not line up exactly. The spring in the temple is not stretched to allow the hole in the temple barrel to line up with the holes in the barrels on the frame front.

There are two parts to this particular spring hinge alignment tool. One part is a tiny "wrench" with a small tip on the end (Figure 10-12). The tip fits into the temple barrel hole to pull the barrel and extend the spring, as shown in Figure 10-13, *A* and *B*. (These two figures are for demonstration purposes only and are not a part of the screw replacement process.)

The second part of the tool is shown in Figure 10-14. It has a slide that will lock it in place after the tool has a grip on the temple. There is also the small "tooth" on the angled head of the tool. Here is the procedure:

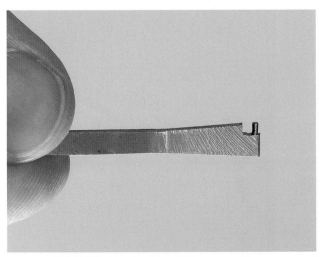

Figure 10-12. This is the "wrench" used with one type of spring hinge alignment tool. The small tip on the end slips into the spring hinge barrel.

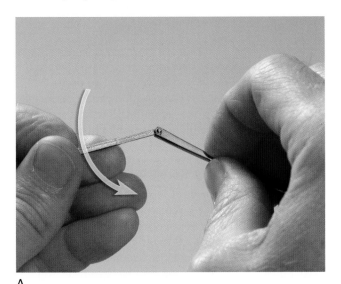

A

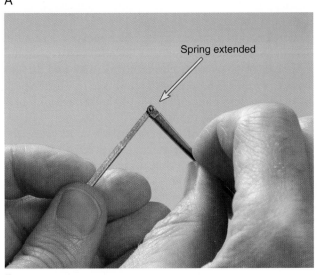

B

Figure 10-13. A, The "wrench" slips into the temple barrel and will extend the spring. **B,** Here the spring in a spring hinge temple has been extended. Note how far it has been pulled out compared with the previous figure.

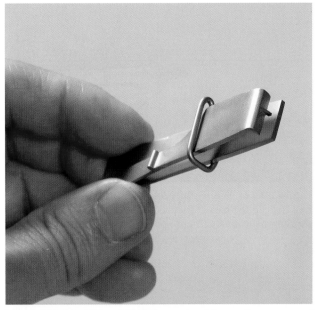

Figure 10-14. This part of the spring hinge alignment tool grasps the temple. The "tooth" on the end will slip into the notch on a notched spring hinge casing and holds the spring in the extended position. For spring hinge casings without a notch (called flat front casings), the angled head of the tool holds the barrel in the extended position.

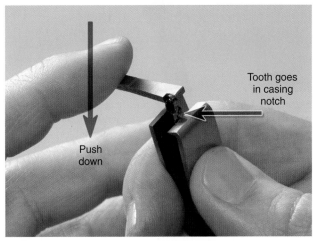

Figure 10-15. The temple is gripped with the spring hinge alignment tool, the "wrench" extends the barrel outward, and the "tooth" slips into the notch in the casing to hold the barrel in the extended position.

1. Put the temple in the tool with the head of the tool behind the barrel and at the front of the casing that surrounds the spring hinge.
2. Place the wrench in the barrel hole and extend the barrel (Figure 10-15). When the spring hinge casing is notched (as shown in the figure) the "tooth" slips into the notch. This holds the barrel in its extended position.
3. Hold the tool tightly and move the slide forward to maintain a solid grip on the temple (Figure 10-16).

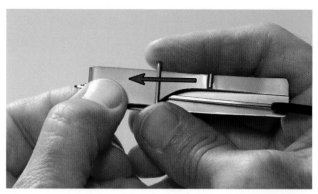

Figure 10-16. While squeezing the spring hinge alignment tool to keep the barrel extended, slip the slide forward so that the alignment tool will not open.

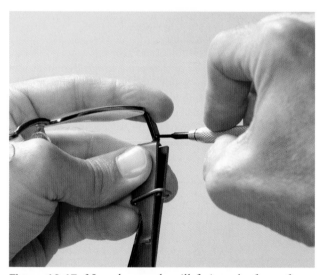

Figure 10-17. Now the temple will fit into the frame front, and all of the barrels will line up. The screw should now go in as if the frame had a normal temple barrel configuration.

4. Now the temple barrel can be slipped into the barrels on the frame front. They will line up as a regular temple would.
5. The screw may now be placed into the barrels and tightened (Figure 10-17).
   (NOTE: Some casings do not have a notch. For this kind of temple, the angled head of the tool is used to grip the flat front of the casing and not the "tooth.")

Misaligned Hinge Barrels

When a temple is still loose even after tightening the screw, the problem may be that the barrels of the frame and temple hinges are mismatched. To correct this problem, remove the screw and the temple and note which hinge has the greater number of barrels (usually the front). Apply parallel-jawed pliers, such as hollow-snipe pliers, to this hinge. Compress the barrels of this front hinge to narrow the spaces into which the barrels of the other hinge fit (Figure 10-18). Take care not to compress the barrels too much; otherwise they must be

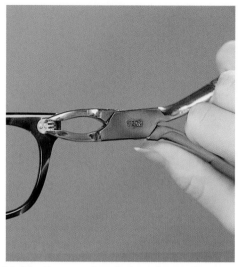

Figure 10-18. Compressing the barrels together somewhat to help tighten up a loose temple is best done with pliers whose jaws are parallel when open. In this instance, hollow snipe-nosed pliers are being used.

pried apart (sometimes breaking a barrel off) before the other part of the hinge can be returned to position.

In some instances this compression can be performed with both hinges in place, actually allowing the barrels to be fitted together while in position. This, however, is usually more difficult.

Replacing a Missing Screw

The most difficult aspect of replacing a missing screw is finding the right sized replacement. Fortunately the industry is gravitating to a common screw diameter of 1.4 mm and a length of 3.0 to 4.0 mm.

Table 10-1 shows the most common sizes of currently used replacement screws for regular spectacle frames, quality sunglasses, over-the-counter sunglasses, nose-pads, and trim.

For the more unusual sizes, Hilco makes a Fast-Find Screw and Hole Gauge Kit that includes two gauges and a booklet or chart with numerous pictures and dimensions of screws. These gauges allow one to easily match an existing screw or quickly find the dimensions of a missing screw using the frame.

To find the size of an existing screw, measure the diameter. This is done by putting the screw through the presized holes on the rulerlike device, as shown in Figure 10-19. Next, measure the overall length of the screw, including the head, using the slots on the same device.

To find the length of a missing screw, use the slots on the ruler-type device to measure the depth of the barrels as shown in Figure 10-20, compensating an additional amount for the screw head. To find the diameter of the missing screw, use the round, spoked tool. Each spoke has a different diameter. These spokes are inserted into the empty barrel of the frame to find the unknown diameter, as shown in Figure 10-21.

TABLE 10-1
Common Replacement Screw Diameter Sizes for Spectacle Frames

Type of Screws	Most Common Replacement Screw Size
Screws for regular spectacle frames, including both hinges and barrel-closing screws	1.4 mm
Screws for quality sunglass frames	1.6 mm
Screws for cheap, over-the-counter sunglasses	1.8 mm
Screws for nosepads	1.0 mm (If this will not fit, a 1.1-mm or 0.8-mm diameter will)
Screws for spectacle frame trim	1.2 mm, 1.4 mm (sometimes 2.0 mm) (lengths from 2.9 mm-3.6 mm)

Data obtained from Woyton R: "How can I find a replacement screw quickly when a customer comes in with a frame that needs one?" Hilco, Plainville, Mass, undated.

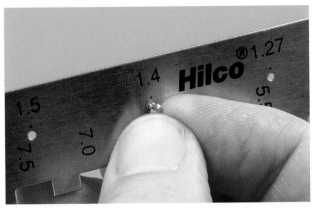

Figure 10-19. To find the diameter of the screw, slip the screw through each hole until a match is found. Incidentally, this 1.4 mm diameter is the most commonly used diameter for optical screws.

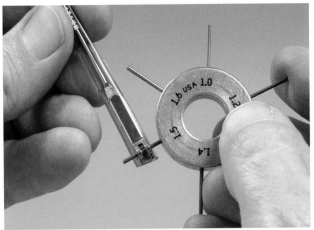

Figure 10-21. To find the diameter of a missing screw, slide the different sized spokes of the hole gauge through the barrels until the correct fit is found.

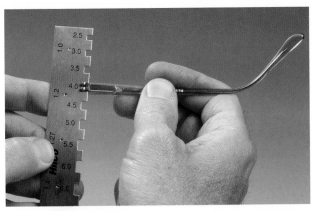

Figure 10-20. To find the screw length for a missing screw, measure the depth of the barrels and compensate an additional amount for the screw head. (Note: In other areas of industry, the head of the screw may not be included in its length.)

Finding a Screw From Inventory

One of the more frustrating aspects of screw replacement is just finding a matching screw. Without an organized system, the dispenser is reduced to searching through a tray or jar full of extremely small screws, all of which begin to look like one another. A person with

a gift for organization can generate their own system of vials or drawers. Or one can buy a system that has the most commonly needed parts, such as the one shown in Figure 10-22, and replenish it as necessary.

Titanium Screws

Because titanium is so strong, the threads on a titanium screw do not give. So if a titanium screw enters the barrels at even a slight angle, it will bind. If this happens, do not force the screw. Just back the screw out and start over. If it continues to bind after several attempts, put a drop of cutting oil into the barrel. (In the absence of cutting oil, which works best, use household oil such 3-in-1.)[1]

Broken and Stuck Screws

Sometimes a screw will not come out or breaks off in the barrels of the frame. Suggestions on how these problems may be corrected are outlined here and summarized in Box 10-2.

Removing Stuck Screws

If the entire screw is still in place but cannot be turned with a screwdriver, either the screw may have corroded

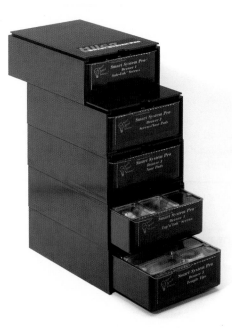

Figure 10-22. Much searching time will be saved if an organized system for storing small frame parts is in place. This is a commercially available example of a stackable system that can be added to as needed.

in the barrel or the screw slot may have been destroyed.

If corrosion is the problem, the screw can be loosened by immersing the affected area in an *ultrasonic cleaner* (Figure 10-23) or by treating it with a *penetrating oil* (Figure 10-24).

Some dispensers remove frozen screws by supporting the tip of the screw on the edge of a small anvil or vise. After placing an optical screwdriver in the screw slot, the *screwdriver is gently tapped with a hammer* once or twice, breaking corrosion or adhesive. (This method may require three hands.)

One idea for removing screws that have been previously bonded in the barrels with an adhesive is to *use a soldering iron set on low.** The iron is held on the tip of the screw for 10 to 20 seconds until the hardened adhesive melts, allowing the screw to be removed normally. (Caution: Do not use this method on plastic frames.)

The Hot Fingers unit works just as well as a soldering iron, if not better. Grasp the top and bottom of the screw with the Hot Finger tips (Figure 10-25). Heat the screw for 10 to 15 seconds. The metal expands when heated and contracts as it cools, helping to break the screw loose. The high heat also burns away any remaining adhesive. (Caution: Do not use this method on a plastic frame.)

To make both the soldering iron and Hot Fingers work even better, as soon as the screw area has been

---

*Thanks to John Moulton, Sarnia, Ontario, for this idea.

<table>
<tr><td>

BOX 10-2

How to Remove Stuck or Broken-Off Screws

TO REMOVE A STUCK SCREW:
1. Immerse in an ultrasonic unit.
2. Use penetrating oil.
3. Place screwdriver in slot and lightly tap the screwdriver with a hammer.
4. Use a soldering iron or Hot Fingers unit.
5. Deepen the slot or cut a new slot at right angles to the old slot.
6. Drive the screw out.
   a. Use press-out, punch-out, or shoot-out type of punch pliers or
   b. Use a Bull's-Eye Screw Extractor or
   c. Use a pointed tool and anvil.
7. Drill the screw out.
   a. Rethread with tap or
   b. Use a self-tapping replacement screw or
   c. Use a screw with a hex nut.
8. Replace the part.

TO REMOVE A BROKEN-OFF SCREW:
1. Use a screw extractor.
2. Slot the tip of the screw.
3. Drive the screw out.
   a. Use press-out, punch-out, or shoot-out type of punch pliers or
   b. Use a Bull's-Eye Screw Extractor or
   c. Use a pointed tool and anvil.
4. Drill the screw out.
   a. Rethread with tap or
   b. Use a self-tapping replacement screw or
   c. Use a screw with a hex nut.
5. Replace the part.

</td></tr>
</table>

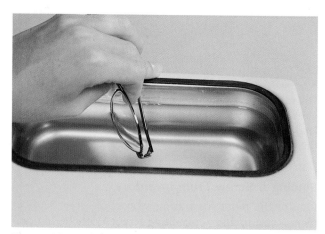

Figure 10-23. Ultrasonic cleaners will loosen frame screws while the frame is being cleaned. This can be used to advantage in loosening an especially stubborn screw.

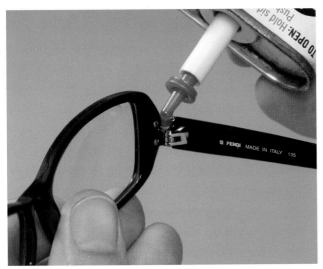

Figure 10-24. Penetrating oil, such as "Liquid Wrench" automotive penetrating oil, helps cut corrosion and loosen stuck screws.

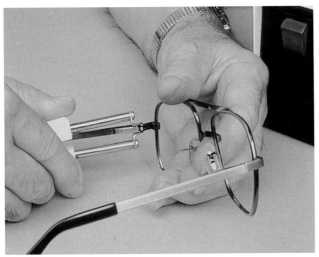

Figure 10-25. A soldering iron or Hot Fingers unit held on the tip of a previously sealed screw will often allow the screw to be removed normally. (Courtesy Hilco, Plainville, Mass.)

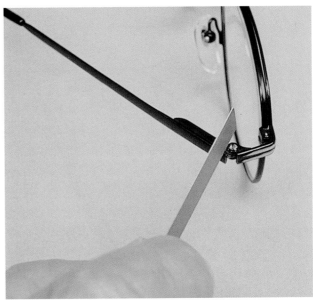

Figure 10-26. When the slot in the head of a screw has been destroyed, a new one can be created using a thin file known as a slotting or ribbon file. (It is sometimes possible to slot the tip of a broken screw as well. This allows a screwdriver to be used to turn the remaining part of the screw out of the bottom of the hinge.) (Courtesy Hilco, Plainville, Mass.)

heated, quickly put a drop of oil on the screw. The heat thins the oil, and the oil is drawn between the threads, dissolving corrosion and lubricating the interface.[2] If neither a soldering iron nor a Hot Fingers unit are available, even heating the screw area with a frame warmer and then applying oil should help.

If the slot of the screw has been worn away, use a *flat slotting file to restore and deepen the slot* so the blade of the screwdriver can again turn the screw (Figure 10-26). If the slot is widened and damaged, try filing a new slot in the screw head. The new slot should be at right angles to the original slot.

If the screw is so corroded that it cannot be loosened and removed by any of the above methods, it can be punched out. This is done with *a small hand pliers* variously called "punch-out," "knock-out," or "shoot-out"

pliers that will punch out broken and stripped screws. (The pin in the pliers is replaceable.)

It is also possible to *drill the screw out*. This is described in the following section.

Removing Broken Screws

Occasionally a screw will break into two parts. The head can easily be removed if the slot is still usable, or it may fall out by itself. The other part of the screw remains stuck in the barrels.

The best tool for this job is a *screw extractor* (Figure 10-27). This device resembles a screwdriver, but has a barbed end that digs into the stem of the screw and turns it. The extractor comes in a variety of sizes to suit the variations in screw diameters.

To use a screw extractor, attack the screw from the bottom (Figure 10-28). Apply hard downward pressure. If the broken-off portion remaining in the barrels is long enough, turn the screw clockwise. This will drive the screw out through the top barrel. If the broken-off portion is not long enough to go back out the top, turn the screw counterclockwise to bring it on out of the bottom. Hint: The screw extractor tip can be mounted in a Dremel tool having a standard Jacob's chuck or in a hanging drill. (The Hilco Hanging Motor Drill is shown in Figure 10-29. The extractor mounted in the chuck of the drill is shown in Figure 10-30.)

There is a device called the Bull's-Eye Screw Extractor (Figure 10-31), which can be very helpful and remove the screw without having to drill it out. This exerts a large amount of turning power in a controlled manner.

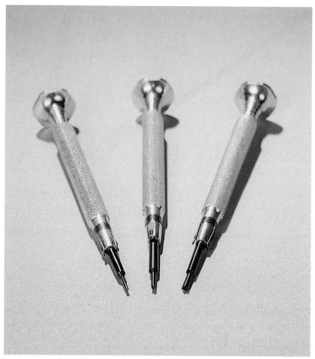

Figure 10-27. In a set of screw extractors, each extractor insert has two tips of different sizes. The extractor tip may be reversed in the same manner as with a two-ended screwdriver blade.

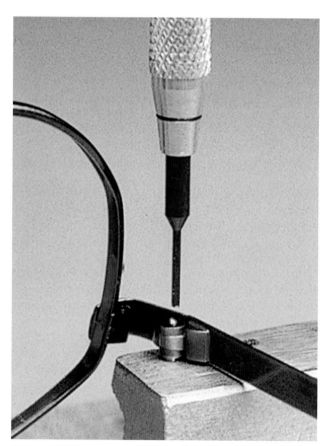

Figure 10-28. A screw extractor is used to gouge and grasp the tip of a broken-off screw so that it may be turned. (Courtesy Hilco, Plainville, Mass.)

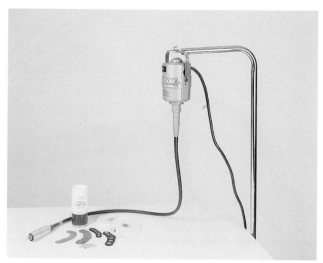

Figure 10-29. A drill with a hanging motor allows for more flexibility. It can be used for purposes other than drilling. Pictured here are attachments for grinding, sanding, cutting, and polishing. (Courtesy Hilco, Plainville, Mass.)

If this tool is unavailable or cannot be used and if a portion of the screw protrudes at the end, use the *slotting or ribbon file* to make a slot in the tip of the screw and then turn the screw out with a screwdriver.

If none of these methods work, it may be feasible to *drive out* the remaining portion of the screw.

If all else fails, *drill out* the screw or its remaining portion (Figure 10-32). Use a drill bit slightly smaller than the diameter of the screw. Most screws in hinges and closing barrels are 1.4 mm in diameter. The drill size most commonly used for these screws is a 0.0430 (No. 57) bit.

Drill from the *bottom* of the screw. (The lower portion of the barrel is the threaded portion.) The conventional way of drilling starts by filing the screw flush with the barrel. Make a punch mark in the center of the screw to act as a guide in drilling. Center the drill carefully on the screw so as not to drill away the metal of the barrel surrounding the screw. Drill the screw out slowly, drilling and pausing to keep from overheating and ruining the drill bit. Always use a cutting or a household oil as a lubricant and/or coolant when drilling.

There is a drilling guide made special for the purpose of keeping the drill bit on course so that it drills just the screw and not the hinge next to the screw. This is called the *Bull's-Eye Screw Drilling Guide*. The guide is clamped to the barrels with the bottom jaw of the guide over the head of the screw (if the head is still there). After clamped in place, put a drop or two of oil into the top of the guide. Use a 0.043 (No. 57) drill bit. The drill bit fits into the top of the drill guide, as shown in Figure 10-33 and drills out the screw.

The threads are destroyed whenever a drill bit or punch pliers is used to drive out a screw. *Use a tap to*

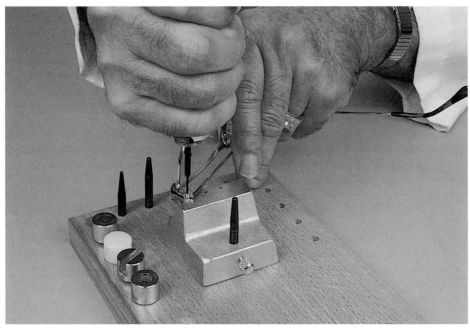

Figure 10-30. Mounting a screw extractor blade in a drill will allow extra torque to be applied when trying to remove a broken-off screw. (Courtesy Hilco, Plainville, Mass.)

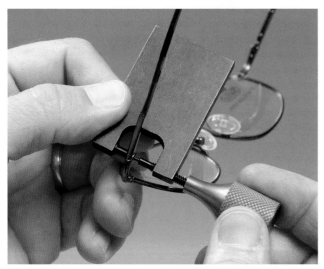

Figure 10-31. This simple device will place a lot of pressure on a broken-off screw and accomplish the same thing that a regular screwdriver-like screw extractor may not be able to do.

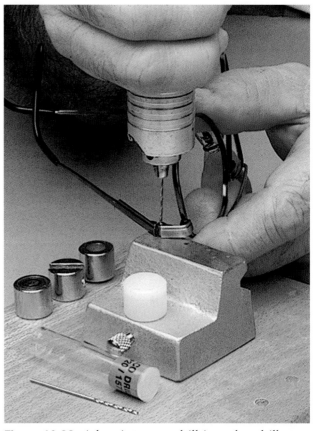

Figure 10-32. A hanging motor drill is used to drill out a broken screw. The frame is being braced against an optician's anvil.

restore the threads (Figures 10-34 and 10-35). The tap can be either regular or oversized, depending on the hole drilled. A standard screw can be reapplied if a regular tap is used, but a special oversized screw must be used if an oversized tap is used.

When a tap cannot be used to restore the threads or is not desired, here are two alternatives:

1. *Use a self-tapping screw.* (This is explained in more detail in the next section.)

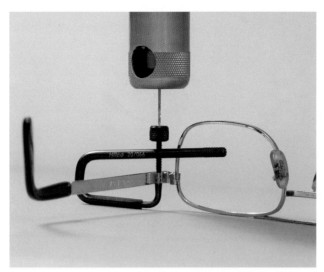

Figure 10-33. The Bull's-Eye Screw Drilling Guide is clamped to the screw. The drill is guided exactly onto the screw by going through a hole in the drilling guide.

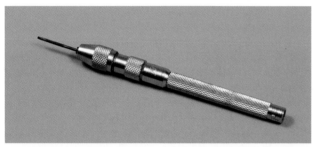

Figure 10-34. A tap is a screw threader. It is held in a chuck with a handle. Threaders of varying size may be mounted in the chuck. The same handle can be used to mount a small drill bit for hand drilling plastic.

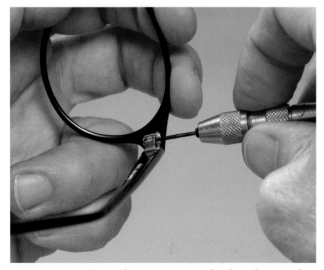

Figure 10-35. Using the tap to restore the threading involves nothing more than turning the tap clockwise into the barrels.

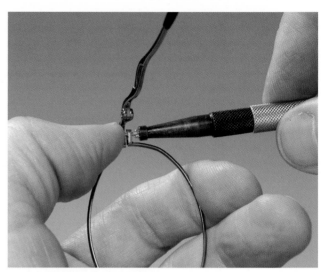

Figure 10-36. A "glass" screw and hex nut will serve when rethreading is no longer feasible. It is not always an attractive option. Look at the construction of the frame to see whether the nut should be at the top or bottom. The position that conceals the nut best is the preferred choice.

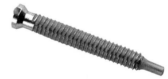

Figure 10-37. A self-tapping screw cuts its own threading. After the screw is fully in place, the excess is broken off with pliers. (Courtesy Hilco, Plainville, Mass.)

2. *Use a longer boltlike screw, often referred to as a glass screw,* in combination with a hex nut* on the end to hold it tight (Figure 10-36).

   Glass screws are longer than temple screws. They were made to pass through thick lenses and hold them in place in a rimless mounting. While tightening such a screw with a screwdriver, hold the hex nut with a hex wrench. Clip off the portion of the screw that protrudes beyond the hex nut and file the end of the screw smooth to the surface of the nut.

Self-Tapping Screws

Self-tapping screws offer a simple alternative to rethreading (Figure 10-37). In most cases they are superior to using glass screws with hex nuts.

Self-threading screws are longer than common screws. After being screwed into place, any excess length extending beyond the end of the barrel should be removed. Self-tapping screws are not cut off with cutting pliers,

---

*Glass screws are, of course, not made of glass, but were used to mount a lens in a rimless mounting. Because the screw went through a glass lens, it is called a "glass" screw.

but snapped off using regular pliers, such as flat-round or needle-nose pliers.

When replacing screws with an oversized or a large self-tapping screw, make sure the screw will freely pass through all the upper barrels that are not supposed to have threads in them. If the self-tapping screw is too large, it can break off before it is screwed in all the way, forcing the dispenser to start the process from the beginning. If the screw is too big to pass through the upper barrel, it is possible to enlarge the hole with either a drill bit or a rattail file.

Replacing Rimless Screws

Sometimes a screw that holds the lens in place in a rimless mounting will break, loosen, or have to be replaced. There are a large variety of mounting methods for rimless eyewear, making it difficult to describe repairs on every conceivable type. However, when lenses are held in place with screws, there are three basic types of assemblies. Each of these assemblies has more than just a screw with a nut. There are a combination of bushings and washers that protect the lens surfaces and remove some of the stress from the screw and nut.

Here are the basic components commonly used in the rimless assembly:

- *A screw*— The screw must be long enough to go through the mounting and full thickness of the lens. The thickness of the lens varies, so after assembly the screw is cut off flush with the nut and filed smooth.
- *A nut*— The nut used can be either a hex nut or a star nut. The hex nut is screwed on to the screw with a nut driver (hex wrench); the star nut requires a star nut driver.
- *Washers*— There are both nylon and metal washers used. The nylon washer goes up against the lens surface and cushions the lens. The metal washer is the last thing between the nut and the rest of the assembly. The metal washer stabilizes the stress around the holes and acts as a barrier between the nut and the softer nylon washer or bushing surface.
- *Bushings*— Bushings are small, hollow cylinders that fit into the hole in the lens. The screw passes through the bushing instead of directly through the lens and cushions the lens. "Top hat" bushings are commonly used for rimless assemblies. These have a "rim" on the bushing that both holds the bushing in place near the surface of the lens and works like a nylon washer. Top hat bushings are the type of bushings normally used for rimless mountings.

Figure 10-38 shows how three common rimless screw assemblies are put together using these components. *Note:* Even if the existing assembly on the wearer's old frame was put together with only a screw and a nut, when making a change, add a nylon washer between the lens and the nut. Better still, use a nylon bushing to protect the lens from the screw.

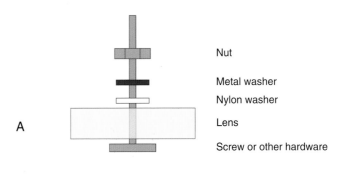

A — Nut / Metal washer / Nylon washer / Lens / Screw or other hardware

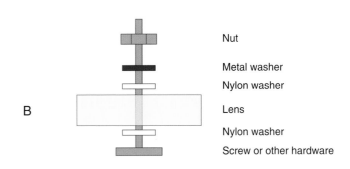

B — Nut / Metal washer / Nylon washer / Lens / Nylon washer / Screw or other hardware

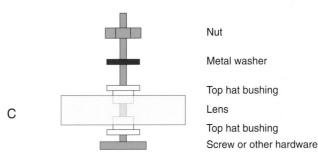

C — Nut / Metal washer / Top hat bushing / Lens / Top hat bushing / Screw or other hardware

Figure 10-38. Here are three basic rimless assembly designs that might be used. Which is used will depend upon the frame design. Some designs use an entirely different method of securing the lens in place. **A,** A simple rimless screw assembly consists of a regular or decorative screw, a nylon washer on the back to protect the lens, a metal washer to stabilize the stress areas, and the nut. The nut may be a hex or a star nut. **B,** A common assembly cushioning both the front and back of the lens with nylon washers. **C,** Top hat bushings replace nylon washers, protect the hole in the lens, and add stability to the assembly.

NOSEPAD REPLACEMENTS

There are many different types of nosepad assemblies. The screw-on and push-on type nosepad assemblies are the most dominant. Every eyecare professional must carry both versions. The most common types are described here. Some of the more uncommon and antique styles are discussed in Appendix 10-A at the end of this chapter. These include clip-on, twist-on, Zeiss bayonet, split-clamp, stirrup, and rivet types.

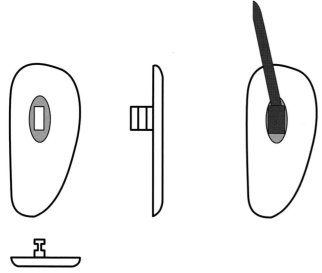

Figure 10-39. The *push-on* nosepad design slips into an indented box on the pad arm.

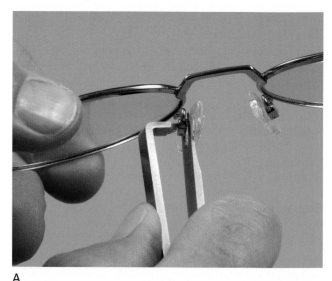

A

B

Figure 10-41. A, The thin edge is slipped between the pad and the pad arm. **B,** The back of the pad has been pressed out of the box on the pad arm.

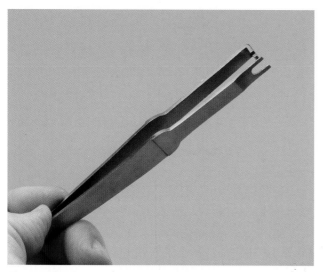

Figure 10-40. A pad popper is used to remove push-on pads without affecting the pad arm alignment.

Push-On

The *push-on pad* is one of the easiest pads to remove and replace. It has a small I-beamlike shape that snaps into an indented box on the pad arm (Figure 10-39). The part of the pad that slips into the box may be either metal or hard plastic.

Although a push-on pad can be removed without the aid of tools, it is possible to use a small device called a *pad popper*. This device is slipped between the pad and the pad arm attachment, as shown in Figures 10-40 and 10-41.

There are pliers specifically designed to aid in attaching a push-on pad to the pad arm. Known as *Push-On Pad Pliers*, they have a curved nylon jaw on one side that cradles the pad face and a flat, metal jaw on the other side to hold the pad arm in place.

If a push-on pad will not stay in the box securely, use a pair of pliers to squeeze and narrow the horizontal dimension of the box slightly.

Screw-On

The *screw-on type* of attachment has a small post on the back of the pad with a horizontal hole in the post. The post slips into either a boxlike assembly or a rounded piece on the pad arm (Figure 10-42). A screw is threaded from one side of the box to the other, passing through the hole in the pad post. The screw is so small that a special screwdriver is usually required.

The greatest problem with the screw-on pad design is having a properly fitting replacement screw available. If someone has the unmounted pad but not the screw, it may be difficult to find a suitable replacement screw. The most common nosepad screw diameter is 1.0 mm. If this

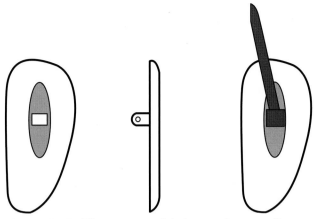

Figure 10-42. The *screw-on* pad design requires a small screw to secure it to the pad arm.

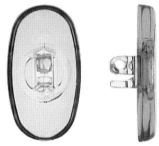

Figure 10-43. This Logic nosepad serves as a replacement for either the screw-on or the push-on type of nosepads.

screw is too small, a 1.1-mm screw should do the job. Since most companies list screw diameters, getting to know the most common sizes can really be helpful in finding replacement screws.

As a last resort, if no replacement screw is available, the nosepad can be temporarily "tied" on using the same type of nylon line as is used to "string mount" lenses. The excess line is cut off using cutting pliers or a razor blade.

Logic

There is a specialty replacement nosepad with an insert that fits both push-on and screw-on types of pad arms. This pad, called the Logic pad, comes in round or oval shapes and is symmetrical, making left and right pads interchangeable. This reduces the need to keep as many pads in inventory (Figure 10-43).

Pad Sizes

Pads are manufactured in various sizes. Sizes can be changed to match the nasal area available or to increase the bearing area when the pressure from the weight of the frame on the nose is too concentrated. Oval pads measuring 13, 15, 17, and 20 mm in their vertical axes and round pads measuring 9 and 11 mm are the most common sizes, though other sizes are available.

Types of Pad Materials

Replacement pads are available in a number of different materials, having more or less flexibility. Here are the three most common materials:

- *Acetate pads*— Pads made from cellulose acetate material (sometimes just called acetate) are hard and do not flex. Cellulose acetate is the same material used for a great many plastic frames.
- *Vinyl pads*— There are also pads made from a soft, vinyl material. Although these pads are flexible, they do not "grab" the nose, but will slide on the nose more easily than a silicone pad.
- *Silicone pads*— Silicone pads do not have a tendency to slide down the nose, even when perspiration or skin oil are present. This is not to say that the pads do not slide at all, but rather they slide much less. Although this is advantageous, it may irritate some people's skin because they may feel a pulling sensation on the skin. If an individual complains that the nosepads seem to pull and irritate the skin, it may be helpful to switch to an acetate or vinyl pad. (The wearer should, of course, be made aware that the glasses will slide more easily. The solution is a trade-off.) Silicone pads come in a "soft silicone," "firm silicone," and "flex silicone." The softness or firmness of the pad does not depend on the basic material, but rather on the mounting insert that is molded into the silicone pad. Soft silicone pads have a small metal mounting inside the pad, whereas firm silicone pads have a metal insert imbedded in a nylon core within the pad. Flex silicone pads do not have a metal insert, but rather a thin nylon core.

Hypoallergenic Nosepad Materials

There are wearers who are sensitive to standard nosepad materials, such as silicone, vinyl, and acetate. Some pads may also contain latex or other materials that cause an irritation around the nasal area. Here are some options that usually satisfy these wearers:

- *Gold-plated metal pads*— There are pads made from gold-plated nickel silver. The gold plating comes in yellow-gold (gold colored) or white-gold (silver colored) and, although nickel is problematic if directly against the skin, the gold plating becomes a barrier that prevents an allergic skin reaction.
- *Titanium pads*— Titanium is extremely well tolerated by those with skin allergies. These nosepads are made of 100% titanium.
- *Crystal pads*— There are pads made of crystal. These look more like regular nosepads and solve the problem of allergic reactions.

Replacing Adjustable Pads with Strap Bridges

A *strap bridge* is like two adjustable pads whose tops are linked together with a "strap." The strap is of the same

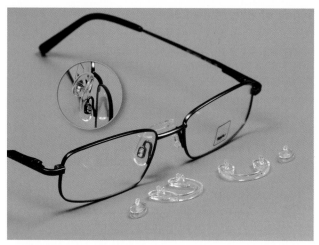

Figure 10-44. A *strap bridge* replaces two adjustable pads. It distributes frame weight over both the traditional nosepad areas and across the crest of the nose. The flexibility of the material allows both pads to still be adjusted separately.

material as the pads and is really an extension of them; the pads and strap are one unit (Figure 10-44). A strap bridge increases the pad bearing area to include the crest of the nose. Strap bridges are attached to the pad arms in exactly the same manner as are adjustable pads. They are also fit to the nose in the same manner. Since the whole piece is flexible, left and right halves adjust independently.

TEMPLE REPAIRS

Replacing Missing or Broken Temples

If a pair of glasses has an irreparably broken temple, it must be replaced. The first choice is to replace it with a new, identical temple. Unfortunately a new, matching temple will not always be available. The frame style may have been discontinued, and it may be impossible to obtain a matching replacement.

Replacing With an Old Temple

Most dispensaries keep a selection of old temples that can be used for temporary replacement purposes. The most difficult task is to find a temple that both looks good and has a hinge with a barrel configuration that matches the frame front. If no match is found, it may be feasible to modify the temple barrels. The end result may be less than ideal but functional.

For example, suppose one barrel is a single, thick barrel and slightly large for the other two matching barrels. In such a case, it may be possible to file either or both the top and bottom of the large, single barrel down so that it fits into the smaller space between the other two barrels.

Eyeglass frame temples come as either a right or a left. Sometimes a left temple is necessary and all that is available is a right temple. For some hinges, it is possible to

mount the right temple on the left side, or vice versa. If this is done, the bent-down portion will turn up instead of down. If the temple will look acceptable, heat the temple bend and bend the earpiece down.

Replacing from a Set of Replacement Temples

A variety of plastic and metal replacement temples can be purchased through an optical accessories supplier. To ensure that the temple will match the front, the butt portion of the temple is longer than necessary. This portion is cut off at the proper angle with a file or coping saw. The angle will depend on the type of endpiece or temple abutment as seen in Figure 1-16.

Replacing the Plastic Earpiece Covers on Metal Temples

Most metal temples are made so that the end of the temple is plastic covered. This allows for greater comfort. If the plastic temple cover becomes damaged, it may be replaced. Plastic replacement temple tips come in a large variety of colors and shapes. They are also available in silicone material to help decrease slippage. The most popular core diameters are 1.4 mm and 1.6 mm.

To replace a temple tip,[3] heat the plastic end of the temple, straighten it out completely, and pull the plastic cover off.

Determine the size of the metal core by measuring or using actual-size diagrams provided by the manufacturer of the replacement tips. (One way to quickly find the diameter of the core wire is to use the same type of gauge used to measure screw diameters.) Match the shape and color of the tip as closely as possible.

Push the replacement tip onto the metal core. (If the core is round instead of rectangular, it is easier to use a back-and-forth twisting motion to get the replacement tip on the temple.) It may be necessary to heat the replacement tip.

The temple may now be rebent so that the bend is just posterior to the top of the ear as described in Chapter 9.

Adding Covers to Cable Temple Earpieces

Some people who need cable temples may be bothered because they find the cable uncomfortable or because they have an allergic reaction to the metal cable. An allergic response is usually caused by the nickel content in the frame material. Signs of this reaction are a rash behind the ear or the cable turning green.

It is possible to cover the end of a cable temple with a plastic cover. Covers for cable temples are available through optical supply houses. They come in plastic, vinyl, and silicone materials. There is also "heat-shrink" tubing sold for this purpose.

Shrink tubing is a simple solution to covering the end of a cable. The inside diameter of a heat-shrink temple cover is larger than the diameter of the cable temple. To apply this tubing, do the following:

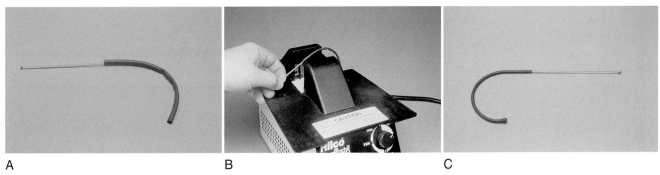

A   B   C

Figure 10-45. It is possible to cover the end of a cable temple with heat-shrink cable tip covers. Find the correct diameter, cut to length, and slip over the end of the cable temple, as shown in **A**. Heat using a frame warmer on the highest setting, as shown in **B**. Heat-shrink cable tips tighten up snugly, as seen on the temple shown in **C**. (Courtesy Hilco, Plainville, Mass.)

1. Determine the diameter size of the shrink tubing needed so it will slip over the end of the cable.
2. Measure how much length is needed. (Allow 10% over the measured length to allow for shrinkage.)
3. Cut a strip to length and slide the cover over the end of the cable temple (Figure 10-45, *A*).
4. Heat both temple and cover with a hot air frame warmer at the hottest setting (Figure 10-45, *B*) until the tubing shrinks to fit the temple snugly (Figure 10-45, *C*).
5. Trim off any excess material.
6. Heat the trimmed area to smooth the edges.

Covering the Temples to Reduce Allergic Reactions

If a wearer has an allergic reaction to the temple along the side of the head, the frame may be sent out to a frame repair center to be entirely coated.

A second option is to use clear, ultrathin shrink tubing that places a thin, clear barrier over the temple. This is done by sliding the tubing over the temple and then heating both tubing and temple with a hot air frame warmer.

Lengthening and Shortening of Metal Temples

Metal temples usually come with bent-down portions that have a metal core, but a plastic outer portion. These types of temples are unique in that they may be shortened or lengthened beyond what would be expected.

To lengthen—Sometimes the desired frame is not made with temples that are long enough for the wearer. Even if the bend is moved by heating and rebending, there is insufficient length for a suitable fit. If this is the case, there are two alternatives:

1. The first alternative is to heat and straighten the temple. Then pull on the temple cover as if to remove it, but only let it slide off part of the way. For example, if the temple is 5 mm too short, pull the temple cover so that it slides 5 mm out. Now rebend the temple so that it is of the proper size.

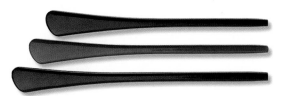

Figure 10-46. Resizing a metal temple using plastic temple tip sizers is no harder than simply replacing the plastic ends. All three of these temple ends will interchange to fit the same temple. (Courtesy Hilco, Plainville, Mass.)

This method does not provide as much support and makes the end of the temple weaker than it would be otherwise.

2. The second alternative is to replace the plastic temple ends. Optical suppliers have temple sizer kits that will allow adding 5 to 15 mm in length to the size of a metal temple just by changing the plastic temple ends (Figure 10-46).

To shorten—If the temple is too long (Figure 10-47, *A*) and cannot be made sufficiently short by moving the temple bend, the temple must be shortened. To shorten the temple, heat the temple end, straighten it (Figure 10-47, *B*), and pull the plastic cover completely off. Clip off the end of the metal core (Figure 10-47, *C*). (The amount clipped should equal the amount the temple must be shortened.) Slip the plastic cover back on; it will now go on farther than it did before, making the temple shorter (Figure 10-47, *D*). Complete the adjustment by rebending the temple to the appropriate length.

Sometimes it is necessary to file down a temple "shoulder" if the cover will not go on past the shoulder without splitting. (That part of the metal temple that is still flat, just before the temple narrows down to a small, round diameter, is called the shoulder.) If this is the case, file either or both the top and bottom of the shoulder (Figure 10-48). The shoulder must be thin enough to allow the temple cover to slide all the way up without splitting.

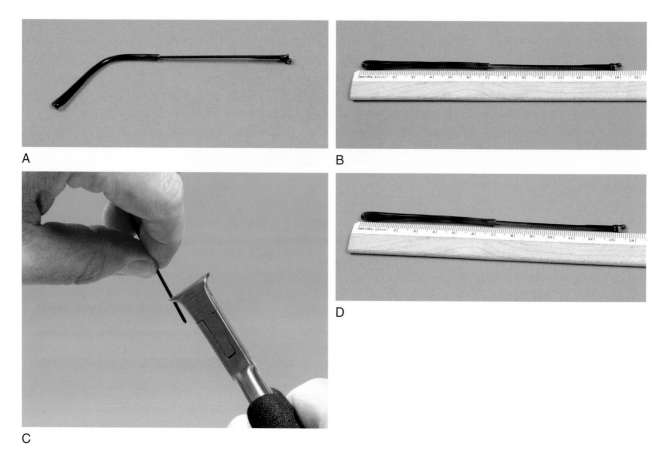

A B

C D

Figure 10-47. Sometimes just moving the location of the bend will not make a temple short enough without leaving an excessively long and unsightly bent-down portion. **A,** Metal temples with plastic temple ends, such as the one shown, can be shortened another way. **B,** To shorten this type of temple, the bend is straightened, and the plastic cover pulled off. This temple has an overall length of 145 mm. **C,** Once the plastic cover is removed, the tip of the metal core is clipped. **D,** The temple cover is replaced and is measurably shorter.

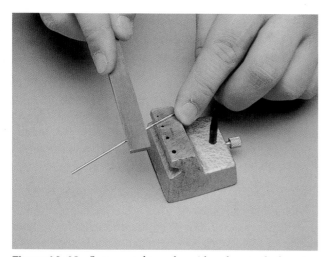

Figure 10-48. Some metal temples widen close to the location of the plastic end cover. The place where the temple widens is called the shoulder. If a temple has been clipped short and the plastic end cannot be put back on without splitting the plastic, the shoulder must be filed.

When the plastic cover is slipped back on, it will now go on farther than it did before, making the temple shorter.

Help in Making Temple Tip Changes Easier
There can be some challenges when changing temple tips. Here are some hints to make the job easier[4]:
- If the old, damaged temple cover will not come off just by heating and sliding it off, use pliers to crush the old plastic until it does come off.
- File any rough places off the metal core of the temple, making certain that the end is filed smooth and rounded.
- Before trying to slide the new temple cover on, heat up the metal core. Slide the temple tip on as far as it will go, then heat the tip with the frame warmer until it will slide on the rest of the way.

Changing Cable Temple Lengths
Cable temples may be shortened by clipping, and either lengthened or shortened by replacing the curled end.

Shortening Cable Temples

If it becomes necessary to shorten a cable temple that is too long, shortening is done by simply clipping off the excess portion of the cable with cutting pliers. The rolled metal cable must be sealed so it will not unravel. To seal the cable, touch the cut end with a soldering iron, apply a small amount of solder, and allow the solder to form a small ball at the end. (It may be desirable to combine this with a heat-shrink cable tip cover.)

Lengthening, Shortening, or Replacing Cable Temple Ends with Silicone Cable

Hilco makes a silicone replacement cable end that may be used to either lengthen or shorten a cable temple. The curled silicone does not have a metal core, but rather one made of acetate. To replace the curled end, use the following sequence of steps:

1. Determine the desired overall temple length.
2. Determine what length of curled cable is to be replaced and get the pair of replacement cable ends in the desired size and color.
3. Subtract the length of the temple to be replaced from the overall temple length.
4. Measure from the hinge center along the temple until the length determined in step 3 is reached. Mark the temple at this point.
5. Measure back an additional 8 mm and mark the temple a second time. This is the cutoff point.
6. Cut the temple off at the second mark and discard the cutoff portion.
7. Heat the replacement cable with a hot air frame warmer for 20 to 30 seconds.
8. Slide the replacement cable onto the core wire until the front of the replacement cable reaches the first mark measured.
9. Cool the whole temple in water to contract the replacement cable for a firm hold.

Example **10-1**

A cable temple is too short. It is 160 mm long and needs to be 170 mm in length. Replacement cable ends come in a variety of sizes. The appropriate length is the length that will allow a proper fit around the back of the ear (shown earlier in Figure 9-27, A) and end at a logical point of attachment to the straight portion of the temple. In this case we will say that our replacement cable end length is 90 mm. To what length should the cable temple be cut to achieve the new length?

Solution

If the overall desired length is 170 mm, we subtract 90 from 170, which equals 80 mm (170 mm − 90 mm = 80 mm). This 80-mm length is measured back from the center of the hinge barrel and marked. Then an additional 8 mm is measured (at 88 mm) and also marked. The temple is cut at the second mark, and the 90-mm replacement part attached.

Converting Standard Plastic Temples to Cable-Style Temples

The same replacement cable ends that were used for the procedure just described above can also be used to convert a standard plastic temple to a cable-style temple. The procedure is very similar to that of changing the length of a cable temple and replacing it with a silicone cable.

First, determine the desired overall cable temple length and the length of the curled replacement cable end that will fit correctly. Match size of the replacement cable end to the wearer's ear and the color of the replacement to the original plastic temple.

Subtract the length of the replacement cable end from the desired overall cable temple length. Measure from the center of the plastic temple hinge until that length is reached. Mark the plastic temple at this point and also at a second point 8 mm farther down the temple (Figure 10-49, A).

Cut the temple off at the second mark (Figure 10-49, B) and throw out the cutoff end (Figure 10-49, C). Using a razor blade or exacto knife, cut through the plastic at the first mark to the depth of the metal core all the way around the temple (Figure 10-49, D). Slip the 8-mm piece of plastic off (Figure 10-49, E). It may be necessary to file and buff the plastic around the core wire to a smooth and somewhat tapered shape so that the transition between plastic temple and replacement cable appears natural.

The replacement cable should be heated with a hot air frame warmer for 20 to 30 seconds and slipped onto the exposed 8-mm temple core wire (Figure 10-49, F). When the replacement cable completely covers the core wire, the whole temple should be cooled in water to contract the replacement cable firmly around the core wire. Assuming the appropriate color match has been made, the finished product should look as if it were originally intended to be a cable-style temple (Figure 10-49, G).

Shortening Plastic Temples

It may be possible to special order a shorter pair of temples from the manufacturer if the current pair for a plastic frame is unacceptably long. This option should not be overlooked. Another option is to check for a suitable replacement pair. (See section "Replacing from a Set of Replacement Temples" earlier in this chapter.)

Should neither option be viable, there is a method that can be used to shorten the length of plastic temples.* It requires care, or the results may reveal the modification. This technique is used when no other satisfactory frame is available and is done with the full knowledge and consent of the wearer. The procedure parallels that used to shorten the length of a metal temple having a plastic cover.

---

*Contributed by Dr. Jerry Bizer, Jeffersonville, Ind.

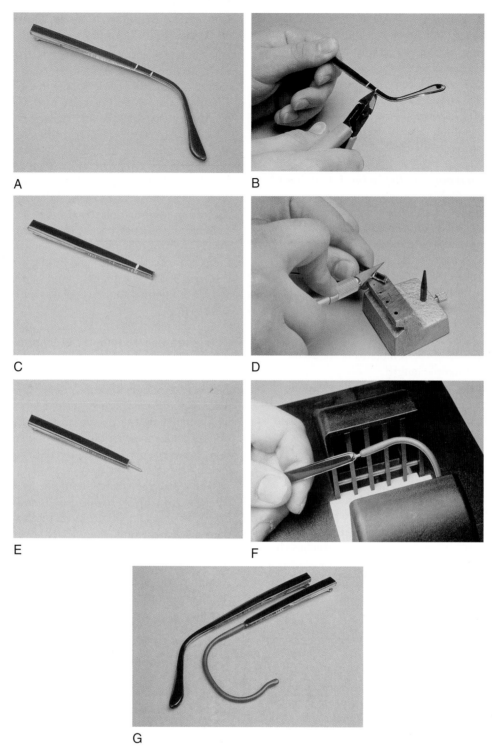

Figure 10-49. **A,** Converting a plastic skull temple to a cable-style temple begins by making two marks on the temple. The position of the first mark in millimeters equals the desired cable temple length minus the length of the replacement cable end. The position of the second mark equals first mark location plus 8 mm. **B,** The plastic temple is cut off at the location of the second mark. **C,** The temple has been cut at the second mark. **D,** The plastic between the first mark and the cut end is cut then stripped from the core wire. **E,** This shows the exposed core wire as it appears before adding the replacement cable end. **F,** After tapering and polishing the cut area of the plastic temple, the replacement cable end is slipped over the exposed 8 mm of core wire and heated. **G,** The skull-to-cable conversion is complete.

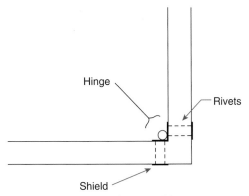

Figure 10-50. Top view of a riveted hinge construction.

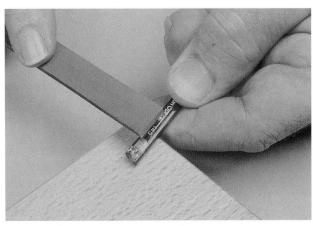

Figure 10-51. To remove a riveted hinge, it is necessary to file the rivets almost flush with the inside of the hinge, leaving only enough rivet visible to act as a guide when pressing them out. (Courtesy Hilco, Plainville, Mass.)

To begin, heat and straighten the plastic temple. With a sharp knife or razor blade, cut around the metal core of the temple about ½ inch in front of where the temple bend should be positioned. If the cut is made to the depth of the metal reinforcing wire, the end of the temple may be pulled off the wire. If it does not pull off easily, heat the temple again.

Next, cut off a section of plastic from the loose temple end adjacent to the first cut. The amount removed should equal the amount that the temple needs to be shortened. Now cut off the end of the metal reinforcing wire. (The amount of wire cut away should be slightly longer than the amount that the temple needs to be shortened.)

Slip the plastic end of the temple back on the wire. Reseal the two pieces with acetone. After the area has dried and hardened, it may be filed and buffed.

REPAIRING THE HINGES

The hinge area of a frame is especially susceptible to damage. A blow or other impact to the side of the head can break the hinge area by forcing the joint between the temple and the front to open farther than it was designed to.

Riveted Hinges

The structure that usually gives way in a plastic frame with riveted hinges is not the hinge, but the rivets that hold the hinge to the frame. A riveted hinge is identifiable by a visible shield on the outside of the endpiece. Since the rivets are attached to the shield, a new shield is required when the rivets break (Figure 10-50). When the barrels of the hinge break, both hinge and shield must be replaced. Before any repairs are made to riveted hinges, the temple must be removed.

Removing the Rivets and Shield

First file the rivets on the inside of the hinge (Figure 10-51) until they are almost flush with the metal, leaving only a small amount of the rivets visible to act as a guide for pushing out the rivet. Then remove them, using one of the following methods:

- *Punch pliers*— Punch pliers have a fine, rounded, rodlike projection that is placed against the filed end of the rivet. The pliers are squeezed to push the rivet out of the plastic.
- *Anvil and punch*— To use the anvil and punch method, brace the endpiece or temple (filed rivet ends up) on an optician's anvil or on the base of a hinge punch set. If no anvil or punch base is available, brace the temple on some other flat surface in such a way that the movement of the rivet out of the plastic is not obstructed. Next, place a punch on the filed end of the rivet. Tap the end of the punch with a small hammer until the rivet moves out of the endpiece (Figure 10-52).
- *Staking tool*— A staking tool may also be used to punch out old rivets (Figure 10-53). Most staking tools come with both a single and a double punch. The single punch is safer to use; the double punch may put too much pressure on the part all at once and damage it. To remove the rivets with a single punch, first push a little on one rivet, then a little on the other. Alternate back and forth between the two, working them free gradually.

Once the rivets are free from the hinge, the hinge comes off the temple or front. The rivets are attached to the shield and are still in the plastic.

- *Cutting pliers*— Cutting pliers serve well for pulling out the shield because the jaws are narrow and can get behind the shield (Figure 10-54, *A* and *B*). They must be held without squeezing and used only for pulling. Inadvertently squeezing the pliers will cut the shield from the rivets.

(As an aside, it should be noted that some cutting pliers are not able to cut especially hard materials, such as stainless steel or titanium. Using the wrong pliers on these materials can ruin the pliers.)

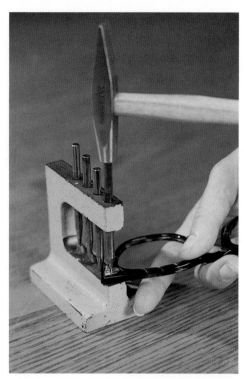

Figure 10-52. One method for removing rivets is tapping the old rivet out with a hammer and punch.

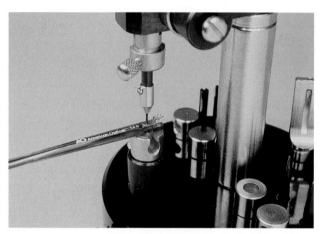

Figure 10-53. A staking tool with interchangeable attachments may be used to press the old rivets out. (Courtesy Hilco, Plainville, Mass.)

Replacing the Shield

Use a shield that matches the old shield that has been removed as nearly as possible. Since an exact duplicate may not always be available, it may be necessary to use a shield that fits but does not look exactly the same. In these cases it is best to have the wearer approve the substitute shield before proceeding with the repair.

For the new shield to fit, the spacing between the rivets of the new shield must be identical to the spacing in the old shield. When the hinges themselves need replacing, the number of barrels and the spacing and type of rivet holes must match the original hinge. Most

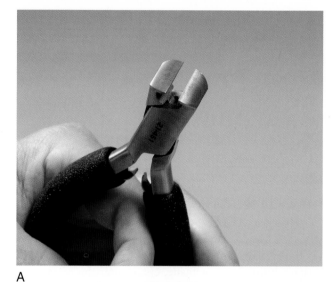

A

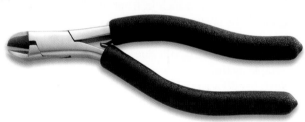

B

Figure 10-54. The most common type of cutting pliers is shown in **A**. There are other designs that cut from the side of the pliers' jaw area, rather than the top, as shown in **B**.

hinges are made for either the left or the right side, but check to be sure that this is the case.

Place the new shield on the outside of the endpiece or temple so the rivets pass through the plastic or metal. Affix the hinge to these protruding rivets and reduce the excess rivet length to about 1 mm using cutting pliers (Figure 10-55).

Round these excess rivet ends into firmly holding "heads," using either peening pliers or a staking set with a peening tool. (The peening tool has a concave, cupped end.) When using peening pliers, one jaw rests on the shield while the other presses and rounds the rivet head. This operation can also be accomplished by placing the shield firmly on a flat surface or anvil, with the exposed rivet ends up, and tapping the ends into a rounded "head" with a hammer (Figure 10-56).

For a summary of how to repair riveted hinges, see Box 10-3.

Rivets can loosen over a period of time, allowing the temple to wobble even when the screw is tight. The rivets can be retightened by hammering or repeening them.

Hidden Hinges

Most plastic frames have a hinge anchored directly in the plastic instead of being fastened with rivets and a

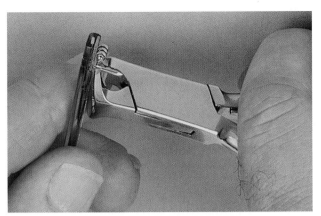

Figure 10-55. Reducing rivet length too much will not allow for a sufficient hold, whereas cutting rivets too long causes them to bend over when compressed rather than form a head.

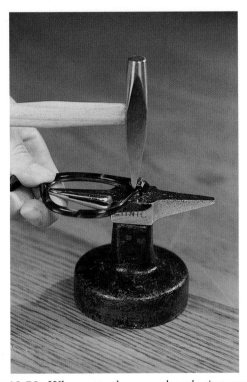

Figure 10-56. When cut to the proper length, rivets are easily hammered to form a rounded head. If the lens is in the frame, the thumb should be placed over the lens near the hinge so that the lens is protected from the hammer.

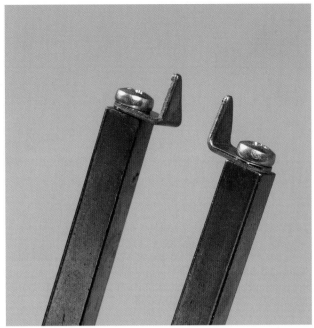

Figure 10-57. The probe of the Hot Fingers unit allows the object being heated to be grasped easily. The Hot Fingers unit may be used to replace or repair hidden hinges, do repairs on plastic frame breaks, and to add adjustable nosepads to plastic frames.

BOX 10-3

Repairing Riveted Hinges

1. Remove the temple.
2. File the rivets.
3. Press the rivets out.
4. Pull the shield off.
5. Put a new shield on.
6. Put the hinge back on.
7. Clip off the rivets.
8. Peen the rivets down.

---

shield. Such a construction is referred to as a "hidden hinge" since no shield is visible from the front.

To repair a damaged hidden hinge, it is necessary to have a soldering iron, or better still, a unit made especially for this purpose, such as a *hidden hinge repair kit* (several types are available from a number of optical suppliers) or Hilco's Hot Fingers. A moderately priced hidden hinge repair kit is considerably easier to use than a soldering iron because it has tips included to allow better contact between the hinge and the hot metal. The

Hot Fingers unit is more expensive, but offers convenience, including the ability to pick up small parts with the tip of the probe (Figure 10-57) and a foot switch for instant heat when necessary.

Repairing a Loose Hidden Hinge
To repair a loose hidden hinge, begin by removing the temple. Hold the tip of the heating unit to the loose hinge until the hinge becomes hot enough to begin to melt the surrounding plastic. Make certain that the hinge is not crooked and plunge the hot area into cold water (Box 10-4).

Repairing a Hidden Hinge That is Completely Torn Out of the Frame
If a hinge has torn completely out of the frame, it may be repaired using the sequence given here and summarized in Box 10-5:

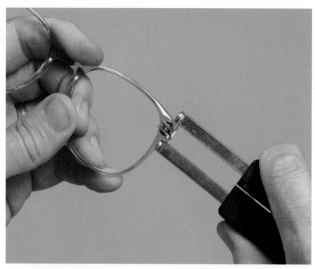

Figure 10-58. The Hot Fingers is used to grasp a torn out hidden hinge, put it back in the frame front, and heat it so that the plastic will be remolded around it.

BOX 10-4

How to Repair a Loose Hidden Hinge

1. Remove the temple.
2. Hold the tip of a hot instrument on the hinge until surrounding plastic softens.
3. Check for hinge straightness.
4. Plunge hinge area in cold water.

BOX 10-5

How to Repair a Torn-Out Hidden Hinge

1. Cut off tiny pieces of a junk frame, make filings from a junk frame, or use virgin plastic pellets.
2. Put a few junk plastic pieces, a plastic pellet, or plastic filings in the hinge hole.
3. Place the hinge squarely in the hole.
4. Hold the tip of a hot instrument on the hinge until surrounding plastic softens.
5. Recheck the hinge for straightness.
6. Plunge hinge area in cold water.
7. Trim away excess plastic.

---

1. First cut off very small pieces, or using a coarse file, produce a quantity of loose plastic filings from an old junk frame made of the same type of plastic as the one being repaired. Alternatively, use virgin plastic pellets available from an optical supplier.
2. Put a few small pieces or filings into the hole where the hinge belongs. Replace the hinge in the hole, making absolutely certain that it is straight. Hold it in place with the Hot Fingers tool (Figure 10-58) or touch it with a soldering iron until the metal becomes hot enough to cause the plastic around it to remold itself to the hinge.

3. Plunge the whole area into cold water to set the plastic.
4. Trim any excess plastic off using a razor blade.

Repairing a Hidden Hinge That is Damaged or Broken Off*

If the barrels of the hidden hinge are split or broken, the old hinge must be removed and replaced with a new hinge. This is most easily done using the Hot Fingers unit because it allows a protruding hinge part to be grasped with the pincerlike end of the heated tool or, if the hinge is broken off flush with the frame, to be pried out with the picklike edge of the tool.

To make the repair, place the Hot Finger tips on the top of the hinge base and depress the foot pedal to heat the hinge. Once the surrounding plastic begins to soften, the hinge will start to rise out of the plastic. When this happens, take one point of the Hot Fingers and pry the hinge out. Use the pincers of the tool to grasp a new hinge by the barrel. The new hinge will have an "anchor" or wider area at the bottom to help hold the hinge in the frame. Heat the new hinge. Then take a pellet of new acetate or a piece of plastic from the scrap frame. Since the hinge is hot, the plastic should stick to the hinge (Figure 10-59). Place the hinge base with the scrap plastic into the hole in the frame. Heat the hinge. As it is heated, it will begin to sink into the plastic. Continue heating until the base of the hinge is flush with the surface (Figure 10-60). Remove your foot from the foot switch to turn off the heat, but do not let go of the hinge. Hold it steady for about 10 seconds to let the frame and hinge cool without moving. This will help set the hinge more securely in the frame. Last, plunge the frame in cold water.

After repairing a hidden hinge, the temple is put back on the frame front. Check that the temple spread is correct. *If the temple is spread too far,* the hinge has not been sunk deeply enough into the plastic. Remove the temple and reheat the hinge until it sinks a little deeper. *If the temple will not open far enough,* the hinge is sunk too deep. Instead of trying to pull the hinge out to some degree, simply file the butt portion of the temple as during standard alignment of a frame.

A note on frame materials—This method works for frames made from cellulose acetate, propionate, polyamide, nylon, and carbon fiber. It will not work on Optyl. The filler material used to secure the hinge must be the same material as the frame being repaired. In other words, if the frame is made of nylon, use only nylon scrap for filler, acetate for acetate, and so forth.

Repairing an Optyl Hidden Hinge

At the time of this writing, it is almost impossible to repair a hidden hinge on an Optyl frame without a Hot

---

*Special thanks to Robert Woyton and Ted Rzemien of Hilco, A Division of the Hilsinger Corp., Plainville, Mass., for information contained in this and the Optyl hinge repair section.

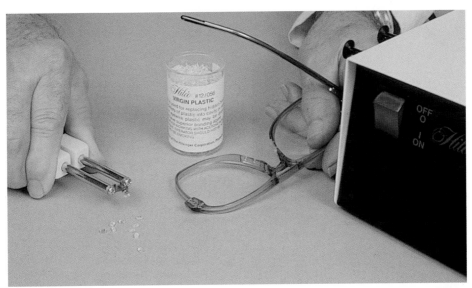

Figure 10-59. Instead of using plastic filings or cut-up pieces from an old frame, it may be helpful to purchase virgin plastic pellets to fill in the extra space when replacing or repairing a hidden hinge. (Courtesy Hilco, Plainville, Mass.)

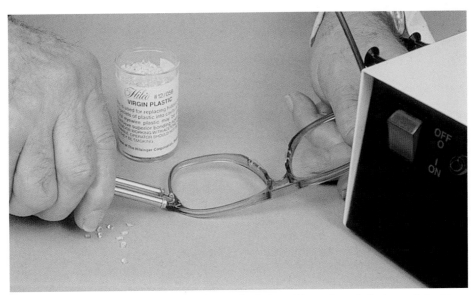

Figure 10-60. The hinge is placed back into the hole and heated until the base of the hinge sinks into the plastic and is flush with the surface. (Courtesy Hilco, Plainville, Mass.)

Fingers unit. This unit is the only piece of equipment that appears to be capable of getting the hinge hot enough to melt Optyl.

To make the repair, grasp the broken hinge with the Hot Fingers and suspend the frame in midair. Use the other hand to lightly hold the other side of the frame so the frame will not fall when the hinge comes out. Begin heating the hinge.

After about 20 seconds, the material around the hinge will start to smoke (Figure 10-61, *A*). Let the frame drop away from the hinge without applying pressure. Trying to pry a hinge out of an Optyl material frame will cause the material to shatter. It should be burned out instead

of pried out. Once the hinge is out, cool the cavity in cold water.

Next, clean out the cavity (Figure 10-61, *B*). This is done with a small burr using a Dremel hand tool (available in hobby shops or hardware stores) or a hanging motor tool (available from optical suppliers). Be sure all burnt material is removed and the hole is deep enough for the new replacement hinge. (Try putting the new hinge in the hole ahead of time to make sure the hole is deep enough.)

When the hole is deep enough, put two or three drops of strong adhesive or epoxy in the hole. Place the new hinge in the hole so that it is seated properly and at the correct angle. Allow the adhesive to dry overnight.

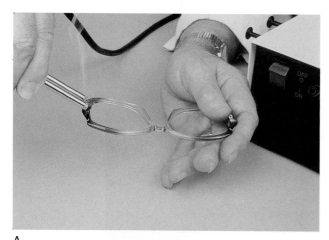

A

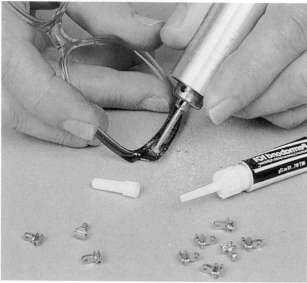

B

Figure 10-61. A, When removing a hidden hinge from an Optyl frame, the hinge must get hot enough to burn its way out. It is already possible to see smoke leaving the hinge area. **B,** After the hinge has been burned out of an Optyl frame, the hole that remains should be cleaned out with a small burr so that the hinge will bond well when glued in place. (Courtesy Hilco, Plainville, Mass.)

BRIDGE REPAIRS

Ordinarily, if a frame has a broken bridge, it takes less effort and looks better to replace the entire frame front than to repair the bridge. On occasion a different frame can be used, if perhaps only temporarily, until a proper replacement is secured. Sometimes, however, either by the wearer's choice or because no other expedient solution is possible, it is necessary to attempt to attach the broken halves of the bridge to each other.

Broken Plastic Bridges

Broken plastic bridges can be repaired using a variety of glues, several forms of wire braces, or several possible combinations of materials and methods. Unfortu-

nately, none of these methods guarantees an attractive repair.

Glues

There are several types of glue that can be used to cement the broken parts of bridges back together. Some of these can also be used in conjunction with wire braces; these applications will be discussed in the following sections.

Epoxy. The use of epoxy glue will result in a strong repair. There are a number of different types of epoxy on the market. Using a type especially designed for plastic will help. One such epoxy is a superadhesive called Plastic Welder and dries to 80% strength in 15 minutes and full bond strength in 1 to 2 hours. Plastic Welder is made by Devcon Corp., Danvers, Mass.

Although different types of epoxy glues require varying amounts of time to dry, the major problem is holding the two parts together properly until the epoxy is set. A special dual-spring vise, used by jewelers, is especially effective for this task. If this vise is not available, make a holding apparatus from modeling clay by simply surrounding the parts with enough clay to hold them in alignment.

Acetone. An old-fashioned method for repairing cellulose acetate frames uses acetone to melt or soften the plastic so that the two separated portions unite and adhere when the plastic hardens.

Since some of the plastic is melted during this process, a slightly narrower distance between lenses may result. To prevent this, melt some excess plastic from an old frame chassis (or other part made of clear plastic) in acetone and apply a bit to each end of the broken bridge before uniting the two parts.

Because acetone is absorbed through the skin, use a cotton-tipped applicator or other tool so that direct contact with the skin is avoided. There are other reasons for caution when using acetone. Acetone is an extremely flammable liquid and there are strict regulations for use and storage. This is especially true when storing larger quantities.

"Instant" Cements. There are a number of quick-drying cements suitable for eyeglass frames that are sold in hardware and other stores. Cements marketed specifically for the purpose of repairing eyeglass frames are sold through optical supply houses.

Vigor Super Glue is a quick-drying glue that is sold specifically for ophthalmic frames and is available professionally from Vigor, Austell, Ga. Other super glues are widely available in hardware stores and are also used extensively to repair frames. Only a small amount of glue is required and will repair almost any break as long as the surfaces are clean, dry, and fit absolutely flush. The glue dries in seconds, so no special holding device is necessary. Once bonded, it holds extremely well, although the permanency of the bond over a long period of time is unpredictable.

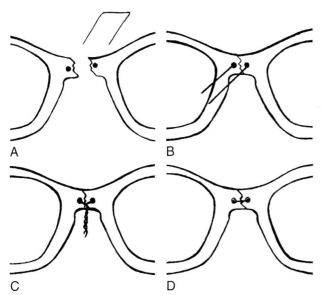

Figure 10-62. A-D, One functional (but unsightly) method of repairing a broken bridge with a wire brace.

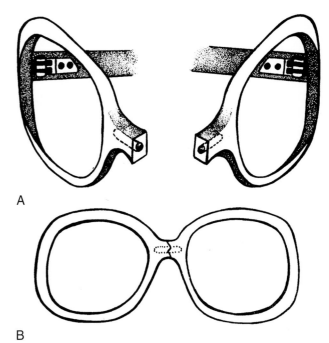

Figure 10-63. A, To repair the bridge, holes are drilled into the broken parts of the bridge parallel to the frame front. **B,** Glue is applied to both halves, and a thin wire (such as a piece of the stiff wire reinforcement used in frame temples) is inserted into the broken parts. The parts are pressed together.

Extreme caution is required to prevent contact with the eyes and to guard against inadvertently gluing the fingers together because these glues bond skin instantly on contact. If this occurs, no attempt should be made to pull the skin apart. There is a debonder made for super glue (also available from Vigor) that is useful. It will clean a broken surface before an application of instant cement, "unglue" a previous repair, clean up excess glue, or unglue fingers. If no debonder is available, glued fingers may be soaked in acetone or nail polish remover.

Note: Individuals with broken frames may order a new pair of glasses, but request that their old frame be repaired temporarily. It may be prudent to require a deposit for the new glasses. With the repaired frame they are no longer in crisis and may not pick up and pay for the new pair.

Wire Braces

Several methods of repairing a broken bridge use wires as braces. The most common method entails drilling holes in each portion of the broken bridge and inserting a thin wire through the holes to hold the two parts together, either using the wire alone or in conjunction with a glue or cement material. An alternate method pushes the wire brace directly into the plastic.

The plastic is best drilled by using a small drill bit in either a hand or variable-speed drill; a high-speed electric drill tends to melt the plastic.

Twisted Wire. Drill a hole *perpendicular* to the frame front in each broken half of the bridge. Cut a U-shaped piece of a wire brace or paper clip and insert one end through each hole (Figure 10-62, *A* and *B*). Twist the protruding portions of the clip about each other with small pliers until the bridge is held securely together (Figure 10-62, *C*). Clip away the excess wire and file the sharp edges smooth (Figure 10-62, *D*).

This method works best when used in combination with glue, acetone, or epoxy resin.

Imbedded Core Wire. A hole is drilled into the center of each half of the broken surface *parallel* to the frame front (Figure 10-63, *A*). The two halves of the bridge are pushed together over a small, thin, stiff piece of wire reinforcement, such as is used in frame temples. The holes should have the same diameter as the wire (Figure 10-63, *B*).

This method works best when used in combination with glue or epoxy resin.

Stainless Steel Screws and Super Glue.* An improved version of the imbedded core wire that was shown in Figure 10-63 is accomplished with stainless steel screws and super glue.

Using a 0.0430 (No. 57) drill bit, drill two holes into one broken end of the bridge. Next, screw a 1.4-mm diameter stainless steel screw into each hole, but not all the way in. Leave enough of the screw sticking out so that the screw head can be clipped off and still have 3 to 4 mm of threaded screw sticking out. With the screws securely in the drilled half of the bridge, clip the end off so that 3 to 4 mm of the screws are left protruding.

---

*Thanks to Robert Woyton of Hilco, A Division of the Hilsinger Corp., Plainville, Mass., for suggesting this method.

In the other broken half of the bridge, drill two holes in as close to the same location as possible, using a slightly larger drill bit. Try to put the two pieces together to see if they will fit correctly. It may be necessary to open up the holes slightly larger to ensure a flush, even fit.

When everything fits properly, put a couple of drops of super glue on the screw threads and press the two halves together. The bridge should be allowed to dry overnight before the frame is used.

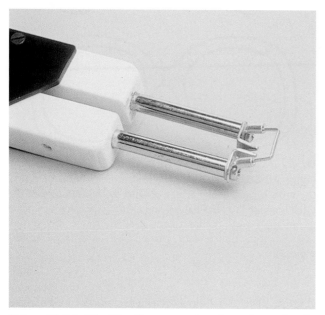

Figure 10-64. The Hot Fingers repair unit can be used to fix a broken bridge with a commercial grade ¼-inch staple. The staple is grasped securely with the staple adapter. (Courtesy Hilco, Plainville, Mass.)

Imbedding Staples Using the Hot Fingers Unit. One effective method uses the Hilco Hot Fingers unit to repair a broken bridge. (For more information on Hot Fingers, see the section on how to repair hidden hinges earlier in this chapter.)

To repair a bridge using the Hot Fingers unit, first repair the break using glue. The Hot Fingers unit has a staple adapter that allows for easy insertion of a ¼-inch industrial staple. Place the staple ends into the adapter holes (Figure 10-64). Depress the foot pedal to heat the staple. Because the staple is thin, it will heat quickly. Slowly and firmly press the staple into the back of the frame bridge so that one staple leg is on either side of the break (Figure 10-65). Do not stop pressing the staple into the frame when the staple top is flush with the surface of the frame bridge. Instead, keep pressing the staple into the bridge. The staple should be imbedded approximately halfway through the thickness of the bridge. This will give extra stability to the broken area and hide the staple somewhat better.

Once the correct depth is achieved, take your foot off the foot pedal and hold the staple in place approximately 10 seconds. Next, cool the bridge area in water and clip off the protruding ends of the staple. The ends should be filed smooth. If the design of the bridge allows, a second staple can be inserted through the top of the bridge for added stability (Figure 10-66).

Replacing Nosepads on Plastic Frames
Replacing Broken-Off Plastic Pads
Though less common, some plastic frames have distinct, plastic nosepads that are attached to the frame. (An example may be seen in Chapter 1, Figure 1-14.) If a

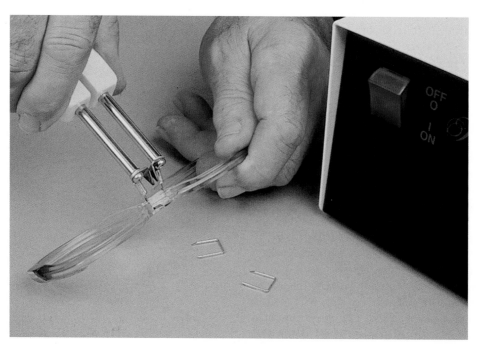

Figure 10-65. Placing the staple on the intended spot, the heat is turned on and the staple pressed into position. (Courtesy Hilco, Plainville, Mass.)

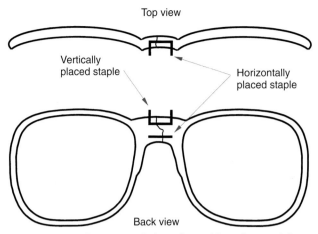

Figure 10-66. Recommended staple positions for repairing a plastic bridge. It is possible to repair a plastic bridge with only one staple. However, whenever possible a second stable should be imbedded into the plastic. Afterwards the ends are clipped off using cutting pliers and then filed smooth.

TABLE 10-2
How to Orient Wedge-Shaped Build-Up Pads for the Best Fit

Desired Effect	Recommended Action
Increase frontal angle	Orient pad with thick part up
Decrease frontal angle	Orient pad with thick part down
Increase splay angle	Orient pad with thick edge forward
Decrease splay angle	Orient pad with thick edge toward back of frame
Narrow bridge without changing angles	Use uniform thickness stick-on or press-on pads

Note: Adding pads directly to a plastic bridge will always have the effect of narrowing the bridge.

plastic nosepad of this type breaks off the bridge, it can readily be replaced by simply cementing a replacement pad to the area that held the original pad. Either plastic cement or acetone is used.

To begin the replacement, file the residue of the original nosepad off the frame and smooth the area with fine sandpaper. File a clear plastic replacement nosepad of the proper size at its contact edge. File the edge to the angle that will allow the pad surface to fit the nose correctly. When properly filed, the replacement pad should display the proper splay angle when attached to the frame.

Apply plastic cement or acetone to the area of the frame that will receive the pad and also to the contact edge of the pad until that edge softens. Press the two edges together at the proper splay angle.

After the joint dries, acetone is applied to smooth the nasal surface. For the best results, apply the acetone in combination with a drop of household oil using a cotton swab. The application should be done using small, quick strokes, all in the same direction. Strokes made in varying directions may ball the plastic or imprint the surface.

Adding Cement or Stick-On Pads to a Plastic Bridge

It is possible to modify the shape and "width" of a plastic frame bridge to fit an especially narrow or unusual nose by using cement, stick-on, or otherwise mounted pads (see Chapter 9, Figure 9-64). They can be used to narrow the fit of the bridge or change the frontal and splay angles.

These pads are attached to the area of the frame that would normally rest on the nose and are secured in place with acetone or an adhesive. (Pads being added to Optyl frames are fastened in place with an epoxy resin.)

Such pads come in varying thickness. Some are uniformly thick and others are thicker at the "top" than the

"bottom" and at the "front" than at the "back." Such wedge-shaped pads can be used to change both frontal and splay angles. Therefore how the pads are applied will determine how well the finished product fits. (See Table 10-2 for how to apply such pads.)

If the fit of the bridge needs to be further modified with the new build-up pads in place, acetate pads can be filed to the right shape after they are dry.

Applying Silicone or Acetate Press-On Pads Directly to a Plastic Frame Bridge

If a frame slips or is uncomfortable on the nose, it may be advisable to apply silicone nosepads directly to the frame bridge area. Acetate or silicone pads can be used to build up the frame bridge area to narrow the bridge or change the way the bridge fits. It is possible to purchase a whole kit (Figure 10-67) or pads only.

To put these pads on the frame, use the marking template that comes with the kit. Mark the bridge area where the pads will rest (Figure 10-68, *A*). Next, drill holes where the bridge is marked (Figure 10-68, *B*). The pad comes with two protrusions. These protrusions are pressed into the drilled holes (Figure 10-68, *C*). When finished the pad sits flush with the frame bridge.

Remember, since these added pads have thickness they will cause an effective narrowing of the bridge. How much the bridge is narrowed depends upon the thickness of the pad chosen. Decreasing the distance between pads will raise the frame on the face and increase the vertex distance slightly.

"Retrofitting" Plastic Frames With Adjustable Nosepads

It is possible to put a pair of adjustable nosepads on a plastic frame if there is a sufficient thickness of plastic in the nasal area of the frame. The pad arms come individually or linked together as a pair. Both kinds are shown in Figure 10-69. The single pad arms are available in either low- or high-mount designs. The design chosen depends upon the thickness of the bridge of the plastic

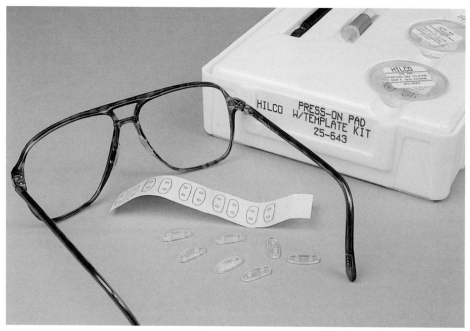

Figure 10-67. Here are the necessary items for mounting press-on build-up pads to a plastic frame. All items are available as a kit. Pads are available in either acetate (regular hard plastic) or silicone (pliable, slip-resistant material). (Courtesy Hilco, Plainville, Mass.)

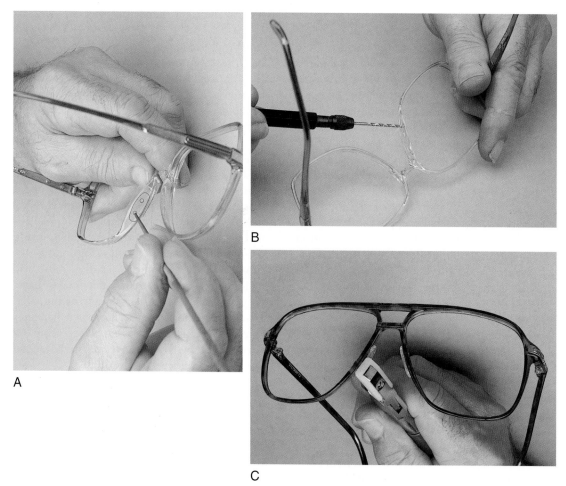

Figure 10-68. A, Either a measuring gauge or clear templates can be used to determine where the bridge area should be drilled. Here the template allows for exact premarking. **B,** A drill bit mounted in a chuck handle is used to bore out the needed holes for a replacement press-on pad. **C,** The protrusions on the backs of the press-on pads are squeezed into the drilled holes, mounting them firmly to the bridge. (Courtesy Hilco, Plainville, Mass.)

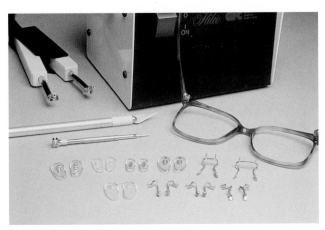

Figure 10-69. Adjustable pads may be added to a plastic frame if the frame has sufficient thickness in the area where the pad arms are to be mounted. Because of design variety in pad arms, chances of finding a suitable match are good. Here are some of the pad arms and pads available, along with tools that are used in mounting. (Courtesy Hilco, Plainville, Mass.)

frame. There must be a sufficient depth of plastic so that the prongs on the pad arms will not hit the lens bevel or go all the way through the plastic. If the frame does not have enough thickness on the rim, then a one-piece bridge can be mounted on the cross portion of the frame bridge. Here is the sequence for mounting the pad arms:

1. First, decide which pad arms are most appropriate.
2. Next, file the existing plastic pads off the frame and smooth the filed area (Figure 10-70, *A*). Even though this area of the frame may not be visible when worn, it may be advisable to buff the area with a buffing wheel and polishing compound to restore the finish.
3. To be certain of getting both pad arms symmetrically placed (or a one-piece bridge properly centered, if this is being done), mark the proposed location of the prongs (Figure 10-70, *B*). Use a template, if provided.
4. Mount the pad arms by either drilling holes in the frame or heating the pad arm and pressing it in place using the Hot Fingers unit. (If the Hot Fingers unit is not available, it is possible to purchase a "Pad Arm Conversion Kit" that contains a small hand drill from Hilco, Plainville, Mass.) Drill the holes and press the pad arm into place.
   a. If the Hot Fingers unit is used, grasp the bridge or individual pad arm using the Hot Fingers tool with the prongs positioned at the previously marked location (Figure 10-70, *C*).
   b. Turn the heat on with the foot switch.
   c. Press the pad arm slowly into the plastic until it is fully seated.
   d. Release the foot switch first, then the pad arm.
   e. Immerse the frame in cold water and check for tightness.

f. It may be necessary to use a razor blade or small surgical knife to cut away excess plastic from around the point of attachment (Figure 10-70, *D*).
5. Last, attach the pads to the pad arms.

NOTE: All of these services are available through Hilco's repair center and through many local laboratories if the dispenser is uncomfortable with attempting them alone.

THE EYEWIRE AND LENS

Attempts to repair a broken plastic eyewire are often unsuccessful since the strain of the lens on such a small area tends to rebreak the repair when the frame is repeatedly taken off and put back on. Some forms of eyewire repair can be attempted in emergencies when it would be extremely difficult for the wearer to do without the glasses.

Repairs to the eyewire that do not relate to an actual break in the eyewire are generally more successful. These procedures concern the fit of the lens in the eyewire of the frame.

Broken Eyewires

The simplest approach is to attempt to repair the eyewire using the methods described for repairing the bridge of a plastic frame—with epoxy and fast-drying glues being the most successful.

The most difficult part of repairing an eyewire is reinserting the lens without rebreaking the frame. Only that portion of the eyewire that is still intact should be heated.

If the repair is to be temporary, it is best to attempt doing the repair with the lens in place.

If all else fails, encircling the lens itself with glue and cementing the frame to the lens provides a temporary means of holding the lens in the frame. This avoids both the necessity of reinserting the lens and of attempting to stretch the frame to encircle the lens.

Epoxy or other glues of that type should not be used; if it will eventually be necessary to remove the lens, scrape off the glue and reinsert the lens in a new frame. Acetone should not be used because it will not adhere to lenses and will damage a polycarbonate lens. An inexpensive model airplane type of glue works best.

Lower Edge Appears Out of the Frame

If the lenses have been inserted unsatisfactorily, particularly in a plastic frame, either the lower or upper portion of the lens may not fit properly in the eyewire and may give the impression that the lens is about to fall out of the frame.

If the lower eyewire of a *plastic frame* has been "rolled" during lens insertion, the lower edge of the lens will appear to be out of the frame. This condition can readily be noted by observing the frame from the side (Figure 10-71).

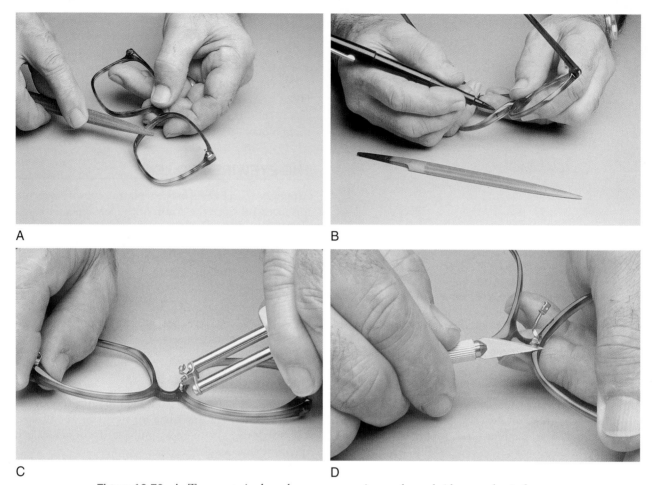

Figure 10-70. A, To mount single pad arms or one-piece pad-arm bridges to plastic frames, begin by filing off any existing plastic pads and file or buff the area clean. **B,** The next step in mounting pad arms to a plastic frame is to mark the proper position for the insertion. **C,** To mount the adjustable arm in the plastic frame, pick up the pad arm with the Hot Fingers tool. Carefully place the pad-arm anchor on the position marks. Firmly, but slowly, let the heated pad arm seat itself in the frame. Release the foot pedal, then the pad arm. Cool the frame in water and check the implant. **D,** After the pad arm has been securely mounted in the plastic frame, trim away any excess plastic with a razor blade or knife. (Courtesy Hilco, Plainville, Mass.)

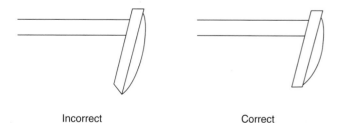

Incorrect   Correct

Figure 10-71. Observing the frame from the side for a lower eyewire that has been "rolled" during lens insertion.

To remedy this situation, remove the lens and reheat the lower portion of the frame. Grasp the eyewire between thumb and forefinger and rotate it back until the bevel again faces directly upward. Shield the fingers, if necessary, with a towel or other protective padding. The eyewire may have to be reheated and turned several times until it is completely aligned. When the eyewire is straight and the bevel directly vertical, the lens is reinserted, taking care not to roll the eyewire again. It might be helpful to insert the lens from the back of the frame if the eyewire was rolled forward if an attempt to put the lens in from the front continues to result in a rolled eyewire.

If the lower edge of a lens in a *metal frame* appears to be out of the frame, the eyewire has not been properly shaped to follow the curvature of the lens edge.

To correct this problem, remove the screw holding the eyewire. Hold the eyewire around the lens so that the bevel of the lens completely fits the groove of the eyewire. Then reinsert the screw. It may be necessary to prebend the eyewire to match the lower curve of the lens edge while the lens is out. This may be done with the fingers or with eyewire shaping pliers. (See Chapter 7.)

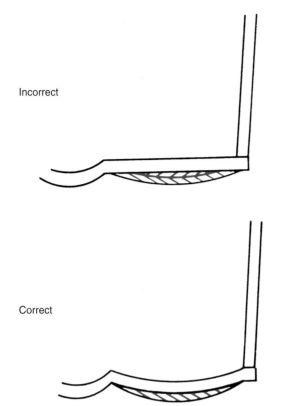

Incorrect

Correct

Figure 10-72. An exposed upper bevel gives an unsightly appearance, but is readily correctable.

Upper Edge Appears Out of the Frame

If the bevel of the lens is excessively visible from the top, the frame probably does not conform to the curvature of the top of the lens (Figure 10-72). This situation is more likely to appear at the top than at the bottom of the eyewire because most lens shapes have a longer, straighter top. The curved front of the lens is more evident at the top, and the frame may not follow the curve as well. This is especially evident with high plus-powered lenses.

With a *plastic frame*, it is sometimes possible to heat the plastic without removing the lens. Pull the eyewire over the bevel, and *while holding it there*, dip the lens and frame into cold water to fix the position.

If this cannot be done, the lens should be removed, the eyewire heated and reshaped to match the lens curvature, and the lens then reinserted.

When the upper bevel of a lens in a *metal frame* sticks out, the lens must be removed, and the eyewire reshaped. The methodology is the same as described in the previous section on reshaping the lower eyewire.

When the Lens Is Too Small for a Plastic Frame

If a lens which fits too loosely has been inserted into a plastic frame, it may rattle or rotate within the frame. When the frame appears to be too large for the lens, the lens must be remounted so it is secure.

Overall looseness is corrected in cellulose acetate and propionate plastic frames by removing the lenses and shrinking the eyewire size by heating and chilling as described in Chapter 7. The process is repeated several times, if necessary. When the eyewire reaches a size that is slightly too small to accept the lens, the frame is again reheated, and the lens is inserted. After the lens has been inserted, immediate chilling of both lens and frame should secure the lens. (For how to "shrink" frames made from other materials, see Chapter 7.)

Occasionally the lens appears secure, but a small gap or space is visible between the lens and the frame. The area standing away from the lens is heated and compressed against the lens bevel. Holding the plastic against the lens while immersing the frame and the lens into very cold water will further shrink the frame around the lens and secure the corrected position of the rim.

Sometimes a lens interliner is used with plastic frames, even though it is intended primarily for metal frames. This is explained in the section below under metal frames.

When the Lens Is Too Small for a Metal Frame

When a lens is loose in a metal frame, the most probable cause is that the screw holding the eyewire together has loosened. As an automatic first measure, check the screw and, if loose, tighten it.

If tightening the screw does not accomplish the desired result, it is probable that the lens has been cut and finished with a circumference slightly too small to firmly fit the eyewire. For a new prescription, this is a quality control issue. The glasses should be returned to the laboratory to be redone. However, if the problem is with an old prescription, there are ways to make the lenses fit better.

Acetate Lens Interliner (Lens Washer)

One method of correcting the problem is to loosen the screw and insert a plastic (acetate) lens liner, commonly referred to as a *lens washer*, in the bevel between the lens and the eyewire. This more common, nonadhesive form of lens liner comes in different thicknesses, is bevel shaped on the outside to fit the eyewire, and contains a bevel on the inside to hold the lens. It is sold in a roll and may be cut to any desired length.

When using acetate liner, it is best to use the 0.010 mm interliner size. It is far less obtrusive than the 0.020 mm interliner. Here are three ways to keep the liner in place while inserting the lens. The first is the currently recommended method:

1. Use a very small amount of super glue to hold the acetate interliner in place. To apply the glue, place a drop on some scrap paper and slide the back side of the interliner through the glue (Figure 10-73). Hold the interliner in the eyewire groove for 20 seconds, and it should stick.

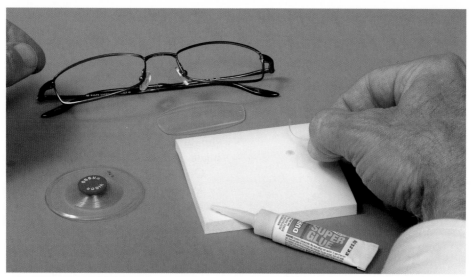

Figure 10-73. To hold acetate interliner in place in the groove while reinserting the lens, drag the outside of the interliner through a drop of super glue.

2. Soak the liner in acetone. When the liner is soft and sticky; place it directly in the bevel of the frame. It will stick in the groove, and the lens can easily be inserted.
3. Tape the liner to the lens with transparent tape and insert the lens in the frame with the tape still in place. When the lens is securely positioned, cut the tape away using a razor or exacto-type knife.

Double-Sided Adhesive

Another form of liner is a double-sided, clear plastic tape. This tape is thin and hence inappropriate when the amount of looseness is considerable. It is much easier to use than the beveled liner, however, because it can be stuck directly to the lens bevel.

If the lens is extremely small for the eyewire and a sufficient amount of room is present, first apply the double-sided adhesive liner to the lens bevel, then fasten the thicker, beveled liner to the double-sided liner. This arrangement provides added bulk and simplifies the task by holding the thicker liner in position.

Latex Liquid Interliner

Instead of using conventional lens liner, there is a liquid liner that can be applied (Figure 10-74). It is dispensed right from the bottle into the "V groove" in the frames' eyewire and can be applied to the entire inside portion of the eyewear, if necessary. Liquid liner dries in about 1 minute and can be used in almost any situation where acetate liner would is used. It may be necessary to use more than one application, depending upon how loose the lens is.

There is one word of caution. Some people are allergic to latex. It should not be used for such individuals.

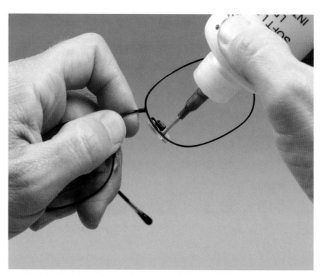

Figure 10-74. Soft Latex Lens Interliner is a liquid latex material that can be applied directly from the bottle to the groove of the frame. It dries is about a minute and, when done properly, is not visible when the glasses are being worn.

Gap or Air Space

If a gap or air space appears in a metal frame between the lens and the eyewire, place a strip of liner between the lens and the eyewire directly *opposite* the gap to force the lens into the gap (Figure 10-75).

A gap is totally unsatisfactory for a new lens. Such repairs should only be used if the glasses were not initially supplied by you. Inform the wearer that although the repair is less than satisfactory, it is the best that can be done without replacing the lenses.

Because of the shape of most lenses, any sizable amount of liner will be far more obvious when placed along the upper bevel of the lens than when used to fill

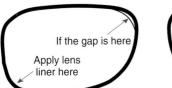
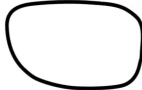

Figure 10-75. To fill an "air hole" between the lens edge and the frame, lens liner is applied in the area *opposite* the position of the gap.

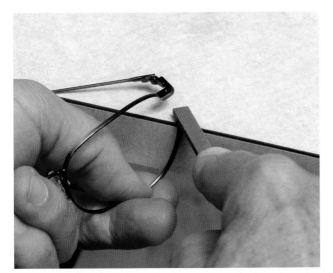

Figure 10-76. Care is taken to file evenly so the barrel section will continue to fit flush as before.

the lower bevel. Consequently, from a cosmetic standpoint, it is less noticeable to place the liner in the lower bevel when only a short strip is necessary.

Any of the previously listed procedures may be used as a temporary measure while a new lens of proper dimensions is made.

Lens Slightly Loose

If the lens is only slightly loose in the frame, reduce the circumference of the metal eyewire itself by removing the eyewire screw and filing the barrel surface. The filing must be done evenly so the barrel sections continue to fit flush (Figure 10-76). This is only possible on barrels that come together flat and not on barrels that have a wedge-shaped abutment (Figure 10-77).

(It is preferable to file the nonthreaded portion of the barrel rather than the side that accepts the tip of the screw.)

The disadvantage of filing is that if the lenses are later changed and the same frame used, the new lenses could appear to be slightly too large for the eyewire, even if actually ground to the original size.

FRAME TRIM

Trim on frames goes in and out of style. Not all trim is attached in just the same way. This section addresses some of the methods for replacing or repairing trim.

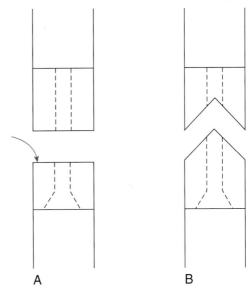

A   B

Figure 10-77. Reducing the circumference of the metal eyewire in the case of a loose lens by filing the barrel is only feasible on type **A**. The surface indicated by the arrow has been filed. Type **B** does not lend itself as readily to filing.

Trim On Plastic Frames

When a plastic frame adorned with metal trim breaks, the plastic chassis can be replaced and the original trim reapplied to the new chassis. The trim is usually attached by screws through holes in the chassis. These screws may have fancy heads that hold the trim or may be part of the trim itself. The screws are fastened in back of the chassis with hex nuts.

To reapply trim, begin by removing the hex nuts and forcing the trim off the old frame by inserting a screwdriver blade between the trim and frame near the screws by pushing on the protruding screws, or both.

Align the trim with the holes in the new chassis and push new screws (where separate) through the trim and the frame with the thumb. Tighten new hex nuts with their rounded surface inside the barrel of the hex wrench onto the ends of the screws (Figure 10-78). The nuts must fit precisely into the wrench and can sometimes be picked up and held in place more easily if the tip of the wrench is moistened as with saliva.

Cut off the excess screw flush with the surface of the nut (Figure 10-79) and file the end smooth with a small, curved, spoon-shaped riffler file (Figure 10-80). If the end is not filed smooth, the rough edges may catch in the patient's brows or prove otherwise irritating.

After the trim has been attached, heat the eyewire and the lens. Apply most of the heat to the portion of the eyewire not covered by trim (usually the lower portion) since heating and stretching the covered portion may raise it above the trim and result in an unsightly appearance. A metal plaque may need to be shielded while heating the frame since it usually becomes too hot to touch.

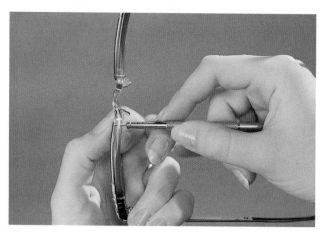

Figure 10-78. Attaching the hex nut to the screw that secures the metal trim to the plastic chassis.

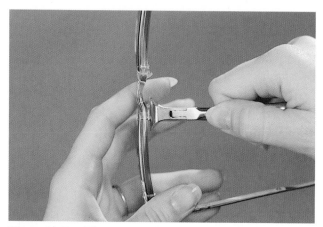

Figure 10-79. The screw is clipped off close since any portion left protruding must be filed.

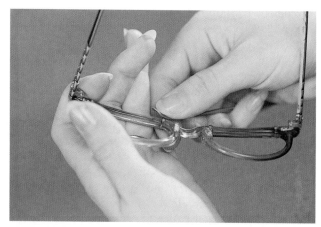

Figure 10-80. The rough end of the clipped-off screw is filed smooth with a riffler file.

Although it may appear easier, inserting the lens before attaching the plaques may stretch the upper part of the eyewire. As a result, the predrilled holes in the chassis separate slightly so that the screws that pass through the plaque no longer pass through the holes in the chassis. In this event, drill one or more new holes to reattach the plaque.

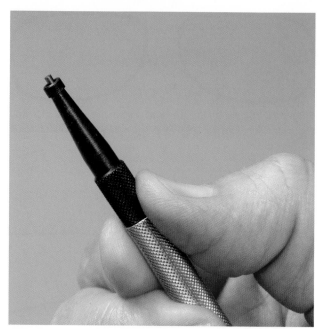

Figure 10-81. This hex wrench has a knock-out pin that ejects a stuck hex nut from the end of a hex wrench.

It is possible that the plastic of the chassis will stretch and become too thin to allow the drilling of such holes. It is also conceivable that the original hole could be moved so far by the stretching process that it would no longer be fully covered by the trim. Even if neither of these situations occurs, the cosmetic effect may be out of balance since one eyewire may stretch somewhat differently from the other.

A Note on Hex Wrenches

Those who have worked with small hex nuts and the optical hex wrench will know that sooner or later a removed hex nut will become lodged in the socket of the wrench and momentarily defy removal. Using a hex wrench with a Teflon-coated socket will help. It should also be noted that there is an optical hex wrench available with a knock-out pin. The pin easily ejects the hex nut from the wrench tip (Figure 10-81).

Metal Plaques on a Metal Chassis

One type of metal frame consists of a metal chassis with a narrow eyewire. Broad plaques are joined to the chassis at the brow area, much like a combination frame. These plaques also contain the endpiece hinges for the temple. They fit over and enclose the upper eyewire of the metal chassis by means of a small, specially-designed screw and a slot attachment.

Frequently, these screws become loose or fall out, causing the frame to disassemble. The size and thread of these screws are of special dimensions. When the screw has simply turned until it has fallen out and the threads in the eyewire are intact, the screw can simply be replaced.

Sometimes this proves difficult to do with the lenses in since the plaques fit at one end in a slot in the chassis with the screw at the other end. If the hole in the plaque does not line up exactly over the hole in the eyewire when the eyewire slot is fitted into the catch in the plaque, there is no alternative but to remove the lens and force the eyewire to line up with the plaque.

It is possible that a new screw will not hold because the threads in the eyewire have been ruined by constant retightening of the screw. In such cases, the plaque must be removed and a larger hole threaded with a tap that is equivalent in diameter to a glass screw. The plaque is replaced (without the lens if necessary, as above) and fastened securely with a glass screw clipped to the length necessary to fit the eyewire thickness.

CLEANING THE FRAME

From time to time, because of repair work or just because of normal wear, frames need to be cleaned. Also, on occasion the action of chemicals in perspiration, the use of tools on the plastic, or the circumstances of overheating a plastic frame, may result in discoloration, blemishes, or marks in or on the plastic. In these instances, the defects need to be removed if the frames are in excellent operational order otherwise.

Cleaning Technique

Frames may be cleaned with ordinary soap and water so long as the soap contains no abrasive pumice material. An old toothbrush serves best for scrubbing hard-to-reach areas, such as the pad arms or trim.

An ultrasonic cleaning unit is a most useful cleaning instrument. Leaving the frame (lens side up) in the small tank loosens dirt that might not otherwise be dislodged. After cleaning a frame in such a unit, be sure to check all screws for tightness since the vibrations tend to loosen them.

The following two types of spectacles should not be cleaned in an ultrasonic unit:
1. Glasses whose lenses are held in place by screws passing through the lenses, such as rimless or semirimless. The intense vibrations of the ultrasonic unit may cause lens breakage.
2. Frames with glued-in rhinestones or other small jewels should not be cleaned ultrasonically because the stones may be dislodged.

It is not advisable to clean antireflection (AR) coated lenses in an ultrasonic unit.

Discoloration

Discoloration usually occurs on the inside of the temples of plastic frames where they contact the hair and the skin and most often appears as a whitish film. With age, cellulose acetate and propionate frames may exhibit a film, which is caused by plasticizers within the material migrating to the surface.[5] In either case, a buffing wheel used with polishing compound will remove the discoloration and will also repolish the plastic.

When a buffing wheel is not available, apply acetone and oil with a cotton-tipped applicator and rub over the entire length of the temple. Dip the applicator in the mixture and run the length of the temple in one direction. Each time the temple is brushed it should be with fresh acetone and oil and in the same direction. Repeat this process as often as necessary until the color is restored. If acetone without oil is used, the brushing action must be rapid to avoid leaving prints in the softened surface. If the wet surface is blown on or exposed to moving air, condensation may again whiten the temple.

Surface Marked by Pliers

If the plastic has been marked by the jaws of pliers, an attempt to restore the surface can be made. Heating the frame at the area of the mark will hopefully cause the compressed portion to expand back to its original dimensions. The area can be reheated repeatedly as long as the plastic is not overheated until it bubbles because this would compound the problem. When it appears that the frame has reexpanded as far as is likely, the area is buffed with buffing compound on a rag wheel.

Restoring Finish on Optyl Frames

The finish of an Optyl frame can be damaged if the frame is inadvertently rubbed against a rough surface. If the frame surface has been marred, remove the defect by buffing the area.

To restore the sheen after buffing, coat the area with polyurethane finish, such as is used in furniture refinishing. Either satin or glossy polyurethane will prove satisfactory.

Bubbles

Bubbles result from overheating the plastic and cannot actually be removed because they ordinarily extend well into the plastic.

An attempt to salvage the aesthetic appearance of the frame can be made, however, by filing the bubbled area smooth and then buffing it to restore the luster.

If the frame looks asymmetric as a result of the one area having obviously been thinned, the mirror portion of the frame is also filed and buffed to match.

SOLDERING

Soldering is the only possible way to repair a broken metal portion of a frame unless the entire front or temple is replaced. The techniques used for soldering spectacles are similar to those used for soldering jewelry and are sometimes performed by jewelers.

Most people hesitate to solder in the office because of the amount of time involved, but since the time involved is still less than would be required to send the frame back

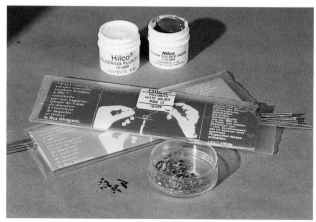

Figure 10-82. Solder comes in a variety of forms and must be used in conjunction with *soldering flux*. Flux is shown in the upper left-hand container. There is a *silver solder paste* that combines both solder and flux. This is seen in the upper right-hand container. Solder is available in *rod form*, as pictured in the plastic envelope in the center of the photo. The *chip form* of solder, at the bottom of the photo, is particularly useful for electric soldering. (Courtesy Hilco, Plainville, Mass.)

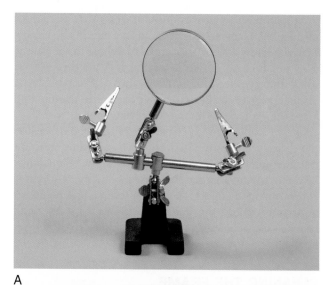

A

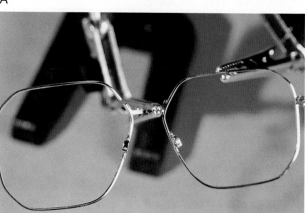

B

Figure 10-83. A, Here is a jig or "third hand" is used to hold the frame in place while soldering. **B,** The jig holds the frame in place during soldering.

to the laboratory or elsewhere for repairs, soldering sometimes provides a definite service to the wearer. It also sets the office apart from others and provides another unique service.

It is a poor risk to solder frames of inferior quality since they tend to come apart at their points of assembly when the frames are heated during the soldering process. It is also difficult to solder metal eyewires because the solder tends to fill the bevel groove into which the lens must fit.

Special solder must be used because of the metals and alloys used to make frames. Only a high quality solder of the type designed for jewelry or frames can be used; normal electrical solder will not work.

Hard solder is available in chip form (to be mixed with liquid or paste flux), paste form (with the flux already mixed in), or rod form (Figure 10-82). Hilco offers a rod form solder called "Pallarium." It melts at a temperature of 1060° F. This temperature may seem high, but compared with other solder melting temperatures is considered very low. Pallarium is a hollow rod with flux running through the center for ease of application. Because it melts at such a low temperature, when used properly it minimizes discoloration of frame components.

It should be noted that titanium frame materials cannot be soldered through conventional frame repair techniques. It is possible to solder the top plating together, but such a repair is usually not strong enough to withstand much use.

Titanium can only be repaired by laser or induction welding machines. It is a very sophisticated process that is dependent on the grade of titanium being welded. The welding process must also be performed in an inert atmosphere, usually an enclosed chamber, to successfully bond the material.

Flame Soldering

Some flame soldering units use one gas, butane. Others use two independently regulated gases, either oxygen and acetylene or oxygen and butane. The oxygen will be used up at twice the rate of either the acetylene or the butane. The single gas unit is less cumbersome to operate. It is recommended when soldering is done in small quantities or only irregularly.

To flame solder, remove the lenses from the frame; if the soldering is to be done near the bridge, remove the nosepads too. If the frame is bent, readjust it before attempting to solder it.

One of the most important aspects of soldering is the proper positioning of the parts. Use a special jig, or "third hand," that consists of adjustable clips mounted on a base to hold the frame in place while soldering (Figure 10-83).

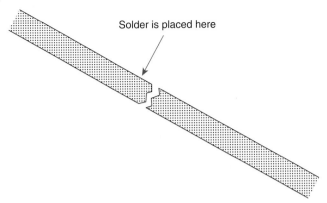

Figure 10-84. The part to be soldered is aligned at somewhat of a slant so that solder will flow over the broken part.

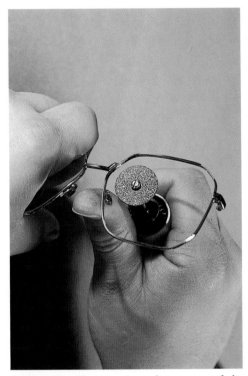

Figure 10-85. If solder gets into the groove of the frame, it must be removed with a grinding disk. (Courtesy Hilco, Plainville, Mass.)

Position the well-cleaned part to be soldered at somewhat of a slant so that the solder, placed slightly above the broken area, will flow downward over the broken part (Figure 10-84). To solder an eyewire, mount the frame so that the broken section is held vertically. This permits the solder, placed on the outside of the bend, to flow down over the break. Place solder *only on the outside of an eyewire*. If solder should get on the inside of the eyewire, it must be removed. This can be done by mounting a separating disk or cutting wheel to a hanging motor tool or hand Dremel to grind away any excess solder (Figure 10-85).

Attach a metal alligator clip to the frame between the solder joint and the next adjacent joint in the frame to

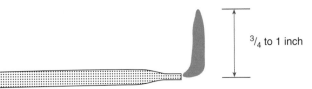

Figure 10-86. When flame soldering with a two-gas system, before the oxygen is turned on, the butane or acetylene flame is regulated to its proper length.

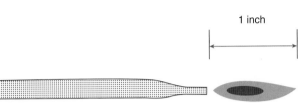

Figure 10-87. For two-gas flame soldering, the oxygen is turned on after the butane or acetylene has been regulated. Oxygen is modified until the total flame is 1 inch long and has a dark blue center.

act as a heat sink and to help absorb the heat. If a great quantity of heat is conducted along the metal to an adjacent joint of the frame, it may loosen the solder of that joint and dismember the frame. The heat sink absorbs the heat before it reaches the area of concern. A commercially available foam to coat the adjacent areas may be used instead.

Place flux on the area to be soldered before applying heat to prevent oxidation and to aid the flow of the solder.

Start the soldering flame by turning on the butane and lighting the torch. If the unit uses two gases, adjust the butane flame to a length of 0.75 to 1.0 inch (Figure 10-86). Then turn on the oxygen and regulate it until the total flame is 1 inch long and reveals a dark blue center (Figure 10-87).

The hottest part of the flame is the tip of the blue center portion, which is applied to the area to be soldered until that area is red hot. Apply solder to the break or slightly above it and remove the heat as soon as the solder flows over the break. If the flame is applied for too long, the solder will melt and finally oxidize away, negating the repair. If the solder does not flow but balls up at the end of the soldering wire, the frame is not hot enough.

Turn off the unit immediately after use. To be sure it is off, since the gases are invisible, immerse the tip of the torch in water so that any escaping gas can be detected.

Electric Soldering

An electric soldering technique to repair frames is preferred by some. Either flame or electricity can produce excellent results, with personal preference and experience the basis for choice.

As with flame soldering, a strong bond requires that the area be brushed clean. After cleaning adjust the

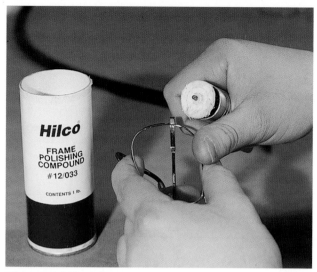

Figure 10-88. Frames are buffed after soldering to remove foreign matter and discoloration. The tiny rag wheel is mounted on a Dremel tool or a hanging motor drill. (Courtesy Hilco, Plainville, Mass.)

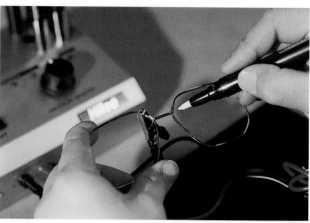

Figure 10-89. It is possible to do touch-up replating after soldering. Plating is applied by first attaching the alligator clip as close to the area to be plated as possible. Plating solution is brushed back and forth across the plating area as shown. Then the unit is turned on. (Courtesy Hilco, Plainville, Mass.)

frame so that it is bent like it should be during normal wear. Then remove the lenses. Once again, hold the parts in contact by means of a soldering jig.

Instead of applying solder after the area is hot, place a small clip of solder on the position of the break while the frame is still cold. The area must be prefluxed as when flame soldering.

Clip a wire from the electric soldering unit to the jig. This will allow an electric current to flow a complete circuit through the frame during the actual soldering.

To do the soldering, touch a carbon rod attached to the soldering unit by a second wire to the solder clip. Depress the foot switch to feed an electric current through the system, bonding the break within 1 or 2 seconds. The strength of the current and karat rating of the solder necessary depends on frame thickness.

Discoloration

Gold- and silver-colored frames can be cleaned quite well after soldering by buffing with a rag wheel and polishing compound. The rag wheel can be a large, bench-mounted wheel or a tiny rag wheel mounted on a hand drill, as shown in Figure 10-88. It is possible, however, that some discoloration may still remain. The wearer should be warned of this consequence ahead of time.

Bronze, pewter, and other colored frames will not buff out.

It the wearer wants the frame soldered with no sign of discoloration, the frame can be completely replated with an electroplating unit and the appropriate solutions. This alternative is seldom used, but is available if needed. An electroplating unit can be used to change a silver frame to a gold or a copper color and vice versa.

Touch-Up Plating

Rather than completely replate an entire frame, it is possible to obtain a unit used for touch-up plating to certain areas of a frame. To plate the part of a frame that has been soldered, polish the discolored area. Then place the frame in an ultrasonic unit to remove all polishing compounds and oils that may be present. (If an ultrasonic unit is not available, clean with warm water and a soft cloth.)

Some plating units come with disposable plating pens. Others come with bottles of plating solutions that are applied with a felt tip. There is a variety of plating colors available, including gold, silver, copper, gunmetal, and nickel or palladium.

To apply the plating, attach the alligator clip as close to the area to be plated as possible. Brush the solution back and forth across the plating area, as shown in Figure 10-89. The color obtained in plating depends on the amount of plating material applied. The more the area is brushed with solution, the deeper the color that will result.

If after plating is initiated no color appears, the alligator clip may not have sufficient contact with the metal of the frame. This can be caused by a clear coating that has been applied to the frame during the manufacturing process. To overcome the problem, move the clip onto a polished area so that the plating will take to the frame.

APPENDIX 10-A

The two most common types of nosepads are **Push-On** and **Screw-On** pads. These are presented beginning on page 229 of this chapter and must not be overlooked. The pad styles presented here are lesser-used styles or antique styles. Even antique styles are still available as replacement parts. When individuals bring in a frame

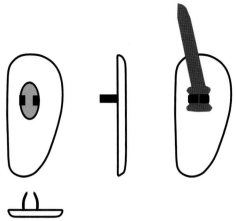

Appendix Figure 10-1. The *clip-on* pad design is also referred to as the *B & L clamp style.*

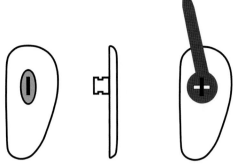

Appendix Figure 10-2. The *twist-on* pad design is sometimes called the *A.O. twist system.*

they want restored to use for their prescription, these pads may need to be replaced.

CLIP-ON

The *clip-on design*, also known as *B & L clamp style*, consists of two curled hooks on the pad, which fit about an indented "waist" in the bearing area of the pad arm (Appendix Figure 10-1). The hooks are passed about this waist and then clamped tight with pliers.

If a broken or corroded pad is to be removed, a special bifurcated tool can be used to separate the hooks to remove them. If this tool is not available, an ordinary optical screwdriver may be used to pry up the hooks by forcing the blade under them. This latter procedure is sometimes difficult to perform, depending on the extent to which the hooks have been compressed and the position of the pad arms in relation to the frame front. It may be more expedient to alter the position of the pad arms so that the hooks can be approached more easily. Care should be taken not to clamp the hooks too tightly. Too tight a clamp totally eliminates the play of the pads at their juncture with the pad arms.

TWIST-ON

One system that twists into place has employed a vertical metal stud that is attached to the pad. This *twist-on method* is sometimes referred to as the *A.O. twist system.* The shaft of the stud itself is indented with two slots that permit it to be inserted, with its long axis horizontal, into a horizontal slot in the pad arm.

When the pad is rotated to a vertical position, the ears on the stud overlap the sides of the slot in the pad arm, preventing the pad from falling off the pad arm (Appendix Figure 10-2). Occasionally, it is necessary to compress the sides of the slots slightly with pliers so that the pad shafts cannot rotate back to a horizontal position.

If a pad is broken, it may be necessary to cut or file away the ears of the stud to remove the old shaft. If the

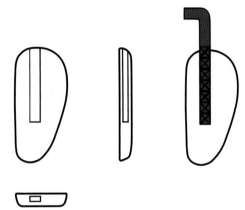

Appendix Figure 10-3. The *Zeiss bayonet* pad design is extremely easy to change and adds the possibility of changing vertex distance and pad separation without moving the basic position of the pad arms.

ears are worn away, the shaft may come out of the slot even though the pads are vertical, in which case an entirely new pad is needed.

ZEISS BAYONET

The *Zeiss bayonet style pad* slips onto a ridged pad arm (Appendix Figure 10-3). It is simple to remove and replace. Some, but not all, types of Zeiss bayonet pads are made so that they will turn around 180 degrees so that they go on either "frontward or backward." When the hole for the pad arm is not exactly centered in reference to the edges of the pad, putting both pads on backward will increase the vertex distance. With some types of Zeiss pads, this is said to change the vertex distance up to 4 mm.

When the hole for the pad arm is not centered in reference to the front and back surfaces of the pad, switching the pads left-for-right and right-for-left will increase the distance between pad surfaces, either making the frame more suitable for a wider nose or causing the frame to sit lower on the face.

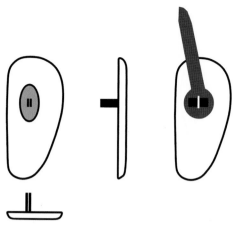

Appendix Figure 10-4. The *split-clamp* pad design is also referred to as the *A.O. split*-type of attachment.

SPLIT-CLAMP

There is a pad with a back that consists of two clasplike pieces of metal, much like the fastener on a large mailing envelope. These two pieces fit through the vertically elongated hole in the pad arm and are spread to hold the frame in place (Appendix Figure 10-4). It is sometimes called the *A.O. split-type* of attachment.

STIRRUP

The *stirrup type* of mechanism consists of a miniature cylinder attached to the back of the pad. (It is similar to the post of the screw-on type pad.) Occasionally the cylinder may have a square or oval cross section rather than a round one.

The pad arm ends in a stirruplike structure that has the "footrest" divided in two. The stirrup is spread apart, using a special tool, a screwdriver blade, or pliers. When half of each stirrup is astride the cylinder, with the ends of the footrest facing the holes, the footrest is then compressed so that each end fits into the corresponding hole.

It is difficult to remove such pads since a special tool is required to spread the stirrup footrest once it has been compressed about a pad. It is possible to remove them using a screwdriver blade, but with more difficulty.

RIVET TYPE

Some older types of pads are attached by means of a loosely fitting rivetlike system that allows rocking of the pads. It is a semipermanent arrangement and cannot be removed unless clipped off. If it becomes necessary to replace this type of pad, the replacement is a split-clamp design and works like the fastener on a large mailing envelope. The replacement pad clips are inserted through this rivet hole in the pad arm and then spread.

REFERENCES

1. Bruneni J, Breheny M: Ask the labs, Eyecare Business, 24, February 2004.
2. Yoho A: Frames: fixing those screwy problems, Eyecare Business, 24-26, July 2000.
3. Hilco 1994 Catalog: Temple tips, Plainville, Mass, Hilco, 2004.
4. Yoho A: Basic repairs, Eyecare Business, *34-36*, May 2005.
5. Fahrner D: Optyl—a new basic material, Norwood, NJ, Optyl Corp.

Proficiency Test

(Answers can be found in the back of the book.)

Screws

If the threads of a barrel are damaged during screw removal:

1. True or false? The hinge must be replaced with a new one.

2. True or false? A self-tapping screw may be used.

3. True or False? Glass screws and hex nuts can be used.

4. True or false? A tap may be used to restore the threads.

For a temple screw that just keeps loosening up, it is possible to:

5. True or false? Seal it in place with a commercially available compound.

6. True or false? File on the head of the screw so it cannot come out.

7. True or false? Hit the tip of the screw with an optician's hammer.

8. When removing a screw that has either broken off or become stuck in the barrel, which of the following possibilities should NOT be used?
   a. File a new slot for the screwdriver in the tip of the remaining portion of a broken screw that protrudes from the barrel and than use a screwdriver to remove that remaining part of the screw.
   b. Soak the endpieces of the plastic frame in acetone and then try to remove the stuck screw with a screwdriver.
   c. Use penetrating oil or an ultrasonic cleaner to loosen the screw and thereafter attempt to remove the stuck screw with a screwdriver.
   d. Use a punch-out pliers to remove the screw.
   e. Drill out the screw.

9. True or false? Self-tapping screws are longer than necessary so that they may be used in frames of different barrel sizes. The extra screw length does not need to be cut with cutting pliers, but simply broken off with any normal thin-nosed pliers that are able to grip the tip of the screw.

10. If a titanium screw starts to bind, what's the best thing to do?
    a. Remove the screw and try again. If this does not work after several tries, use a drop of cutting oil in the barrel.
    b. Remove the screw and try again. If this does not work after several tries, force the screw on in. Titanium is hard enough that it will rethread the barrel itself.

11. When drilling a screw out, from which direction should you drill?
    a. The top (where the head of the screw was or is)
    b. The bottom (where the tip of the screw is)

12. Replacement spring hinge screws:
    a. have hexagonal heads so that it is easier to drive them in.
    b. come with lock nuts so they will not loosen up.
    c. have a tapered tip so they start into the barrels easier.

13. A "top hat bushing" is used with what frame type or frame part?
    a. spring hinges
    b. rimless mountings
    c. combination frame chassis
    d. nylon cord frames
    e. trim on plastic frames

14. True or false? Replacement screws with an epoxy coating on the threads will not back out once they are tightened down. Nor can they ever be removed.

15. What is the most common diameter for optical screws?
    a. 0.5 mm
    b. 0.9 mm
    c. 1.4 mm
    d. 1.7 mm
    e. 2.0 mm

Nosepads

16. Clip-on, screw-on, twist-on, push-on, bayonet, split-clamp, stirrup, and rivet are all terms which apply to:
    a. a type of temple endpiece.
    b. a type of rimless mounting.
    c. a type of nylon cord mounting.
    d. a type of adjustable nosepad.

17. True or false? A frame persists in sliding down the nose even after being properly adjusted for the wearer. If the pads are not silicone, it may be helpful to replace them with silicone pads.

18. What is NOT a possible way to add silicone nosepads to a plastic frame?
    a. Use a silicone pad that has stick-on adhesive.
    b. Drill the nasal area of the frame and press the protrusions of a specially constructed silicone nosepad into the holes.
    c. Mount adjustable pad arms to the frame and put silicone pads on these pad arms.
    d. All of these methods are satisfactory.

19. At the time of this writing, the two most common types of adjustable nosepads are:
    a. push-on and twist-on.
    b. twist-on and screw-on.
    c. rivet and twist-on.
    d. screw-on and bayonet.
    e. screw-on and push-on.

20. What is a good material to use for a nosepad replacement when the wearer is allergic to standard nosepad materials?
    a. nickel
    b. propionate
    c. crystal
    d. acetate

Temples

21. True or false? Some metal temples with plastic coverings over the bent-down portions can be lengthened somewhat by heating and straightening the plastic endpiece, pulling it out the necessary distance, and then rebending it at the proper position.

22. True or false? If a left replacement temple is needed and the only temple available is a right temple, you could try to use the right temple anyway and reverse the direction of the bent-down portion.

23. True or false? It is possible to shorten a metal temple by removing the earpiece, clipping off a piece of the core wire, and putting the earpiece back on again.

Hinges

24. Which tool is used for grasping a shield to pull it out of the frame during hinge repair?
   a. cutting pliers
   b. Numont pliers
   c. half-padded pliers
   d. finger-piece pliers
   e. hollow-snipe pliers

Bridges

25. True or false? There are a number of different ways to repair a broken bridge. However, the best policy is to never attempt to combine two different bridge repair methods.

26. True or false? Without a Hot Fingers unit, it is not possible to mount adjustable pad arms to a plastic frame.

Eyewires

27. When the lens is slightly small for the eyewire of a metal or combination frame, which tool might prove helpful, depending on eyewire closure construction?
   a. optician's hammer
   b. file
   c. half-padded pliers
   d. tap

28. True or false? Marks on a plastic frame made by pliers are never repairable.

29. What could be used to *temporarily* hold a lens in a broken eyewire? (The lens will be reused in a new frame.)
   a. clear nail polish
   b. soldering iron
   c. model airplane glue
   d. lens liner
   e. super glue

30. How can lens liner be made to stay in position while a lens is being reinserted in the frame?
   a. Tape it in place.
   b. Fasten it to the lens with a thin, double-sided material.
   c. Soak it in acetone.
   d. Drag the outside of the liner through a drop of super glue.
   e. All of the above methods may be workable.

31. To eliminate a gap between the lens and a metal eyewire, the best alternative is to:
   a. place a strip of lens liner at a point exactly opposite the gap.
   b. place a strip of lens liner in the gap area.
   c. heat the lens while it is in the frame and then allow it to cool back to room temperature.

32. True or false? One advantage of cellulose acetate and propionate frames is that if the lens is too small, it may be possible to heat the frame and then plunge it in ice-cold water to shrink the frame.

Trim

33. Which of the following is used to smooth off a screw that attaches trim to the frame front?
   a. clear nail polish
   b. a soldering iron
   c. a riffler file
   d. a screw extractor
   e. cutting pliers

Cleaning

34. Which frame type should *not* be cleaned in an ultrasonic unit?
   a. metal frame
   b. jeweled frame
   c. plastic frame
   d. nylon frame

Soldering

35. True or false? Soldering may discolor the frame. Silver frames may be buffed, but buffing gold frames should be avoided since the gold color buffs off, exposing the base metal.

PART II

Ophthalmic Lenses

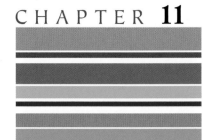

CHAPTER 11

Review of Elementary Mathematical Principles

This chapter reviews the mathematical principles used in basic optics. If you are well versed in mathematics, you may omit this chapter and use it for reference. The Proficiency Test may help you determine your mastery of this subject. If the questions are easy for you, continue on to the next chapter.

THE METRIC SYSTEM

When using the metric system of measurement, it is best to develop such familiarity with it that it is no longer necessary to think of it in relation to the English system. For example, it is much simpler to know how long a centimeter is than to figure out what fraction of an inch it might be. This can be done without much effort since most rulers now have a metric scale on one edge. Additionally the interpupillary distance (PD) rule, which no dispenser can be without for measurement of PD, uses the metric scale exclusively.

The unit of measure upon which the metric system is based is the *meter* (m). All other units are expressed as either multiples or fractions of that unit.

Just as there are 10 *dimes* in a dollar, so also are there 10 *deci*meters (dm) in 1 m. Just as there are 100 *cents* in a dollar, so also are there 100 *centi*meters (cm) in 1 m. And just as the wormlike *milli*pede is reputed to have 1000 legs, so also does 1 m have 1000 *milli*meters (mm).

A kilometer also has reference to a thousand, but this time 1 kilometer = 1000 m.

Therefore:

$$1 \text{ m} = 10 \text{ dm} = 100 \text{ cm} = 1000 \text{ mm}$$

and

$$1 \text{ km} = 1000 \text{ m}$$

(Weight measures are in multiples of 10 as well, retaining the same prefixes as the previously discussed linear measures. The basic unit of metric weight is the *gram*.)

If conversion from metric to English linear measurements becomes necessary, conversion factors are:

$$1 \text{ m} = 39.37 \text{ in}$$
$$1 \text{ cm} = 0.394 \text{ in}$$
$$1 \text{ in.} = 2.54 \text{ cm}$$

REVIEW OF ALGEBRA

Algebra uses positive and negative numbers and letters or other symbols to express mathematical relationships (Table 11-1). These relationships are used in formulas or equations. Letters or systematic symbols take the place of a number that is either unknown or subject to change to allow for dimensional variations.

Algebra offers versatility by allowing an equation to be altered to a new form for a specific need. For example, the formula:

$$a + b = c$$

is in the best order if *a* and *b* are known, and *c* is unknown. (If *a* is equal to 1 and *b* is equal to 2, what is *c*?) This form of the equation is not as easily used if *a* is the unknown. In this case it would be better to transform the equation to make for greater ease in solving for *a*.

Transformation

To transform an equation, the components are moved from one part of the equation to another. If a component is moved across the equal sign, the sign of the number moved must be changed from plus to minus or minus to plus. To follow the logic behind a required change in sign, it is noted that the same number (or symbol for a number) may be added to or subtracted from both sides of an equation. If

$$1 + 2 = 3$$

the two sides of the equation are still equal even if 2 is subtracted from each side:

$$1 + 2 - 2 = 3 - 2$$

TABLE 11-1
Commonly Used Algebraic Symbols

Operation	Symbol
Addition	$a + b$
Subtraction	$a - b$
Multiplication	$a \times b$ or $a \cdot b$ or ab
Division	$a \div b$ or $\dfrac{a}{b}$
Quantity squared	a^2
Square root	$\sqrt{a}$

Therefore if

$$a + b = c,$$

then

$$a + b - b = c - b.$$

Since

$$b - b = 0,$$

then

$$a = c - b,$$

and the transformation is accomplished.

Transforming when multiplication or division is involved is the same as multiplying both sides of the equation by the same number. For example, if

$$2 \cdot 3 = 6$$

Then

$$2 \cdot 2 \cdot 3 = 2 \cdot 6$$

or if

$$2 \cdot 3 = 6$$

then

$$\frac{2 \cdot 3}{2} = \frac{6}{2}$$

In each case the quantities are still equal, and the equation remains valid. Expressed in more generalized terms, if

$$a \cdot b = c$$

then

$$\frac{a \cdot b}{a} = \frac{c}{a}$$

and because

$$\frac{a}{a} = 1$$

then

$$b = \frac{c}{a}$$

The equation is the same as before, but expressed in a different form.

Naturally, if one side of the equation contains more than one term, both terms are affected by the transformation. For example,

$$ab = b + c$$

$$\frac{ab}{b} = \frac{b + c}{b}$$

$$\frac{a\cancel{b}}{\cancel{b}} = \frac{b + c}{b}$$

$$a = \frac{b + c}{b}$$

Use of Parentheses

When symbols are multiplied or divided or otherwise have a mathematical operation performed on them as a group, they are symbolically held together by parentheses. For example,

$$3(a + b) = c$$

means that both a and b are multiplied by 3. In fact another valid way to write this equation would be:

$$3a + 3b = c$$

If the equation were written as

$$3a + b = c$$

without the parentheses, it would not be the same equation at all. Only a would be multiplied by 3, showing the importance of the parentheses. In a transformation, those items within parentheses are treated as a single item. For example,

$$x(a + b) = 2(c + d)$$

then

$$\frac{x(a + b)}{(a + b)} = \frac{2(c + b)}{(a + b)}$$

since

$$\frac{(a + b)}{(a + b)} = 1$$

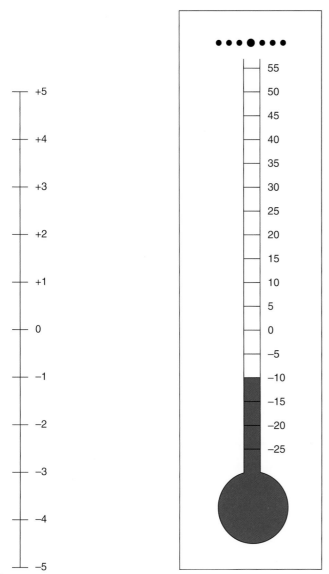

Figure 11-1. The concept of positive and negative numbers is easily illustrated by use of a number line and is seen commonly on instruments, such as a thermometer.

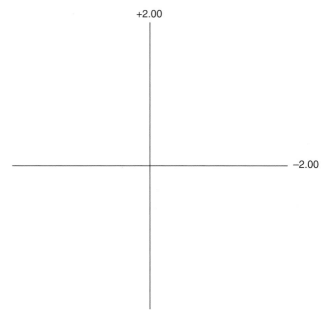

Figure 11-2. Illustrating the relationship between positive and negative numbers, the prescription shown has a value of +2.00 –4.00 × 90. The difference between positive and negative meridian is the value of the cylinder, which is 4.00 D.

then the equation becomes

$$x = \frac{2(c+b)}{(a+b)}$$

Positive and Negative Numbers

Positive and negative numbers are continuous with one another on the same line. Both start at zero but begin "counting" in opposite directions (Figure 11-1). Most everyone uses both positive and negative numbers daily. For example, when the thermometer drops below zero, negative numbers are used to describe the temperature. When something is indicated as being 300 feet below sea level, it can be said to be at –300 feet. In this case sea level is the zero point.

In working with negative numbers, one must remember how they relate in their distance from positive numbers. Again this can be most easily illustrated using the thermometer concept. How many degrees colder is –10° than +10°? When the mercury drops from +10° to –10°, it travels 10 units to reach zero and another 10 units to reach –10°. The drop in temperature is a total of 20°.

In optics this is most directly applicable to cylinder values. If the 90-degree meridian has a power of +2.00 D and the 180-degree meridian a power of –2.00 D, how strong is the cylinder (Figure 11-2)? (The cylinder value is the difference in power between the two major meridians of a lens.) On a number line, such as found on conventional lensmeter scales, it is readily seen that a total of 4 units must be traveled in going from the +2 mark to the –2 mark. Therefore the value of the cylinder is 4.

Use of the Reciprocal

The reciprocal of a number is obtained by dividing that number into 1. For example, the reciprocal of 2 may be written as 1 ÷ 2 , or $^1/_2$, or 0.5. Conversely, then the reciprocal of 0.5 is 1 ÷ 0.5, or $^1/_{0.5}$ or 2.

In optics reciprocals are used to convert focal lengths into dioptric units of lens power. If the focal length of a lens is 0.20 m, the dioptric power of the lens is the reciprocal of that focal length.

$$\frac{1}{0.20\,m} = 5\,D \text{ of lens power}$$

Roots and Powers

When a number is multiplied by itself, it is said to be *squared*. For example, 10 squared = 100, which is another way of saying 10 × 10 = 100. "Squared" is abbreviated mathematically by a superscript 2 written above and to the right of the number. The number indicates that *2* units of that same number are to be multiplied by each other. Ten squared $(10 \cdot 10)$ would be written as 10^2. It may also be spoken of as 10 to the second *power*. If 10^2 equals 100, the "root" from which the result of 100 has "grown" was the quantity 10 squared. Therefore the *square root* of is 100 is 10. To find the square root of a number, the operation is indicated by the symbol $\sqrt{}$ enclosing that number. For example,

$$\sqrt{100} = 10$$

A number can be "raised" to any given power; in other words, a number can be multiplied by itself any number of times. This operation is again indicated by a superscript:

$$10^3 = 10 \cdot 10 \cdot 10 = 1000$$
$$10^4 = 10 \cdot 10 \cdot 10 \cdot 10 = 10,000$$
$$a^5 = aaaaa$$

and so forth.

When indicating that the quantity is multiplied by itself a given number of times, it is also possible to place the superscript outside a parenthesis. This indicates that the whole quantity within the parentheses is multiplied by itself the number of times indicated by the superscript.

For example,

$$(a \cdot b)^2 = (a \cdot b)(a \cdot b)$$

REVIEW OF GEOMETRY

Since geometry is used fairly often in optics, a basic understanding of it is essential. It might be said that the concept of geometry is built on a "triangular foundation," which is to say that understanding the mathematics of a triangle is the basis for understanding geometry.

The Cartesian Coordinate System

The Cartesian coordinate system is a method of graphical localization of a point in space. In two-dimensional space, which is a flat plane, such as a sheet of paper, localization may be done with a paired set of numbers, *x* and *y*. These two numbers symbolize the horizontal and vertical location of a given point with reference to an original point: *x* is the number of units to the right (+) or to the left (−) of the zero point, whereas *y* refers to the localized point above (+) or below (−) this point (Figure 11-3). The reference point, or *origin*, is specified as (0,0). The horizontal location (*x*) is always given as the first number in the pair, and the vertical (*y*), as the second. The Cartesian coordinate system allows for ease and clarity of localization of any point, line, or geometric figure.

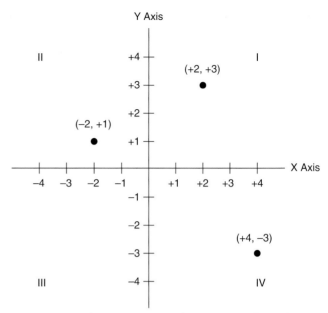

Figure 11-3. The Cartesian coordinate system allows the specific, repeatable localization of points in space. The *x*- and *y*-axes divide an area into four quarters known as *quadrants*. The upper right-hand quadrant is termed the *first quadrant*, or *quadrant I*. *Quadrant II* is the upper left quadrant, *quadrant III* the lower left, and *quadrant IV* the lower right.

Triangular Forms

There are 360 degrees in a complete circle. The wedged end of a pie-shaped piece of the circle contains a given number of these 360 degrees. The number of degrees contained between the two edges of the piece of pie that meet at the point is the degree measure of the angle formed.

A triangle contains three such points, or angles. The sum of the three angles contained within a triangle always equals 180 degrees.

If any one of these three angles is a 90-degree angle, the triangle is known as a *right triangle* (Figure 11-4). It obtains its name from the angle itself since 90-degree angles are known as *right angles*. The side of the triangle *opposite* the right angle is called the *hypotenuse*. If one of the angles of a triangle is 90 degrees, it logically follows that the sum of the two remaining angles must be 90 degrees.

In any right triangle, there is a certain relationship that exists between the lengths of each of the sides. This relationship states that *for a right triangle, the length of the hypotenuse squared is equal to the sum of the squares of the remaining two sides*. This relationship is referred to as the *Pythagorean theorem* (Figure 11-5) and may be abbreviated as $a^2 + b^2 = c^2$ where *c* is the length of the hypotenuse and *a* and *b* the lengths of the two remaining sides.

Triangles even more specific in shape than the right triangle also can have more specific established relationships between their sides. For example, a triangle whose angles are 45 degrees, 45 degrees, and 90 degrees has two

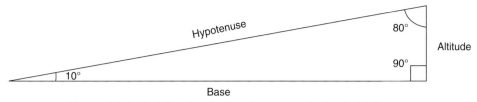

Figure 11-4. A right triangle contains one angle that is 90 degrees.

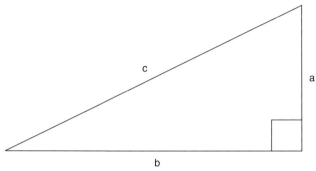

Figure 11-5. The Pythagorean theorem states that $a^2 + b^2 = c^2$. This theorem is valid only for right triangles.

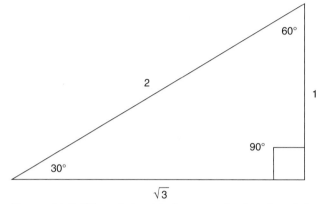

Figure 11-7. The relationship between the lengths of the sides for a 30-degree, 60-degree, and 90-degree triangle.

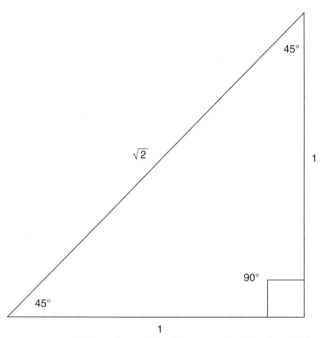

Figure 11-6. The relationship between the lengths of the sides for a 45-degree, 45-degree, and 90-degree triangle.

sides of equal length. If each of these sides is taken as being 1 unit long, then the hypotenuse will be $\sqrt{2}$ units long (Figure 11-6). This follows from the Pythagorean theorem. (If this triangle occurs, algebraic equalities may be used to simplify solutions to a given problem.)

Another triangle with specific side-length relationships is the 30 degrees-60 degrees-90 degrees triangle. In this case if the shortest side is taken as 1 unit of length, the second side will be $\sqrt{3}$ units, and the hypotenuse 2 units (Figure 11-7).

Similar Triangles

When two triangles have exactly the same shape but different sizes, they are said to be *similar triangles*. Similar triangles have (1) corresponding angles that are equal and (2) corresponding sides that are proportional in size (Figure 11-8). This corresponding size relationship helps considerably in finding unknown linear measurements when other corresponding measures in a similar geometrical configuration are known. Simple algebraic equalities may be used to find these unknown dimensions using side-length relationships of

$$\frac{a}{a'} = \frac{b}{b'} = \frac{c}{c'}$$

(See Figure 11-8.)

Example **11-1**

If a vertical stick protruding 0.80 m out of the ground casts a shadow 0.30 m long, how high is a flagpole nearby that casts a shadow 5 m long?

Solution

Referring to Figure 11-8, *a* corresponds to the 0.80 m stick, *b* to the 0.30 m shadow. The 5-m flagpole shadow corresponds to *b'* and the unknown height of the flagpole to *a'*.

In other words,

$$a = 0.80 \text{ m}$$
$$b = 0.30 \text{ m}$$
$$b' = 5 \text{ m}$$

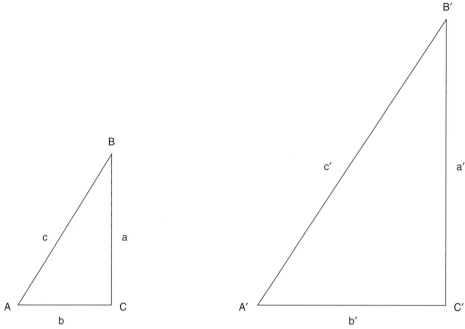

Figure 11-8. Similar triangles facilitate calculation of unknown dimensions from those which are already known. Capital letters represent angular measures; small letters stand for side lengths. In similar triangles, angles $A = A'$, $B = B'$, and $C = C'$.

since

$$\frac{a}{a'} = \frac{b}{b'}$$

$$\frac{0.80}{a'} = \frac{0.30}{5}$$

$$0.80 = \frac{(0.30) \cdot a'}{5}$$

$$\frac{(0.80)(5)}{.30} = a'$$

$$a' = 13.33 \text{ m}$$

This means that the flagpole is $13^1/_3$ m high.

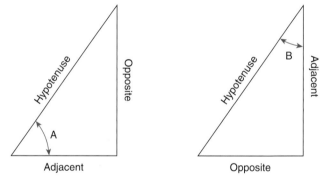

Figure 11-9. Although the position of the hypotenuse remains constant, the sides termed *opposite* and *adjacent* vary as to which of the angles is being referred to.

REVIEW OF TRIGONOMETRY

The section on geometry demonstrated how unknown length dimensions can be found when one dimension of a triangle is known along with the dimensions of a similarly shaped triangle.

This can also be done when only one dimension of a triangle is known using the angular measures of the triangle. This method uses *trigonometry.*

If the specific angles of a given triangle are known, it is possible to predict the ratio of any two sides of a triangle using a concept of similar right triangles. One can determine unknown dimensions of a triangle through the use of these predetermined ratios, which are known as *trigonometric functions.*

For a given angle of a triangle, there are three main ratios of importance. In Figure 11-9, if angle A is the angle being used, then the ratio of

$$\frac{\text{the side opposite angle A}}{\text{hypotenuse}} = \text{the sine of angle A}$$

The ratio of

$$\frac{\text{the side adjacent to angle A}}{\text{hypotenuse}} = \text{the cosine of angle A}$$

And the ratio of

$$\frac{\text{the side opposite angle A}}{\text{this side adjacent to angle A}} = \text{the tangent of angle A}$$

These are abbreviated more commonly as

$$\sin A = \frac{opp}{hyp}$$

$$\cos A = \frac{adj}{hyp}$$

$$\tan A = \frac{opp}{adj}$$

Sine, cosine, and tangent ratios are found by using a calculator preprogrammed for these functions.

Example **11-2**

The image of an object 6 m away from a prism is displaced upwards 10 degrees by that prism. How far above the original position does the image now appear to be? (Figure 11-10 shows this situation.)

Solution

The ratio used for the 10-degree angle must include the known dimension and the dimension that needs to be calculated. In this case the needed dimension is that which is *opposite* the 10-degree angle, and the known dimension is the one *adjacent* to the angle. The proper trigonometric function must contain both of these sides. The function containing both opposite and adjacent sides is the tangent of the angle.
   Therefore if

$$\tan \angle = \frac{opp}{adj}$$

then

$$\tan 10 \text{ degrees} = \frac{opp}{6}$$

A calculator tells us that the tangent of 10 degrees is 0.17632. So tan 10 degrees = 0.17632. This means that

$$0.17632 = \frac{opp}{6}$$

Using algebraic transformation,

$$opp = (0.1763)(6)$$
$$= 1.06 \text{ m}$$

This indicates that the image is displaced 1.06 m from its original position by the prism.

Vector Analysis

A *vector* is a mathematical quantity that conveys both magnitude and direction. It may be represented by a line of a given length pointing in a specific angular direction. Vectors are both additive and subtractive. Two vectors combined produce a resultant *vector sum*, which may be different from the two original vectors in both magnitude and direction. For example, a tractor pulls northward on an object with a force of 300 lb (Figure 11-11, *A*). A second tractor is hooked to the same object and also pulls in the same northward direction with a force of 300 lb (Figure 11-11, *B*). The sum total of pull is 600 lb northward. This can be found with vector analysis by placing the second vector on the first, "tail-to-head" (Figure 11-11, *C*). If drawn to scale, the measured sum of the two vectors gives the resultant vector sum. If the second tractor were pulling south, however, the resultant directional force would be zero. This time when the second vector is placed "tail-to-head" on the first, the head of the second ends up back on the starting point, indicating no net resultant force (Figure 11-11, *D* and *E*).

   Thus far the forces have been entirely complimentary to one another or completely opposing one another. When the vector forces are related to each other at angles other than 0 or 180 degrees, results are somewhat

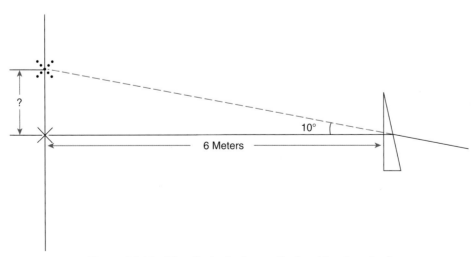

Figure 11-10. How far is the image displaced by the prism?

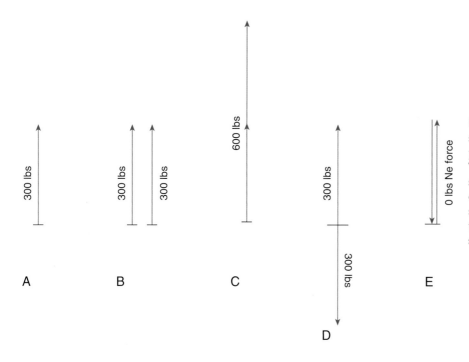

Figure 11-11. Vector analysis is the net sum of forces. **A**, Represents a tractor pulling northward with a force of 300 lb. The two forces **(B)** result in the vector sum **(C)**. If two equal forces pull in opposite directions **(D)** when the vectors are plotted "tail-to-head," the head of the second arrow returns again to zero, showing no net force **(E)**.

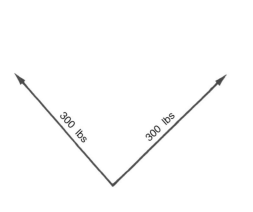

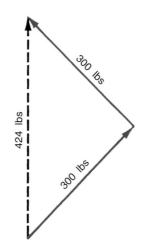

Figure 11-12. When forces are exerted in nonparallel directions, the principle of plotting these forces as "tail-to-head" may yet be used. The result is a straight line from origin to endpoint.

different. To illustrate: If one of these tractors were now pulling northeast and the other northwest, there is a cumulative effect of the two, but it is not as great as if both were pulling in the same direction. (On a 360-degree scale, one of the tractors would be pulling at 45 degrees, the other at 135 degrees.) Vector analysis can be done by again placing the second vector "tail-to-head" on the first, leaving its angular direction unchanged (Figure 11-12). If the two forces are carefully drawn to scale and their angular directions maintained, the resultant vector can be obtained by measurement. In this example, the vector sum is 424 lb of force being exerted in a northward, or 90-degree, direction.

Another way of thinking of vector analysis is in terms of "completing a parallelogram." A *parallelogram* is a

four-sided geometrical figure with opposing sides parallel. Two vectors originating at the same point become the first half of a parallelogram, and it is then completed by drawing in the two missing sides parallel to those already present (Figure 11-13). The vector sum is the diagonal of the parallelogram drawn from the point of origin to the opposite corner.

The solution procedure just described has been *graphical*, in that the vectors are often drawn on a graph to aid in accuracy. It is possible to use trigonometric functions to obtain more accurate results.

Vector analysis may be used in optics to determine the sum of two crossed prisms or two obliquely crossed cylinders.

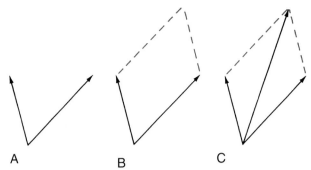

Figure 11-13. A, A representative pair of vector forces. Instead of plotting these vectors "tail-to-head," it is possible to realize their sums by using them to complete a parallelogram **(B)**. The resultant vector may now be drawn from the point of origin to the opposite corner of the parallelogram **(C)**.

Proficiency Test

(Answers can be found in the back of the book.)

1. How many centimeters are there in a meter?
   a. 12
   b. 10
   c. 100
   d. 1000
   e. 0.01

2. The basic metric unit of weight is the:
   a. meter.
   b. centimeter.
   c. cubic centimeter.
   d. gram.
   e. pound.

3. In mathematical transformations, if a complete component is moved across the equal sign to the other side of the equation:
   a. the number is squared.
   b. the number will always become a negative number.
   c. the sign of the number is changed.
   d. the operation cannot be performed.
   e. the operation is possible, but not as described in any of the answers above.

4. The opposite of –4 is:
   a. –4.
   b. Zero.
   c. +4.
   d. –(–4).
   e. both c and d are correct.

5. Solve for *a*:
   a. $a = \dfrac{(3) \cdot (7)}{4 - 1}$
   b. $a = (3 + 7) \cdot (4 - 2)$
   c. $a = \dfrac{(4 \cdot 9) + 2}{8}$
   d. $5 = \dfrac{a + 4}{3}$
   e. $7 = \dfrac{(7 \cdot 3 + 2)}{a}$
   f. $b = \dfrac{(4 \cdot a) - 3}{4}$
   g. $4 = \dfrac{ab}{(3 + 2b)}$
   h. $c = \dfrac{4b - a}{2b}$

6. Which of the following are not equal to $2(a + a)$?
   a. $2a + 2a$
   b. $2a^2$
   c. $(2 + 2)a$
   d. $4a$
   e. All of the above are the same as $2(a + a)$.

7. Find the reciprocal of each of the following numbers.
    a. 20
    b. 1
    c. 4
    d. 100
    e. 0.5
    f. 0.25
    g. $^1/_8$
    h. $^3/_4$

8. Square each of the following.
    a. 10
    b. 2
    c. a
    d. $(10 - 3)$
    e. 12
    f. $(5 \cdot 3)$

9. Find the square root of each of the following.
    a. 121
    b. 64
    c. 484
    d. b^2
    e. $(6 - 4)(6 - 4)$
    f. $(5a) \cdot (5a)$

10. Solve for each of the following.
    a. 7^3
    b. $\sqrt{9}$
    c. $\dfrac{10^2}{10}$
    d. $\left(\dfrac{10}{10}\right)^2$
    e. $\left(\dfrac{10 \cdot 10}{10}\right)^2$
    f. $\sqrt{a^2}$
    g. 2^4

11. In the late afternoon, a stick stuck in the ground vertically casts a shadow 1.36 m long. A telephone pole also casts a shadow that is 22 m long. If the stick is 1 m high, how high is the telephone pole?

12. A board 3 m long is leaned against a wall. The base of the board is 50 cm from the wall. How high up on the wall does the top of the board touch?

13. A ladder is leaned against the side of a house at a 60-degree angle (measured from ground to ladder). If the ladder is 4 m long: *a*. How far away from the house is the base of the ladder, and *b*. How far up the house is the top of the ladder?

14. A point on the Cartesian coordinate system is denoted by the paired (x, y) set as (+8, +3): *a*. How far from the origin in this point? *b*. If a line is drawn from the origin (0, 0) to this point (+8, +3), what angle will this line make with the *x*-axis?

15. A line is drawn from the origin (0, 0) on the Cartesian coordinate system at an angle of 120 degrees. If the line is 12 cm long, at what paired (x, y) coordinate set does the line end?

16. A plane takes off to fly to a destination that is due east, 130 km away. Unfortunately, although flying in a straight line, instead of flying due east it flies east, northeast 10 degrees off course. When due north of its destination, how many kilometers has the plane flown since takeoff?

17. A vacant lot is rectangular in shape, measuring 25 m wide and 73 m long: *a*. If a string is strung diagonally across the lot, how long must the string be? *b*. What are the three angles within the equal triangles now formed?

18. Which of the following is *not* a parallelogram?
    a. square
    b. rectangle
    c. triangle
    d. diamond

19. Bill and Fred attach ropes to a stump in the ground in an attempt to pull it out. Bill pulls in the direction of due north (90 degrees) while Fred pulls due east (0 degrees). Bill, being stronger, pulls to create a force of 175 lb, while Fred pulls with a 110-lb force: *a*. What is the net force applied to the stump? *b*. To the nearest degree, in what direction is that force?

20. In question 19, Bill and Fred were unable to dislodge the stump. In another attempt to dislodge it, Bill moves nearer to Fred so that their ropes are now at a 20-degree angle to each other. Fred does not move from his position. Both men pull their maximum, Bill with 175 lb of force and Fred with 110 lb of force. What is: *a*. The net force applied to the stump? *b*. To the nearest degree, what is its direction?

CHAPTER 12

Characteristics of Ophthalmic Lenses

An understanding of lens optics begins with basic study of the action of a single ray of light and how it is affected when passing into or through a transparent optical surface. Principles of reflection and refraction of light form the basis for understanding the nature of prism.

Vision takes place when rays of light from an object or objects are brought together in focus on the retina of the eye. Once again the process of refraction, or bending of rays, is involved. This time, however, a curved refracting surface is required so multiple rays will all be either directed toward or away from a specific point in space. Understanding the action of a curved surface on more than one ray of light is the basis for comprehending the optics of lenses.

THEORY OF LIGHT

To understand the way light behaves for lenses, we need to look at the nature of light itself. In simplistic terms, when light travels, it behaves in two ways:
1. Like a wave generated by dropping a rock into a pond (Figure 12-1).
2. Like a particle or photon. This could be compared with a controlled and continuing "explosion" of light that might be visualized in Figure 12-2.

For our purposes, we can best understand light as a wave.

Defining Light Waves

A light wave has certain characteristics as shown in Figure 12-3. The highest part of the wave is called the *crest*, and the lowest, the *trough*. The vertical distance from the trough to the crest is called the *amplitude*. The greater the amplitude is, the greater the intensity of the light. The horizontal distance from one crest to the next is called the *wavelength*. As wavelength changes, so does the perceived color of the light.

The Visible Spectrum

The wavelengths of light that are visible to the human eye vary in length from 380 to 760 nm. These are only a small part of what is called the *electromagnetic spectrum*. The electromagnetic spectrum goes from very short cosmic or gamma rays to extremely long radio waves

(Figure 12-4). Human vision is sensitive to only a very small portion of the electromagnetic spectrum.

When the sun radiates visible light, it includes the entire visible spectrum. When we see the whole spectrum of visible wavelengths together, we perceive the light as being white; when we see only one wavelength of light or several wavelengths that are very close to one another in length, we see that light as one specific color.

Colored Light

When white light is broken up into its component colors, it has a specific order of colors. Those colors of the rainbow were memorized by most people in elementary school by using the acronym for the imaginary name "Roy G Biv" (Figure 12-5). The letters refer to the colors red, orange, yellow, green, blue, indigo, and violet. In optics we order colored light according to wavelength, starting with the shortest and going to the longest. The shortest visible wavelength is blue, and the longest is red. Therefore we need to consider the "Roy G Biv" acronym as being spelled backwards (vib g yor).

Technically, each wavelength has its own color. However, the changes in color from one wavelength to the next are so small that we can only discriminate in wavelength areas. Figure 12-6 shows approximate wavelengths and their associated colors. Interestingly enough, different cultures make the color break at different places. For example, at the border between blue and purple, some cultures will identify that "in-between" wavelength area as blue, whereas another will call it purple.

A luminous or primary source is one that generates light. A candle would be an example of a primary source of light. The color of such an object depends upon the wave length(s) of light that the luminous source generates.

A secondary source of light is one that is reflecting light from a primary source. The moon is a secondary source of light, or a sweater would be a secondary source. The color of a secondary source of light depends upon what wavelengths it is reflecting. A white shirt reflects all wavelengths of light. A blue shirt reflects only blue light and absorbs all other wavelengths. A black shirt absorbs all wavelengths of light. With this in mind, it is

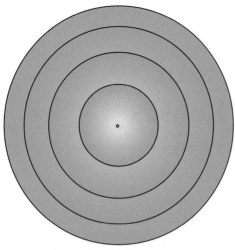

Figure 12-1. Light can be thought of as traveling away from its point of origin in waves, much like what happens when an object is thrown into a smooth pond, causing a wave to travel outward.

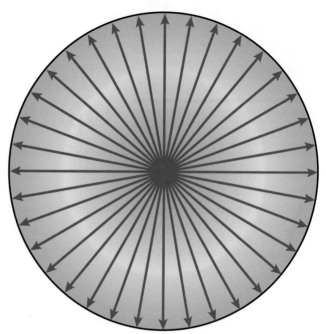

Figure 12-2. Light can also be thought of as particles of energy leaving the source.

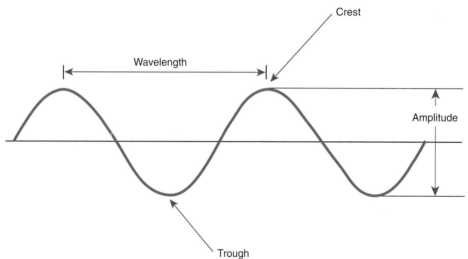

Figure 12-3. Light waves have crests and troughs, with a wavelength being measured from crest to crest.

understandable why white shirts are cooler on hot, sunny days than black shirts.

For more on the visible spectrum, including ultraviolet and infrared radiation, see Chapter 22.

REFLECTION

Unless interrupted, a single ray of light travels in a straight line. Placing a highly reflective object in its path causes the light to bounce back at an angle. This type of reflection is called *regular or specular reflection* (Figure 12-7). The angle at which the light strikes the surface is known as the *angle of incidence* (Figure 12-8). It is mea-

sured from a line perpendicular to the reflecting surface at the point of reflection known as the *normal* to the surface. The angle at which the ray is reflected is known as the *angle of reflection*. This also is measured from the normal.

The angle at which the light is reflected is predictable if the angle at which it strikes the surface is known since the *angle of incidence (i) is always equal to the angle of reflection (r)*.

When light strikes matte or dull (irregular) surfaces, it is still reflected, but variable scattering of the light rays occurs. This type of reflection is called *diffuse reflection* (Figure 12-9).

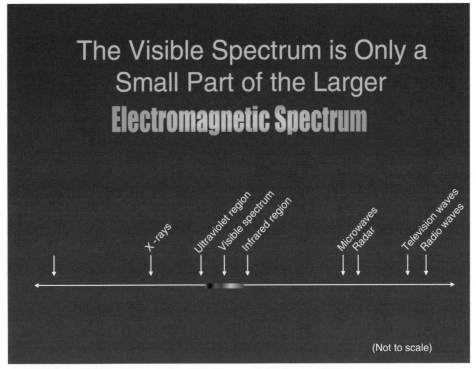

Figure 12-4. Visible light is only a small part of the larger electromagnetic spectrum that includes everything from very short gamma rays to extremely long radio waves.

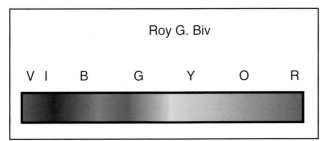

Figure 12-5. When we consider light, we generally go from left to right, starting with the shortest violet wavelengths and ending with the longer red wavelengths. So when looking at the order of the colors, the traditional acronym, "Roy G Biv," will be spelled backwards.

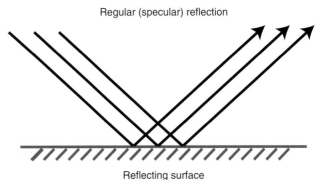

Figure 12-7. Specular or regular reflection occurs with a smooth surface.

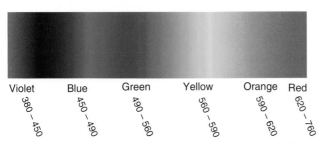

Figure 12-6. How color and wavelength correspond.

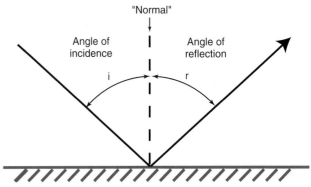

Figure 12-8. For reflected light, the angle of reflection always equals the angle of incidence. Both angles are measured from a line perpendicular to the reflecting surface known as the normal.

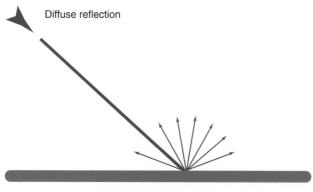

Diffuse reflection

Diffuse reflecting surface

Figure 12-9. Diffuse reflection occurs when light strikes a surface that is matte or irregular.

THE SPEED OF LIGHT AND REFRACTIVE INDEX

Light is able to travel faster through some materials than through others. Simply stated, some materials have more resistance to the speed of light than others. There is no resistance to light in a vacuum because there is nothing in a vacuum. Light travels at its maximum speed of about 186,355 miles/sec (or 299,792,458 m/sec). However, when light enters a clear medium, such as water, there is resistance, and the speed of light slows. The medium of less resistance (such as air) is said to be the *rarer* medium. The medium of more resistance is said to be the *denser* medium.

The amount of resistance to the speed of light that slows it down is represented by a number. This number is referred to as the *refractive index*. The more the material slows the passage of light, the higher is its refractive index.

The number for the refractive index of a given substance is obtained by comparing the speed of light in a vacuum with the speed of light in the new substance. It is written as a fraction. The speed of light in a vacuum is on top (the numerator) and the reduced speed of light in the new substance on the bottom (the denominator). The speed in the denominator is always the slower speed and smaller number; thus the fraction will always come out greater than 1. Here is how it is written:

$$\frac{\text{Speed of Light in a Vacuum}}{\text{Speed of Light in New Substance}}$$
$$= \text{Absolute Refractive Index}$$

Because there cannot be less resistance to the speed of light than nothing at all (a vacuum), this number for the refractive index is called the *absolute refractive index*.

However, we live on earth where most everything is surrounded by air. Since light travels almost as fast in air as in a vacuum, we use air instead of a vacuum as the standard when calculating refractive index. Since the value for refractive index obtained is relative to air instead of to a vacuum, the refractive index obtained in this manner is called the *relative refractive index*. This is expressed as the fraction:

$$\frac{\text{Speed of Light in Air}}{\text{Speed of Light in New Substance}}$$
$$= \text{Relative Refractive Index}$$

Refractive index is commonly abbreviated as *n*, and the number we use when speaking of refractive index is really relative refractive index.

REFRACTION

When light strikes a new, transparent medium straight on (at a 90-degree angle, perpendicular to the surface), the light slows down, but continues on in the same direction.

But when light strikes a new substance or medium at an angle, the change in speed in the new media causes the light to change direction. Consider, for example, the case of light passing from a low refractive index medium, such as air, to a higher refractive index medium, such as water or even glass, which are both denser than air. To understand what is happening and why, consider the analogy of a car traveling on a smooth substance with little resistance, such as a smooth, paved road. In a moment of inattention, the car drifts to the side and encounters a rough substance, such as the gravel shoulder of the road. When the right wheel hits the rough gravel, in which direction does the car want to go? Because the right side of the car slows faster than the left side, the car pulls to the right.

When a light ray passes from a rarer medium (low refractive index) and strikes a denser medium at an angle, the light will be bent, or *refracted*. The direction of the refraction is toward the normal to the surface (Figure 12-10). Remember, the "normal" to the surface is a line perpendicular to the surface at the place where the light strikes the surface.

Snell's Law

If the refractive indices of both media through which light is traveling are known, the angle of refraction for a given angle of incidence is predictable. It may be calculated geometrically using the sines of the angles of incidence and refraction. It is expressed algebraically as:

$$n \sin i = n' \sin i'.$$

This is known as *Snell's law*.

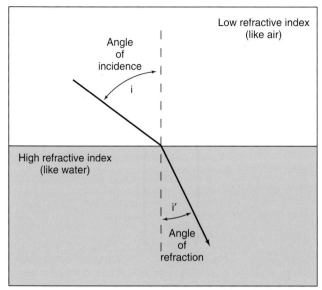

Figure 12-10. The figure shows the bending or refraction of light going from a rarer to a denser medium. To see how light is bent going from a denser to a rarer medium, simply turn the figure upside down and visualize it traveling in the opposite direction.

Example **12-1**

Suppose a ray of light is traveling from air of refractive index 1 to glass of index 1.523. If the ray strikes the glass at an angle of 30 degrees, what will be the angle of refraction?

Solution

We know that:

$$n = 1 \text{ (refractive index of air)}$$
$$n' = 1.523 \text{ (refractive index of glass)}$$
$$i = 30 \text{ degrees (angle of incidence).}$$

But we do not know the angle of refraction.

$$i' = ? \text{ (angle of refraction)}$$

If

$$n \sin i = n' \sin i',$$

then for our example

$$(1) (\sin 30) = (1.523) (\sin i').$$

Since sin i' is the unknown, the above formula can be rearranged algebraically as follows:

$$\frac{(1) (\sin 30)}{1.523} = (\sin i')$$

Using a calculator capable of generating trigonometric functions, it is found that:

$$\sin 30 = 0.5.$$

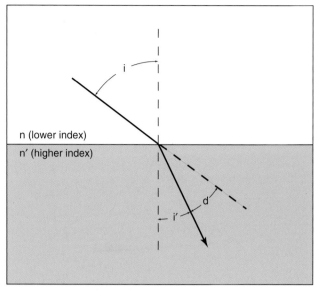

Figure 12-11. The angle of deviation is the angular change in light direction from its original path.

Therefore

$$\sin i' = \frac{(1) (0.5)}{1.523}$$
$$= 0.3283$$

Again using a calculator it is determined that 0.3283 is the sine of 19.2 degrees. (This is done by finding the inverse sin[sin⁻¹] of 0.3283.) Thus the resulting angle of refraction is 19.2 degrees.

Angle of Deviation

The angle of refraction is the angle of the refracted ray with reference to a line perpendicular to (normal to) the refracting surface. It does not directly tell how much the ray has deviated from its original path. This amount of that the light has deviated from its original path is called the *angle of deviation* (d) (Figure 12-11).

It can be seen from the geometry of the figure that for light leaving a rare and entering a dense medium, $i = d + i'$. Therefore the angle of deviation is $d = i - i'$.

Example **12-2**

Example 12-1 asked for the angle of refraction for light entering a new medium at an angle of incidence of 30 degrees. The angle of refraction was found to be 19.2 degrees. Knowing this, what is the angle of deviation?

Solution

We know that the angle of deviation is:

$$d = i - i'.$$

Since the angle of incidence (i) is 30 degrees and the angle of refraction (i') is 19.2 degrees, then:

$$d = 30 - 19.2$$
$$= 10.8 \text{ degrees.}$$

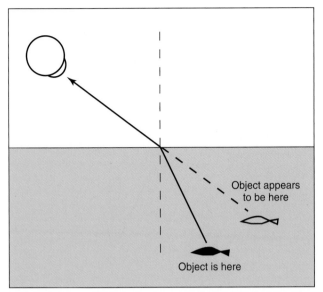

Figure 12-12. When light from an object in another media, such as water, is seen at an angle, the light rays are bent, making the object appear to be somewhere other than its actual location.

The angle of deviation is calculated as d = i – i′ because light is leaving a rare medium and going into a dense one. When the opposite situation exists and light is traveling from a dense medium and entering a rare one, the angle of deviation would become d = i′ – i. An example of light coming from a dense medium, like water, and traveling into a rare medium, like air is shown in Figure 12-12. This figure helps to explain why objects that are viewed below the surface of water are not always where they appear to be. Attempts to spear the fish in figure 12-12 would be unsuccessful unless the spear fisherman compensated for the apparent location of the fish.

PRISM

When Light Goes Straight Through Parallel Surfaces

When light leaves air and enters a slab of glass, the light travels more slowly in the glass. If the two sides of the glass slab are parallel and the light enters perpendicular to the front surface, it does not bend at all. It simply slows down. And when the ray of light strikes the back surface of the glass, it is still perpendicular to the surface and does not bend. It comes out the other side of the slab of glass unchanged in direction. The light leaves the other side of the glass at exactly the same 90-degree angle that it first entered (Figure 12-13). (Incidentally, when the light leaves the glass and goes back into air, it speeds back up to its original, expected speed in air.)

When Light Goes Through Parallel Surfaces at an Angle

If light strikes a parallel-surfaced slab of glass at an angle, the ray will be bent at each surface in accordance with

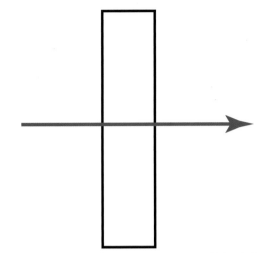

Figure 12-13. A ray of light entering a parallel-sided slab of glass perpendicular to both surfaces will pass through without ever changing direction.

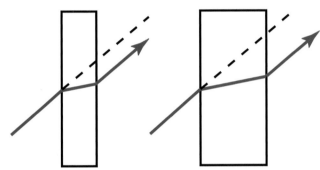

Figure 12-14. Light entering a parallel-sided slab of glass at an angle is bent at both front and back surfaces. If the media on both sides of the material are the same, as when the slab is surrounded by air, the ray of light will leave parallel to its original direction. Although traveling in exactly the same direction, the ray of light will be displaced laterally. The amount of displacement depends on the thickness of the slab.

the rule of refraction. Since the indices of the glass and of air at both surfaces are the same, the emergent ray and the incident ray will be parallel, just as when the ray struck the glass from straight ahead. The only difference is that it will be slightly displaced laterally. The amount of displacement depends upon the angle at which the incident ray struck the glass and the thickness of the glass (Figure 12-14).

When the Two Surfaces Are Not Parallel

Suppose that the two surfaces of glass are not parallel to one another as shown in Figure 12-15. In this figure a ray of light strikes the first surface straight on, at a 90-degree angle. It is not bent from its original path. However, the second surface is at an angle to the first surface, giving the glass a prism shape.

The ray of light continues to pass through the glass and strikes the second (angled) surface at an angle. In

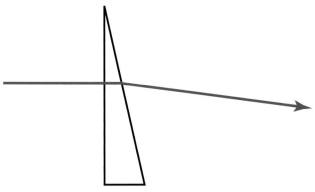

Figure 12-15. Here light strikes the first surface straight on and is not bent until it reaches the second angled surface. Now it is bent and leaves in a different direction.

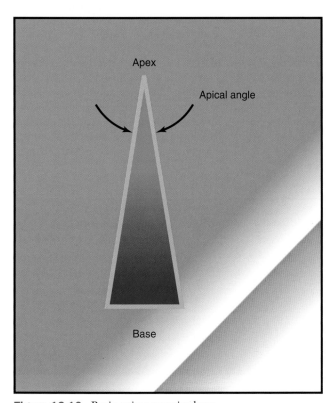

Figure 12-16. Basic prism terminology.

this case the angle that the light strikes the surface is equal to the angle of tilt of the second surface. Because the ray of light is going from a denser to a rarer medium, it will be bent away from the normal to the surface by an amount greater than its angle of incidence. This will cause the light to be bent downward toward the base of the prism. The amount of this deviation is predictable using Snell's law. *Light is always bent toward the base of a prism.*

The tip of a prism is called the *apex*. The wider, bottom part of a prism is called the *base* (Figure 12-16).

More information on how prism works will be found in Chapters 15 and 16.

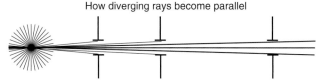

How diverging rays become parallel

Figure 12-17. By looking at light passing through a series of apertures, it is easier to see that the farther from a source light rays travel, the less they diverge from one another. And the less they diverge from one another, the more parallel they become.

HOW CURVED LENSES REFRACT LIGHT

Refraction of Multiple Light Rays

Up to this point, we have seen how light acts when it is viewed as a single ray and strikes a flat surface. However, light does not come as a single ray, but many. And lenses have curved surfaces instead of flat surfaces. With a curved refracting surface, multiple rays will all be either directed toward or away from a specific point in space.

Light rays emanate from a light source or object in an ever-increasing circle similar to the way a ripple goes out from the place where a stone is thrown into water. As these rays go out from their source, they are said to be *diverging.* The outer border of this ever-growing circle of light is called the *wave front.* The farther from the object source this wave front is, the less that light rays passing through an *aperture* or "hole" of a certain size will be diverging. In essence they become more parallel, as seen in Figure 12-17. After traveling far enough away from the object, these light rays no longer appear to be diverging. At an infinite distance from the object, they become parallel.

Focusing Light

Suppose it becomes desirable to divert parallel rays coming from an object at infinity to bring them to focus at one image point. If it were only a question of two parallel rays, the problem could be solved easily using principles explained earlier in the chapter. Since a prism deviates light at a known angle, if two prisms were placed base to base so as to interrupt these two rays, the rays could be caused to meet at a specified point, known as the *focal point* (Figure 12-18). Rays traveling toward one specific point are said to be *converging.* In our example, the position of the focal point can be arbitrarily changed by merely increasing or decreasing the power of the two prisms.

If there were four parallel rays to be focused, however, the two-prism concept would no longer be feasible (Figure 12-19). Stronger prisms would be required to deviate the two outer rays enough to bring them to the same focal point. It would be possible to stretch this system by cutting off the tops of the original prisms and replacing the tops with prisms of stronger power (Figure 12-20). It quickly becomes obvious, however, that the

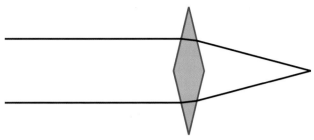

Figure 12-18. If only two parallel rays of light have to be brought to a single point of focus, the job would be fairly simple. Just use two prisms placed base to base.

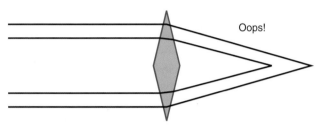

Oops!

Figure 12-19. A two-prism system cannot be expected to bring light to a single point of focus if there are more than two rays of light.

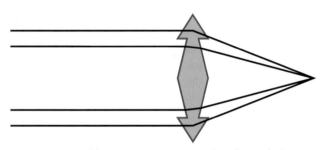

Figure 12-20. If just prisms were used to bring light to a focus, a different prism would be necessary for each incoming parallel ray to form a single point focus.

more parallel rays there are, the more new prisms will be required.

Fortunately the problem may be solved by creating a curved surface to replace the theoretical series of stacked prisms. The curve of the surface is in the form of an arc of a circle (Figure 12-21).

The shorter the radius of curvature, the more light is bent when striking the surface and consequently the closer to the lens the focal point will be.

FOCAL POINTS AND DISTANCES

For a source at infinity, the specific point at which an image will be focused is known as the *second principal focus* (F′) of the lens. The distance from the lens to the second principal focus is known as the *second (or secondary) focal length* of the lens (f′) (Figure 12-22).

The *first principal focus* (F) of a lens is that point at which an object may be placed so that the lens will form an image of that object at infinity. In other words, the

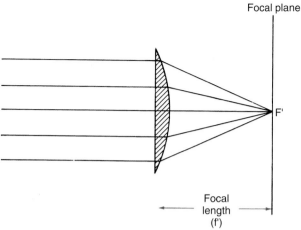

Focal plane

F'

Focal length (f')

Figure 12-21. The point where parallel light entering a lens is brought to focus is known as the second principal focus of the lens. The distance from the center of the lens to this principal focus is the second focal length. In this figure, parallel light rays coming from an object at infinity converge to form a real image of the object. The lens is drawn with the front surface flat so that it is easier to see how the curved back surface has a changing angle. If a ray of light strikes the lens at the exact center, the curved back surface is actually flat, and the light ray passes through without being bent. The farther toward the outside edge of the lens, the more the back surface will be angled. The more the back surface is angled, the more the incoming ray of light will be bent.

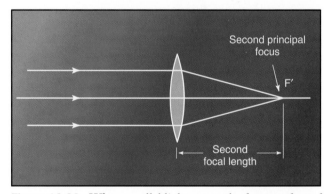

Second principal focus

F'

Second focal length

Figure 12-22. When parallel light enters the front surface of a lens, light is brought to a focus at what is called the *second principal focus* of the lens.

object is placed so that light rays *leaving* the lens are now parallel. The distance from the lens to the first principal focus is the *first (or primary) focal length* of the lens (Figure 12-23.

For spectacle lenses the more important focal point is the second principle focus.

QUANTIFYING LENSES

Sign Convention

Up to this point, when prisms or lenses have been shown, the first surface has usually been a flat surface and perpendicular to the light. (In optics a flat surface is called a *plano* surface.) All light entering the prism or lens has been parallel light. If the first surface is flat and perpendicular to the entering light, then light passes through the first surface undeviated (without being bent). It is not bent until it reaches the tilted or curved second surface. There has therefore been only one factor to consider: the second surface.

To have a common groundwork for understanding the action of a lens on other than parallel light and lenses with both surfaces curved, it is necessary to adhere to accepted conventions.

These *sign conventions* serve to prevent confusion and errors in describing the optics of lenses. Some of these conventions include the following:

1. Light is traditionally represented in optical drawings as traveling from left to right.
2. Any measurements are made with the lens at the center of the system. It is as if the lens is at the zero point of a number line. All distances to the right of the lens are expressed as positive and all distances to the left as negative (Figure 12-24).
3. When measurements must be made anywhere other than left or right of the lens, all positions above a horizontal line passing through the lens center are considered positive; all positions below a horizontal line passing through the lens center are negative.
4. Lenses that cause parallel rays of light to converge are designated as having *plus* power, whereas those causing parallel rays of light to diverge are identified as being *minus*.

Surface Curvature

To enable the steepness of curvature of a surface to be quantified, a unit of measure based on the radius of curvature (abbreviated r) has been chosen (Figure 12-25). So a surface can be quantified by its radius of curvature. But the reciprocal of the radius of curvature in meters

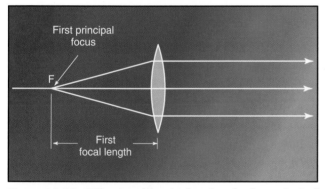

Figure 12-23. When an object is placed at the first principal focus of a lens, light rays will leave the lens parallel to one another.

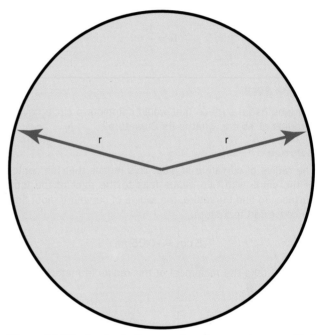

Figure 12-25. A spherically curved surface may be quantified by the radius of curvature of that spherical surface.

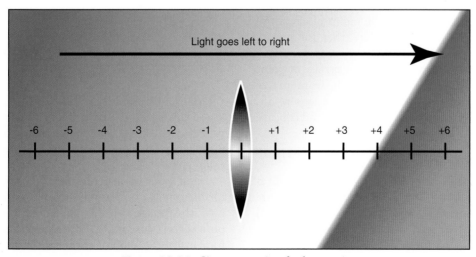

Figure 12-24. Sign convention for lens optics.

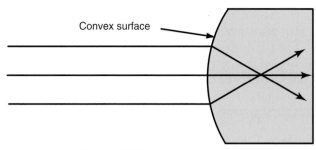

Figure 12-26. A convex surface.

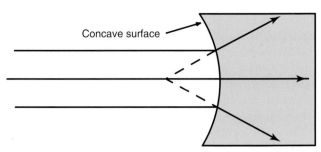

Figure 12-27. A concave surface.

is the measure commonly used and is referred to as *Curvature*. Curvature is expressed in units of reciprocal meters (m^{-1}) and is abbreviated *R*.

$$R = \frac{1}{r}$$

Example **12-3**

If a lens has a surface that would complete a circle having a radius of +5 cm, what is its Curvature?

Solution

The radius of curvature is plus. This means that the center of the circle with this radius falls to the right of the lens surface. To find Curvature, the radius of curvature must first be converted to meters:

$$+5 \text{ cm} = +0.05 \text{ m.}$$

Then we take the reciprocal of the radius in meters to find Curvature (R).

$$R = \frac{1}{+0.05} = +20 \text{ m}^{-1}$$

Convex and Concave Surfaces

Suppose the front surface of a lens has a radius of curvature of 20 cm. If the center of the radius of curvature is to the right of the front lens surface, then the surface is a convex surface (Figure 12-26).

If the radius of curvature of the front surface of a lens is centered to the left of the lens surface, the front surface is a concave surface (Figure 12-27). For a lens in air, convex surfaces are positive (plus) in power, and concave surfaces are negative (minus).

Units of Lens Power

The total power of a lens or lens surface to bend light is referred to as its *focal power*. Units of focal power are expressed as diopters (D) and are related to the focal length of the lens or lens surface. The *focal length* is symbolized by f or f', for primary or secondary focal length, whereas the focal power (in diopters) of the lens

is symbolized by *F*. Because ophthalmic lenses are generally referenced by their second focal length and are worn in air, the relationship between focal length and focal power is expressed by the formula:

$$F = \frac{1}{f'}$$

The focal length (f') must be in meters when calculating lens power.

$$F = \frac{1}{f'}$$

Example **12-4**

If a lens has a secondary focal length of +20 cm, what is the power of the lens?

Solution

Focal length must first be converted to meters:

$$+20 \text{ cm} = +0.20 \text{ m.}$$

Then lens power may be found as:

$$F = \frac{1}{f'}$$
$$= \frac{1}{+0.20}$$
$$= +5.00 \text{ D (diopters of focal power)}$$

Positive Lenses and Real Images

Up to this point, the type of lens spoken of has been the type that causes parallel light rays to converge, or come together. This type of lens is referred to as a *positive* or a *plus* lens.

Light from an object brought to a focus by a lens will form an image of that object. In the case of converging rays, this image can be intercepted, forming an image on a screen, just like a camera forms an image on the film in the back of the camera. This type of image is known as a *real image*.

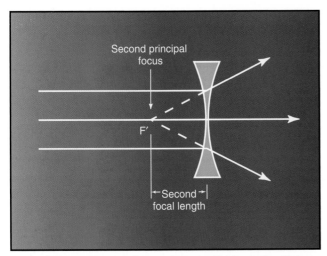

Figure 12-28. A minus lens causes parallel incoming light to diverge. The point from which light appears to diverge is called the second principal focus. The image formed by the backward projection of these diverging rays is a virtual image.

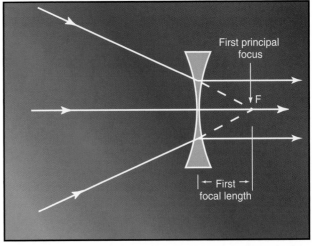

Figure 12-29. For light to leave the second surface of a lens as parallel rays, entering light rays must be converging toward the first principal focus of the lens.

Negative Lenses and Virtual Images

According to sign convention, a lens whose focal point is to the left of the lens will have a negative focal power. When parallel rays enter a lens that has a negative focal length (and therefore also a negative power) rays leaving the lens diverge or spread away from one another instead of converge toward one another.

Whereas a positive lens was described as analogous to prisms placed base to base, a negative lens can he compared with the action of two prisms placed apex to apex. The focal point of a negative lens is found by extending the diverging rays backward to a point from which they appear to originate (Figure 12-28). This is called the *second principal focus* of the lens.

However, if rays of light leave the lens parallel, they must have been converging when entering the lens. The point toward which they are converging is called the *first principal focus* of the lens (Figure 12-29).

When rays diverge on leaving a lens as shown in Figure 12-28, the image of the object cannot be focused on a screen. This is because the image is formed by a backward projection of the diverging rays to their apparent point of origin. Even though they do not originate from that point, they appear as if they do. This type of image is referred to as a *virtual image*.

Example **12-5**

If a lens has a focal point which is 40 cm to the left of the lens (−40 cm from the lens), what focal power does the lens have?

Solution

To solve the problem, the focal length is first converted to meters.

$$-40\text{ cm} = -0.40\text{ m}.$$

Next the focal power is found by taking the reciprocal of the focal length.

$$F = \frac{1}{f'}$$
$$= \frac{1}{-0.40}$$
$$= -2.50\text{ diopters}$$

The lens is found to have a power of −2.50 D.

Surface Power and the Lensmaker's Formula

When a lens is thin, that lens derives its total power from the combined powers of its front and back surfaces.

The amount light is bent by a lens surface depends on the radius of curvature of that surface and on the refractive index of the lens material. The formula taking these two factors into consideration when light is passing into the first surface of a lens is:

$$F_1 = \frac{n' - n}{r}$$

where F_1 = the surface power of the first surface expressed in diopters,

 n' = the refractive index of the lens (i.e., the medium into which the light is entering),
 n = the refractive index of air (the medium the light is leaving), and
 r = the radius of curvature of this first lens surface in meters.

This formula is often referred to as the *Lensmaker's formula*.

It can be seen from this formula that just because two lens surfaces have the same radius of curvature it does not necessarily mean that they will have the same ability to refract (or bend) light. The index of refraction of the material also has an effect. Therefore two surface powers will not be the same if the index of refraction of the two materials is different. Consider, for example, a CR-39 plastic lens of index 1.498 and a higher index plastic lens of index 1.66. Both have a front curve with a radius of curvature of +8.66 cm. Using the Lensmaker's formula, we find the lens surface power of the CR-39 lens to be:

$$F_{1(CR-39)} = \frac{n'-n}{r}$$
$$= \frac{1.498-1}{0.0866\,\text{m}}$$
$$= +5.75\,\text{D}$$

However, the lens surface power of the 1.66 index plastic lens is:

$$F_{1(HI)} = \frac{n'-n}{r}$$
$$= \frac{1.66-1}{0.0866\,\text{m}}$$
$$= +7.62\,\text{D}$$

It can be seen that what may appear to be a small change in refractive index can create a considerable change in surface power.

The surface power for the second surface is calculated in the same manner, except that the values for n' and n are reversed. This time light is leaving the lens and reentering air. Therefore the equation for the second, or rear, lens surface power becomes:

$$F_2 = \frac{n'-n}{r_2}$$

where n' is 1 (air) and n is the index of the lens.

One way to find the power of the lens is to add the powers of the front and back lens surfaces together. When lens power is found in this way, it is called the *nominal power* of the lens. So

$$\text{Nominal power} = F_1 + F_2$$

For low-powered thin lenses, this proves to be a fairly accurate measure of lens power. But for thick lenses, the thickness of the lens also influences lens power. Most low-powered ophthalmic lenses can be considered thin lenses. Thick lenses will be considered in Chapter 14.

THE ACTION OF A LENS ON OTHER THAN PARALLEL LIGHT

The Concept of Vergence

Up to this point, only parallel light that is entering the lens from straight ahead has been considered. Such light is brought to a focus at the focal point of the lens. If light entering the lens is *not* parallel, light leaving the lens will

no longer come to a focus at the secondary focal point of the lens, but at some other point. That point may be determined by using both:

1. A quantitative value for the vergence of light entering the lens and
2. The power of the lens.

Finding a Value for Converging and Diverging Light

The quantitative unit value for vergence is expressed in diopters in the same way that lens focal powers are. When light is converging, it is converging to a certain point in space. When it is diverging, it appears to be coming from a given point in space. There is a specific distance from this image or object point to the lens. This distance is abbreviated using the symbol l or l'. The dioptric value of the vergence itself is abbreviated by L or L'. The relationship between the two is:

$$\frac{n}{l} = L$$

and

$$\frac{n'}{l'} = L'$$

How do we distinguish between references to object or image points? When referring to the object, symbols l and L are used; when referring to the image, symbols l' and L' are used (Figure 12-30). In air the relationship simplifies to:

$$\frac{1}{l} = L$$

and

$$\frac{1}{l'} = L'$$

There is a relationship between the entering vergence of light and the exiting vergence of light. It is as follows: The vergence of the light entering the lens added to the dioptric value of the lens is found to equal the vergence of the light leaving the lens. This can be expressed in the form of an equation:

$$L + F = L'$$

This equation is commonly expressed in transposed form as $F = L' - L$, called the Fundamental Paraxial Equation. For single refractive surfaces it is written in the more basic form:

$$F = \frac{n'}{l'} - \frac{n}{l}$$

where n' is the refractive index of the second media into which light is entering and n is the refractive index of

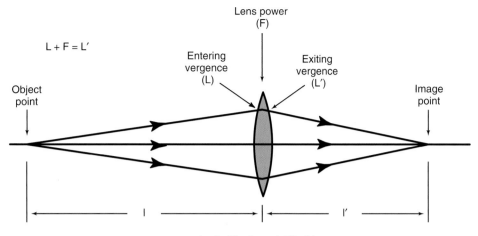

In air, $1/l = L$, and $1/l' = L'$.

Figure 12-30. Diverging or converging light may be quantified using vergence. Object and image points that correspond (as shown here) are referred to as *conjugate foci*.

the first or primary media. For spectacle lenses that will be worn in air, this simplifies to:

$$F = \frac{1}{l'} - \frac{1}{l}$$

What is the situation when talking about lens surfaces only, instead of whole lenses? In the instance of a single surface that separates two media, the relationship between object and image distance is determined in basically the same manner. If

$$\frac{n' - n}{r}$$

is substituted for the surface power *F*, then the equation for vergence becomes:

$$\frac{n' - n}{r} = \frac{n'}{l'} - \frac{n}{l}$$

This *fundamental paraxial equation* is a *paraxial* equation because it remains valid for those rays in the paraxial or central region of the refracting surface. (Rays that are a great distance away from the center of the lens are affected by lens aberrations. They no longer fall exactly at the focal point.)

Example **12-6, A**

Use vergence concepts to find the convergence of light leaving a +10.00 D lens if the light entering the lens is parallel.

Solution

Since parallel light neither diverges nor converges, its vergence value is zero. Therefore in the case of parallel light entering a +10 D lens, we can find the vergence of light leaving the lens as follows:

The vergence of light entering the lens is zero. Therefore

$$L = 0.00 \text{ D.}$$

The power of the lens is +10.00 D so:

$$F = +10.00 \text{ D}$$

If

$$L + F = L'$$

then

$$0.00 \text{ D} + 10.00 \text{ D} = L'$$

and

$$L' = +10.00 \text{ D}$$

Therefore the vergence of the light leaving the lens equals +10.00 D, which as expected corresponds to the focal power of the lens. Because the vergence of the light leaving the lens is plus in power, we know that it must be *converging* light. By sign convention a "+" connotes a point of focus to the right of the lens.

Example **12-6, B**

What is the distance from the lens to the point of focus for this +10.00 D lens if the light entering the lens is parallel?

Solution

Using vergence concepts, the distance from the lens to the point of focus is determined by:

$$L' = \frac{1}{l'}$$

And we know that

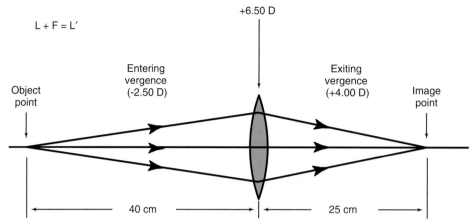

Figure 12-31. This diagram shows how vergence may be used to find the image point for an object that is at a known distance from the lens.

$$+10.00 \text{ D} = \frac{1}{l'}$$

which transposes to

$$l' = \frac{1}{+10.00} = +0.10 \text{ m} = +10 \text{ cm}$$

So the point of focus is 10 cm to the right of the lens. Because the entering light was parallel, this corresponds to the focal point of that lens.

Example **12-7**

Light is coming from a point 40 cm in front of a +6.50 D lens. Use vergence concepts to determine where the image of the object formed.

Solution

We can solve the problem with vergence using the fundamental paraxial equation.

$$L + F = L'$$

We know that, in air

$$L = \frac{1}{l}$$

(Now as the answer progresses, follow along using Figure 12-31.)

In the example problem, the distance from the lens to the object is 40 cm. So *l* is −40 cm. It is negative because it is to the left of the lens, and sign convention makes it negative. It also needs to be in meters for the equation, making *l* equal to −0.40 m.

$$L = \frac{1}{l}$$
$$= \frac{1}{-0.40 \text{ m}}$$
$$= -2.50 \text{ D}$$

Now we can use the fundamental paraxial equation to solve for the vergence of light leaving the lens.

$$L' = L + F$$
$$= -2.50 + 6.50$$
$$= +4.00 \text{ D}$$

If the vergence of light leaving the lens is +4.00 D, we can now find the distance from the lens to the image point. That distance is symbolized by *l'*. Therefore

$$L' = \frac{1}{l'}$$

or in transposed form

$$l' = \frac{1}{L'}$$
$$= \frac{1}{4.00}$$
$$= 0.25 \text{ m}$$

Converting 0.25 m into centimeters tells us that the distance of the image point from the lens is 25 cm.

Example **12-8**

Light is diverging from an object 50 cm to the left of a +10.00 D lens. Use vergence concepts to determine where light will come to focus to produce an image of the object?

Solution

First we need to find the vergence of light entering the lens. We can find that vergence because we know the light's point of origin; it is 50 cm to the left of the lens.

$$l = -50 \text{ cm} = -0.50 \text{ m}$$

The value is negative since the point of reference is to the left of the lens. As a result, light diverges from this point. Now we can find the dioptric value of that divergence.

$$L = \frac{1}{-0.50 \text{ m}} = -2.00 \text{ D}$$

So the divergence is −2.00 D. To complete the problem, we know that $F = +10.00$ D. We use the equation:

$$L + F = L'$$

and find that

$$-2.00 \text{ D} + 10.00 \text{ D} = L'$$

and

$$L' = +8.00 \text{ D}$$

So the vergence leaving the lens has a value of +8.00 D.

Now we can find the distance from the lens to the focal point. This is done by taking the reciprocal value of the vergence.

$$l' = \frac{1}{+8.00 \text{ D}}$$
$$= +1.25 \text{ m}$$
$$= +12.5 \text{ cm}$$

It can be seen that if light leaves an object that is 50 cm to the left of a +10.00 D lens, it will not come to a focus at the normal focal point of the lens. Instead, light coming from an object closer to the lens than infinity will focus farther to the right of the defined focal point of the lens than it normally would for parallel incoming light.

Example **12-9**

We know that a minus lens causes incoming parallel light to diverge. This places the focal point to the left of the lens, making the lens value negative and the image of the object virtual. Now for the problem:

We have the same situation as described in the previous example. However, the +10.00 D lens is replaced with a −10.00 D lens. Now where will the image point be for an object point 50 cm to the left of the lens?

Solution

Since the object is still 50 cm to the left, L still equals −2.00 D.

The basic equation remains

$$L + F = L'$$

In the case of the −10.00 D lens, the appropriate substitutions are

$$-2.00 \text{ D} + (-10.00 \text{ D}) = L'$$

so

$$L' = -12.00 \text{ D}$$

The vergence of light leaving the lens has a dioptric value of −12.00 D. Knowing this we can find the image point. Knowing that

$$L' = \frac{l}{l'}$$

and substituting −12.00 D for L', we get

$$-12.00 = \frac{l}{l'}$$

resulting in

$$l' = -0.083 \text{ m}$$
$$= -8.3 \text{ cm}$$

This tells us that light leaving the minus-powered lens diverges as if it were coming from a point 8.3 cm to the left of the lens.

SPHERES, CYLINDERS, AND SPHEROCYLINDERS

Spheres

All lenses considered thus far have a single point where light is brought to a focus. This is true even if that point must be found by extending diverging rays backward as in the case of minus lenses. When a lens has a single point focus, it is referred to as a *spherical* lens.

The surface curvature of a spherical lens duplicates the surface curvature of a sphere, or ball. A plus spherical surface can be compared with a slice off the side of a glass ball, whereas a minus spherical surface would form an exact mold for a ball of equal radius of curvature (Figure 12-32).

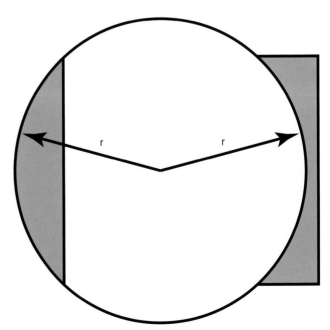

Figure 12-32. A plus spherical surface has a shape as if cut from the side of a sphere, whereas a minus spherical surface is shaped as though molded from a sphere.

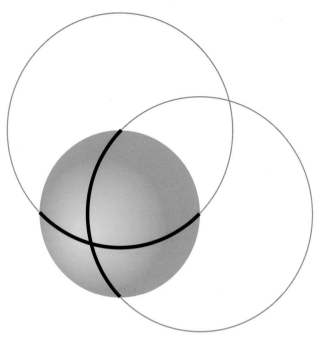

Figure 12-33. A spherical surface has the same radius of curvature in every meridian.

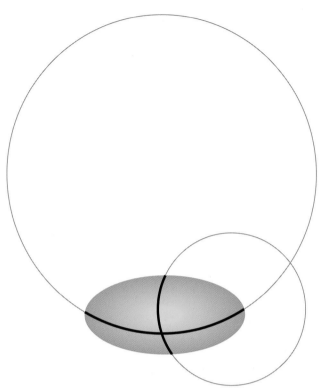

Figure 12-34. A toric surface has different radii of curvature in each of two major meridians.

Spheres Correct for Nearsightedness and Farsightedness

The *sphere* is the most basic type of ophthalmic lens used and is used to correct both nearsightedness and farsightedness.

Plus spheres are used for the correction of *hyperopia*, or *farsightedness*. This occurs when light focuses behind the retina of the eye. A plus lens adds more convergence to incoming light and draws the focus point up onto the retina.

Minus spheres correct for *myopia*, or *nearsightedness*. Myopia occurs when light focuses in front of the retina. A minus lens causes the light to diverge (or converge less) before entering the eye and allows the focal point to drop back onto the retina.

The Problem of Astigmatism

If a refracting surface of the eye is not spherical, the eye cannot bring light to a single point focus on the retina. For example, the front surface of the eye (the cornea) should have a front surface that is spherical, like a spherical ball, such as a basketball (Figure 12-33). But instead it may be shaped more like the surface of a football. There are now two different curves to consider: one being from tip to tip of the football and the other running around the central part at right angles to the first curve (Figure 12-34). Each of these two curves has its own radius of curvature. When this happens, a single point focus is no longer possible.

When an eye has two different curves on a single refracting surface, the condition is known as *astigma-*

tism. A situation can occur that may require a correction in only one of those two refracting meridians.

Cylinder Lenses

A lens that only has power in one meridian can be visualized as one that is cut from the side of a clear glass cylinder (Figure 12-35). A commonly occurring example of something cylindrical in shape is a pillar used to support the porch of a house. A rod is also cylindrical in shape. The lens that optically behaves as if it were cut from the side of a glass cylinder takes on the name of the structure from which it is cut. It is therefore known as a *cylinder*.

Because a cylinder lens can be turned from an up-and-down to a sideways position (or to any orientation between the two), a method for specifying its exact orientation must be chosen. That method is to specify the *axis* direction. The axis of a cylinder can be thought of as being equivalent to the string threaded through the center of a cylindrical bead (Figure 12-36). As this "string" is tilted, the angle of tilt is specified by degrees. Horizontal is considered zero. The angle in degrees the "string" or cylinder axis makes with this horizontal line specifies orientation (Figure 12-37). When the cylinder axis is horizontal, instead of writing 0 degrees, it is conventional to write 180 degrees. Zero and 180 are both on the same horizontal line and, for cylinder axes, are the same. Only degrees 0 through 180 are necessary for complete specification because, as in the example of Figure 12-37, 210 degrees is the same as 30 degrees.

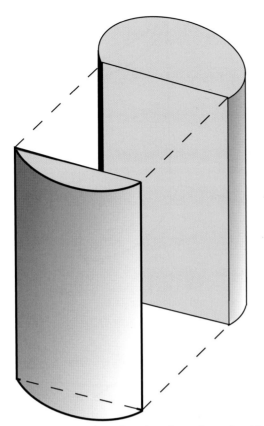

Figure 12-35. A lens shaped as though cut from the side of a clear glass cylinder is referred to as a *cylinder lens*.

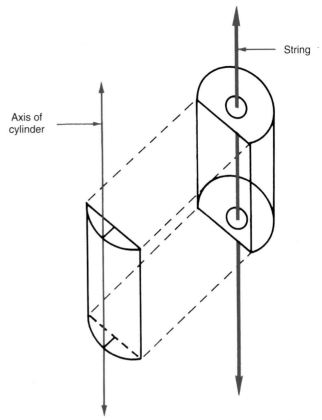

Figure 12-36. The axis of a cylinder is the reference for determining its orientation. The axis of a cylinder parallels an imaginary string running through the center of a cylindrical bead.

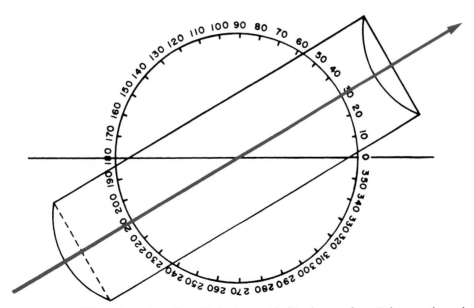

Figure 12-37. The orientation of a cylinder is specified in degrees from 0 degrees through 180 degrees. Specifying beyond 180 degrees is unnecessary because it duplicates 0 degrees through 180. (Zero degrees and 180 degrees are really the same axis. By convention 180 is used instead of 0.) In this figure, the axis of the cylinder shown is oriented at 30 degrees.

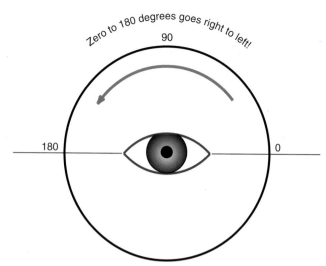

Figure 12-38. When looking at the person wearing spectacle lenses, the cylinder axis degree scale goes counterclockwise, from right to left. This is the same for both right and left eyes.

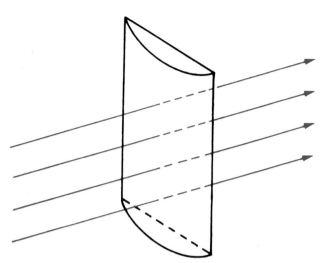

Figure 12-39. Light striking a cylinder along the cylinder axis is not bent. For a plano cylinder, such as the one shown, both surfaces are flat along the axis.

If a person is wearing a cylinder lens in a pair of glasses, the scale is always counterclockwise, or right to left, as shown in Figure 12-38. It is as if the wearer's eye was directly *behind* the scale, looking *through* it. This is true for both right and left lenses.

Optics of a Cylinder Lens

As previously stated, a cylinder can be used to compensate for the eye that does not bring light to a point focus. This can happen if the shape of the cornea in the 90-degree meridian is more curved than it is in the 180-degree meridian. A cylinder lens is suited for correcting this difference because light that strikes the lens along the axis of the lens will pass through that lens undeviated (Figure 12-39).

The meridian of the lens paralleling the cylinder axis is called the *axis meridian*. Along the cylinder axis, both the front and back surfaces of the cylinder are flat. So the cylinder lens has no light refracting power along the axis of the cylinder.

Light striking the cylinder at any other point on the lens will be bent in accordance with the power the curved meridian of the cylinder has (Figure 12-40).

The meridian of the cylinder lens at right angles to its axis has one flat surface and one curved surface. This means the lens has power in this meridian. This meridian is called the *power meridian* of the cylinder. *The axis of a cylinder is always at right angles to the power meridian of the cylinder* (Figure 12-41).

Writing Cylinder Power

As with spherical lenses, the power of a cylinder is also specified in dioptric units. Remember that the full power of the cylinder is only in the meridian opposite the axis

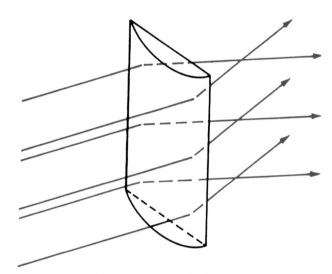

Figure 12-40. Light striking a cylinder at any other location than on the axis will be focused along a line parallel to the cylinder axis and at a constant distance from the lens.

of the cylinder. As a result, when quantifying a cylinder lens, not only must a dioptric power be specified, but also the orientation of the lens axis. For instance, a cylinder may have +3.00 D of power in the horizontal meridian and zero power in the vertical meridian. The specification would therefore be +3.00 D cylinder power with axis at 90 degrees. This may be abbreviated +3.00 × 90, with the x being short for "axis." Because any lens with an axis orientation *must* be a cylinder, it is unnecessary to write "cylinder" or "cyl."

Spherocylindrical Combinations

A cylinder lens compensates for the astigmatic eye that does not bring light to a single point focus. The proper cylinder lens will fully compensate for astigmatism. Unfortunately, much of the time astigmatism may not

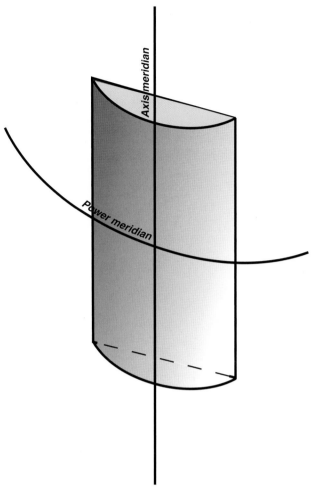

Figure 12-41. For a plano plus cylinder with a flat rear surface, imagine placing a pencil on the front surface of the lens on the cylinder axis. It rests flat on the lens. Because the back of the lens is also flat, it is easy to see that there is no power in the axis meridian. In the power meridian, however, a pencil would not sit flat on the front surface. The pencil would rock because the lens surface is curved. There is power created by the lens curve.

be the only deficiency. Once the light entering an astigmatic eye is corrected to a point focus, it may be found that the point focus is still not on the retina where it should be. The eye may still manifest myopia (nearsightedness) or hyperopia (farsightedness) and additionally need correcting with either a plus or a minus sphere lens. When this happens it becomes necessary to use both sphere and cylinder lenses to correct the person's refractive error. When both sphere and cylinder lenses are required, the result is referred to as a *spherocylinder combination* (Figure 12-42, *A*).

In the case of a spherocylindrical combination, the effect of the two lenses together may be duplicated in the form of a single lens (Figure 12-42, *B*). For example, if both the cylinder and the spherical lenses were plus, such a lens could be ground in a form as if it were cut from the side of a barrel. It can be seen from this that,

as in the football example, there are two separate curves on the same lens surface.

With the addition of a sphere to the cylinder, rays traveling through the axis meridian no longer remain unbent in parallel paths as was shown in Figure 12-39, but now are caused to converge or diverge by the power of the added sphere lens (Figure 12-43, *A*). The rays striking the lens, as was shown in Figure 12-40, will be caused to focus on a line even closer to the lens than before if the added sphere is plus in power as in Figure 12-43, *B*. The combined effect is shown schematically in Figure 12-43, *C*.

Writing Spherocylinder Power

To write the power and orientation characteristics of a spherocylinder combination lens so as to be understandable, it becomes necessary to include sphere power, cylinder power, and cylinder axis. Such a combination is written in exactly this order: sphere, cylinder, and axis orientation in degrees.

If the sphere lens used was +5.00 D in power and the cylinder a +3.00 D lens with the orientation of its axis at 90 degrees, the lens combination could be written as follows:

$$+5.00 \text{ D sph.} \supset +3.00 \text{ D cyl} \times 90$$

(The symbol "$\supset$" means "in combination with.")
The above combination can be further shortened to

$$+5.00 +3.00 \times 90$$

Minus Cylinder Lenses

Cylinder lenses previously described and used in examples have all been plus in power. It is also possible to have a cylinder lens that is minus in power. As with a minus sphere, a minus cylinder lens has an oppositely curved, or concave, refracting surface. The surface is such that it would cradle a cylindrical rod of equal radius (Figure 12-44). It is as if it were molded from a cylindrical rod.

As with the plus cylinder lens, the axis of a minus cylinder parallels the area of equal lens thickness. On a plus cylinder, this is along the line of maximum lens thickness; with the minus cylinder, the axis runs along the line of minimum lens thickness. To continue the analogy, a minus cylinder axis can be thought of as the imaginary string through the center of a cylindrical rod or bead against which a minus cylinder lens could rest. This meridian on the lens where the axis is found is referred to as the *axis meridian*.

There is also no power found in the axis meridian of a minus cylinder; maximum power is found 90 degrees away from it. The meridian of maximum power in a minus cylinder is still referred to as the *power meridian* (Figure 12-45).

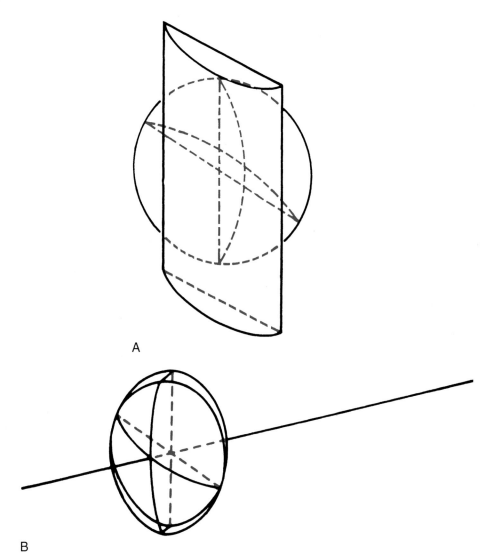

A

B

Figure 12-42. A spherocylinder combination can be thought of as just that—a sphere lens and a cylinder lens placed together **(A).** This combined power combination may be constructed as a single lens with two curves on one surface **(B).**

LENS FORM

Lenses can be made in a variety of forms, with many forms possible for a lens of the same power. One lens form may be steeply curved, whereas another of identical power may appear quite flat. It is also possible to manufacture a lens of a specified power with a cylinder component on either the front or back surface.

Lens Forms a Sphere May Take

The *nominal power* of a lens is the sum of its front and back surface powers. When expressed as an equation, this is $F_1 + F_2 = F_{TOTAL}$. Up to this point, most lenses have been shown with one flat surface of no power and one curved surface. The curved surface makes the lens either plus or minus in power. The flat surface is referred to as *plano*, or without power.

If one surface is plano and the other an outward-curved plus surface (i.e., a *convex* surface), the lens is

referred to as *planoconvex*. If one surface is plano and the other curved inward for minus power (i.e., a *concave* surface), the lens is *planoconcave* (Figure 12-46). If both surfaces are convex or both concave, the lens is *biconvex* or *biconcave* (Figure 12-47). This form does not specify that both surfaces necessarily be equal in power. If this were the case, the lens could be further classified as *equiconvex* or *equiconcave* (Figure 12-48). For example, a biconvex lens of +4.00 D of power could have surface powers, such as the following:

$$F_1 + F_2 = F_T$$
$$(+2.00 \text{ D}) + (+2.00 \text{ D}) = +4.00 \text{ D}$$
$$(+3.00 \text{ D}) + (+1.00 \text{ D}) = +4.00 \text{ D}$$
$$(+0.50 \text{ D}) + (+3.50 \text{ D}) = +4.00 \text{ D}$$

It is also possible to have a lens with one side convex (plus) and the other concave (minus). This is the most

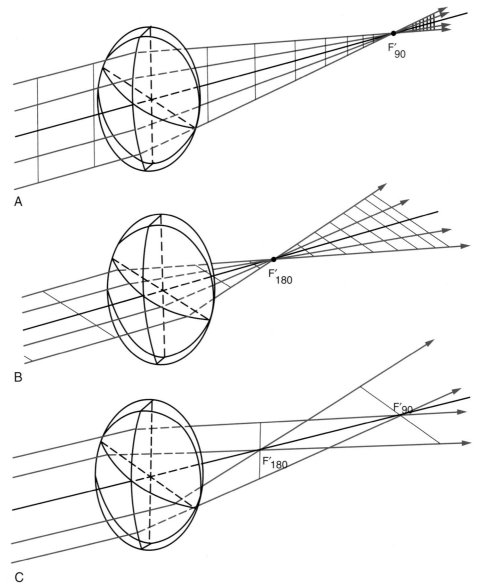

Figure 12-43. This lens is the same spherocylinder lens combination as was shown in Figure 12-42. **A,** Rays previously unbent in the 90-degree cylinder axis meridian are now brought to a focus because of the addition of a plus sphere component. **B,** Rays in the 180-degree power meridian of the cylinder that were previously brought to a line focus by the cylinder are now refracted more by the additional plus sphere power. **C,** The net effect of both sphere and cylinder components results in two line foci.

common ophthalmic lens and is referred to as a *meniscus** lens (Figure 12-49). The same +4.00 D lens power might then have any one of the following forms, which represent only a fraction of the possibilities.

$$F_1 + F_2 = F_T$$
$$(+7.00\ D) + (-3.00\ D) = +4.00\ D$$
$$(+8.00\ D) + (-4.00\ D) = +4.00\ D$$
$$(+10.00\ D) + (-6.00\ D) = +4.00\ D$$

---

* Originally a meniscus lens was one that had a 6.00 D surface curve either on the front (+6.00 D) or on the back (−6.00 D). Now it has come to mean a lens with a convex front surface and a concave minus surface.

Lens Forms a Cylinder May Take

Even a pure cylinder may take several forms. These forms are limited only in that one meridian must have a net power of zero and the other a net power equal to the cylinder value. To keep the two meridians of a cylinder separate, it is helpful to use the concept of a power cross. A *power cross* is a schematic representation of the two major meridians of a lens or lens surface. For a pure cylinder, these two meridians, at right angles to each other, are the axis meridian and the power meridian. A +4.00 D × 90 cylinder is schematically represented on a power cross in Figure 12-50.

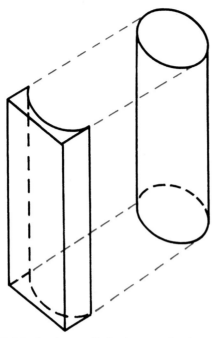

Figure 12-44. A minus cylinder lens can be thought of as if molded from a cylindrical rod.

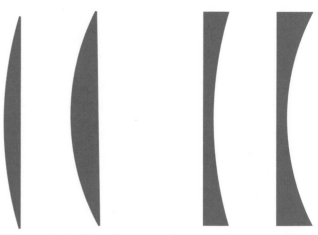

Figure 12-46. Two planoconvex lenses are shown on the left, two planoconcave on the right.

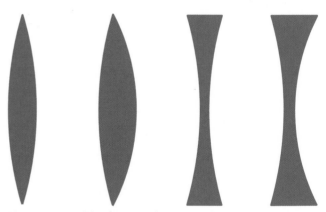

Figure 12-47. Two biconvex lenses are shown on the left, two biconcave on the right.

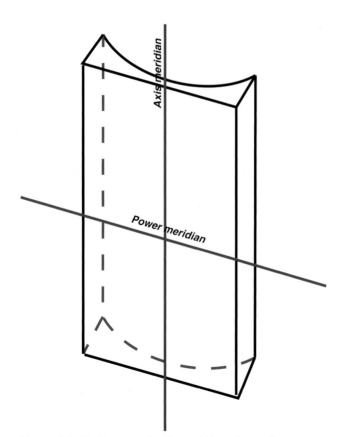

Figure 12-45. Power and axis meridians shown for a minus cylinder.

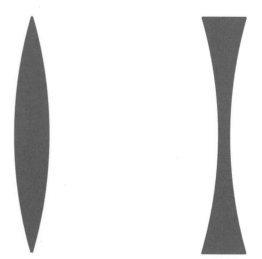

Figure 12-48. Equiconvex and equiconcave lenses must have the same curvature on both front and back surfaces.

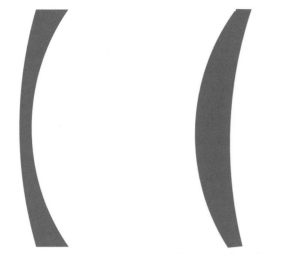

Figure 12-49. A meniscus lens has a plus (convex) surface on the front and a concave (minus) surface on the back.

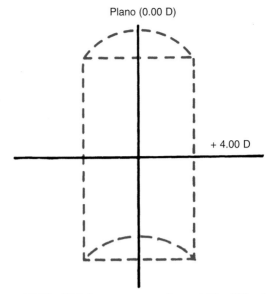

Figure 12-50. This is a power cross for a +4.00 × 090 cylinder lens. The outlined cylinder is for reference only, never appearing on an actual power cross.

Figure 12-51. For this lens, the front surface is the toric surface with two different lens powers. The back surface is spherical, so both 90-degree and 180-degree back surface meridians have the same power. The total power of the lens can be found by adding corresponding surface meridians together—90 with 90 and 180 with 180.

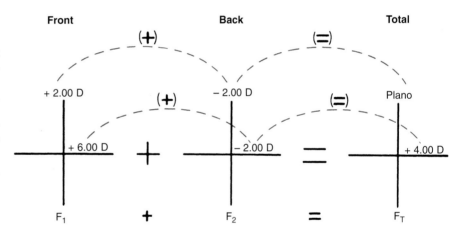

In the "original," or most easily visualized form, this lens has two front curves. One is a plano surface "curve" of zero power in the 90-degree meridian, the other a +4.00 D powered curve in the 180-degree meridian. The back surface is flat, or plano, in both meridians. In this lens form, since the back surface has zero power, the front surface creates the total power of the lens.

Suppose, however, that the back surface of the lens has a power of –2.00 D in both meridians. It is still possible to construct a cylinder lens with the same total power.

For example, suppose the front surface powers are as follows:

$$F_1 \text{ at } 90 = +2.00 \text{ D}$$
$$F_1 \text{ at } 180 = +6.00 \text{ D}$$

With the back surface power of $F_2 = -2.00$ D, the total lens power is still +4.00 × 90. Figure 12-51 shows a series of three power crosses—one for the front surface, one for the back surface, and a third power cross for the total lens power. Both 90-degree surface meridians are added together to obtain the total lens power in the 90-degree meridian, and both 180-degree meridians are added together to obtain the total lens power in the 180-degree meridian.

When a lens has two separate curves on a surface, neither being plano but both having power, the surface is said to be *toric*.

Example **12-10**

Suppose a lens has a toric front surface. F_1 at 90 is +4.00 D, and F_1 at 180 is +6.00 D. If the back surface has a surface power of –4.00 D, what is the total power of the lens?

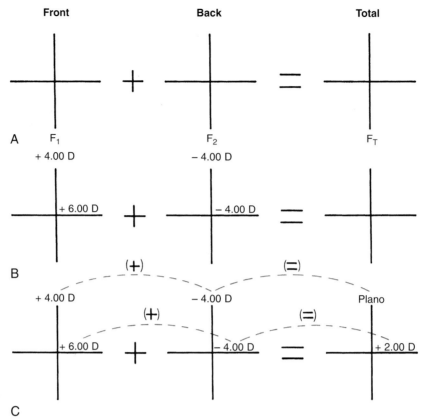

Front	Back	Total

A F_1 +4.00 D F_2 −4.00 D F_T

B   +6.00 D   +4.00 D   (+)   −4.00 D   −4.00 D   (=)   Plano

C   +6.00 D   (+)   −4.00 D   (=)   +2.00 D

Figure 12-52. Steps in solving lens form power problems consist of: **A,** drawing the appropriate series of crosses; **B,** writing all known lens powers on the crosses; and **C,** solving for the remaining unknown factors.

Solution

The simplest method of solving the problem is to first draw three empty power crosses representing F_1, F_2, and F_T (Figure 12-52, *A*). Next the known component may be written in at the proper meridians for F_1 and F_2 (Figure 12-52, *B*). Surface powers are then added together to obtain the total power of the lens (Figure 12-52, *C*). Last, these powers are taken off the power cross and written in abbreviated form. In this case a +2.00 × 90 cylinder is obtained.

Plus and Minus Cylinder Form Lenses

When the lens obtains its cylinder power from a difference in power between two *front* surface meridians (i.e., a toric front surface lens), the lens is said to be ground in *plus cylinder form.* If, on the other hand, a lens has a cylinder component, but the cylinder power is a result of a difference in power between two *back* surface meridians (i.e., a toric rear surface lens), it is a *minus cylinder form lens.* In other words, the plus cylinder form lens has two curves on the front and one spherical curve on the back, whereas a minus cylinder form lens has one spherical curve on the front and two curves, making up the cylinder component, on the back.

Example **12-11**

If a lens has dimensions of F_1 = +6.00 D, F_2 at 90 = −8.00 D, and F_2 at 180 = −6.00 D, what form does the lens have and what is its total power?

Solution

Because the cylinder component is on F_2, the back surface, by definition the lens is minus cylinder in form. To find the total lens power, the front and back surface power crosses are mapped out and added together (Figure 12-53).

F_1 at 90 = +6.00 D	F_1 at 180 = +6.00 D
F_2 at 90 = −8.00 D	F_2 at 180 = −6.00 D
F_T at 90 = −2.00 D	F_T at 180 = 0.00 D (plano)

The power of this cylinder is at 90, which means that the axis is at 180. In abbreviated form the lens may be written −2.00 × 180.

Lens Forms a Spherocylinder May Take

Minus Cylinder Form

As seen earlier, either a sphere or a cylinder lens may be constructed in several different forms, all having the

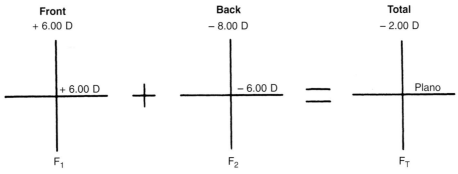

Figure 12-53. The lens represented on this power cross series is minus cylinder in form since the toric surface is on the back of the lens.

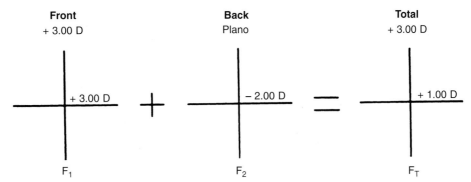

Figure 12-54. Front and back curves and total lens power for a spherocylinder lens.

same total power (F_T). In the same way it is also possible to construct a spherocylinder lens in several different forms, all having the same total spherocylinder power.

Example **12-12**

A lens has the following form:

A spherical front surface power (F_1) of +3.00
A cylindrical back surface where
F_2 at 90 equals 0 and
F_2 at 180 equals −2.00 D

Is the lens constructed in plus or minus cylinder form? What is the power of the lens?

Solution

To tell if the lens is constructed in plus or minus cylinder form, we need only look to see which surface has two powers. If the cylinder power comes from the front surface, the lens is plus cylinder in form. If the cylinder power is on the back of the lens, the lens is minus cylinder in form. This lens has the cylinder on the back and is a minus cylinder form lens.

To find the power of the lens, draw three sets of power crosses—one for the front surface, one for the back surface, and one for the total power of the lens. Enter the front and back surface powers on the front and back surface power crosses as shown in Figure 12-54.

Just looking at the powers entered on the first and second power crosses tell us that this spherocylinder lens will have a sphere power of +3.00 D and a cylinder power of −2.00 × 90. This becomes apparent because the lens form is constructed as if a plano convex sphere lens of +3.00 D front surface power with a flat back surface were placed flush against the flat front surface of a plano minus cylinder lens. So the spherocylinder combination could be written as +3.00 sph −2.00 cyl × 90, or in the more commonly used abbreviated form, as +3.00 −2.00 × 90.

However, very few problems lend themselves to such obvious interpretation. So now the same problem will be done in the more conventional manner.

Once front and back surface powers are entered on the power crosses, add the front and back surface 90-degree meridians together.

$$(+3.00) + 0.00 = +3.00$$

The +3.00 D power is entered on the 90-degree meridian for the total lens power.

The same is done for the 180-degree meridian.

$$(+3.00) + (−2.00) = +1.00$$

The +1.00 D power is entered on the 180-degree meridian for the total lens power.

In a pure cylinder lens having no spherical component, since one meridian is zero, the other meridian shows

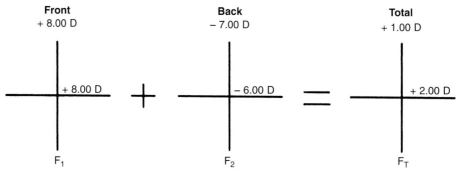

Figure 12-55. This spherocylinder lens is a minus cylinder form lens.

the exact cylinder power. The cylinder power is then the difference between the two meridians. In the case of a spherocylinder lens where *both* meridians have power, the cylinder power is still the numerical difference between the two meridians. In the example, the difference between +1.00 and +3.00 is 2.00. This means that the cylinder power is 2.00 D. It may be either a +2.00 D or a –2.00 D cylinder, depending upon how the prescription is to be written.

Power can be interpreted from information given on a power cross as follows: If the prescription is to be written with the cylinder as a minus cylinder (in minus cylinder form), the greater plus (or least minus) value is the sphere power. In this case the +3.00 is the sphere power because it is the most plus.

Since the cylinder value is 2.00 D less than the +3.00 D sphere, the *difference* is the power of the cylinder (–2.00). The abbreviated minus cylinder form for this lens combination then becomes +3.00 –2.00 × 90. It is helpful to remember that *the cylinder axis always falls in the meridian that represents the spherical power of the lens.*

___

Example **12-13**

Suppose a lens has a front surface power of +8.00 D. The back surface power is –7.00 D in the 90-degree meridian and –6.00 D in the 180-degree meridian. What is the total power of the lens when written in minus cylinder form?

Solution

Again, draw three power crosses for front surface, back surface, and total lens power. Enter the +8.00 D on both meridians of the front surface power cross. A spherical surface always has the same power in every meridian.

Enter the back surface values on the second surface power cross as shown in Figure 12-55.

Now add the 90-degree powers together and the 180-degree powers together to get the total as again shown in Figure 12-55.

To write the resultant lens formula in minus cylinder form, the most plus meridian becomes the sphere component (+2.00). The difference between the two meridians is l.00. The prescription, written in minus cylinder form, becomes +2.00 –1.00 × 180.

Plus Cylinder Form

A minus cylinder form lens gets the cylinder power from the back surface of the lens. A plus cylinder form lens has the cylinder power difference on the front surface. So a plus cylinder form lens may be constructed such that the front surface is toric and the back surface spherical. A lens with the same power may be constructed in plus cylinder form or minus cylinder form.

___

Example **12-14**

Find the power of a lens having a toric front surface of F_1 at 90 equal to +7.00 D and F_1 at 180 equal to +8.00 D. The power of the back surface is –6.00 D. Write the results in plus cylinder form.

Solution

The data are entered on a set of power crosses shown in Figure 12-56, and total power (F_T) is calculated. Notice that the power cross reflects the same results as were found for the minus cylinder lens of Figure 12-55, even though the lens has a different form.

The difference between the two power meridians for the total lens power is 1.00 D. However, if we are to write this lens as a plus cylinder lens, we need to write the cylinder power as +1.00 instead of –1.00. So which power on the power cross is the sphere power? Is it the +1.00 D power or the +2.00 D power?

Expressing the written lens power in plus cylinder form means that the cylinder value is "in addition to" the value of the sphere. The value of the sphere is therefore the *least plus* (or most minus) of the two values. In Figure 12-56 this is the +1.00 D. The second meridian is 1.00 D greater than the sphere value, so the cylinder is +1.00 D.

By definition the axis of a cylinder is 90 degrees away from the cylinder power meridian (i.e., in the sphere power meridian). In our example, the plus cylinder axis is at 90 degrees. The lens prescription written in plus cylinder form will therefore be

+1.00 D sph in combination with +1.00 cyl × 90

or

+1.00 +1.00 × 90.

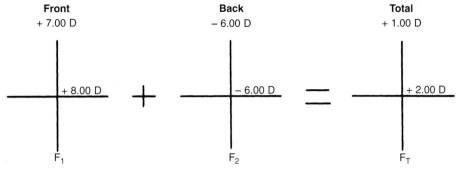

Figure 12-56. The spherocylinder lens shown here is in plus cylinder form. Notice that this figure and Figure 12-55 have the same F_T values despite differences in cylinder form.

Toric Transposition

It has been shown that it is possible to have a spherocylindrical lens of the same power expressed in at least two different lens forms and written in two different ways, either the plus or the minus cylinder form of prescription writing. Most logically one would assume that the plus cylinder form of prescription writing would be used exclusively for lenses with a toric front surface and the minus cylinder form of prescription writing for lenses with the toric surface on the back. This, however, is not the case. Instead of indicating the location of the toric surface for the prescribed lens, the written form usually only indicates the type of lenses used during the examination process. In the past, optometrists wrote prescriptions in minus cylinder form, and ophthalmologists wrote prescriptions in plus cylinder form. This is no longer universally true. However, prescriptions of both forms are commonly seen.

However, there is a high consistency in how spectacle lenses are made. Almost every lens used for prescription eyewear in the United States has the toric surface on the back and is thus a minus cylinder form lens.

Because lens prescriptions may be written in either plus or minus cylinder form, it is necessary to be able to convert or *transpose* from one form to another. This process is known as *toric transposition*.

Steps for transposing from one form to the other are as follows:
1. Add the sphere and cylinder values to obtain the new sphere value.
2. Change the sign of the cylinder (plus to minus or minus to plus).
3. Change the axis by 90 degrees. (This can be done by addition *or* subtraction since the end result is the same. The answer for the axis, however, must be from 1 to 180 degrees. An answer of 190 degrees, for example, is not acceptable.)

Example **12-15**

Transpose the written minus cylinder lens prescription of +2.00 −1.00 × 180 into plus cylinder form.

Solution

1. The sphere and cyl values are added: (+2.00) + (−1.00) = +1.00. The new sphere value is +1.00 D.
2. Change the sign of the cyl. The new cyl becomes +1.00 D.
3. Change the axis by 90 degrees. If 90 degrees is added to 180 degrees, a value of 270 degrees is obtained. If 90 degrees is subtracted from 180 degrees a value of 90 degrees is obtained. It can be seen that a cylinder axis actually runs through *both* 90 and 270. By convention only values between 0 and 180 are used, making 90 the appropriate value. The new cyl axis is 90.
4. The new written lens form is +1.00 +1.00 × 90.

Crossed-Cylinder Form

Another possible abbreviated form of prescription writing is the *crossed-cylinder form*. This form is never used to write a prescription for spectacle lenses. However, an understanding of this form of prescription writing aids in a more complete understanding of lenses. The crossed-cylinder form of prescription writing is also the way that keratometer readings are written when measuring the front surface power of the cornea for contact lens purposes.

To understand the crossed-cylinder form of prescription writing, think through the following:
- If two spherical lenses are placed together, a new sphere power results from the sum of the two.
- If a sphere and a cylinder are placed together, a spherocylinder results.
- If two cylinders are placed together with axes 90 degrees apart from one another, a sphere, a cylinder, or a spherocylinder may result.

Suppose, for example, +1.00 × 180 and +2.00 × 90 lenses are placed together. These are both cylinders and their axes are "crossed" in relationship to one another. In abbreviated crossed-cylinder form this reads

$$+1.00 \times 180 \supset +2.00 \times 090$$

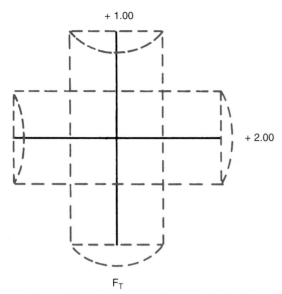

+ 1.00

+ 2.00

F_T

Figure 12-57. Writing lens power in crossed-cylinder form is easier when the cylinder components are visualized on a power cross. In crossed-cylinder form, the prescription represented would be +2.00 × 090/+1.00 × 180.

or

$$+1.00 \times 180/+2.00 \times 090$$

This would be spoken as "plus one axis one-eighty in combination with plus two axis ninety." On a power cross this would appear as shown in Figure 12-57. Note that the combination of these two crossed cylinders results in the same total power as shown in Figures 12-55 and 12-56. Because all three of these lenses have the same total power, these two crossed cylinders can be written in crossed-cylinder form, plus cylinder form, or minus cylinder form.

The simplest and most direct method of transposing from plus or minus cylinder form into crossed-cylinder form is to first place the powers on a power cross. In that form, the power observed for each major meridian is the power of one of the two "crossed cylinders." The location of the axis for each of these two cylinders is 90 degrees away from its meridian of power.

An Alternate Crossed-Cylinder Form
The normal way of writing a lens prescription in crossed-cylinder form is done just like writing a plano cylinder. When the +1.00 × 180 and +2.00 × 90 lenses were placed together in the example just given, the crossed-cylinder combination was written as

$$+1.00 \times 180/+2.00 \times 090$$

The powers were referenced to the axis meridians because the lens was considered as if it was two plus cylinders combined as was shown in Figure 12-57. Some-

times the powers are referenced to their own meridians instead. The +1.00 cylinder has power at or in the 90-degree meridian. The +2.00 cylinder has power at or in the 180-degree meridian. So the power could be written as

$$+1.00 @ 090/+2.00 @ 180$$

This is spoken as "plus one at ninety in combination with plus two at one-eighty." This form is seen in contact lens practice when reading or writing the keratometer reading of the front surface of the cornea. Of course the powers are considerably higher and might look something like this:

$$+42.50 @ 090/+43.75 @ 180$$

The Spherical Equivalent
A spherocylinder lens will correct for astigmatism and myopia or hyperopia. If it was necessary to correct a nearsighted or farsighted person who also has astigmatism, but there were no cylinder lenses available, what would be the best correction using only a sphere lens? Looking back to Figure 12-43, *C*, we see how a spherocylinder lens has two focal lines. If only a sphere lens is to be used, the best lens will be one that has a focal point at a dioptric value that is halfway* between these two focal lines. (The location that is halfway between the two dioptric values of the spherocylinder lens is called the *circle of least confusion*. The rays of light do not come to a point focus, but instead form a circle at this location.) That compromise sphere lens is called the *spherical equivalent*.

How to Find the Spherical Equivalent
To find the spherical equivalent of a spherocylinder lens:
1. Take half the value of the cylinder and
2. Add it to the sphere power.
   In other words, as a formula the spherical equivalent is

$$\text{Sphere} + \frac{\text{Cylinder}}{2} = \text{Spherical Equivalent}$$

---

*The halfway location is not at the physical halfway point between the two focal lines. Instead it will be at a point that is based on the dioptric value halfway in between. For example, a lens with a power of +1.00 +2.00 x 180 has two focal lines—one for the +1.00 D power meridian, the other for the +3.00 D power meridian. These lines are at 100 cm and 33.3 cm from the lens. The physical halfway point would be 66.7 cm from the lens. However, the location of the circle of least confusion is determined by the spherical equivalent of the lens. The spherical equivalent is +2.00 D. The focal point of +2.00 is at 50 cm, not 66.7 cm. Therefore the circle of least confusion is at 50 cm.

Example **12-16**

What is the spherical equivalent for this lens?

$$+3.00 - 1.00 \times 180$$

Solution

Using the formula for the spherical equivalent we have:

$$\text{Spherical Equivalent} = (+3.00) + \frac{-1.00}{2}$$
$$= (+3.00) + (-0.50)$$
$$= +2.50\,\text{D}$$

Example **12-17**

What is the spherical equivalent for a lens having a power of −4.25 −1.25 × 135?

Solution

Again using the formula we find the spherical equivalent as:

$$\text{Spherical Equivalent} = (-4.25) + \frac{-1.25}{2}$$
$$= (-4.25) + (-0.625)$$
$$= -3.625\,\text{D}$$

Proficiency Test

(Answers can be found in the back of the book.)

1. A flashlight is shone on a pond at an angle. The angle of incidence of the beam is 40 degrees. Some of the light is reflected by the surface, and some is refracted. To the nearest degree, what are the angles of reflection and refraction? (Water has a refractive index of 4/3, or 1.33.)
    a. angle of reflection = 59 degrees; angle of refraction = 40 degrees
    b. angle of reflection = 50 degrees; angle of refraction = 29 degrees
    c. angle of reflection = 40 degrees; angle of refraction = 59 degrees
    d. angle of reflection = 40 degrees; angle of refraction = 29 degrees

2. A scuba diver swimming underwater shines a flashlight up out of the water (refractive index of 4/3, or 1.33). The beam of light strikes the surface at an angle of incidence of 37 degrees. Is the beam bent toward or away from the normal (perpendicular) to the surface? Just what is the angle of refraction (to the nearest degree)?
    a. away, 27 degrees
    b. toward, 53 degrees
    c. toward, 27 degrees
    d. away, 53 degrees

3. A ray of light strikes a slab of clear plastic at an angle of incidence of 8 degrees. The plastic has an index of refraction of 1.5. If the plastic slab is 5 cm thick with parallel sides, assuming the surrounding medium is air, with what angle does the light leave the plastic after passing through it?
    a. 5.0 degrees
    b. 5.3 degrees
    c. 8.0 degrees
    d. 12.0 degrees

4. A lens has a focal length of +66.67 cm. What is its power?
    a. +1.50 D
    b. +3.00 D
    c. +6.67 D
    d. +0.02 D

5. If a lens has a power −7.12 D, what is its focal length?
    a. +13 cm
    b. −0.1404 m
    c. +14.04 cm
    d. 5 in

6. A +2.50 D lens has a focal length of +40 cm. In this particular instance, if the power of the lens is doubled, the focal length:
    a. is doubled.
    b. is halved.
    c. is quartered.
    d. remains the same.

7. Light that enters a lens in parallel rays produces a virtual image 0.50 m in front of the lens. What is the power of the lens?
   a. +0.50 D
   b. –0.50 D
   c. –2.00 D
   d. +2.00 D
   e. +5.00 D

8. A lens of refractive index 1.50 has a radius of curvature of +8.00 cm. To the nearest 0.125 D, what power does the lens surface have in air?
   a. +0.50 D
   b. +6.25 D
   c. –0.62 D
   d. –3.25 D

9. An object is located –15 cm from a –15.00 D lens. How far from the lens is the image point located?
   a. +1 cm
   b. –1.2 cm
   c. +12 cm
   d. –1 cm
   e. –12.00 cm

10. A lens has a surface power in air of +3.50 D. If the radius of curvature is 20 cm, what index of refraction does the lens have?
    a. 1.33
    b. 1.50
    c. 1.60
    d. 1.70
    e. 1.80

11. An object is positioned 50 cm in front of a –4.00 D lens. How far from the lens will the image of this object be?
    a. +50 cm
    b. –50 cm
    c. –16.67 cm
    d. –19.33 cm

12. A lens has +2.50 D of power and causes an image to form at +33.33 cm. Where is the object point located?
    a. +2.00 m
    b. –50 cm
    c. –18 cm
    d. +18 cm

13. A cylinder lens has a power of +2.00 D and an axis orientation of 25 degrees. Where is the meridian of minimum power?
    a. 25 degrees
    b. 115 degrees
    c. 70 degrees
    d. 160 degrees

14. For a plano cylinder, light passes through the _____ meridian undeviated.
    a. power
    b. axis
    c. major
    d. minor

15. An object is situated at normal reading distance (i.e., –40 cm away from the lens.) If this lens has a power of –2.25 D, with what vergence will the light leave the lens?
    a. +2.25 D
    b. –0.25 D
    c. +0.25 D
    d. –4.75 D

16. If an object is –33.33 cm from a +4.50 D lens, where will the light come to a focus?
    a. 66.67 cm to the right of the lens
    b. 13.33 cm to the right of the lens
    c. 33.33 cm to the right of the lens
    d. 33.33 cm to the left of the lens

17. An image forms 50 cm to the right of a +10.00 D lens. Where was the object?
    a. –8.33 cm from the lens
    b. +8.33 cm from the lens
    c. –12.5 cm from the lens
    d. –10 cm from the lens
    e. At the plane of the lens

18. A lens surface has a power of –5.00 D in air. What power does the lens surface have in water? (Index of lens = 1.523; index of water = 1.333.)
    a. –1.81 D
    b. –1.94 D
    c. +1.94 D
    d. –0.02 D

19. A lens has a refractive index of 1.523. If the front surface has a radius of curvature of 22 cm, what is the Curvature of the surface?
    a. 2.38 m^{-1}
    b. 4.55 m^{-1}
    c. 0.02 m^{-1}
    d. 0.05 m^{-1}

20. F_1 of a lens is +3.25 D, and F_2 is +3.25 D. The lens may be said to be:
    a. biconvex.
    b. meniscus.
    c. equiconvex.
    d. both a and c.
    e. both b and c.

21. If F_1 = +8.00 D and F_2 = –8.00 D, the lens is:
    a. equiconvex.
    b. equiconcave.
    c. planoconvex.
    d. biconvex.
    e. meniscus.

22. A –2.00 D thin lens having a front surface power equal to +6.00 D could be described as:
    a. equiconcave.
    b. biconvex.
    c. meniscus.
    d. planoconcave.
    e. planoconvex.

23. In the transposition process, which of the following is an *incorrect* step?
    a. Subtract the sphere from the cylinder value to obtain the new sphere value.
    b. Change the sign of the cylinder (plus to minus, minus to plus).
    c. Change the axis by 90 degrees.
    d. None of the above.
    e. Two of the choices in *a*, *b*, and *c* are *incorrect* steps.

24. Transpose the following prescriptions as indicated:
    a. +3.50 –1.25 × 012 into *plus* cylinder form.
    b. –0.50 +1.00 × 075 into *minus* cylinder form.
    c. –0.50 +1.00 × 075 into crossed-cylinder form.

25. A power cross has a power of –4.00 D in the 90-degree meridian and –1.00 D in the 180-degree meridian. This lens can be written in prescription form as:
    a. –4.00 –1.00 × 180.
    b. –3.00 –1.00 × 090.
    c. –4.00 –3.00 × 080.
    d. –1.00 –3.00 × 180.

26. The prescription pl –3.00 × 010 can also be written as:
    a. pl +3.00 × 100.
    b. +3.00 –3.00 × 100.
    c. –3.00 +3.00 × 100.
    d. +3.00 × 10/–3.00 × 100.
    e. None of the above.

27. Transpose the following Rx to two other forms:

    +l.25 × 165/–3.00 × 075.

28. Transpose the following Rx to two other forms:

    +0.75 –1.25 × 013.

29. What is the spherical equivalent for a spherocylinder lens with a power of –6.00 –1.00 × 180?
    a. –5.50 D
    b. –6.50 D
    c. –6.00 D
    d. –7.00 D
    e. –7.50 D

Challenge Question

30. Two thin lenses in air are separated by a distance of 80 cm. Both are +5.00 D in power. An image point formed by the first lens becomes the object point for the second. If an object is –40 cm from the first lens, where will the image point for the second lens be?
    a. +40 cm to the right of the second lens
    b. +13.33 cm to the right of the second lens
    c. –66.67 cm to the left of the second lens
    d. +28.57 cm to the right of the second lens

CHAPTER **13**

Lens Curvature and Thickness

A major factor in how a lens will perform depends upon how the lens is shaped. Shape is defined by how the lens is curved, starting with the base curve. The chapter begins by looking at how lenses are shaped, and how that shape, or curvature, is measured. Lens curvature and lens thickness are related. To know how a lens with a given prescription will look in a frame, an understanding of lens thickness is needed. The latter part of the chapter explains how lens thickness can be predicted from lens power.

CATEGORIES OF OPHTHALMIC LENSES

Ophthalmic lenses may be divided into the following three broad categories:
- Single vision lenses
- Segmented multifocal lenses
- Progressive addition lenses

Single Vision Lenses

Single vision lenses are the most basic type of lens. These lenses have the same power over the entire surface of the lens. Single vision lenses are used when the same optical power is needed for both distance and near vision. They are also used when a person requires no prescription for distance, but needs reading glasses. Whenever possible single vision lenses are edged from lenses kept in stock at the laboratory. Because these lenses are finished optically to the correct power on both the front and back surfaces, they are called *finished lenses*. Finished lenses are also referred to as *uncuts* because they have not yet been "cut" to the correct shape and size (Figure 13-1, *A*). When single vision lenses are in uncut form and do not require that a surface power be ground onto the lens, they are called *stock single vision lenses*.

A stock single vision uncut lens is less expensive than a custom surfaced lens. However, if the stock lens is too small for the frame, then a stock single vision lens will not work. Instead the lens must be produced in the surfacing section of the optical laboratory. The surfacing laboratory puts surface power on the lens. They start with a lens having only one surface that is ready to use, or "finished." This is usually the front surface. The laboratory must grind and polish the second surface to the required power. A lens with only one of the two surfaces

finished is called a *semifinished* lens because it is only half finished. The prefix *semi-* means half (Figure 13-1, *B*).

Finished uncut and semifinished lenses have not been edged. Before a lens has been edged, it is called a *lens blank*.

Segmented Multifocal Lenses

Segmented multifocal lenses have more than one power. Each power is located in a distinct area of the lens bordered clearly by a visible demarcation line. When two different areas exist, the lens is called a *bifocal* (Figure 13-2, *A*). When three areas exist, the lens is called a *trifocal** (Figure 13-2, *B*).

Multifocal lenses may be created in one of several ways. Here are the two ways most often used:
1. Multifocals may be individually ground and polished to power by a surfacing laboratory from a semifinished lens blank.
2. Multifocals may be individually cast molded to the prescribed power. Cast molding creates the lens from a liquid resin material. It is the same process used to make both plastic semifinished lenses and stock single vision plastic lenses. Cast molding multifocal lenses to power skips the semifinished lens stage. Cast molding to power may be done by a larger wholesale facility or, if equipment is available, on a small scale in conjunction with a finishing laboratory.

Progressive Addition Lenses

Progressive addition lenses are used as an alternative to a segmented multifocal lens. They have distance power in the upper half of the lens. Lens power gradually increases as the wearer looks down and inward to view near objects.

With exception of some high-end product, progressive addition lenses are prepared for the finishing laboratory in the same way as segmented multifocal lenses.

---

*There are a few exceptions. For example, a lens with a near section at the bottom and a second near section at the top will have three sections, but is a double segment occupational lens and not a trifocal.

304

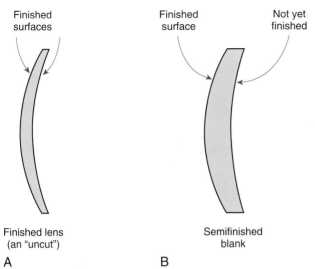

Figure 13-1. **A,** A finished lens is also referred to as an *uncut*. Most single vision lenses are premanufactured to power as finished lenses and are also referred to as *stock single vision lenses*. **B,** Most any type of lens of any material may be made beginning with a semifinished lens.

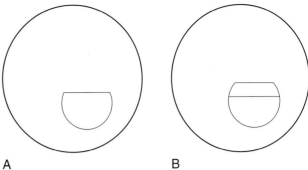

Figure 13-2. When a lens has a different power for near vision than distance vision, the lens area is divided between distance and near powers. **A,** A segment area for near vision is placed within the distance power lens. A lens with two different powers is a bifocal lens. **B,** Two segment areas are included: one for intermediate viewing and one for near viewing. This type of lens is a trifocal lens. Both lenses are flat-top-style multifocals.

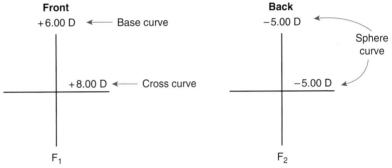

Figure 13-3. The base curve of a plus cylinder form single vision lens is the weaker curve on the front surface.

BASE CURVES

Single Vision Lens Curves

In constructing an ophthalmic lens, one of the lens curves of one surface becomes the basis from which the others are determined. This beginning curve, on which the lens power is based, is called the *base curve*. In single vision prescription ophthalmic lenses, the base curve is always found on the front surface.

- *For spherical lenses:* In the case of spherical lenses, the front sphere curve is the base curve.
- *For plus cylinder form spherocylinder lenses:* If the lens is in plus cylinder form, there are two curves on the front. The base curve is the weaker, or flatter, of the two curves. The other curve becomes the *cross curve* (Figure 13-3). The back surface is quite naturally referred to as the *sphere curve* since it is spherical.
- *For minus cylinder form spherocylinder lenses:* If the lens is in minus cylinder form, the front spherical curve is the base curve. The weaker back-

surface curve is known as the *toric base curve;* the stronger back-surface curve is known as the *cross curve* (Figure 13-4). Optical laboratories refer to the toric base curve of a minus cylinder form lens as the *back base curve.* (On a plus cylinder form lens the "base curve" and "toric base curve" are the same curve.)

Example **13-1**

If a lens has a power of +3.00 − 2.00 × 180 and is to be ground in plus cylinder form, what front and back curves would be used if a base curve of +6.00 D were chosen?

Solution

The way to solve this is summarized in Box 13-1. We will solve the problem using these steps for plus cylinder form lenses.

1. A series of power crosses should be drawn. The first power cross is for the front surface, the second power cross for the back surface, and the third power cross for

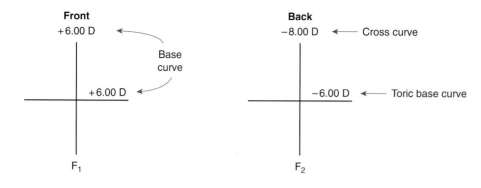

Figure 13-4. For a minus cylinder form single vision lens, the base curve is the front sphere curve.

How to Find Lens Curves if Lens Power and Base Curve Are Known

FINDING LENS CURVES IN PLUS CYLINDER FORM
1. Make front surface, back surface, and total lens power crosses.
2. Put the total lens power on the power cross.
3. Locate the base curve meridian. (Look on the F_T power cross. Find the least plus meridian. If the front surface has plus power, this least plus meridian will correspond to the base curve meridian on the front surface.)
4. Find the back curve power for that same meridian.
5. The other back surface meridian will be the same power.
6. Find the front cross curve power from the total power and the back surface power. ($F_1 + F_2 = F_T$)
7. Check for cylinder accuracy on the front surface to be sure you chose the correct base curve meridian.

FINDING LENS CURVES IN MINUS CYLINDER FORM
1. Make front surface, back surface, and total lens power crosses.
2. Put the total lens power on the power cross.
3. Put the base curve on the front surface power cross.
4. Algebraically find the back surface curves.

---

the total lens power. All initially given data should be entered on the power crosses. Here is how it is done.

2. The total lens power can be placed on the last of the three power crosses. This is the F_T or total lens power cross shown in Figure 13-5, *A*. Here the sphere power corresponds to the 180-degree axis meridian since there is no cylinder power in the cylinder axis meridian. When writing spherocylinder lens power on a power cross, enter the sphere power on the axis meridian. Then add the cylinder power to the sphere. In this case we add a −2.00 to a +3.00 to get +1.00.

3. Now we can enter the base curve on the front surface. But because the cylinder power is on the front, on which meridian will the +6.00 D curve be found? The base curve is, by definition, the *weaker* of the two front

curves. Therefore it corresponds to the meridian of least plus power. In the example, we look at the powers on the last power cross and find that the least plus is in the 90-degree meridian. Therefore +6.00 D is entered on the F_1 power cross at 90, as shown in Figure 13-5, *A*.

4. Now both F_1 at 180 and F_2 may be calculated by simple algebra. If F_1 at 90 is +6.00 D and F_T at 90 is +1.00 D, then

$$F_{1(90)} + F_{2(90)} = F_{T(90)}$$

In this example

$$+6.00\ D + F_{2(90)} = +1.00\ D$$
$$F_{2(90)} = +1.00\ D - 6.00\ D = -5.00\ D$$

The value −5.00 D may now be entered on the power cross at $F_{2(90)}$.

5. Since F_2 is spherical, not only is $F_{2(90)}$ −5.00 D in power, so is $F_{2(180)}$.

6. This leaves only the cross curve as an unknown. This can be solved in either of two ways. The first is to use the system:

$$F_{1(180)} + F_{2(180)} = F_{T(180)}$$

which gives

$$(F_{1(180)}) + (-5.00D) = (+3.00)$$

Transposed this is the same as:

$$(F_{1(180)}) = (+3.00D) - (-5.00D)$$
$$= (+3.00D) + (5.00D)$$
$$= +8.00D$$

7. We can check our work by using a second method of solving this problem. We see that the power of the cylinder is 2 D. Knowing this and realizing that the entire cylinder is on the front curve, it becomes apparent that the cross curve must be 2.00 D stronger than +6.00 D, which results in +8.00 D. Since this is the same value we found in step 6, the answer checks.

Figure 13-5. For plus cylinder form lenses, to find the unknown curves, first enter the known values **(A)**. The base curve can only go on the 90-degree meridian for this lens, because the weaker power is in the 90-degree meridian. The remaining curves **(B)** may be found by algebraic additions. The base curve (and toric base curve) is +6.00 D. The cross curve is +8.00 D. The sphere curve is –5.00 D.

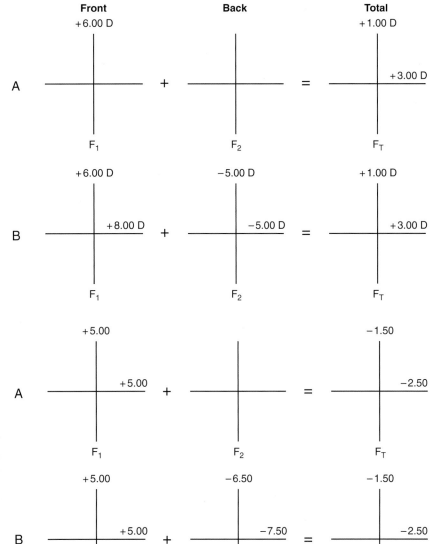

Figure 13-6. For minus cylinder form lenses, enter the known values on the power crosses first **(A)**. Then calculate the unknown values **(B)**. The base curve (and sphere curve) is +5.00 D. The toric base curve (sometimes called the back base) is –6.50 D. The cross curve is –7.50 D.

Example **13-2**

If a lens has a power of –1.50 –1.00 × 090 and is to be ground in minus cylinder form, what front and back curves would be used if a base curve of +5.00 D were chosen?

Solution

The way to solve this minus cylinder base curve problem is also summarized in Box 13-1 and will be solved using these steps for minus cylinder form lenses.

1. The three power crosses are drawn.
2. The sphere power is written on the 90-degree cylinder axis meridian of the last power cross as –1.50 D. The power in the 180-degree meridian is:

$$(-1.50) + (-1.00) = (-2.50)$$

3. The base curve is +5.00 D and is entered on both curves of the front surface power cross. This is

because the lens is a minus cylinder form lens and the front curve is spherical, having the same power in all meridians (Figure 13-6).

4. Lastly, we find the second surface powers algebraically. For the 90-degree meridian this is:

$$(+5.00) + (F_{2(90)}) = (-1.50)$$
$$(F_{2(90)}) = (-1.50) - (+5.00)$$
$$(F_{2(90)}) = -6.50 \text{ D}$$

For the 180-degree meridian we find

$$(+5.00) + (F_{2(180)}) = (-2.50)$$
$$(F_{2(90)}) = (-2.50) - (+5.00)$$
$$(F_{2(90)}) = -7.50 \text{ D}$$

The toric base curve is the weaker of the two curves. The weaker of the two curves is the –6.50 D curve in the

90-degree meridian. The cross curve is "across" from the base curve. It is the −7.50 D curve in the 180-degree meridian.

Multifocal Lens Base Curves

The base curve of a segmented multifocal lens is always on the same side of the lens as the segment. If the bifocal or trifocal segment is on the front, so is the base curve. If on the back, the base curve will be on the back as well, contrary to single vision lenses. Because a toric surface will not be ground on the same side as the multifocal seg, the base curve is always a sphere curve.

MEASUREMENT OF LENS CURVATURE

When ordering a replacement lens or supplying the wearer with a duplicate second pair of glasses some time after the initial order, one factor in wearer acceptance of the new glasses is consistent duplication of base curves. A change in base curve will change the way peripherally viewed objects are perceived, even though lens power may be identical. To measure a preexisting lens curve for accurate duplication or verification, a *lens measure* (sometimes referred to as a *lens clock*), is used (Figure 13-7).

The Lens Measure

The lens measure operates on the principle of the *sagittal depth* (sag) formula. The sagittal depth, or "sag," is the height or depth of a given segment of a circle (Figure 13-8). If both the sag of a lens surface and the index of refraction of the lens material are known, the surface power may be calculated.

The lens measure has three "legs," or points of contact with the lens surface. The outer two are stationary, and the center contact point moves in and out. The vertical difference between the positions of the two outer contact points in reference to the position of the center contact point is the sag for the arc of a circle. This circle can be thought of as having a chord, the length of which is the distance between the outer contact points of the lens measure (Figure 13-9).

The lens measure does not have a scale showing a direct measure of the sag, but rather shows dioptric value for the surface power. This power is based on an assumed index of refraction of 1.53. (Most tools found in a U.S. optical laboratory are based on an assumed index of 1.53.) The power shown on the lens measure is obtained by using the sagittal depth of the surface.

The Sagittal Depth Formula

Steps for finding the dioptric value for a lens surface begin with a geometric construction, as shown in Figure 13-9. We need to know r, the radius of the circle, to find the front or back surface powers of a lens (F_1 or F_2).

From the geometry of right triangles, the triangle FGC has a relationship between its three sides that,

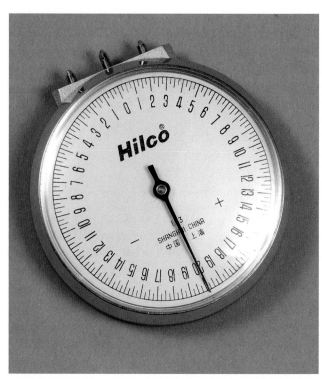

Figure 13-7. A lens measure may use direct plus and minus scales as shown here, or an outer minus scale for concave surfaces and an inner plus scale for convex surfaces.

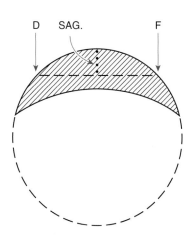

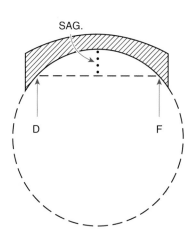

Figure 13-8. The sagittal depth or height of the chord of a circle is shown as it applies to lens surface measurements. The chord of the circle is represented by lines DF.

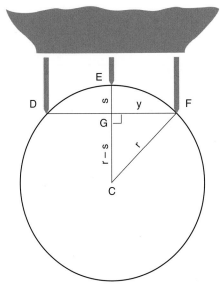

Figure 13-9. A lens clock works by mechanically determining the sagittal depth of a chord, the length of which is equal to the distance between the outer contact points of the lens clock.

because of the Pythagorean theorem, can be written as:

$$y^2 + (r - s)^2 = r^2$$

This is the same as:

$$y^2 + r^2 - 2rs + s^2 = r^2$$

By transposition:

$$y^2 + s^2 = r^2 - r^2 + 2rs$$

And again by transposition:

$$\frac{y^2 + s^2}{2s} = r$$

and

$$r = \frac{y^2}{2s} + \frac{s^2}{2s}$$

giving one form of an equation referred to as the *sagittal depth* or *sag formula**

$$r = \frac{y^2}{2s} + \frac{s}{2}$$

---

*The more commonly seen form of the sag formula is $s = r - \sqrt{(r^2 - y^2)}$, which finds the sagittal depth when radius and chord semidiameter are known. This is exactly the same equation, but in transposed form. This transposed form of the equation is introduced later in the chapter when discussing lens thickness.

Once r is determined using the sag formula, then the lens maker's formula for surface power may be used to solve for F_1 or F_2 in air.

$$F_1 = \frac{n' - n}{r_1} = \frac{n_{(lens)} - 1}{r_1}$$

$$F_2 = \frac{n' - n}{r_2} = \frac{1 - n_{(lens)}}{r_2}$$

A lens measure is calibrated for an index of 1.530, which becomes the n of the lens value in the above formulas. (Commonly used crown glass material has an index of 1.523. When used on crown glass lenses with low surface powers, the lens measure still gives fairly accurate surface power results. However, most lenses are plastic and have a variety of different refractive indices.)

So

$$F_1 = \frac{1.530 - 1}{r_1}$$

and

$$F_2 = \frac{1 - 1.530}{r_2}$$

For now we will ignore the lens measure and its assumed 1.53 index, and just use sagittal depth and the lens maker's formula to find lens surface power.

Example **13-3**

A certain lens of index 1.523 has a convex spherical front surface. The sag of the front surface is 1 mm for a chord whose length is 20 mm. What is the power of the front surface?

Solution
Using the sag formula,

$$r = \frac{y^2}{2s} + \frac{s}{2}$$

$$y = \frac{chord\ length}{2} = \frac{20\ mm}{2} = 10\ mm$$

$$s = 1\ mm$$

Since

$$r = \frac{y^2}{2s} + \frac{s}{2}$$

We can use this equation and find that

$$r = \frac{10^2}{2(1)} + \frac{1}{2} = \frac{100}{2} + \frac{1}{2}$$

and
$$r = 50.5 \text{ mm} = 0.0505 \text{ m}$$

Therefore
$$F_1 = \frac{1.523 - 1}{r_1}$$
$$= \frac{0.523}{0.0505}$$
$$= 10.36 \text{ D}$$

The front surface power of the lens is +10.36 D.

Using the Lens Measure to Find the Nominal Power of a Lens

Because it is possible to measure lens surface values directly for materials at or near an index of 1.53 using a lens measure, it is also possible to use a lens measure for finding the nominal or approximate power of such lenses. Examples of lenses with an index of 1.53 would be the plastic materials Spectralite and Trivex. Crown glass has an index of 1.523. (Remember, the nominal power of a lens is the sum of the front and back surface powers. Nominal lens power ignores the effect lens thickness may have on lens power.)

For example, if a spherical lens has a measured front curve (F_1) of +6.00 D and a measured back curve (F_2) of −4.00 D, then the nominal power of the lens will be +2.00 D.

Not all lenses are spherical. This makes it necessary to check more than one lens surface meridian for differences in power. To do this, hold the lens measure such that the center contact point of the lens measure is at the center of the lens and is perpendicular to the lens surface (Figure 13-10). The lens measure is rotated around this center contact point with all three contact points against the lens.* If the indicator on the lens measure dial remains stationary, the surface is spherical. The spherical surface value is as shown on the lens measure. If the indicator shows a changing value, the surface is toric, with two separate curves. The values of these curves are indicated when the lens measure shows its maximum and minimum values. The orientation of the three contact points on the lens at maximum and minimum readings corresponds to the major meridians of lens power.

Example **13-**4

When rotating the lens measure on the front surface of a crown glass lens, it is found that all meridians read +6.50 D. On the back surface, if the three contact points are horizontally aligned exactly along the 180-degree meridian, a maximum value of −7.50 D is found. When the three contact points are oriented in the vertical (90-degree) meridian, a minimum value of −6.00 D is found. What is the

---

*If there is a chance that the lens or lens surface may be scratched by rotating the lens measure on the surface of the lens, alternately lift and reposition the lens measure instead.

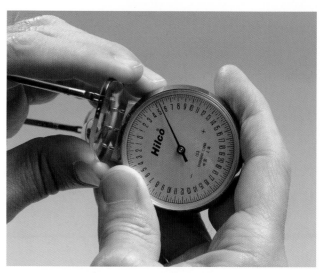

Figure 13-10. A lens measure is held perpendicular to the lens surface with the center contact point at the optical center. Tilting of the lens measure results in a variation in the measured power.

nominal power of the lens? Is the lens made in plus cylinder form or minus cylinder form?

Solution

The lens measure has found the major meridians of the lens. The values read may be transferred directly to power crosses for calculation of the total nominal lens power (Figure 13-11).

Using methods previously discussed, the total lens power could be written in one of three possible forms:
1. +0.50 − 1.50 × 090
2. −1.00 + 1.50 × 180
3. +0.50 × 180 / −1.00 × 090

Because the toric surface is the back surface, the lens is minus cylinder in form.

Use of the Lens Measure With Multifocals

When the lens measure is used on a segmented multifocal lens, positioning of the contact points depends on lens construction. Multifocals may be fused or one piece.

The *fused* multifocal segment uses glass of a different refractive index from that in the rest of the lens. The junction between distance and near portions is visible, but cannot be felt since the glass segment is fused into the lens such that there is no change in lens surface curvature. A lens measure may therefore be used normally on the lens surface. Its reading will indicate only the surface power for the main lens. It does not read segment power.

A *one-piece* multifocal lens construction uses the same lens material for distance and near portions. Power differences between distance and near portions are brought about by a change in lens curvature. One-piece bifocals may be identified by either a ledge or by a change in the surface curve. The change may be felt by rubbing the

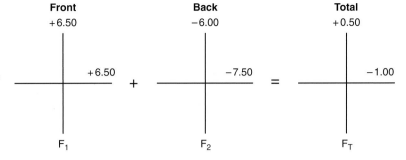

Figure 13-11. Lens clock readings may be transferred directly to power crosses for lens power calculation.

finger over the juncture. In this case to determine lens surface power for the main lens accurately, none of the three contact points must rest on the segment portion. To measure a one-piece bifocal, the lens measure is placed on the lens with all three contact points horizontally positioned in the center of the lens and above the multifocal line.

Why Measured Base Curves Do Not Always Come Out As Expected

When using a lens clock to measure the base curve of a lens, the values measured do not always come out the same as the manufacturer's stated value. A semifinished glass lens may arrive at the optical laboratory with a base curve of +8.25 D marked on the box. But when the front lens surface is measured, it may be slightly less than +8.25 D. Or a plastic lens could be marked as having a base curve of +10.25 D, but measure as +10.50 D. Some assume that the lens measure is inaccurate; others assume that variations are due to differences in the index of refraction of the lens and the lens measure scale. Actually, neither assumption is correct.

The real reason for the mismatch stems from the fact that there are several different front-surface lens curve terms used to describe the same lens surface curve. These terms are:
1. The nominal base curve
2. The true base curve (or so-called true power)
3. The refractive power

The Nominal Base Curve

The *nominal base curve* was originally established as a reference number for the convenience of the optical laboratory. When low-powered crown glass lenses had their surfaces ground to power without the help of computerized lens surfacing programs, the correct back curve was found by subtracting the front surface from the needed lens power. For example, if the lens is supposed to have a power of +1.25 D and the base curve of the lens is +6.50, then the back surface curve should be:

$$+1.25 - 6.50 = -5.25 \text{ D}$$

As the plus power of the lens increases, however, so does its thickness. Because of increased thickness, simple subtraction will not work. To make it possible for laboratory personnel to continue using the same simple calculation, lens manufacturers changed the front curve of the lens slightly to compensate for the effect of increasing thickness; but they left the listed base curve as the same number. When this is done, the value of the base curve is not the real power of the surface. Thus it is called the nominal base curve. (This is not to be confused with nominal lens power, which is the sum of the first and second surface powers.)

With plastic lenses, the base curves vary from their marked values for a different reason. Plastic lenses start out as liquid resin and are molded. When their surfaces cure during manufacture, once removed from the mold, the final curve of the surface may vary from the curve of the mold. Initially, it was difficult to predict the exact final lens curve value. Although the final curve of the lens after being removed from the mold is now predictable, the difference between marked surface power (the nominal base curve) of a plastic lens and measured surface power remains.

True Base Curve ("True Power")

The so-called *true base curve* of a lens is the value of the front surface as measured using a lens measure. Synonyms for true base curve are "*true power*" and "*actual power*." This lens clock used to measure surface curvature is calibrated for an index of 1.53. Lenses at or close to this refractive index are Spectralite and Trivex plastic at 1.53, and crown glass, having an index of 1.523. The *true base curve* is the 1.53 indexed value. Many, or perhaps even most, lenses are not at all close to an index of 1.53. Because of differences in refractive indices, it is easy to see that the "true" base curve measured with a lens clock is unlikely to be the refractive power of the lens surface.

The Refractive Power of the Lens Surface

The *refractive power* controls what happens to light at the surface of the lens. It will be recalled that surface power is dependent on three factors. These are:
1. The refractive index of the lens surface
2. The refractive index of the media surrounding the lens
3. The radius of curvature of the lens surface

For the front surface of the lens this refractive power is found using the lens maker's formula:

$$F_1 = \frac{n' - n}{r_1}$$

As previously stated, lens clocks are calibrated for lens material having a refractive index of 1.53. If a lens made from material of a different refractive index is used, compensation must be made so that surface refractive power can be found using a lens clock.

Finding the Refractive Power of a Lens Surface Using a Lens Measure

To find the refractive power of a lens surface using a lens clock, the "true power" reading from the lens clock must be converted to refractive power. This is done with the help of the lens maker's formula shown above.

When using the lens clock, we are indirectly determining the radius of curvature of the surface in question, regardless of its refractive index.

Example **13-5**

The front surface of a lens is measured with a lens clock. The lens clock shows a value of +6.00 D based on an assumed index of 1.530. What is the radius of curvature of the lens surface?

Solution

The information given allows all terms of the lens maker's formula to be filled in except r_1 .

$$F_1 = \frac{n' - n}{r_1}$$

$$+6.00 = \frac{1.53 - 1}{r_1}$$

Therefore,

$$r_1 = \frac{1.53 - 1}{+6.00}$$
$$= \frac{0.53}{+6.00}$$
$$= 0.0883$$

The lens surface has a radius of curvature of 0.0883 m.

Example **13-6**

Suppose that instead of having an index 1.530, the above lens material is CR-39 plastic with an index of 1.498. What front surface refractive power does this lens have?

Solution

Again the basic surface power equation may be used and the known values substituted to find the unknown value for $F_{1(CR\text{-}39)}$.

$$F_{1(CR\text{-}39)} = \frac{n' - n}{r_1}$$
$$= \frac{1.498 - 1}{0.0883}$$
$$= 5.64\,D$$

The front surface refractive power for the CR-39 lens is +5.64 D. Because the lens has a lower refractive index, the lens surface does not have as much refractive power as shown by the lens clock.

Using a Conversion Factor

It is possible to reduce the process of converting from lens clock readings to surface refractive power by using a formula-generated conversion factor. This is done as follows:

If, for the lens measure,

$$F_{(lens\ measure)} = \frac{1.53 - 1}{r}$$

then

$$r = \frac{0.53}{F_{(lm)}}$$

and if, for the surface of different index material

$$F_{(new\ material)} = \frac{n' - 1}{r}$$

then

$$r = \frac{n' - 1}{F_{(nm)}}$$

Since both equations are referring to the same lens surface, then both r values are the same. As a result we can combine the two equations, giving the following:

$$\frac{0.53}{F_{(lm)}} = \frac{n' - 1}{F_{(nm)}}$$

Transposing gives the refractive power for the new material.

$$F_{(nm)} = \frac{(n' - 1)F_{(lm)}}{0.53}$$

This means that for any given lens material, we can substitute the refractive index of the new material for n′ into the formula and obtain a conversion factor.

Example **13-7**

What is the conversion factor for converting the lens measure reading to refractive power for a lens surface made from 1.586 polycarbonate material?

Solution

Substituting 1.586 into the formula for n' results in the following:

$$F_{(nm)} = \frac{(n'-1)F_{(lm)}}{0.53}$$
$$= \frac{(1.586-1)F_{(lm)}}{0.53}$$
$$= \frac{(0.586)F_{(lm)}}{0.53}$$
$$= (1.106)F_{(lm)}$$

The conversion factor is 1.106.

Example **13**-8

Use the conversion factor for polycarbonate to find the surface refractive power for the front surface of a polycarbonate lens. The lens clock measures a "true power" of +8.12 D for the lens.

Solution

We use the conversion formula with the 1.106 conversion factor to find:

$$F_{(nm)} = (1.106)F_{(lm)}$$
$$= (1.106)(8.12)$$
$$= +8.98 \text{ D}$$

The surface of the lens is +8.98 D or, if rounded, is +9.00 D of refractive power.

Using the Lens Measure to Find Lens Power for Lenses of Different Refractive Indices

If it is possible to use the lens measure to find front surface refractive power, it is also possible to measure both front and back surfaces in an attempt to find a nominal lens power. It should be noted that for a thick lens, the lens power found may still not be exact. Remember, the lens power obtained by adding front and back surfaces is called the "nominal power" of the lens and should not be confused with the nominal base curve.

Example **13**-9

A lens clock is used on the front and back surfaces of a lens. The front surface value found is +2.00 D. The back surface measures −6.87 D in the 90-degree meridian and −6.00 D in the 180-degree meridian. The lens has an index of refraction of 1.66. What is the power of the lens expressed in minus cylinder form?

Solution

To answer the question, we first need a conversion factor.

$$F_{(nm)} = \frac{(n'-1)F_{(lm)}}{0.53}$$
$$= \frac{(1.66-1)F_{(lm)}}{0.53}$$
$$= (1.245)F_{(lm)}$$

The conversion factor is 1.245.

Applying the conversion factor to the first surface we find:

$$F_{(nm)} = (1.245)(+2.00)$$
$$= +2.49 \text{ D}$$

Applying the conversion factor to the back surface in the 90-degree meridian results in:

$$F_{(nm)} = (1.245)(-6.87)$$
$$= -8.55 \text{ D}$$

and in the 180-degree meridian we get:

$$F_{(nm)} = (1.245)(-6.00)$$
$$= -7.47 \text{ D}$$

Adding front and back surface powers together gives:

$$F_{\text{Nominal}} = F_1 + F_2$$
$$F_{90} = (+2.49) + (-8.55) = -6.06 \text{ D}$$
$$F_{180} = (+2.49) + (-7.47) = -4.98 \text{ D}$$

This is shown in Figure 13-12. Rounding to more realistic values gives −6.00 D in the 90 and −5.00 D in the 180. In minus cylinder form, the lens power is written as

$$-5.00 \; -1.00 \times 180.$$

The Compensated Power Method

It is possible to find the power of the lens by adding front and back surface lens-clock-measured values *before* multiplying by the conversion factor. This will save a step and give the same results.

In the previous example, adding together front and back surface lens measure values gives:

$$F_{\text{Nominal}} = F_1 + F_2$$
$$F_{90} = (+2.00) + (-6.87) = -4.87 \text{ D}$$
$$F_{180} = (+2.00) + (-6.00) = -4.00 \text{ D}$$

These two values are called *compensated powers*.* Multiplying the compensated powers (−4.87 D and −4.00 D) by the 1.245 conversion factor gives −6.06 D and −4.98 D in the 90- and 180-degree meridians, respectively. These are the same values as found by the first method. The logic of the process is shown by noticing the arrows drawn in Figure 13-12.

Using the Lens Measure on Plastic Surfaces

It should be mentioned that when a lens measure is being used on a plastic lens, care should be taken to prevent

---

*Before computer software programs became readily available, the optical laboratory used the compensated power concept to determine the back surface powers needed to surface minus lenses. The ordered back vertex power was converted into a 1.53-based "compensated power." Then the correct 1.53-indexed surfacing tools were found by subtracting the 1.53-referenced front-surface power from the compensated power.

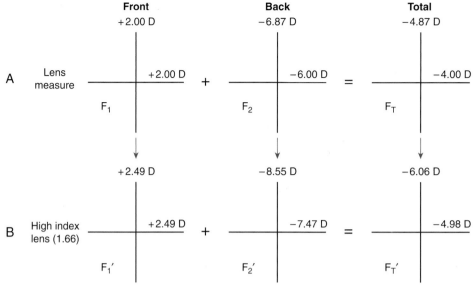

Figure 13-12. A lens measure is used on a lens having an index of refraction of 1.66. The lens measure readings for the front and back surfaces are entered on the first and second power crosses **(A)**. The actual lens power may be found in one of two ways. The first way is to correct both front and back surface powers for refractive index and then add them together. This is shown in the figure by converting the numbers for the front and back surfaces **(A)** and entering them on the power crosses directly below **(B)**. Then the new front and back surface powers **(B)** are added together and entered on the F_T' power cross **(B)**. The second, easier way to find actual lens power is to first add the original lens measure readings for the front and back surfaces together. This total is shown as the third F_T' power cross **(A)**. Then these values are corrected for index of refraction. The results are entered directly on the third F_T' power cross **(B)**.

scratching the surface. Instead of simply twisting the lens measure with the contact points directly on the lens surface, lift the lens measure and place in a new location. Turning the lens measure and dragging the contact points over the surface may damage the surface material. Lens measures are designed with rounded points to reduce this possibility, but care should nonetheless be taken during the measuring process.

When to Specify Base Curve[1]

There are certain situations where base curve should be specified when ordering a prescription. These are:
- *When replacing one lens in a pair:* Base curve choices are made as a pair. When only one lens is ordered, the laboratory will not know what the other lens is if the old lenses do not accompany the order. And even if they do accompany the order, they might not be checked.
- *When ordering an identically powered second pair:* Base curve should also be specified when ordering an identically powered second pair of glasses. This second pair of glasses will be worn interchangeably with the first pair. The curve of a lens affects how shapes and straight lines appear. Two pair of glasses made using different base curves will cause shapes to distort differently. Some individuals are more sensitive to this than others. To prevent the

possibility of difficulty when changing back and forth with different pairs of glasses, the safest policy is to keep the base curve powers of the two lens pairs as close to one another as possible.

When specifying a certain base curve, remember that semifinished lenses come in only so many base curves. Ordering a +8.00 base curve may result in one that is close, but not exactly +8.00. ANSI Z80.1 Prescription Standards allow a base curve tolerance of ±0.75 D. To help in getting a lens with the exact same base curve, try ordering from the same optical laboratory that was used for the first pair. The brand of lenses they use is more likely to allow an exact match.

When Not to Specify Base Curve

There are some situations where a base curve should not be specified so that the laboratory can pick the best base curve for the prescription ordered.
- *Do not insist on matching the base curve of the new glasses to the wearer's previous lenses.* Prescriptions change. And as the power of the lens changes, to prevent unwanted lens aberrations, the power of the base curve should be expected to change too. A base curve should not be expected to perpetually be the same for the life of the wearer.
- *Do not request a flatter base curve to get a thinner, better-looking lens.* Flattening a base curve will

often make a plus lens look much better. It will usually reduce magnification, decrease thickness, and even reduce the weight a bit. However, there will be an increase in unwanted aberration in the periphery of the lens because of using a base curve that is not correct for the power of the lens.

- ***Do not change the base curve to solve ghost-image internal lens reflection problems.*** Before antireflection coating, the common solution for getting rid of ghost images was to change the base curve. Changing the base curve will shift the size and location of those ghost images, but will not drop them out like an antireflection coating will. Only use a base curve change to help with ghost images if an antireflection coating is not an option.
- ***Do not automatically steepen the base curve for people with long eyelashes.*** Try to solve the problem of lashes touching the lens with a good frame selection. It is true that steepening the base curve by 2 D will give about 1.2 mm of extra lash clearance. But it will mean that optimal optics from a good base curve selection will be lacking.

ADDING CYLINDERS

Lenses are able to be added together. This is done routinely during the eye examination. Small spherically powered lenses are added to large spherically powered lenses. For example,

$$(+3.00 \text{ D sphere}) + (+0.25 \text{ D sphere})$$
$$= +3.25 \text{ D sphere.}$$

Sphere lenses are added to cylinder lenses, resulting in spherocylinder lens combinations, as with these two lenses.

$$(+3.00 \text{ D sphere}) + (\text{pl} - 1.50 \times 180 \text{ cylinder})$$
$$= (+3.00 - 1.50 \times 180)$$

In the same way that power crosses are used when adding front and back lens *surfaces* together to find total lens power, so also may power crosses be used as a help when adding two or more *lenses* together. To visualize how lens meridians add together for the sphere and cylinder lenses in the above example, see Figure 13-13.

Adding Cylinders Having the Same Axis or With Axes 90 Degrees Apart

Just as spheres and spheres and spheres and cylinders may be added, so also may cylinders and cylinders be added. Here we will be looking at adding cylinders whose axes are either the same, or 90 degrees away from each other.

Example **13-10**

What is the resulting sum of two cylinder lenses, both having a power of pl − 2.00 × 180?

Solution

To find the solution, make three power crosses, with the first two adding to equal the third. Place the powers of the two cylinder lenses on the first two power crosses. Because both lenses are identical, they will look the same on the first two power crosses. The axis is 180, so there is zero power in the 180-degree axis meridian. The power is −2.00, so −2.00 is written on the 90-degree power meridian. This is shown in Figure 13-14.

Next the powers in the 180 are summed. Zero plus zero equals zero. Then the 90-degree powers are summed. (−2.00) + (−2.00) = (−4.00).

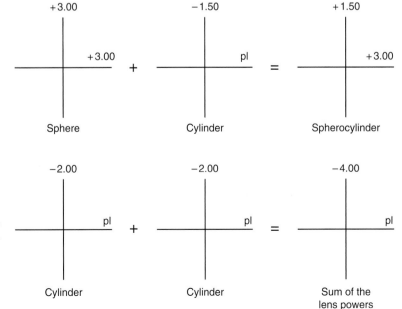

Figure 13-13. Power crosses allow a sphere and cylinder to be added together to form a spherocylinder.

Figure 13-14. When two plano-cylinder lenses are placed together axis-to-axis, the resulting cylinder power is the sum of the cylinder powers.

The resulting power cross may be written in minus cylinder form as pl − 4.00 × 180.

Example **13-11**

We will now take the same two cylinder lenses, but with axes oriented differently, and sum them. What is the sum of a pl − 2.00 × 180 lens and a pl − 2.00 × 090 lens?

Solution

Again placing these two lenses on power crosses helps in visualizing what is happening. The first lens has zero on the 180-degree meridian and −2.00 on the 90-degree meridian. The second lens has zero on the 90-degree meridian and −2.00 on the 180-degree meridian. When the two lenses are added together in each meridian, as shown in Figure 13-15, the result is a −2.00 D sphere.

Example **13-12**

Add these two lenses to find the resulting spherocylinder lens.

$$pl - 1.25 \times 090$$

$$pl - 2.25 \times 180$$

Solution

Draw three power crosses and enter the cylinder lenses shown above on the first two, as shown in Figure 13-16. Sum the 90-degree meridians, then the 180-degree meridians. The result is a lens with a power of −1.25 − 1.00 × 180.

Jackson Crossed Cylinders

A *Jackson crossed cylinder* (JCC) is a lens used in the eye examination process to help in determining cylinder axis and cylinder power. It has plus power in one meridian

and an equal and opposite amount of minus power in the other. An example of a Jackson crossed cylinder is shown in Figure 13-17.

A Jackson crossed cylinder is written as if the lens were two cylinders of equal and opposite powers.

Example **13-13**

What would a ±1.00 JCC look like on a power cross? From what two plano cylinders is it derived?

Solution

A ±1.00 JCC has a power of +1.00 in one meridian and −1.00 in the opposite meridian. Figure 13-18 shows what this could look like if the +1.00 were in the 90-degree meridian. It is the same as crossing two cylinders of equal and opposite value. In this case these two cylinders would be

$$pl + 1.00 \times 180/pl - 1.00 \times 090.$$

By flipping the cylinder over using its handle positioned halfway between the major meridians of the JCC lens, the minus and plus powers trade places. When looking through first one orientation of the lens, then flipping the JCC by 90 degrees to the opposite orientation, exaggerated views through the opposing cylinders are seen. Exaggerating the differences makes it easier to know the answer to the familiar question asked during refraction, "Which (view) is better, one or two?"

Example **13-14**

A ±1.00 JCC is held so that the plus power is in the 90-degree meridian. This was the situation shown in Figure 13–18. A JCC lens can also be written as if it were an ordinary spherocylinder lens combination. If ±1.00 JCC lens

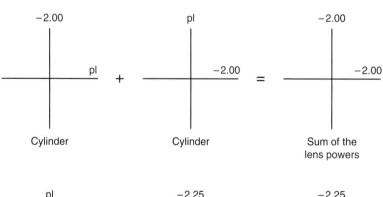

Cylinder   Cylinder   Sum of the
lens powers

Figure 13-15. When two equal powered plano cylinders are placed together with axes 90 degrees away from one another, the resulting lens is a sphere.

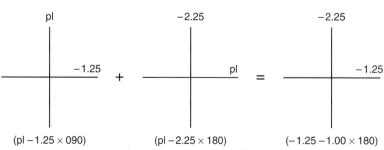

(pl −1.25 × 090)   (pl −2.25 × 180)   (−1.25 −1.00 × 180)

Figure 13-16. When two unequally powered plano cylinders are placed together with axes 90 degrees away from one another, the result is a spherocylinder lens.

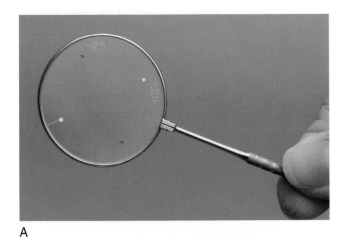

A

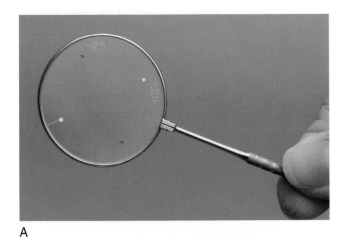

B

Figure 13-17. Jackson crossed cylinders are used during lens refraction to find cylinder power and cylinder axis.

were to be written as a spherocylinder lens combination, how would it be written?

Solution

If written in minus cylinder form, the meridian of highest plus or least minus is the sphere power. The difference between the two meridians is the cylinder power, and the axis location is the meridian of sphere power. Therefore this ±1.00 JCC has a spherocylindrical power of +1.00 − 2.00 × 90.

Obliquely Crossed Cylinders

It is considerably harder to add two cylinders or spherocylinder lenses together whose axes are neither the same, nor at 90 degrees away from one another, but are crossed obliquely. For example, one may have an axis of 35 and another may have an axis of 65.

Obliquely crossed cylinders can occur clinically. From a spectacle lens standpoint, when a person is wearing an existing pair of glasses and, for some reason, a refraction is done over the existing lenses, there may be a spherocylinder in the original glasses and a second spherocylinder lens combination in the overrefraction. These auxiliary lenses may be clipped to the wearer's glasses with a refracting cell to hold the lenses. From a practical standpoint, the easiest way to find the resultant combination is to take the wearer's glasses with the cell and auxiliary lenses in place to the lensmeter and simply read the total lens combination.

Another clinical situation occurs when a person is wearing a toric contact lens that contains a cylinder power. The power may not quite be right. The examiner refracts over the contact lenses. The overrefraction must be combined with the existing spherocylinder contact lens power to find the needed contact lens power.

In doing an obliquely crossed cylinder calculation, there are three ways that are used to arrive at an accurate answer. These are:

- Use a graphical method.
- Use a formula method.
- Use a computer program.

The graphical method is helpful in that it not only is able to furnish a usable answer, but will help in conceptually understanding how obliquely crossed cylinders interact to give a resultant spherocylinder lens power. It is the basis for the formula method. The formula method is complex, but favored by those who love math. It is the basis for writing a simple computer program.

Figure 13-18. A ±1.00 Jackson crossed cylinder is the same as a plano +1.00 cylinder and a plano − 1.00 cylinder with axes 90 degrees apart. If this particular lens were written as a spherocylinder lens, it would have a power of +1.00 − 2.00 × 090.

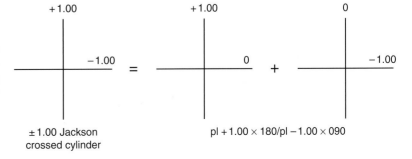

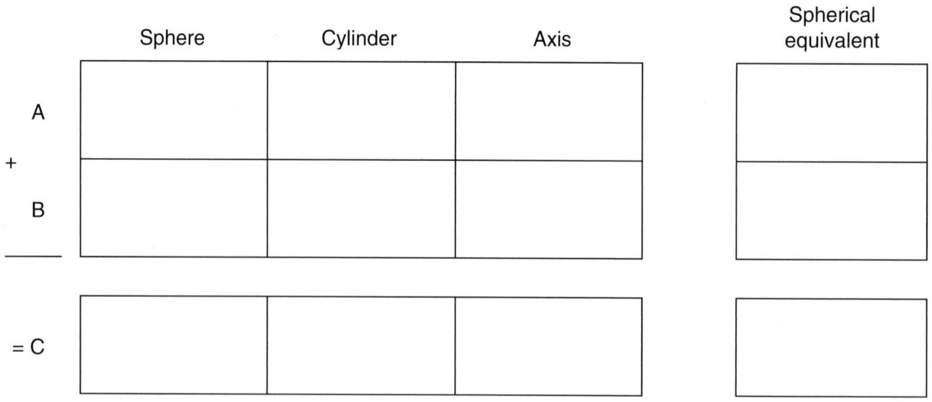

	Sphere	Cylinder	Axis
A			
+			
B			
= C			

Spherical equivalent

Figure 13-19. A template to help in calculating the resultant of two obliquely crossed cylinder lenses.

The Graphical Method

The graphical method uses vectors to find the power and axis direction of the combined cylinder lenses. However, it is not exactly like normal vector problems, but requires some modification. The reason for this is because a cylinder of power -2.00×000 is not equal and opposite of a cylinder of power -2.00×180 degrees. If these are added together, the resulting cylinder would be -4.00×180. This is because axis 0 is the same as axis 180.

The two degree values that are opposite from a vector stand point are 0 (or 180) and 090. In other words, if -2.00×000 and -2.00×090 are added, the cylinders cancel out. The result is a -2.00 D sphere. Therefore if a problem like this is to be solved with vectors, the cylinder axes need to be doubled.

With that in mind, here is a graphical method for finding the resulting power of two obliquely crossed plano cylinders or spherocylinders.

1. Convert the two cylinders to be consistent with one another. In other words, both must be written as plus cylinders or both written as minus cylinders.
2. Construct a set of boxes for ease of calculation (Figure 13-19). Write the lens powers of the two spherocylinder lenses in the appropriate boxes.
3. Compute equivalent spheres for the two lenses and add them together, entering the sum in the "spherical equivalent C box." (If two spherocylinder lenses are combined, the resulting lens has the same spherical equivalent as the sum of the spherical equivalents.)
4. Plot and construct vectors of the two cylinder values and find the resulting vector sum and axis. Here's how it's done.
   a. Double the axes of the cylinders for vector drawing purposes. (This is because a cylinder axis of 90 is opposite from a cylinder axis of 180.)
   b. Draw the cylinder powers to scale as written, but draw the axis as doubled.
   c. Draw out the resultant vector and measure its length. This is the resultant cylinder power.
   d. Read off the angle of the new cylinder vector and divide by two. This value is the new cylinder axis.

5. Enter the new cylinder power and axis in section C of Figure 13-19.
6. Take the spherical equivalent of the new cylinder power and *subtract** it from the equivalent sphere power found in "spherical equivalent C box." This gives the new sphere power of the resultant spherocylinder lens.

Example **13-15**

Use the graphical method just described to find the resultant spherocylinder lens power when these two obliquely crossed cylinders are combined.

$$pl - 2.00 \times 180$$

$$-2.00 + 2.00 \times 135$$

Solution

1. One lens is a minus cylinder, the other a plus cylinder. Converting them both to minus cylinders results in:

$$pl - 2.00 \times 180$$

$$pl - 2.00 \times 045$$

2. The lens powers are written in the box shown in Figure 13-20.
3. The spherical equivalent of pl -2.00×180 is -1.00 D sphere. This is also the spherical equivalent of the other lens. So -1.00 is entered into the first two spherical equivalent boxes for A and B. These are then added together and -2.00 is entered into the C spherical equivalent box.
   a. To plot these cylinder values, we need to double each axis. Doubling axis 180 gives 360. (Since axis 180 is the same as axis 0, this is the same as saying 0 doubled is 0.) Doubling axis 45 gives 90.
   b. The cylinder power vectors are entered at 0 and at 90, as shown in Figure 13-21. (When drawing cylinder powers, negative signs are ignored.)
   c. The new cylinder power is measured out to be 2.83. (Actually we cannot measure to this degree of

---

*If the lens is minus cylinder in power, you will be "minusing" a minus value.

		Sphere	Cylinder	Axis		Spherical equivalent
	A	0.00	−2.00	180		−1.00
+	B	0.00	−2.00	45		−1.00
= C		−0.58	−2.83	22.5		−2.00

Figure 13-20. The template for finding the result of two obliquely crossed cylinders crossed at a 45-degree angle.

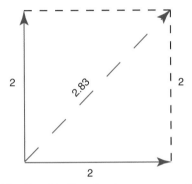

Figure 13-21. Graphically plotting two equally powered obliquely crossed cylinders:
For pl − 2.00 × 180 the axis is doubled and drawn at axis zero.
For pl − 2.00 × 45 the axis is doubled and drawn as 90.
The resultant power is −2.83 along the 45-degree meridian.
The resultant axis is $^{45}/_2$ or 22.5 degrees.

accuracy, but we can be close.) So the cylinder power is −2.83.

d. The new cylinder axis measures 45 degrees. We divide 45 by 2. This result of 22.5 degrees is the axis of the new cylinder.

4. The new cylinder power and axis values are written in section C of Figure 13-20.

5. Now we know everything except the new sphere power. Since we know the spherical equivalent of the new lens, we can find the sphere value by taking half of the new cylinder power and subtracting it from the spherical equivalent. In other words, if:

$$\text{Spherical Equivalent} = \text{sphere} + \frac{\text{cylinder}}{2}$$

Then

$$\text{sphere} = \text{spherical equivalent} - \left(\frac{\text{cylinder}}{2}\right)$$

So, for the problem at hand,

$$\text{sphere} = \text{spherical equivalent} - \left(\frac{\text{cylinder}}{2}\right)$$
$$= -2.00 - \frac{-2.83}{2}$$
$$= -2.00 - (-1.42\,\text{D})$$
$$= -0.58\,\text{D}$$

The new spherocylinder lens power will be −0.58 −2.83 × 22.5.

Example **13-16**

Use the graphical method to find the resultant spherocylinder lens power when these two obliquely crossed spherocylinder lenses are combined.

$$-1.00 - 2.00 \times 020$$

$$-2.50 - 3.00 \times 080$$

Solution

1. Since both these lenses have the same sign for the cylinder, neither needs to be converted.
2. The powers of these two lenses are entered into Figure 13-22.
3. Since

$$\text{Spherical Equivalent} = \text{sphere} + \frac{\text{cylinder}}{2}$$

then for the first lens

$$\text{Spherical Equivalent} = -1.00 + \frac{-2.00}{2}$$
$$= -1.00 - 1.00$$
$$= -2.00$$

And for the second lens

$$\text{Spherical Equivalent} = -2.50 + \frac{-3.00}{2}$$
$$= -2.50 - 1.50$$
$$= -4.00$$

	Sphere	Cylinder	Axis
A	−1.00	−2.00	20
+ B	−2.50	−3.00	80
= C	−4.68	−2.64	60

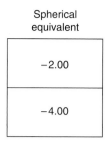

Spherical equivalent

−2.00

−4.00

−6.00

Figure 13-22. The template with two obliquely crossed spherocylinder lens powers entered.

These are entered into the A and B spherical equivalent boxes, then added together. The −6.00 D spherical equivalent sum is entered into box C.

4a. The cylinder axes are doubled so that the first will be 40 and the second 160.

4b. The cylinder powers are left as is, and vectors are constructed as shown in Figure 13-23.

4c. The resultant vector is measured to be 2.64 units long.

4d. The axis read is 120. This value is divided by 2, making the new cylinder have a cylinder axis of 60 degrees.

5. The value −2.64 × 060 is entered into section C of Figure 13-22.

6. The new sphere power is found as:

$$\text{sphere} = \text{spherical equivalent} - \left(\frac{\text{cylinder}}{2}\right)$$

$$= -6.00 - \frac{-2.64}{2}$$
$$= -6.00 - (-1.32)$$
$$= -4.68$$

The new spherocylinder lens is then −4.68 −2.64 × 060.

The Formula Method

By using the graphical method, it is possible to develop a formula for finding the resultant of two obliquely crossed cylinders. This formula can be used to solve the problem or to construct a computer-based program to solve obliquely crossed cylinder problems. Without going into the derivation, the formula method is as follows:

1. If both cylinders are not in the same form, transpose one lens so that both are plus or both minus.

2. Find the difference between the two cylinder axis angles. The angular difference in degrees between F_{cyl1} and F_{cyl2} will be called a. We will call the cylinder with the smaller axis F_{cyl1} and the cylinder with the larger axis value, F_{cyl2}.

3. Find how far the new cylinder axis is from the cylinder with the smaller axis value (F_{cyl1}) by using the formula:

$$\tan 2\theta = \frac{F_{cyl2} \sin 2a}{F_{cyl1} + F_{cyl2} \cos 2a}$$

Where:

F_{cyl1} = the power of the first cylinder
F_{cyl2} = the power of the second cylinder
a = the difference between the two cylinder axes in degrees, and
θ = how far the axis of the new cylinder is from the first cylinder axis

4. Find the axis of the new cylinder. This is done by adding θ to the axis of the first cylinder (the cylinder with the smaller axis).

5. Find the sphere power (S) resulting from the two cylinders crossing. This is done using the formula:

$$S = F_{cyl1} \sin^2 \theta + F_{cyl2} \sin^2 (a - \theta)$$

(NOTE: This is only the power of the new spherocylinder combination *if* the lenses being combined are just *plano* cylinders. If there are sphere components to the combining lenses, these will be added in later.)

6. Find the new cylinder power (C), using the formula:

$$C = F_{cyl1} + F_{cyl2} - 2S$$

7. Find the new total sphere power (S_{Total}) by adding the sphere powers in the original two lenses (S_1 and S_2) to the sphere power (S) resulting from the crossing of the cylinders.

$$S_{Total} = S + S_1 + S_2$$

Example **13-17**

Use the formula method to find the resultant spherocylinder lens power when these two obliquely crossed spherocylinder lenses are combined. (These are the same lenses as used in Example 13-16 that were combined using the graphical method earlier.)

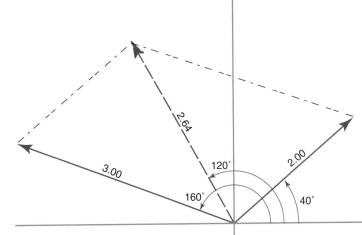

Figure 13-23. Graphically plotting two unequally powered obliquely crossed cylinders.
For −2.00 × 20, the axis is doubled and the power drawn at 40.
For −3.00 × 80, the axis is doubled and the power drawn at 160.
The resultant power is −2.64 along the 120-degree meridian.
The resultant axis is $^{120}/_2$ or 60 degrees.

$$-1.00 - 2.00 \times 020$$

$$-2.50 - 3.00 \times 080$$

Solution

1. Both cylinders are minus cylinder form lenses and do not need to be transposed.
2. The difference between the two cylinder axis angles is:

$$80 - 20 = 60 \text{ degrees}$$

3. The distance from the smaller cylinder axis to the new cylinder axis is:

$$\tan 2\theta = \frac{F_{cyl2} \sin 2a}{F_{cyl1} + F_{cyl2} \cos 2a}$$

$$= \frac{3 \sin (2 \bullet 60)}{2 + 3 \cos (2 \bullet 60)}$$

$$= \frac{3 \sin 120}{2 + 3 \cos 120}$$

$$= \frac{3 (0.866)}{2 + 3 (-0.5)}$$

$$= \frac{2.60}{0.5}$$

$$\tan 2\theta = 5.2$$
$$2\theta = 79.1 \text{ degrees}$$
$$\theta = 39.6 \text{ degrees}$$

4. The new cylinder axis is 20 + 39.6 = 59.6 degrees. Rounded to the nearest degree, the new axis is 60 degrees.
5. The sphere power resulting from the crossing of the cylinders (and not including the sphere powers of the combining spherocylinder lenses) is

$$S = F_{cyl1} \sin^2 \theta + F_{cyl2} \sin^2 (a - \theta)$$
$$= -2.00 \sin^2 39.6 + -3 \sin^2 (60 - 39.6)$$
$$= -2.00 (0.41) + -3.00 (0.12)$$
$$= -0.82 - 0.36$$
$$= -1.18 \text{ D sphere}$$

6. The new cylinder power is:

$$C = F_{cyl1} + F_{cyl2} - 2S$$
$$= -2.00 + -3.00 - 2(-1.18)$$
$$= -2.64 \text{ D cyl}$$

7. The new total sphere power is:

$$S_{Total} = S + S_1 + S_2$$
$$= -1.18 + (-1.00) + (-2.50)$$
$$= -4.68 \text{ D sphere}$$

Therefore the new spherocylinder lens resulting from the obliquely crossed spherocylinder lenses is −4.68 − 2.64 × 060.

Conceptual Questions for Anticipating the Sum of Two Obliquely Crossed Cylinder Lenses

In reality few people will be using either the formula method or the graphical method to find the result of two obliquely crossed cylinders. Instead a computer program will be used. However, it is useful to understand enough about lenses to know how two obliquely crossed cylinders or spherocylinders will interact. Here are some conceptual questions to help in understanding how two cylinder lenses will sum. Examples are included for two cylinders that are not at oblique angles with one another. Each question represents an important aspect in understanding how cylinders add together. The answers were obtained by exact calculations. Exact calculations are not important, however. The important thing to notice is the relative power of the cylinder and position of the new axis.

Question 1. True or false? The sum of the spherical equivalents of the two obliquely crossed spherocylinders will always equal the spherical equivalent of the resultant lens.

Answer: True

Question 2. True or false? If the axes of either two plus cylinder or two minus cylinder lenses are the same, then the resultant cylinder power will be the sum of the two cylinders.

Answer: True

For example, if a pl − 2.00 × 180 is combined with pl − 2.00 × 180, the result equals pl − 4.00 × 180.

Question 3. If the axes of two cylinders are very close to one another, what can be said about the power of the new cylinder?

Answer: The resultant cylinder power will closely approach the sum of the two cylinders. The sphere power will increase only slightly, closely approaching no change.

For example, pl − 2.00 × 002 combined with pl − 2.00 × 178 equals −0.02 − 3.96 × 180.

Question 4. If the axes of two equally powered cylinders are 90 degrees away from one another, what will be the result?

Answer: The cylinder power will be zero, and the sphere power resulting from the two combined cylinder components will change by the full power of the cylinder.

For example, pl − 2.00 × 090 combined with pl − 2.00 × 180 equals −2.00 sphere.

Question 5. True or false? If the powers of two obliquely crossed cylinders are equal, the axis of the new cylinder will be halfway in between the two.

Answer: True

For example, pl − 2.00 × 030 combined with pl − 2.00 × 070 results in −0.47 − 3.06 × 050.

Question 6. If the cylinder powers of two obliquely crossed cylinders are *un*equal, what happens to the axis of the cylinder?

Answer: The resulting cylinder axis will be pulled in the direction of the axis of the stronger cylinder.

For example, pl − 2.00 × 030 combined with pl − 1.00 × 070 results in −0.31 − 2.39 × 042.

Question 7. If the axes of two equally powered plano cylinders are very close to being 90 degrees away from one another, what will be the result in terms of sphere and cylinder powers?

Answer: The cylinder power will be close to zero, and the sphere power change resulting from the two combined cylinder components will change by nearly the full power of the cylinder. The cylinder axis of the resultant cylinder will be halfway between the axes of the original cylinders.

For example, pl − 2.00 × 088 combined with pl − 2.00 × 002 equals −1.86 − 0.28 × 45.

Question 8. If the axes of two *un*equally powered cylinders are 90 degrees away from one another, what happens to the resulting sphere and cylinder powers?

Answer: The new cylinder power will be the difference between the two cylinder powers, and the sphere power will increase by the amount of the smaller cylinder.

For example, pl − 2.00 × 090 combined with pl − 1.00 × 180 equals −1.00 − 1.00 × 090.

Question 9. If the axes of two *un*equally powered plano cylinders are very close to being 90 degrees away from one another, what happens to the resulting sphere and cylinder powers?

Answer: The cylinder power will be close to the difference between the two cylinder powers. The sphere power will increase by close to the amount of the smaller cylinder. (The axis will be close to the axis of the lens with the higher powered cylinder.)

For example, pl − 2.00 × 088 combined with pl − 1.00 × 002 equals −0.99 − 1.02 × 084.

Conceptually Understanding Obliquely Crossed Spherocylinder Lenses

By using the concept questions for adding cylinder lenses just presented in the previous section, it is relatively easy to apply these concepts to spherocylinders. To anticipate the resulting spherocylinder powers and axis when adding two spherocylinders together without doing actual calculations. Start with just the cylinders and ignore the spheres. First estimate the sum of the cylinders. Afterwards add back the sphere powers.

For example, in Question 5, when a pl − 2.00 × 030 is combined with a pl − 2.00 × 070, the exact result is a lens with a power of −0.47 − 3.06 × 050. Since the cylinder powers are equal, the resulting axis will be exactly halfway in between. (The resulting cylinder power could be estimated as greater than either cylinder alone, but less than both together. The new sphere would then be halfway between the sum of the two original cylinders and the new resultant cylinder.)

If the two lenses where spherocylinders with powers of −1.50 − 2.00 × 030 and −1.25 − 2.00 × 070, remove the spheres, then sum the cylinders. The cylinders by themselves sum to −0.47 − 3.06 × 050. Now add the old spheres together [(−1.50) + (−1.25) = (−2.75)] and combine them with the new sphere [(−2.75) + (−0.47) = (−3.22)]. The new spherocylinder power is −3.22 − 3.06 × 050.

LENS THICKNESS

Sagittal Depth

The formula that is the basis for determining lens thickness is the *sagittal depth*, or *sag formula*, which was introduced previously in the chapter. Sagittal depth is the depth of the lens surface curve and is shown in Figure 13-24. Remember that a chord is a straight line joining two points on a curve. In Figure 13-24, the two points on the curve are at the edges of the lens, and the length of the chord equals the diameter of the lens.

To find the sagittal depth, it is necessary to know the length of the chord and the radius of curvature of the lens surface. Figure 13-25 shows the radius (*r*) as the hypotenuse of a right triangle. (Notice that this uses the same principles as were discussed for the lens clock previously in the chapter. Figure 13-25 is another view of what was shown in Figure 13-9.) The other two sides are y, which is one half of the chord (or ½ the lens diameter), and (*r* − *s*), which is the radius minus the sag. Because this triangle is a right triangle, the Pythagorean theorem can be used to find the sag: (When discussing the lens measure we used the Pythagorean theorem to find the radius of curvature [*r*].)

$$y^2 + (r-s)^2 = r^2$$

By transposition,

$$(r-s)^2 = r^2 - y^2$$

and

$$r - s = \sqrt{(r^2 - y^2)}$$

which simplifies to

$$-s = -r + \sqrt{(r^2 - y^2)}$$

and results in

$$s = r - \sqrt{(r^2 - y^2)}$$

This last equation is called the *accurate sag formula*.

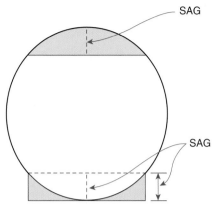

Figure 13-24. A knife-edged plus lens has the same center thickness that the edge of an infinitely thin minus lens would have when both diameters and curvatures are the same.

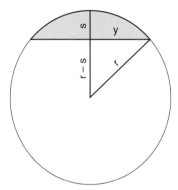

Figure 13-25. The geometry of the figure shows how the sag formula is derived from the Pythagorean theorem. Here $y^2 + (r-s)^2 = r^2$.

The Approximate Sag Formula

Before the advent of hand calculators, simplified formulas yielding an approximate result were used to find the sag of a curved surface. To simplify calculations, the more complex formula of $s = r - \sqrt{(r^2 - y^2)}$ was simplified to

$$s = \frac{y^2}{2r} \quad \text{(the approximate sag formula)}$$

The *approximate sag formula* only works when the diameter is small and the radius of curvature is long. In other words, it only approximates well for small lenses with low-powered surfaces. Because it enjoyed such widespread usage, it is still seen and referred to. However, using the accurate sag formula is no longer as difficult and yields accurate results over the whole range of lens sizes and powers.

Example **13-18**

A certain lens surface has a radius of curvature of 83.7 mm. The lens has a diameter of 50 mm. What is the sag of the front surface of the lens?

Solution

Using the accurate sag formula,

$$s = r - \sqrt{(r^2 - y^2)}$$

The value for r has been given as 83.7 mm. The *value of y* is half of the lens diameter. Since the lens has a diameter of 50 mm, y is 25 mm. Therefore

$$s = 83.7 - \sqrt{(83.7)^2 - (25)^2}$$
$$= 83.7 - 79.9$$
$$= 3.8 \text{ mm}$$

The s, r, and y can be expressed in meters or millimeters, as long as all are in the same units. In this case all three are expressed in millimeters. The sag of this surface is 3.8 mm.

Example **13-19**

Suppose a lens has a true base curve (TBC) of +7.19 D. If the diameter of the lens is 52 mm, what is the sag of the front surface at the full 52-mm diameter?

Solution

To find the sag of the surface, we need to know r and y. The y value is easy to find, since it is half of the 52-mm (chord) diameter. In other words, $y = 26$ mm. However, to find the radius, we must use the *lens maker's formula*:

$$r = \frac{n-1}{F}$$

Because the true base curve is based on a lens clock value and the lens clock uses an assumed index of refraction of 1.53, then n = 1.53, or

$$r = \frac{1.53 - 1}{F}$$

To find r for a +7.19 D TBC surface, we use:

$$r = \frac{1.53 - 1}{+7.19}$$
$$= \frac{0.53}{+7.19}$$
$$= 0.0737 \text{ m}$$

The sag formula requires that all the terms in the equation be expressed in the same units. Converting 0.0737 m to millimeters makes $r = 73.7$ mm. Now we can use the sag formula:

$$s = r - \sqrt{(r^2 - y^2)}$$
$$= 73.7 - \sqrt{(73.7)^2 - (26)^2}$$
$$= 73.7 - \sqrt{5431.7 - 676}$$
$$= 73.7 - \sqrt{4755.7}$$
$$= 73.7 - 69.0$$
$$= 4.7 \text{ mm}$$

The sag of a +7.19 D TBC surface on a 52-mm lens is 4.7 mm.

Example **13-20**

A lens has a true base curve (TBC) of +7.19, a diameter of 52 mm, a plano back surface, and an edge thickness of 1.6 mm. What is the center thickness (CT) of the lens?

Solution

We have already calculated the sag of the front surface of this lens in Example 13-19. To visualize what this plano-convex lens looks like, see Figure 13-26, *A*. From the figure we can see that the *CT* of the lens will be equal to the sag of the front surface (s_1), plus the edge thickness (*ET*). Therefore the *CT* of this lens is:

$$CT = s_1 + ET$$
$$CT = 4.7 \text{ mm} + 1.6 \text{ mm}$$
$$= 6.3 \text{ mm}$$

In Figure 13-26, the edge thickness has been drawn exceptionally thick to keep front and back surface sagittal depth labels (s_1 and s_2) from overlapping. If drawn to scale, the edge would be much thinner and would correspond more accurately to the example.

Thickness of Meniscus Lenses

Although a few ophthalmic lenses worn today may be plano concave or plano convex, most lenses have a convex front surface and a concave back surface. These lenses are referred to as *meniscus lenses*. To determine the thickness of a meniscus lens, calculations must be made for both the front and back surfaces.

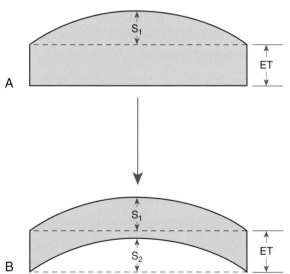

Figure 13-26. A, For a plus lens with a convex front surface and plano (flat) back surface, lens center thickness is equal to the edge thickness plus the sagittal depth of the front surface (s_1). **B,** A meniscus lens has a convex front surface and a concave back surface. The center thickness of a meniscus lens is equal to the edge thickness plus the sagittal depth of the front surface (s_1) minus the sagittal depth of the second surface (s_2).

To better understand the construction of such a lens and how calculations are carried out, think of the meniscus lens as being two lenses glued together. A meniscus lens can first be thought of as a plano-convex lens, as shown in Figure 13-26, *A*. For a plano-convex lens, center thickness is equal to the sagittal depth of the first surface (s_1) plus the edge thickness, or:

$$CT = s_1 + ET$$

After center thickness calculations have been carried out for a plano-convex lens, imagine grinding a minus curve on the back of the lens, as shown in Figure 13-26, *B*. This reduces the CT by the sag of this freshly ground concave surface. The CT then becomes:

$$CT = s_1 + ET - s_2$$

or

$$CT = s_1 - s_2 + ET$$

where s_2 is the sag of the second surface.

Sagittal depths are found using the accurate sag formula:

$$s = r - \sqrt{r^2 - y^2}$$

as previously described.

Concepts in Understanding Lens Thickness

One of the motivations for understanding lens thickness concepts is so that it is easy to visualize how a given prescription will look in different types of frames. In fact knowing thickness concepts will keep one from ordering a lens prescription for a frame that is either unsightly or even unsuitable. In going through the next section, here is a quick review of the formulas needed for working the problems in the sequence they will normally be used.

$$1.\ y = \frac{chord\ diameter}{2}$$
$$2.\ r = \frac{n-1}{F}$$
$$3.\ s = r - \sqrt{r^2 - y^2}$$
$$4.\ CT = s_1 - s_2 + ET$$

As we progress through this section, some of the examples may seem overly simplistic. This is done intentionally to make certain that each conceptual step is understood.

Center Thickness for a Plano-Convex Lens

Example **13-21**

What is the center thickness for a lens with the following dimensions?

Lens power = +3.00 D

Index of refraction = 1.53

Lens diameter = 50 mm

Lens form is plano convex (+3.00 D front curve and a plano back surface).

Edge thickness is zero. (A lens with a zero edge thickness is said to be knife edged.)

The lens has no decentration. (The optical center is exactly in the middle of the edged shape.)

Solution

In learning to conceptualize lens thickness, it is helpful to try to draw a picture of the lens as soon as possible. In this case because the lens is round and the optical center is in the middle of the lens, the chord diameter is the same as the eye size or the A dimension of the frame.

This information will allow us to draw a cross section of the lens, as shown in Figure 13-27. This makes the semidiameter (*y*) equal to:

$$y = \frac{chord\ diameter}{2}$$
$$= \frac{50}{2}$$
$$= 25\ mm$$

The radius of curvature is found using the lens maker's formula where:

$$r = \frac{n-1}{F}$$
$$= \frac{1.53-1}{3.00}$$
$$= \frac{0.53}{3}$$
$$= 0.1766\ m\ or\ 176.7\ mm$$

The sagittal depth of the lens surface is:

$$s_1 = r - \sqrt{r^2 - y^2}$$
$$= 176.7 - \sqrt{(176.7)^2 - (25)^2}$$
$$= 176.7 - \sqrt{31223 - 625}$$
$$= 176.7 - \sqrt{30598}$$
$$= 176.7 - 174.9$$
$$= 1.8\ mm$$

We can use the formula for center thickness. But even before using the formula, we know that the center thickness will be 1.8 mm. This is because there is no edge thickness, and the back of the lens is flat. Because the lens is flat, the

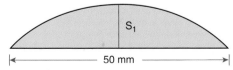

Figure 13-27. The center thickness of a plano-convex lens with a zero edge thickness is equal to the sagittal depth of the convex surface.

sagittal depth of the second surface (s_2) is equal to zero. Here is the formula solution:

$$CT = s_1 - s_2 + ET$$
$$= 1.8 - 0 + 0$$
$$= 1.8 \text{ mm}$$

Before finishing the problem, we need to look at the whole lens—center, left edge, right edge, and top and bottom edges. To look at the lens in horizontal and vertical cross sections, see Figure 13-28.

Example **13-22**

A lens is a +3.00 D sphere with the same dimensions as the previous lens, except that this lens is ground so that the resulting edge is 1.0 mm thick. What is the center thickness of the lens?

Solution

The answer here is intuitive. If the previous lens has an edge thickness of zero and is 1.8 mm thick in the center, then this lens with a 1.0 mm edge thickness will be 1.0 mm thicker everywhere, resulting in a lens of 2.8 mm center thickness. But the example was introduced to further the reasoning in finding lens thickness.

The lens is drawn as shown in Figure 13-29. We find s_1, the sagittal depth of the first surface, exactly as before. The figure shows us (and the formula tells us) that:

center thickness = the sag of the front surface + edge thickness

In other words,

$$CT = 1.8 \text{ mm} + 1.0 \text{ mm}$$
$$= 2.8 \text{ mm}$$

The sag of the second surface is zero, so it does not factor in. (Incidentally, when drawing figures like the one shown in Figure 13-29, the center thickness in both horizontal and vertical cross sections will always be the same because both are part of the same lens.)

Example **13-23**

A. What is the center thickness of a cylinder lens with a power of pl +3.00 × 090 that is edged to a 50-mm round shape and has no decentration? The thinnest edge of the lens is zero. In other words, at its thinnest point the lens is "knife edged." This lens has a plano back surface, and the index of refraction is 1.53.
B. Where are the thin knife edges located?
C. How thick are the thickest edges?

Solution

A. If this lens is drawn, as shown in Figure 13-30, we see that the axis meridian is at 90 and the power meridian at 180. The lens has the same +3.00 D power and 50-mm chord size as the +3.00 D sphere in the previous example. Therefore since it is knife edged and plano convex, the sagittal depth is the same 1.8 mm that we found in the previous example. This equals the center thickness of the lens.
B. The knife edges are on the left and right sides of the lens in the 180-degree horizontal power meridian. This is shown in Figure 13-30.
C. Because the lens is plano in the 90-degree axis meridian, the thickness remains the same all along the axis. If this plano cylinder lens is 1.8 mm thick in the center, it is also 1.8 mm thick at the top and bottom edges.

Edge Thickness for a Plano-Concave Lens

The methodology used for finding edge thickness of minus lenses is practically the same as that used to find the center thickness for plus lenses.

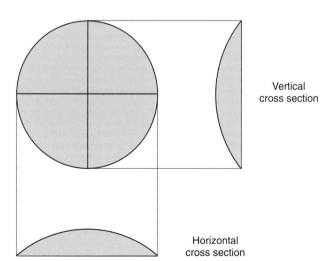

Figure 13-28. Cross sections of a knife-edged plano-convex lens.

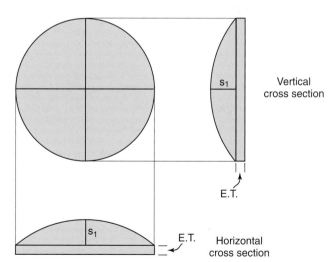

Figure 13-29. When a plano-convex lens (with no decentration) has edge thickness, the center thickness of the lens equals the sagittal depth of the convex surface plus the edge thickness.

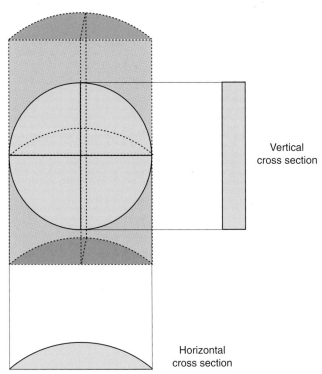

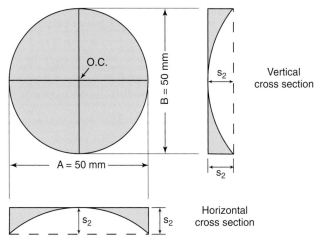

Figure 13-31. Horizontal and vertical cross sections of a plano-concave lens with an infinitely thin center. With zero center thickness, the edge thickness equals the sagittal depth of the concave (minus) surface.

Figure 13-30. Cross sections of a plano-convex cylinder lens in the major meridians of the lens. When the plano-convex cylinder (shown with axis at 90 degrees) is edged to a round shape, the horizontal cross section in the power meridian looks like a normal plus lens. The center is thick, and the edges on either side are thin. In the vertical (axis) meridian, the thickness of the lens is the same at center and edges.

If we were to use the formula to find edge thickness, we would use:

$$CT = s_1 - s_2 + ET$$

or

$$ET = CT - s_1 + s_2$$
$$ET = 0 - 0 + 1.8 \text{ mm}$$
$$ET = 1.8 \text{ mm}$$

Example **13-24**

What is the edge thickness for this minus lens that has been edged to a 50-mm round shape if the optical center is exactly at the center of the edged shape? Here are the lens parameters:

The front surface curve is flat ($F_1 = 0$).

The back surface curve has a power of -3.00 D ($F_2 = -3.00$ D).

The refractive index is 1.53.

The lens is infinitely thin in the center. In other words, the lens has a center thickness of zero.

Solution

Set the problem up with a drawing. That drawing is shown in Figure 13-31. Here we see the round lens with horizontal and vertical cross sections. Because the lens is round, with the optical center in the middle of the lens shape, both horizontal and vertical cross sections are identical. Because the lens has zero center thickness and the front of the lens is flat, the sagittal depth of the back surface equals the edge thickness of the lens.

The sagittal depth of the back surface is found in the same manner as was done for front surface sagittal depth. The same dimensions have been chosen as in earlier examples, conveniently allowing us to know that $s_2 = 1.8$ mm.

Example **13-25**

A lens is a -3.00 D lens with the same dimensions as the previous lens, except that it has a 1.0 mm center thickness. How thick are the lens edges in the horizontal and vertical meridians?

Solution

As the center increases in thickness, so does the edge. So if the sagittal depth of the second surface in 1.8 mm, and the center thickness is 1.0 mm, then the edge thickness will be 2.8 mm (Figure 13-32). This should be intuitive. However, the formula sequence is:

$$ET = CT - s_1 + s_2$$
$$= 1.0 - 0 + 1.8$$
$$= 2.8 \text{ mm}$$

The object here is to intuitively know how center and edge thickness work, not to work a formula. It is highly unlikely that someone will sit down in an optical dispensary and calculate center or edge thickness. However, it is very important to conceptually know what an ophthalmic lens prescription will look like in a given frame shape and lens material when completed, even before it is ever ordered.

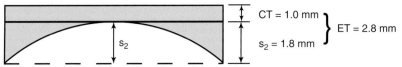

Figure 13-32. The edge thickness of a plano-concave (minus) lens is the sum of the center thickness and the sagittal depth of the concave surface.

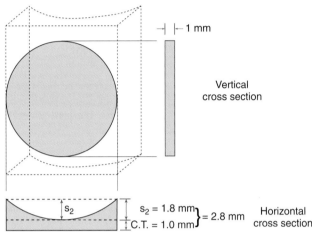

Vertical
cross section

$s_2 = 1.8$ mm
C.T. = 1.0 mm $\Big\}$ = 2.8 mm   Horizontal
cross section

Figure 13-33. Horizontal and vertical cross sections of a plano-concave cylinder with center thickness. The thickness along the cylinder axis does not change.

Example **13-26**

A lens has the following parameters:
- Power = pl − 3.00 × 090
- Lens form: a plano-concave cylinder
- The lens is edged 50 mm round.
- The optics of the lens are centered in the edged shape (i.e., there is no decentration).
- Index of refraction is 1.53.
- The center thickness of the lens is 1.0 mm.

What are the edge thicknesses in the horizontal and vertical meridians?

Solution

Begin by setting up the problem as a drawing. Figure 13-33 shows a plano minus cylinder oriented at axis 90 degrees. Now imagine edging that cylinder to a 50-mm round shape by drawing a circle over it. (The flat plane drawing of the circle will not exactly mesh with the three-dimensional aspects of the plano cylinder drawing, but should be understandable.)

Now draw horizontal and vertical cross sections of the lens. A plano minus cylinder lens has the same thickness along its axis meridian. Therefore the top and bottom edges of the lens have the same thickness as the center of the lens (1.0 mm).

The plano minus cylinder lens thickens toward the edge in the power meridian. Edge thickness along the power meridian is equal to the center thickness plus the sagittal depth of the second surface in the meridian. In this case as before, the sagittal depth is 1.8 mm. So the edge thick-

---

nesses on both sides of the 180-degree meridian are 2.8 mm. As before:

$$ET_{180} = CT - s_1 + s_2$$
$$= 1.0 - 0 + 1.8$$
$$= 2.8 \text{ mm}$$

Center and Edge Thicknesses for Meniscus Lenses

Here are some example problems for plus and minus meniscus lenses using the same principles that have already been covered up to this point.

Example **13-27**

What is the center thickness for this +2.00 D lens that is edged to a horizontally oval shape? The lens parameters needed to solve the problem are:
$F_1 = +8.00$ D (front surface power)
$F_2 = -6.00$ D (back surface power)
$n = 1.53$
   Minimum edge thickness = 1.5 mm
A = 50 mm (This is the horizontal dimension of the oval shape.)
B = 30 mm (This is the vertical dimension of the oval shape.)
The optical center of the lens is in the center of the lens shape.

Solution

Before we start any calculations, we need to know where the thinnest edge(s) of the lens are found. The easiest way to find the location of the thinnest edge(s) is to conceptualize the lens. To do this, ignore the fact that the lens is a meniscus lens. Imagine it as a plano-convex lens of power +2.00 D. If we draw it out this way, it would appear as shown in Figure 13-34. We know that a plus lens is thickest in the middle and thins gradually as the distance from the center increases. Therefore the thinnest edge of a plus sphere lens will be the edge farthest from the lens optical center.

Both left and right edges are equally far from the optical center and are the points that are farthest from the optical center. The top and bottom edges are closer to the optical center and are thicker.

Knowing this we can redraw the horizontal cross section as shown in Figure 13-35. If we can find the sagittal depths for the first and second surfaces, we will know what the center thickness is.

For the first surface:

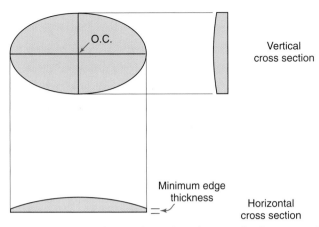

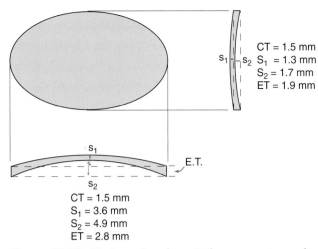

Figure 13-34. When a plus sphere lens is edged to an oval shape, edge thickness will be greatest for the edge closest to the optical center of the lens.

Vertical
cross section

Minimum edge
thickness

Horizontal
cross section

CT = 1.5 mm
S₁ = 1.3 mm
S₂ = 1.7 mm
ET = 1.9 mm

CT = 1.5 mm
S₁ = 3.6 mm
S₂ = 4.9 mm
ET = 2.8 mm

Figure 13-36. Horizontal and vertical cross sections of a minus sphere meniscus lens that has been edged oval.

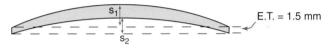

E.T. = 1.5 mm

Figure 13-35. The center thickness of a meniscus lens is equal to the sagittal depth of the first surface (s_1), minus the sagittal depth of the second surface (s_2) plus the edge thickness ($CT = s_1 - s_2 + ET$).

$$r = \frac{n-1}{F_1} = \frac{1.53-1}{8.00}$$
$$= 0.06625 \, m = 66.25 \, mm$$

$$s_1 = r - \sqrt{(r)^2 - (y)^2}$$
$$= 66.25 - \sqrt{(66.25)^2 - (25)^2}$$
$$= 66.25 - \sqrt{4389 - 625}$$
$$= 66.25 - 61.35$$
$$= 4.9 \, mm$$

For the second surface:

$$r = \frac{1-n}{F_2} = \frac{1-1.53}{-6}$$
$$= 0.08833 \, m = 88.33 \, mm$$

$$s_2 = r - \sqrt{(r)^2 - (y)^2}$$
$$= 88.33 - \sqrt{(88.33)^2 - (25)^2}$$
$$= 88.33 - \sqrt{7803 - 625}$$
$$= 88.33 - 84.72$$
$$= 3.6 \, mm$$

Therefore center thickness of this lens is:

$$CT = s_1 - s_2 + ET$$
$$= 4.9 - 3.6 + 1.5$$
$$= 2.8 \, mm$$

Example **13-28**

A −2.00 D lens has the following parameters:
- F_1 = +6.00 D
- F_2 = −8.00 D
- n = 1.53
- Center thickness = 1.5 mm
- It is edged to a horizontal oval shape, where
- A = 50 mm (horizontal dimension)
- B = 30 mm (vertical dimension)

How thick are the lens edges in both the horizontal and the vertical meridians?

Solution

Notice first of all that the lens in this example and the plus lens in the previous example have much in common. Even their surface curves are the same, except that now the 6 diopter curve is on the front and the 8 diopter curve on the back. Remember that a minus lens is thinnest in the center and gradually increases in thickness toward the edges. The edge closest to the center is thinnest; the farthest edge thickest. To solve the problem, begin by drawing it out. This is shown completed in Figure 13-36.

For the horizontal meridian:

To find the edge thickness of the horizontal meridian, we know the chord diameter is 50 mm. The index and surface curves are the same as in the previous problem. Therefore for the +6.00 front curve, the sagittal depth (s_1) is 3.6 mm. The second surface of −8.00 has a sagittal depth (s_2) of 4.9 mm. This gives an edge thickness of:

$$ET = CT - s_1 + s_2$$
$$= 1.5 - 3.6 + 4.9$$
$$= 2.8 \, mm$$

For the vertical meridian:

Even though the curves in the vertical meridian are the same as the horizontal meridian, the sagittal depths will be different because the chord diameter (or chord length) is smaller. For the +6.00 D surface, we already know that the surface radius is 8.33 mm. The semidiameter of the vertical chord diameter is:

$$y = \frac{chord\ diameter\ (or\ length)}{2}$$
$$= \frac{30\ mm}{2}$$
$$= 15\ mm$$

So sagittal depth for the first surface in the 90-degree meridian is:

$$s_1 = r - \sqrt{r^2 - y^2}$$
$$= 88.33 - \sqrt{(88.33)^2 - (15)^2}$$
$$= 88.33 - \sqrt{7803 - 225}$$
$$= 88.33 - 87.05$$
$$= 1.3\ mm$$

The sagittal depth for the second surface in the 90-degree meridian is:

$$s_2 = r - \sqrt{r^2 - y^2}$$
$$= 66.25 - \sqrt{(66.25)^2 - (15)^2}$$
$$= 66.25 - \sqrt{4389 - 225}$$
$$= 66.25 - 64.53$$
$$= 1.7\ mm$$

This makes the top and bottom edge thickness equal to:

$$ET = CT - s_1 + s_2$$
$$= 1.5 - 1.3 + 1.7$$
$$= 1.9\ mm$$

So the horizontal edge thicknesses of this lens are 2.8 mm and the vertical edge thicknesses are 1.9 mm.

Determining Lens Diameter for Noncentered Lenses

The lens diameter needed to find the correct sag value depends on both the frame size and the location of the optical center. Normally the optical center is not in the middle of the lens once it has been edged. To visualize the situation, mark the point on an edged lens where the optical center will fall. Next draw a line from the optical center (OC) to the point on the lens edge that is farthest from the OC (Figure 13-37). The resulting line is the y value we are interested in. Twice y is very close to the *minimum blank size* (MBS).* In fact when considering single vision uncut lenses, the diameter we are interested in is equal to the minimum blank size, but it does not include the 2-mm safety factor for lens chipping that is included in the MBS formula.† The formula for this diameter, which we will call the *chord diameter*, is:

$$Chord\ diameter = ED + (A + DBL - Far\ PD)$$

---

*For more on Minimum Blank Size, see Chapter 5.

†The MBS formula for single vision lenses is MBS = ED + (A + DBL − PD) + 2 = ED + (decentration per lens) × 2 + 2

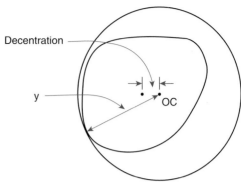

Figure 13-37. The diameter used in calculating lens thickness is basically the same as that used for minimum blank size. The only difference is that the chipping factor is ignored.

where

ED = the effective diameter of a lens*
A = the boxing eye size
DBL = the distance between lenses
Far PD = the wearer's interpupillary distance for distance viewing

This chord diameter formula may be used for both single vision and multifocal lenses.

Estimating Edge Thickness

It can be very useful to be able to estimate edge thickness quickly. Such estimates are useful when asked, "How thick will my lenses be?" It is not possible to accurately know edge or center thickness without calculating chord diameter and sag values. To make estimations easier, calculations can be dropped by assuming equal decentration for all cases and by using the effective diameter (ED) of the frame instead of chord diameter. This means that for a lens having an ED of 50 mm we can use a constant (K) of 0.7 and multiply it by the power of the lens. The constant used for lenses with an ED of 50 mm is 0.7. Lenses with a 58-mm ED call for a constant of 1.0. If the numbers (50, 0.7) and (58, 1.0) can be remembered, constants other than 0.7 and 1.0 can be estimated, depending upon how close the ED of the frame is to 50 or 58. (These estimations are for low-index glass or plastic lenses. To estimate thickness for higher index materials, it is feasible to reduce the constants of 0.7 and 1.0 to somewhat smaller values. The higher the index of refraction is, the lower the value of the constant will be.)

Example **13-29**

Estimate the edge thickness of a −6.00 D lens that has a center thickness of 2.2 mm and is to be placed in a frame with an ED of 55 mm.

---

*For more on effective diameter, see Chapter 2.

Solution

A 55-mm E D is more than halfway between 50 and 58. This means that the constant chosen will be more than halfway between 0.7 and 1.0. (Halfway is 0.85.) The constant chosen will be 0.9. Edge thickness is:

$$\text{Edge Thickness} = K(F) + \text{center thickness}$$
$$= 0.9\ (6.00) + 2.2$$
$$= 5.4 + 2.2$$
$$= 7.6\ \text{mm}$$

The lens has an estimated edge thickness of 7.6 mm.

When a lens has prism as part of the prescription, for estimation purposes one half of the prescribed prism amount is added to lens thickness. (The reason why prism changes the thickness of a lens will be explained more fully later in the chapter on prism.)

Thus the rule of thumb can be expressed as:

Center or edge thickness = K(F) + (edge or center thickness) + P/2

where
K = the constant
F = the power of the lens
P = the power of the prism

Example **13-30**

Estimate the edge thickness of the lens in Example 13-29 if it is also to have 3 prism diopters of base-out prism.

Solution

The thickness factor for prism is an estimated 0.5 mm for every diopter of prism. This increases the estimated thickness by 1.5 mm. Therefore the estimated edge thickness is:

$$\text{Edge thickness} = K(F) + CT + \frac{P}{2}$$
$$= 0.9\ (6.00) + 2.2 + 1.5$$
$$= 9.1\ \text{mm}$$

It should be understood that this method of estimation is intended to provide only a rough estimation and cannot be unerringly depended on.

CURVATURE IN AN OBLIQUE MERIDIAN

When specifying lens curvature, the curve can be denoted by either its radius of curvature (*r*) or by the unit "Curvature."

A spherically curved surface has a specific *radius* of curvature, *r*. By definition, the *Curvature* of a surface, specified with *R*, is the inverse of the radius of curvature in meters, or reciprocal meters (m⁻¹). In other words,

$$R = \frac{1}{r}$$

A plano plus cylinder appears as shown in Figure 13-38. In the figure, there is no curve to the lens surface in

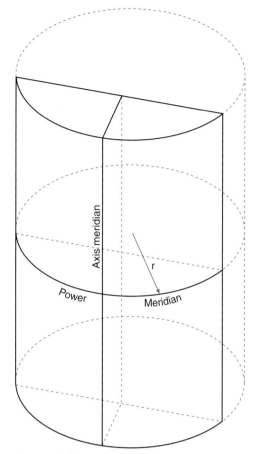

Figure 13-38. A plano, plus cylinder has no power in the axis meridian. The refractive power in the power meridian depends on the index of refraction of the material and the radius of curvature.

the axis meridian. The surface is flat. In the power meridian, the surface has maximum curvature. Therefore there is zero curvature along the axis of the plano-cylinder lens surface. Along the power meridian, the curvature is *R*. In between the axis meridian and the power meridian, curvature will increase by degree. (Figure 13-39). The specific curvature of the surface may be found using the equation:

$$R_\theta = R_{cyl} \sin^2 \theta$$

where

R_θ = Curvature in the oblique meridian
R_{cyl} = Curvature in the power meridian

and

θ = the angle between the oblique meridian and the cylinder axis.

The short-cut method says that since, for a lens surface in air,

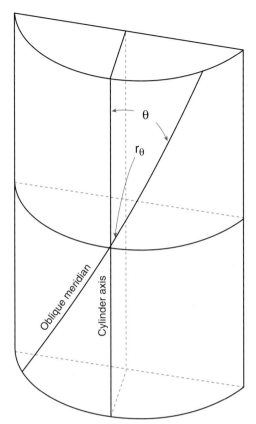

Figure 13-39. The radius of curvature, r_θ, in an oblique meridian of a plano, plus cylinder lens will vary depending upon the power of the cylinder curve and the angle (θ) of the oblique meridian.

$$F = \frac{n-1}{r}$$

or

$$F = (n-1)R$$

then

$$R = \frac{F}{n-1}$$

It would seem logical then that if

$$R_\theta = R_{cyl} \sin^2 \theta,$$

then we should be able to say that

$$\frac{F_\theta}{n-1} = \frac{F_{cyl}}{n-1} \sin^2 \theta$$

and

$$F_\theta = F_{cyl} \sin^2 \theta.$$

Unfortunately, this assumption is not entirely correct. Although the curvature of a cross section changes, and "power" in an oblique cylinder meridian may be read using a lens clock on the surface, technically a plano cylinder does not vary in power along an oblique meridian, only in curvature. This sine-squared approximation method can be helpful in certain circumstances, however.

Using Sine-Squared θ to Find the "Power" of the Cylinder in an Oblique Meridian

To use the sine-squared approximation method for finding the "power" of a cylinder in an oblique meridian, use the following steps:
1. Find "theta."
   Theta (θ) is the difference between the meridian in question and the axis of the cylinder.
2. Apply the sine-squared formula ($F_\theta = F_{cyl} \sin^2\theta$) to the cylinder power.

Example **13-31**

What is the "power" of a pl + 2.00 × 030 cylinder in the 180-degree meridian?

Solution

To find theta, we find the difference between the cylinder axis and the 180-degree meridian. This difference is the same as the axis of the cylinder (Figure 13-40). To find the "power" of the cylinder in the 180-degree meridian, we use the formula $F_\theta = F_{cyl} \sin^2 \theta$.
   By substitution we have:

$$F_\theta = F_{cyl} \sin^2 \theta$$
$$= (+2.00)\sin^2 30$$
$$= (+2.00)(0.25)$$
$$= +0.50 \, D$$

Therefore, the "power" of the cylinder in the 180-degree meridian is +0.50 D.

Thickness in an Oblique Meridian

The sine-squared method for finding the curvature of a lens in an oblique meridian means we can find the radius of curvature in an oblique meridian. With radius of curvature and chord diameter it is now possible to find sagittal depth in an oblique meridian. Sagittal depth in an oblique meridian leads directly to lens thickness in that oblique meridian. Thus using sine-squared principles, we should be able to find lens thickness for any point on a lens. It is left to the reader to take this concept further and find lens thickness for any given point on a lens.

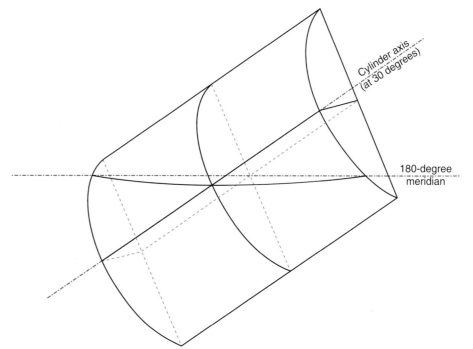

Figure 13-40. Finding the "power" of a plus cylinder lens in the 180-degree meridian can be visualized as shown in the figure.

Cylinder axis (at 30 degrees)

180-degree meridian

REFERENCES

1. Brooks C: Specifying base curves: the dos and don't, Rev Optom 45-48, 1996.

Proficiency Test

(Answers can be found in the back of the book.)

Lens Surface Powers and Base Curves

1. A lens has the following specifications
   $F_1 = +7.25$ D
   F_2 at 90 = -6.00 D
   F_2 at 180 = -8.00 D
   What is the base curve?
   a. -6.00 D
   b. -8.00 D
   c. $+7.25$ D

2. A lens has the following specifications:
   F_1 at 90 = $+6.00$ D
   F_1 at 180 = $+8.00$ D
   $F_2 = -7.00$ D
   What is the base curve?
   a. $+6.00$ D
   b. $+8.00$ D
   c. -7.00 D
   d. -1.00 D
   e. $+1.00$ D

3. If the lens $+2.00 + 1.00 \times 090$ is ground in minus cylinder form with the following dimensions, what is the toric or back base curve?
   $F_1 = +8.00$ D
   F_2 at 90 = -6.00 D
   F_2 at 180 = -5.00 D
   a. $+8.00$ D
   b. -6.00 D
   c. -5.00 D

4. If the lens +2.00 + 1.00 × 090 is ground in plus cylinder form with the F_2 surface being −4.00 D, what is the base curve?
   a. +6.00 D
   b. +7.00 D
   c. −4.00 D
   d. +2.00 D
   e. none of the above

5. True or false? *Base curve* and *toric base curve* are always synonymous terms.

6. True or false? The toric base curve is on the back of a minus cylinder lens.

7. A lens prescription of −3.25 D cylinder is made up on a +6.00 D base curve. The ocular surface could be:
   a. −3.25 D sph
   b. −6.00 D/−9.25 D
   c. −6.00 D sph
   d. −9.25 D sph
   e. either b or d

8. True or false? It is highly unlikely that lenses today will be made in plus cylinder form. At present, almost all lenses are made in minus cylinder form.

9. A single vision lens has a power of +3.00 + 2.25 × 030. If the lens is ground in minus cylinder form having a base curve of 6.00 D, what are the remaining two curves?
   a. +3.75 D and −0.75 D
   b. −0.75 D and −3.00 D
   c. +8.25 D and −3.00 D
   d. −3.75 D and −3.00 D
   e. none of the above

10. A lens has a power of +1.25 − 2.00 × 180. If it is ground in plus cylinder form on an 8.00 D base curve, what are the surface powers and in which meridians are they?

11. A lens has a power of +3.00 − 1.00 × 180 and a +8.00 D base curve. What are the possible lens dimensions?
    a. F_1 at 180 = +8.00 D
       F_1 at 90 = +7.00 D
       F_2 = −5.00 D
    b. F_1 = +8.00 D
       F_2 at 180 = −5.00 D
       F_2 at 90 = −6.00 D
    c. F_1 at 90 = +8.00 D
       F_1 at 180 = +9.00 D
       F_2 = −6.00 D
    d. both b and c
    e. all of the above

12. A lens has a 6.00 D base curve. The Rx is +1.25 −2.00 × 090. What are the two possible forms the lens may have? (Give front and back curves in their proper meridians for both lenses.)

13. On the back surface of a lens having a plano front surface, a lens clock shows +1.25 in the 67-degree meridian and −1.75 in the 157-degree meridian. Assuming that the lens is made from a material with an index close to 1.53, what is the lens prescription?
    a. +1.25 − 1.75 × 067
    b. −1.75 + 3.00 × 157
    c. −1.75 − 3.00 × 067
    d. +1.25 − 3.00 × 157
    e. none of the above

14. A lens clock reads as follows in the major meridians:

	Front Surface	Back Surface
In the 10-degree meridian	+7.12 D	−7.50 D
In the 100-degree meridian	+8.25 D	−7.50 D

    Assuming that the lens material has an index close to 1.53, what is the prescription in minus cylinder form?

15. A lens clock reads as follows on the major meridians:

	Front Surface	Back Surface
In the 20-degree meridian	+8.00 D	−6.00 D
In the 110-degree meridian	+8.00 D	−7.00 D

    Assuming that the lens material has an index close to 1.53, what is the prescription in minus cylinder form?

16. A lens surface has a refractive power of +8.25 D. If the lens is made from material having an index of 1.53, what is the radius of curvature of the lens surface?

17. A lens surface has a refractive power of +8.25 D. If the lens is made from material having an index of 1.74, what is the radius of curvature of the lens surface?

18. If a plus lens surface has a radius of curvature of 64.24 mm, what surface power would it have if made from a 1.74-index material?

19. A certain lens of index 1.66 has a concave back surface. The lens is small and has a diameter of 40 mm. The sagittal depth of this back surface is 0.8 mm. What is the power of the back surface of the lens?

20. A lens clock calibrated for index 1.53 is used on a lens of index 1.70.

The front surface of the lens is measured on the major meridians as follows:

Measured Front Surface:

90-degree meridian   4.54 D

180-degree meridian   3.79 D

   a. What are the refractive powers for the front surface of the lens?

   b. What is the value of the cylinder, assuming the back surface to be spherical?

21. A lens clock measures F_1 at 90 = +8.00 D, F_1 at 180 = +5.00 D, $F_2 = -4.00$ D.

   a. If the lens clock is calibrated for 1.53, what is the nominal lens power of the lens measured?

   b. What would the power be if the lens were made from plastic of index = 1.49?

22. A lens clock calibrated for index 1.53 is used on a lens with an index of refraction of 1.80. The lens clock measures the surface as follows:

F_1 at 90 = +10.33 D

F_1 at 180 = +9.00 D

$F_2 = -3.00$ D

Assume the lens to be a thin lens. Without taking lens thickness into consideration, what is the lens prescription?

   a. +11.25 − 2.25 × 180

   b. +11.05 − 1.33 × 090

   c. +9.06 + 1.33 × 090

   d. +9.06 + 2.00 × 180

   e. none of the above

23. A lens of index 1.70 is ordered, and the base curve specified. The specified base curve is +8.25 D. When it arrives, the base curve is checked with a lens clock and is found to be +8.17 D. What are the nominal, true, and refractive powers for this lens surface?

24. You measure the front surface of a spherical polycarbonate lens with a lens clock. What are you measuring?

   a. the nominal base curve

   b. the true base curve

   c. the refractive power of the surface

   d. It is not possible to tell from the information given.

25. A lens has an index a refraction of 1.498 and a nominal base curve of +6.25. What is the true base curve?

   a. +6.13

   b. +6.20

   c. +6.25

   d. +6.33

   e. cannot be determined from the information given

26. You would like to find the refractive power of a number of lens surfaces. All of the surfaces are on lenses of index 1.67. You use a lens clock (lens measure) on the surface. This gives you a reference surface power, but not the refractive power you are looking for. You could find the refractive power by multiplying your lens clock power by:

   a. 0.791.

   b. 0.916.

   c. 1.092.

   d. 1.264.

   e. It is not possible to find surface refractive power in this manner.

27. True or false? A person comes in for an eye exam, and the prescription has increased slightly. When ordering the new pair of glasses, one should always check the base curve of the old glasses and order the same base curve for the new glasses.

28. True or false? When ordering an identically powered pair of glasses as a second pair, it is advisable to check the base curve of the first pair and order the same base curve for the new glasses.

Crossing Cylinders and Spherocylinders

29. A ±1.00 D Jackson crossed cylinder is placed in front of a −2.50 sphere lens. You read this lens combination in a lensmeter. What power would you expect to find?

   a. −2.00 − 1.00 × something

   b. −3.50 − 2.00 × something

   c. −2.50 − 2.00 × something

   d. −3.00 − 1.00 × something

   e. −1.50 − 2.00 × something

30. A ±1.00 D Jackson crossed cylinder lens oriented 90/180 is placed in front of a +2.00 D sphere lens. Which spherocylinder lens power could be a resultant of these two lenses?

   a. +3.00 − 1.00 × 090 or 180

   b. +2.00 − 2.00 × 090 or 180

   c. +4.00 − 2.00 × 090 or 180

   d. +2.00 − 1.00 × 090 or 180

   e. +3.00 − 2.00 × 090 or 180

31. Give the sum of these two lenses: +2.00 − 2.00 × 090 and pl − 2.00 × 180. (Give your answer to the nearest quarter diopter.)

   a. +2.00 − 4.00 × 045

   b. +2.00 − 3.00 ×045

   c. +2.00 sphere

   d. pl − 2.00 × 090

   e. 0.00

32. Give the sum of these two lenses: pl − 3.00 × 015 and pl − 3.00 × 165. (Give your answer to the nearest eighth diopter.)
    a. pl − 5.25 × 090
    b. −0.50 − 5.25 × 180
    c. −0.50 − 5.25 × 090
    d. pl −3.25 × 180

33. Give the sum of these two lenses: +3.00 + 1.50 × 110 and +2.00 + 2.25 × 130. (Give your answer to the nearest eighth diopter.)
    a. +7.00 + 2.12 × 126
    b. +5.00 + 3.62 × 119
    c. +4.62 + 3.25 × 124
    d. +5.00 + 3.75 × 118
    e. +5.12 + 3.50 × 122

The next three questions (Questions 34, 35, and, 36) are based on the following text.
You order a toric soft contact lens having a power of

−3.50 − 2.00 × 015.

The contact lens stabilizes and orients exactly as you expected it would. It is not rotated.
You do an overrefraction. Your results yield a power of

+0.50 − 1.25 × 075.

You need to order another contact lens incorporating your overrefraction. What contact lens should you order? For sphere and cylinder power, order to the nearest quarter diopter, for cylinder axis, order to the nearest 5 degrees.

34. To the nearest quarter diopter, the correct sphere power is:
    a. −2.75.
    b. −3.25.
    c. −3.75.
    d. −4.25.

35. To the nearest quarter diopter, the correct cylinder power is:
    a. −1.00.
    b. −1.50.
    c. −1.75.
    d. −2.75.

36. The correct cylinder axis is:
    a. 35.
    b. 40.
    c. 60.
    d. 70.

37. Give the sum of these two lenses: pl − 3.25 × 180 and pl − 3.25 × 045. (Give your answer to the nearest quarter diopter.)
    a. −1.00 − 4.50 × 023
    b. pl − 6.50 × 068
    c. pl − 4.50 × 068
    d. pl − 4.50 × 023

You should not have to do any hard calculations for any of the following five questions (Questions 38-42). They are concept questions and should not require a calculator.

38. What would the resulting lens power be for a −2.00 − 1.00 × 090 lens and a −2.50 − 1.00 × 180 lens placed one on top of the other in a lensmeter?
    a. −2.25 − 1.00 × 045
    b. −4.50 − 2.00 × 045
    c. −4.50 DS
    d. −5.50 DS
    e. None of the above are correct responses.

39. What would the resulting lens power be for a −1.50 − 1.50 × 085 lens and a −3.00 − 1.50 × 005 lens placed one on top of the other in a lensmeter? Give the answer rounded to the nearest 1/8 diopter that will be closest to the actual calculated values.
    a. −4.50 − 3.00 × 045
    b. −4.50 − 1.50 × 045
    c. −5.75 − 0.50 × 045
    d. −6.00 − 1.50 × 045
    e. −6.00 DS

40. What would the resulting lens power be for a −1.50 − 1.50 × 050 lens and a −3.00 − 1.50 × 040 lens placed one on top of the other in a lensmeter? Give the answer rounded to the nearest 1/8 diopter that will be closest to the actual calculated values.
    a. −4.50 − 3.00 × 045
    b. −4.50 − 1.50 × 045
    c. −5.75 − 0.50 × 045
    d. −6.00 − 1.50 × 045
    e. −6.00 DS

41. What would the resulting lens power be for a −1.50 − 1.00 × 010 lens and a −2.50 − 1.50 × 020 lens placed one on top of the other in a lensmeter? Give the answer rounded to the nearest 1/8 diopter that will be closest to the actual calculated values.
    a. −4.00 − 2.50 × 016
    b. −4.00 − 2.50 × 015
    c. −4.00 − 2.50 × 014
    d. −2.00 − 1.25 × 015

42. What would the resulting lens power be for a
−1.00 − 0.50 × 085 lens and a −3.00 − 2.00 × 005
lens placed one on top of the other in a lensmeter?
a. −4.00 − 2.50 × 045
b. −4.50 − 1.50 × 010
c. −4.50 − 1.50 × 035
d. −4.50 − 1.50 × 045
e. −4.50 − 1.50 × 075

Lens Thicknesses

*(Read the next three questions [Questions 43, 44, and
45] carefully. They are not trick questions, but you do
have to pay attention.)*

43. A lens has a power of pl − 2.00 × 090. It is
decentered 2 mm nasally and edged 50 mm round.
Which edge is thickest?
a. top and bottom
b. nasal
c. temporal

44. A lens has a power of +2.00 D sphere. It is
decentered 2 mm nasally and edged 50 mm round.
Which edge is thickest?
a. top and bottom
b. nasal
c. temporal

45. A lens has a power of pl + 2.00 × 090. It is
decentered 2 mm nasally and edged 50 mm round.
Which edge is thickest?
a. top and bottom
b. nasal
c. temporal

46. A lens has an index of refraction of 1.67. The lens
is plano concave in form. The power of the lens is
−2.75 D sphere. The lens is to go into a
horizontally oval frame with an A dimension of
48 mm and a DBL of 20 mm. The wearer's PD is
66 mm. If the center thickness of the lens is 1 mm,
what is the thickness of the thickest edge? Choose
the answer that is closest to the correct answer,
even if you cannot find your exact answer.
a. 2.3 mm
b. 2.9 mm
c. 3.7 mm
d. 4.2 mm
e. 5.0 mm

47. A lens has a power of +2.00 − 4.00 × 180. It is
edged 50 mm round and decentered 2 mm nasally.
Which edge is thickest?
a. top and bottom
b. nasal
c. temporal

48. A plano-convex, round lens with no decentration is
surfaced to a 50-mm diameter. It is surfaced until
the edge has no thickness (a knife edge). The lens
is made from polycarbonate (index 1.586). If the
front surface of the lens has a radius of curvature
of 95.1 mm, what is the center thickness of the
lens?
a. 1.87 mm
b. 14.2 mm
c. 3.23 mm
d. 3.34 mm

49. Using the Rule of Thumb for estimating lens
thickness, estimate the expected edge thickness for
the lens below. Assume the lens to be crown glass
or CR–39 lenses. (There is more information given
than is needed to answer the question.)
Power = −9.00 D sphere
A = 50
DBL = 18
ED = 56
PD = 62
center thickness = 2.0
a. 6.3 mm
b. 6.9 mm
c. 8.1 mm
d. 8.3 mm
e. 10.1 mm

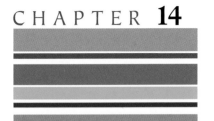

CHAPTER 14

Optical Considerations With Increasing Lens Power

As lens power increases, previously insignificant factors such as thickness and positioning before the eye affect lens power. Unless compensation for these influences is made, the finished product fails to perform as anticipated.

LENS POWER AS RELATED TO POSITION

The principal point of focus of a lens is always the same distance from the lens. So when the lens is moved, the point of focus moves as well. If the lens position has to be changed, but the focal point must stay in the same place, a new lens power is required.

For example, if a camera has a distance of +10 cm from the lens to the film, there is only one power of lens that will cause an object at infinity to focus on the film. The proper lens power may be calculated knowing that the focal length of the lens must be +10 cm or +0.10 m.

Since

$$F = \frac{1}{f'}$$

then

$$F = \frac{1}{+0.10 \text{ m}} = +10.00 \text{ D}$$

If, however, the camera has a distance of +12.5 cm from lens to film, the +10.00 D lens is inappropriate, since it would focus light 2½ cm in front of the film, producing a blurry image. This is true whether the film moves or the lens moves. As long as the distance between lens and film changes from +10 to +12.5 cm, the power of the lens must be changed. To focus on the film at a distance of +12.5 cm, a power of +8.00 D is required—less power than for the shorter distance (Figure 14-1).

Positional Lens Power Problems

Example **14-1**

If a lens of power +5.00 D is mounted so as to focus light on a small screen, what new power lens will be required if the lens mounting is moved 5 cm farther away from the screen?

Solution

A +5.00 D lens has a focal length of +20 cm. We know then that the mounting was originally 20 cm away from the screen. If the mounting is moved 5 cm farther from the screen, it is now 25 cm away. To cause parallel rays of light to focus on the screen, a lens with a focal length of +25 cm must be chosen. The reciprocal of 0.25 m is 4. Therefore a +4.00 D lens must be chosen.

Example **14-2**

Parallel light enters an optical system and must be made to diverge. A −12.50 D lens gives the correct amount of divergence. The system is redesigned, and this lens must be moved 2 cm to the right (light is assumed to be traveling from left to right). According to the new system, the light must still diverge as if from the same point. What new lens power must be used at the new location to give the same effect?

Solution

The situation described is shown in Figure 14-2. In the old system, since the focal length of a −12.50 D lens is −8 cm, light appeared as if it were coming from a point 8 cm to the left of the lens. The new system requires that this point be maintained, but the lens must now be 2 cm farther from it. The old lens may not be used since moving it 2 cm to the right would also move the focal point 2 cm to the right. To maintain the integrity of the system, the focal length of the new lens must be 2 cm longer than that of the old, which is 8 cm +2 cm, or 10 cm to the left of the lens. The diverging lens that has a focal length of −10 cm has a refractive power of

$$\frac{1}{-0.10 \text{ m}} = -10 \text{ D}$$

Effective Power

The power of a lens is normally designated by its dioptric power. Dioptric power depends on focal length. When light leaves the lens, the exiting light rays are either parallel, converging, or diverging. The amount of convergence or divergence of light rays is a dioptric value. Lenses get their dioptric power based on the reciprocal of the distance from the lens to the point of focus. However, as the light travels closer to the point of focus, its vergence value changes.

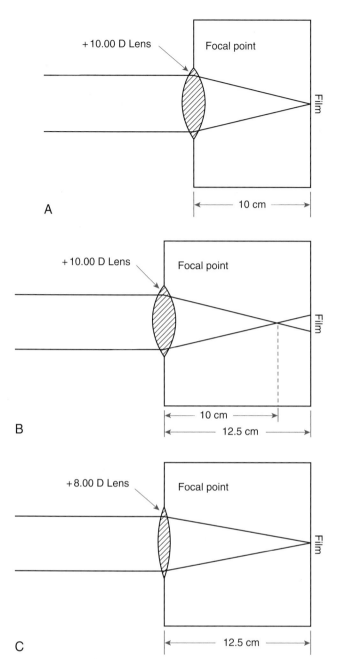

A

B

C

Figure 14-1. The relationship between lens power and desired focal plane may be illustrated using the example of a camera. In (**A**) the +10.00 D lens is correct for the camera's 10-cm depth. Placing that same lens in a deeper camera (**B**) however, results in a blurred image. The lens is farther from the film, and the image falls short. Choosing a lens of longer focal length (**C**) resolves the problem.

The vergence power a lens produces at a position other than that occupied by the lens itself is known as the *effective power* of the lens for that particular reference plane. The effective power of a given lens in air may be obtained by taking the reciprocal of the distance in air from the new reference plane to the focal point of the lens (Figure 14-3).

For example, if light rays are converging towards a given point in air, when these rays are 10 cm away from

the point of focus, they have a vergence of +10.00 D. At a reference plane one centimeter closer, the same rays now have a vergence of:

$$\frac{1}{0.09\text{m}} \text{ or } +11.11 \text{ D}$$

Still another centimeter closer and the vergence will be:

$$\frac{1}{0.08\text{m}} \text{ or } +12.50 \text{ D}$$

To help in understanding effective power, suppose a +10.00 D lens is to be replaced by a different lens positioned 2 cm to the right of the original +10.00 D lens. Remember, the same focal point must be maintained. Therefore to have the same effective power as the +10.00 D lens, the replacement lens must be a +12.50 D lens.

As a second example, suppose a +10.00 D is to be replaced by a different lens positioned 5 cm to the right. To have the same effective power as the +10.00 D, but at a position 5 cm to the right, a +20.00 D lens would be required (Figure 14-4).

Effective Power as Related To Vertex Distance Changes

The distance from the back surface of the spectacle lens to the front surface of the wearer's eye is known as the *vertex distance*. Traditionally, for purposes of calculation, a distance of 13.5 mm was considered average. In actual practice, vertex distances vary considerably. Positioning the glasses at a vertex distance other than that used during the refraction means that the effective power at the refracting distance is now different from that originally intended. For a low-powered lens whose focal length is long in comparison with the vertex distance, there is very little difference. But for higher powered lenses, a small change in vertex distance can make a considerable change in effective power.

Example **14-3**

A person is refracted at a 12.0-mm vertex distance and found to need a +8.50 D lens. A frame selection is made and the lenses fitted at a 17-mm vertex distance. (Incidentally, this is *not* a good frame selection for this prescription.) What power lens must be used at 17 mm to give the same effective power recorded for the refracting distance?

Solution

A +8.50 D lens has a focal length of +11.765 cm. If the new lens has a vertex distance of 17 mm, this is 5 mm to the left of the original position. To achieve the same refractive effect for the wearer, the focal length of the lens dispensed must be 5 mm longer than for the refracting lens.

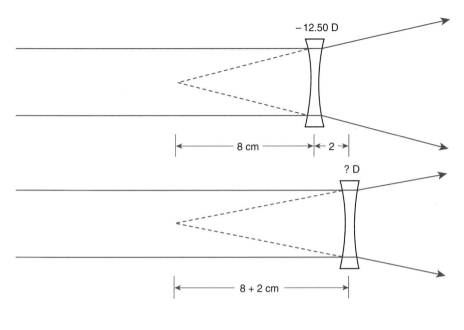

Figure 14-2. If the position of a lens changes, to maintain the same effect, a lens of a different power must be chosen.

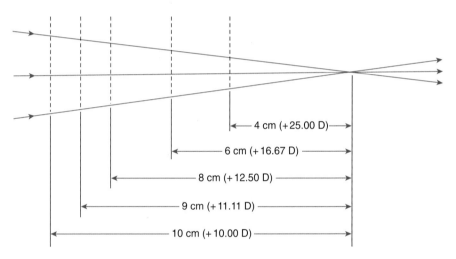

Figure 14-3. Vergence of light in air is the reciprocal of the distance from the reference plane to the point of focus.

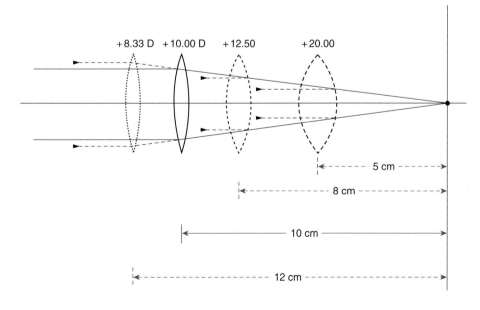

Figure 14-4. It can be seen that for different planes of reference, the effective power of the original lens is different from the marked value. Thus the effective power of a +10.00 D lens at a point 2 cm to the left of where it actually stands is +8.33 D. In other words, the lens that would be used to replace a +10.00 D lens at a point 2 cm to the left of it would be a +8.33 D lens.

+11.765 cm + 0.5 cm = +12.265 cm

If the new focal length must be +12.265 cm, the new lens power must be:

$$\frac{1}{+0.12265 \text{ m}} = +8.15 \text{ D}$$

Effective Power of a Spherocylinder Lens

When calculating the new power needed for a spherocylinder lens at an altered vertex distance, the power in each major meridian must be considered separately.

Example **14-4**

If a +14.00 −3.00 × 090 lens is prescribed at 12-mm vertex distance and the frame selected is positioned at 15 mm, what will the new prescription be?

Solution

The major meridians are:

$$F_{180} = +11.00 \text{ D}$$
$$F_{90} = +14.00 \text{ D}$$

The new effective power for the 180-degree meridian is calculated by first finding the focal length:

$$f'_{180} = \frac{1}{+11.00} = +9.09 \text{ cm}$$

The new lens will be 15 − 12 or 3 mm farther from the line foci of the lens. Therefore since the lens is plus, the focal lengths will be 3 mm longer.

$$\text{New } f'_{180} = +9.09 \text{ cm} + 0.3 \text{ cm} = +9.39 \text{ cm}$$

So the new $F_{180} = \dfrac{1}{+0.0939 \text{ m}} = +10.65 \text{ D}$

To find the new power in the 90-degree meridian:

$$\text{since } F_{90} = +14.00,$$
$$\text{then } f'_{90} = +7.14 \text{ cm}$$
$$\text{New } f'_{90} = +7.14 + 0.3 = +7.44 \text{ cm}$$

Therefore

$$\text{New } F_{90} = \frac{1}{+0.0744 \text{ m}} = +13.44 \text{ D}$$

If new $F_{180} = +10.65$ D and new $F_{90} = +13.44$ D, then the new lens power will be +13.44 −2.79 × 090. Not only has the sphere power changed, but also the power of the cylinder.

In this case it is *not* valid to calculate the power of the sphere (+14.00 D), then calculate the power of the cylinder (−3.00) independently. The cylinder value is the *difference* between two meridians and not an independent entity.

Effective Power Written as a Formula

Effective power can be written as a formula. As a formula, effective power is as follows:

$$F_{\text{eff}} = \frac{1}{\dfrac{1}{F'_v} - d}$$

where F_{eff} is the effective power, F'_v is the back vertex power of the lens, and d is the distance in meters from the original position of the lens to the new position of the lens. It is not advisable to memorize the formula instead of trying to understand the concept of effective power.

AS LENS THICKNESS INCREASES

As a lens becomes thicker, there is an increase in distance between front and back surfaces. Changing the position of the first lens surface with respect to the second means that the effective power of the first surface at the plane of the second surface is no longer the same. This in turn causes a change in total lens power. The actual amount of change may be calculated using vergences.

Vergence of Light As It Travels Through a Lens

When light strikes a lens, it is refracted at the front surface and then travels through the thickness of the lens. It is again refracted when reaching the back lens surface. For thin lenses, the distance traveled from front to back surfaces makes no appreciable change in total lens power. The thicker the lens becomes, however, the more of a discrepancy there is between nominal or approximate power ($F_1 + F_2$) and the actual measured power of the lens. As light strikes the first surface of the lens (F_1), its vergence is changed, converging or diverging to a greater or lesser extent than previously. It has an additional vergence change when reaching the second surface (F_2).

Vergence for Thin Lenses
For a thin lens, when the vergence of the entering light is zero (parallel rays), the light exiting the lens has a vergence equal to the dioptric powers of the first and second surfaces ($F_1 + F_2$).

For example, if $F_1 = +5.00$ D and $F_2 = +1.00$ D, when light strikes F_1 it is caused to converge. It now has a vergence of +5.00 D. Because the lens is thin, it immediately strikes the back surface before its vergence changes. Now the back surface (F_2) causes light to converge an additional +1.00 diopter. So on leaving the second surface of the lens (F_2), the light now has a vergence of +6.00 D.

Vergence for Thick Lenses
For a thick lens, the converging light leaving the first surface would have a chance to travel a significant

distance before reaching the second surface (F_2). As will be recalled from the previous section on effective power, as converging or diverging light travels through the lens, by the time it reaches the second surface, F_2, it will have a slightly different vergence value from what it had when it left the first surface, F_1. This is because it is now a different distance from its plane of reference. It is this *new* vergence (the effective power of F_1 at F_2) that is altered to produce a different vergence leaving the lens. However, with thick lenses, vergence is affected not only by the thickness of the lens, but by the refractive index of the lens material.

Reduced Thickness and Refractive Index

Light passing from one medium to another through a curved surface experiences a change in vergence, which, expressed as shown previously, is quantified by the equation:

$$F = L' - L$$

This equation, called the *fundamental paraxial equation*, may also be written as:

$$F = \frac{n'}{l'} - \frac{n}{l}$$

To see the interrelationship between distance (l or l') and refractive index (n or n'), consider the familiar situation of looking into an aquarium filled with water.

Suppose the aquarium is 100 cm from front to back. The observer is standing in front of the aquarium observing a snail on the back surface (Figure 14-5). How far away from the front surface will the snail appear to be?

(The question really asks, "What effect will the refractive index of water have on the distance perceived compared with what it would otherwise appear to be in air?")

We can assume that the glass separating the air and water is thin enough to be of no concern in calculations. The situation is one in which light leaves the object (a snail), and diverges for 100 cm until it reaches a refractive surface (the front of the aquarium). Therefore since the side of the aquarium is flat:

$$F = 0.00 \text{ D,}$$
$$l' = -100 \text{ cm or } -1.0 \text{ m,}$$
$$n = 1.33, \text{ and}$$
$$n' = 1.00$$

(The distance l' is taken as minus, since the surface of the tank is the refracting surface and light is traveling first through water before it reaches the surface of the tank.)

The equation

$$F = \frac{n'}{l'} - \frac{n}{l}$$

results in

$$0 = \frac{1}{l'} - \frac{1.33}{-1.0}$$

which algebraically transforms to:

$$\frac{1.33}{-1.0} = \frac{1}{l'}$$

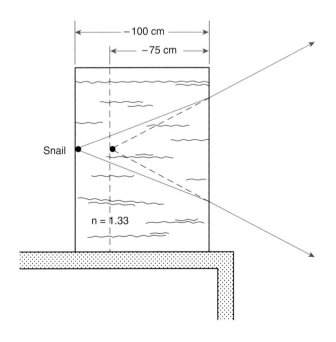

Snail

−100 cm
−75 cm

n = 1.33

Figure 14-5. The most familiar example of reduced thickness is seen with an ordinary aquarium. Looking at the contents through water makes individual objects seem to be closer than they would otherwise appear if viewed only through air.

$$l' = \frac{-1.0}{1.33}$$
$$= -0.75 \text{ mm}$$

So the snail and the back surface of the tank appear to be −0.75 m or −75 cm from the front surface.

Interestingly enough, this example clearly shows that the light entering and leaving the front surface of the front glass has exactly the same vergence, for if $F = 0$, then $L = L'$. The distance in water as compared with that in air is reduced because the light is traveling more slowly in water than in air. This concept is referred to as *reduced thickness* because objects of a higher refractive index than air appear thinner than they actually are when compared with the equivalent air distance. The relationship between the *reduced thickness,* the actual thickness (t), and the index of the medium in question (n) can be stated simply as:

$$\text{reduced thickness} = \frac{t}{n}$$

Vergence of Light Striking the Second Surface of a Thick Lens

For a thick lens, after light has left the first surface, F_1, it travels for a time inside the lens. The lens has a refractive index that is higher than that of air. Because vergence depends on the relationship between refractive index and distance:

$$L = \frac{n}{l}$$

the vergence of light leaving F_1 and striking F_2 may not be calculated in terms of distance alone.

Initially, one would think that the new vergence would be found by directly adding or subtracting lens thickness from the image distance of light leaving the first surface (l'). This was the case in previous effective power problems because in air this proves true. But here it is necessary to find the new vergence at F_2 by adding or subtracting the *reduced thickness* of the lens from the reciprocal of the vergence. This keeps the reference medium as air. This is the better choice since calculations are easier when the final results are for rays converging or diverging in air.

Example **14-5**

Parallel light enters a 7-mm thick crown glass lens that has a front surface power of +12.00 D and a refractive index of 1.523. What vergence will the light have by the time it reaches the back surface (F_2)?

Solution

After leaving F_1, the light has a vergence that can be calculated from:

$$F_1 = L_1' - L_1$$

Substituting the correct numerical values, we find that:

$$+12.00 \text{ D} = L_1' - 0$$

or

$$L_1' = +12.00 \text{ D}$$

Light leaving F_1 has a vergence of +12.00 D.

The light is now converging toward a point to the right of the front surface. That point in air would be found by taking the reciprocal of the vergence.

$$L_1' = \frac{l}{l_1'}$$

and

$$+12.00 = \frac{l}{l_1'}$$

$$l_1' = +0.0833 \text{ m}$$

The distance in question is +0.0833 m.

The light must travel through glass for 7 mm before reaching air, however. To find the vergence of light at F_2, the *reduced thickness* of this lens must be subtracted from l_1' because the point of focus is now closer to the new plane of reference, which is the back surface of the lens. Therefore the new distance (l_2) is:

$$l_2 = l_1' - \frac{t}{n}$$

where $\frac{t}{n}$ is the reduced thickness of the lens. (Thickness must be expressed in the same units as l_1'.)

$$l_2 = 0.0833 \text{ m} - \frac{0.007 \text{ m}}{1.523}$$
$$= 0.0833 \text{ m} - 0.0046 \text{ m}$$
$$= 0.0787 \text{ m}$$

The vergence of the light entering F_2 is the reciprocal of 0.0787 m.

$$L_2 = \frac{1}{l_2}$$
$$= \frac{1}{0.0787 \text{ m}}$$
$$= +12.71 \text{ D}$$

The vergence of light entering F_2 is +12.71 D. It can be seen from the above example that if F_2 were plano, the vergence of light leaving F_2 would also be +12.71 D. This is *not* the result that would be expected if lens power were assumed to be the sum of the two lens surface powers.

FRONT AND BACK VERTEX POWERS

It has been shown that because of lens thickness the nominal or approximate power of a lens does not accurately predict the actual power of the lens. It will be recalled that when parallel light enters the front of a lens, it is refracted and exits from the rear surface of the lens. The image, be it real or virtual, falls at the *second principal focus*.

The reciprocal of the distance in air from the rear surface of the lens to the second principal focus is a specific measure of the power of this lens and is known as the *back vertex power* (F_v'). (This is the measure of power of most importance in ophthalmic lenses.)

(NOTE: Chapter 6 has information on how to measure lens power using the lensmeter. The material found there is relevant to this section as well.)

If parallel light enters from the rear surface, the place where the image forms is known as the *first principal focus*. The reciprocal of the distance in air from the front surface of the lens to the first principal focus is another measure of the power of the lens. This measure is referred to as the *front vertex power* (F_v) (Figure 14-6). It is not unusual to find front and back vertex powers to be different. If the lens is equiconcave or equiconvex, the front and back vertex powers will be the same. If the lens has any other form and is thick, there may be a measurable difference between front and back vertex power.

Calculating Front and Back Vertex Powers

Front and back vertex powers may be found by finding vergence as light approaches and leaves each lens surface. They may also be found using a formula summarizing the necessary vergence factors. By following the vergence methods for solving this type of problem, it will result in a much better understanding of the action of a lens on light than will simple formula memorization. Both methods are described.

Solving for Front and Back Vertex Powers Using Vergence

If light enters the front surface of a lens as parallel rays, the back vertex power of a lens will be equal to the vergence these light rays have when leaving the back surface of the lens. If the form, thickness, and refractive index of that lens are known, the back vertex power may be found by systematically tracing the path light rays take through the lens.

Example **14-6**

A lens has the following dimensions:

$$F_1 = +8.00 \text{ D}$$
$$F_2 = -2.00 \text{ D}$$
$$t = 5 \text{ mm}$$
$$n = 1.523$$

What is the back vertex power of the lens?

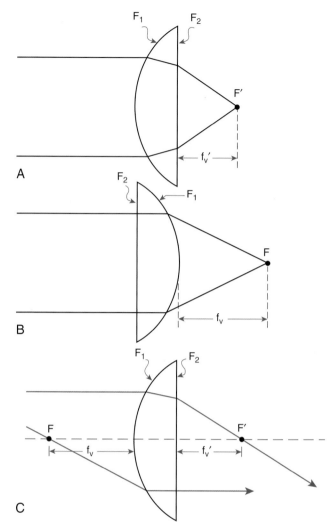

Figure 14-6. When light enters a lens from the front, the focal length, and consequently the measured focal power, can be different from when light enters a lens from the back. **A** and **B** show the difference between front vertex and back vertex focal lengths (f_v and f_v'). These focal lengths will directly determine front and back vertex focal powers (F_v and F_v'). (**B**, drawn with the lens backward to allow better visual comparison between the front and back vertex focal lengths.) **C**, The conventional manner of representing front and back vertex focal lengths diagrammatically. (F = first principal focal point; F' = second principal focal point; f_v = front vertex focal length; f_v' = second vertex focal length.)

Solution

Light entering the lens must be from an object at infinity to determine back vertex lens power. The rays entering the front surface of the lens will then be parallel, having a vergence of zero (Figure 14-7). Since

$$L_1' = F_1 + L_1$$

and

$$L_1 = 0.00 \text{ D}$$

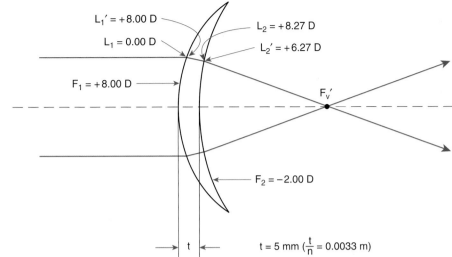

Figure 14-7. Lens curvature and thickness have a definite bearing on the final back vertex power of a lens.

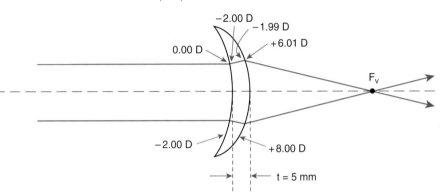

Figure 14-8. Reversing a lens may change the position of the image. For some lenses, front and back vertex power may be quite different. Here, the lens shown in Figure 14-7 has been reversed to more easily use a vergence method of finding its vertex power.

then

$$L_1' = +8.00 \text{ D} + 0.00 \text{ D}$$

or

$$L_1' = +8.00 \text{ D}$$

To find the vergence of light at F_2, the reduced thickness is subtracted from l_1'.

$$l_2 = l_1' - \frac{t}{n}$$
$$= \frac{1}{+8.00} - \frac{0.005 \text{ m}}{1.523}$$
$$= 0.125 \text{ m} - 0.0033 \text{ m}$$
$$= 0.1217 \text{ m}$$

Therefore the vergence of light at F_2 is:

$$L_2 = \frac{1}{l_2} = \frac{1}{0.1217} = +8.22 \text{ D}$$

(This is the same procedure as finding the effective power of F_1 at F_2.)
Now since

$$L_2' = F_2 + L_2$$

then in this case,

$$L_2' = -2.00 + 8.22$$
$$= +6.22$$

Since back vertex power is the vergence with which light from an object at infinity leaves a lens, the back vertex power (F_v') for this lens is +6.22 D. This is noticeably different from the nominal power of the lens, which equals +6.00 D.

Example **14-7**

What would the front vertex power be for the lens described in the previous problem?

Solution

To simplify the construction, it is easier to find the front vertex power by turning the lens around and considering light to be entering from the back as was shown in Figure 14-6, B. In this manner then, sign conventions are maintained and less confusion results. The same methodology may be used as in finding the back vertex power, F_v'. To prevent confusion in terminology, the back surface of the lens now becomes F_1 (since light now enters it as if it were the front surface), and the front surface will become F_2 (Figure 14-8).
Now since

$$L_1' = F_1 + L_1$$

and

$$L_1 = 0.00 \text{ D}$$

with the new

$$F_1 = -2.00 \text{ D}$$

then

$$L_1' = -2.00 \text{ D} + 0.00 \text{ D}$$
$$= -2.00 \text{ D}$$

Again, the vergence of light at F_2 is found as reduced thickness subtracted from l_1'.

$$l_2 = l_1' - \frac{t}{n}$$
$$= \frac{1}{-2.00} - \frac{0.005 \text{ m}}{1.523}$$
$$= -0.50\text{m} - 0.0033\text{m}$$
$$= -0.05033\text{m}$$
$$L_2 = \frac{1}{l_2} = \frac{1}{-0.5033 \text{ m}} = -1.99 \text{ D}$$

Now

$$L_2' = F_2 + L_2$$
$$= +8.00 \text{ D} - 1.99 \text{ D}$$
$$= +6.01 \text{ D}$$

The front vertex power for this lens is +6.01 D, which is extremely close to the nominal power of the lens. If the surface of the lens that light was entering had been plano, this vertex power would have been equal to the nominal power. The more curved the entering surface, the more the vertex power of the lens will differ from its nominal power.

Solving for Front and Back Vertex Powers Using Formulas

The previous vergence methods may be summarized into formulas. The formula for back vertex power is:

$$F_v' = \frac{F_1}{1 - \frac{t}{n}F_1} + F_2$$

And the formula for front vertex power is:

$$F_v' = \frac{F_2}{1 - \frac{t}{n}F_2} + F_1$$

The above formulas give results that are accurate and identical to those found by the vergence method. Simplified formulas that approximate F_v and F_v' front and back vertex powers and have been derived from the above formulas by using higher mathematics are:

$$F_v' = F_1 + F_2 + \frac{t}{n}(F_1)^2$$

and

$$F_v = F_1 + F_2 + \frac{t}{n}(F_2)^2$$

These formulas are approximations and, although somewhat easier to work, are not expected to give the accuracy of the more exact forms. The approximations were more widely used before small calculators became available.

Proficiency Test

(Answers can be found in the back of the book.)

1. If a +11.00 D lens is worn at a 13-mm vertex distance, what must the Rx be changed to if it is to be worn at an 10-mm vertex distance?

2. A prescription for a myodisc reads:

   O.D. −27.50 DS
   O.S. −24.00 DS
   Refracting distance 14 mm.
   If the Rx were to be worn at 11 mm, what would the necessary lens powers be?

3. If a person with a high minus spectacle Rx switches to contact lenses, the power in the contact lens would be _____ the power in the spectacle lens.
   a. greater than
   b. less than
   c. the same as

4. A person's eyes were examined at a vertex distance of 14 mm and found to require +8.50 D sphere power. A frame having a vertex distance of 11 mm is desired. If the Rx is to be worn at 11 mm, what must the power of the lens be to give the same visual correction? (Round off to the nearest $^1/_8$ D.)

5. A prescription of +6.00 +3.25 × 15 is determined using a vertex distance of 14 mm. If the frame is unwisely fit for a 22-mm vertex distance, what must the theoretical power of the lens be?
   a. +9.99 −3.69 × 105
   b. +8.61 −2.88 × 105
   c. +5.73 +3.25 × 15
   d. +7.69 −2.39 × 105
   e. none of the above

6. A +13.25 −1.75 × 180 lens is worn at a 13-mm vertex distance. What is the equivalent prescription for a zero vertex distance contact lens?
   a. +16.00 -l.75 × 180
   b. +11.25 −1.25 × 180
   c. +11.25 −1.75 × 180
   d. +16.00 −2.50 × 180
   e. none of the above

7. A prescription lens has a high plus sphere component and a moderate cylinder component. If the vertex distance is increased, what would have to happen to retain the correct optical effect before the eyes?
   a. The sphere component must increase, and the cylinder component decrease.
   b. The sphere component must decrease, and the cylinder component decrease.
   c. The sphere component must decrease, and the cylinder component increase.
   d. The sphere component must increase, and the cylinder component remain the same.
   e. The sphere component must increase, and the cylinder component increase.

8. If a single-vision lens is placed in the lensmeter in the reverse position (concave side toward the observer), the power value obtained is a measure of:
   a. equivalent power.
   b. effective power.
   c. back vertex power.
   d. front vertex power.
   e. true power.

9. A thick lens has a convex front surface and a plano back surface. Which of the following statements about this lens is true?
   a. The front vertex power is greater than the back vertex power.
   b. The back vertex power is greater than the front vertex power.
   c. Front and back vertex powers will be equal.
   d. Such a lens will always have the seg on the back surface.
   e. None of the above are true.

10. What is the back vertex power for a lens ground to these specifications?
    Front surface curve +13.00 D
    Back surface curve plano
    Center thickness 10 mm
    Index of the lens 1.5
    a. +11.87 D
    b. +13.00 D
    c. +13.50 D
    d. +13.87 D
    e. +14.12 D

11. A lens has the following dimensions:
    $F_1 = +8.00$ D
    $F_2 = -1.00$ D
    $n = 1.70$
    $t = 5$ mm
    What is the *front* vertex power of the lens?

12. When measured with a lens clock, a lens having an index of 1.53 measures as +10.00 D on the front surface and plano on the back surface. The lens is 4 mm thick.
    a. What is the nominal power?
    b. What is the back vertex power?

13. A lens has a front surface power of +8.00 D. It must be ground 5 mm thick from material of refractive index 1.5. To obtain a *back vertex power* (F_v') of −2.00 D, what power must the back surface of the lens have?

14. A minus cylinder form lens has a base curve of +6.00 D and is to be ground 5 mm thick from material of index 1.523. For the lens to have an F_v' of +6.00 −1.00 × 180, what must the back surface curvature be?
    a. $F_2 = -0.25$ D at 90, $F_2 = -1.25$ D at 180
    b. $F_2 = -l.25$ D at 90, $F_2 = -0.12$ D at 180
    c. $F_2 = 0.08$ D at 180, $F_2 = -1.00$ D at 90
    d. $F_1 = +5.00$ D at 90, $F_2 = -0.12$ D sphere

15. A lens is thick, high plus in power, and meniscus in form. It also has a cylinder component. To obtain the same back vertex power as indicated by the prescription:

a. if the cylinder is ground on F_1 it must be greater in power than the cylinder value indicated in the prescription.

b. if the cylinder is ground on F_2 it must be less in power than the cylinder value indicated in the prescription.

c. if the cylinder is ground on F_1 it must be less in power than the cylinder value indicated in the prescription.

d. if the cylinder is ground on F_1 it must be the same power as the cylinder value indicated in the prescription.

e. Two of the above are correct.

CHAPTER 15

Optical Prism: Power and Base Direction

A lens causes incoming light to change in its vergence by making that light converge or diverge. A prism causes light to change direction without changing its vergence. The image of an object can be optically repositioned with a prism. People who have problems with how their eyes work together as a team can be helped by the use of prism. In this chapter we look at what a prism is and how it is used in eye care.

OPHTHALMIC PRISMS

A prism consists of two angled refracting surfaces. The simplest form of a prism is two flat surfaces that come together at an angle at the top. The point is called the *apex* of the prism; the wider bottom of the prism is called the *base*.

The Relationship Between Prism Apical Angle and Deviation of Light

Suppose a prism is oriented so that incoming light strikes the first surface perpendicularly. When light strikes the first surface it is going from a low refractive index material (air) into a higher refractive index material (the prism). However, it does not change direction because it enters the surface straight on. Light will continue to travel through the prism without being bent until it reaches the second surface (Figure 15-1). This ray of light then strikes the second surface at an angle. *Because the light has not been bent by the first surface, the angle at which it strikes the second surface is equal to the apical angle of the prism* (Figure 15-2). As this ray of light approaches the second surface of the prism, it is traveling from the denser (high refractive index) medium of the prism to a less dense medium (air) and will be bent away from the normal* to the surface. Light is always bent toward the base of a prism.

What is the relationship between the apical angle of a prism and the amount of deviation of the light produced by that prism?

*Remember, "normal" to the surface means perpendicular to the surface.

Example **15-1**

If a prism has an apical angle of 8 degrees and is made from CR-39 plastic with a refractive index of 1.498, how many degrees will the prism deviate the light ray from its original path?

Solution

When working through this example problem, refer to Figure 15-2. Notice that light entering the first surface is perpendicular to the surface and is not bent. It is bent at the second surface and, according to Snell's law,

$$n \sin i = n' \sin i'$$
$$\text{where } n = 1.498$$
$$n' = 1.0,$$
$$\sin 8 = 0.1392$$

So by substituting,

$$(1.498)(0.1392) = (1.0)(\sin i')$$
$$\sin i' = 0.2085$$

Next using a calculator we find the inverse sine ($\sin^{-1}$) of 0.2085 to be:

$$i' = 12.03 \text{ degrees}$$

The angle of refraction is the angle at which the light ray leaves the second surface. To find the angle of deviation (i.e., how many degrees the light is deviated from its original path), subtract the angle of incidence from the angle of refraction.

$$\text{(angle of deviation)} = \text{(angle of refraction)}$$
$$- \text{(angle of incidence)}$$
$$d = i' - i$$
$$= 12.03 - 8.00$$
$$= 4.03 \text{ degrees}$$

In this instance, the resulting angle of deviation is 4.03 degrees, or rounded off, 4.0 degrees.

Example **15-2**

A prism is made from polycarbonate material having an index of 1.586. It has an apical angle of 5 degrees. What is the angle of deviation that it produces in air?

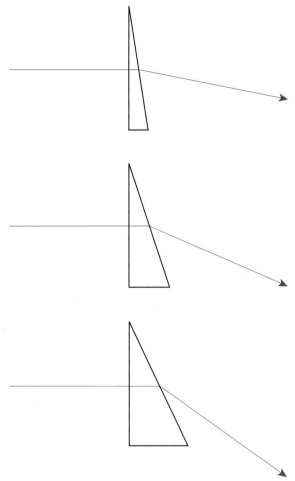

Figure 15-1. The more wedge shaped a prism is, the greater is its ability to divert light in another direction.

Solution

Again using Snell's law,

$$n \sin i = n' \sin i'$$

We can substitute and find:

$$(1.586)(\sin 5) = (1.0)\,(\sin i')$$
$$(1.586)\,(0.0872) = \sin i'$$
$$\sin i' = 0.1382$$

Next the inverse sine of 0.1382 is found.

$$i' = 7.95 \text{ degrees}$$

The angle of deviation is:

$$d = i' - i$$
$$= 7.95 - 5$$
$$= 2.95 \text{ degrees}$$

So the angle of deviation is 2.95 degrees.

Simplifying for Thin Prisms

In an effort to simplify, there is a shortcut for finding the angle of deviation that may be applied for thin prisms.

We know by looking at Figure 15-2 that:

• The angle of incidence (i_2) equals the apical angle of the prism (*a*), or ($i_2 = a$)

The angle of refraction (i_2') is the sum of the apical angle (*a*) plus the angle of deviation (*d*), or

$$(i_2' = a + d)$$

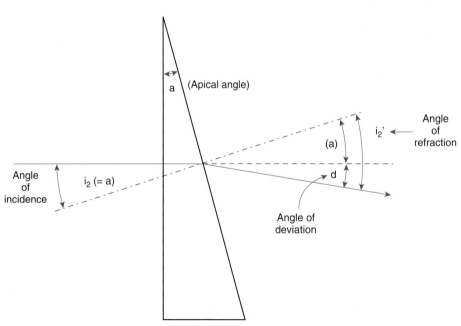

Figure 15-2. This prism is oriented with the first surface perpendicular to the incoming light ray. This means that the angle of incidence at the second surface (i_2) is equal to the apical angle of the prism. Note also that the angle of refraction (i_2') equals the apical angle (*a*) plus the angle of deviation (*d*).

This means if we begin with:

$$n \sin i_2 = n' \sin i_2'$$

We can substitute and get:

$$n \sin a = n' \sin (a + d)$$

When angles are small (10 degrees or less), the sine of the angle is the same as the angle measured in radians. If this is the case, it is possible to say that:

$$(n)\,(a) = (n')\,(a + d)$$

Because the prism is in air, $n' = 1$, and the equation becomes:

$$(n)\,(a) = (a + d)$$

To find d, we can transpose the equation and get:

$$d = (n)\,(a) - a$$

or, written another way,

$$d = a(n - 1)$$

For this equation, it does not matter if the angle is in radians or degrees. It still works. So for prisms with an apical angle of less than 10 degrees, the angle of deviation equals the apical angle times the quantity "index minus 1." (Remember that this formula is an accurate approximation for thin prisms only, but quickly loses accuracy once a prism increases in thickness.)

For material with an index of 1.5, the calculation is even easier and reduces to:

$$\begin{aligned} d &= a(n-1) \\ &= a(1.5-1) \\ &= a(0.5) \\ d &= \frac{a}{2} \end{aligned}$$

In other words, when the lens is made from index 1.5 material (CR-39 plastic has an index of 1.498), then the angle of deviation is equal to half the apical angle.

Example **15-3**

A prism with an index of refraction of 1.70 has an apical angle of 9 degrees. Using the thin prism approximation, what is the angle of deviation?

Solution

Because the prism index is far from 1.5, we cannot use the very simple approximation and just divide the apical angle by 2. Instead we use:

$$d = a(n - 1)$$

In this case by substituting we get:

$$\begin{aligned} d &= a(n-1) \\ &= 9(1.7-1) \\ &= 9(0.7) \\ d &= 6.3 \text{ degrees} \end{aligned}$$

The angle of deviation is 6.3 degrees.

Example **15-4**

A prism made from CR-39 plastic has an apical angle of 8 degrees. Using the thin prism approximation, what is the angle of deviation?

Solution

This is the same problem as given in Example 15-1. This time, however, we can use the most simplified form of the thin prism approximation since CR-39 plastic is so close to 1.5 index. Therefore

$$\begin{aligned} d &= \frac{a}{2} \\ &= \frac{8}{2} \\ &= 4 \text{ degrees} \end{aligned}$$

Finding Apical Angle from Degrees of Deviation

It is possible to find the apical angle from degrees of deviation by transposing the same thin prism simplified equation of:

$$d = a(n - 1)$$

that was described previously to:

$$a = \frac{d}{n-1}$$

Example **15-5**

A prism made from 1.66 index material is shown to deviate light 6 degrees. What is its apical angle?

Solution

Using the equation:

$$a = \frac{d}{n-1}$$

We can substitute and find:

$$\begin{aligned} a &= \frac{6}{1.66-1} \\ &= \frac{6}{0.66} \\ &= 9.09 \text{ degrees} \end{aligned}$$

So the apical angle of the prism is approximately 9.1 degrees.

The Prism Diopter (Δ)

The power of a prism could be quantified in terms of apical angle. The problem is that prism power would vary depending upon the refractive index of the prism. So this does not work very well.

A prism could also be quantified in terms of the angle of deviation in degrees that it produces. This is better because it is independent of index. However, angle of deviation is not as easy to work with for ophthalmic purposes.

A third way of quantifying prism power is to express it in terms of how far it displaces light when measured on a flat screen. In other words, how far was light displaced from the point it would otherwise have struck at a given distance from the prism had it not first been bent by the prism. This type of unit is called the *prism diopter* and is abbreviated by the Greek delta symbol (Δ). The prism diopter is an angular measure derived by using the tangent of the angle of deviation. The prism diopter is the unit of angular measure whose tangent is 0.01 or $\left(\frac{1}{100}\right)$.

Remember, in trigonometry the tangent of an angle is the opposite over the adjacent $\left(\tan d = \frac{opp}{adj}\right)$ (Figure 15-3). This means that for a screen 100 cm away, if a prism displaces the image 1 cm, the prism has a power of 1 prism diopter. So from the geometry of Figure 15-4 we see that:

$$\tan d = \frac{P}{100}$$

where P is the number of centimeters that the image is displaced at a distance of 100 cm (1 m). By definition P will also be the number of prism diopters (Δ) of prism displacement power.

Finding Prism Displacement for Any Distance

If prism displacement can be written as

$$\tan d = \frac{P}{100}$$

we can also determine prism diopters if we know the amount of displacement of the ray for any given distance from the prism. If the displacement is x units on a flat plane that is located y units from the prism, then:

$$\tan d = \frac{x}{y}$$

This means that:

$$\tan d = \frac{P}{100} = \frac{x}{y}$$

or

$$\frac{P}{100} = \frac{x}{y}$$

Notice that both x and y must be the same units of measure. If x is centimeters, then y must also be centimeters (See Figure 15-4, *B*.)

Example **15-6**

A prism displaces light a lateral distance of 9 cm at a plane 300 cm from the prism. What is the power of the prism in prism diopters?

Solution
Using the equation:

$$\frac{P}{100} = \frac{x}{y}$$

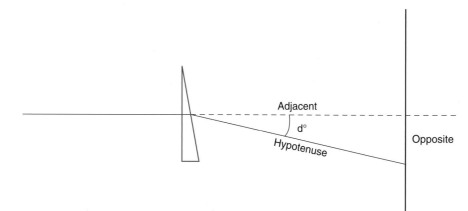

Adjacent

d°

Hypotenuse

Opposite

Figure 15-3. A trigonometric rationale for converting degrees of deviation to prism diopters.

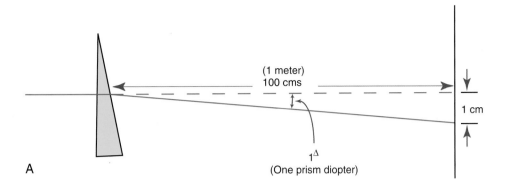

A

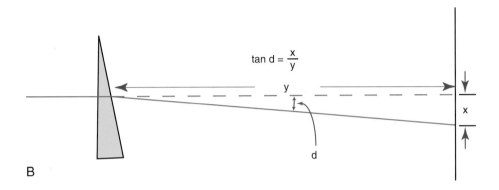

B

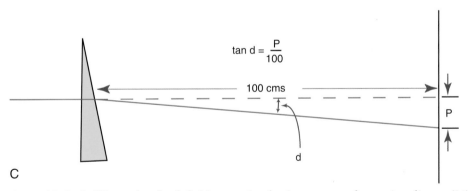

C

Figure 15-4. **A,** We see that, by definition, a prism having a power of one prism diopter (1Δ) will displace a ray 1 cm at a distance of 100 cm. **B,** We notice that the angle of deviation caused by the prism (d), and the amount of displacement (x) on a plane at a given distance (y) from the prism can be described by $\tan d = \dfrac{x}{y}$. **C,** Knowing what we see in **B,** we can relate prism diopters to the angle of deviation with the relationship: $\tan d = \dfrac{P}{100}$

and knowing that $x = 9$ cm and $y = 300$ cm, then:

$$\frac{P}{100} = \frac{9}{300}$$
$$P = \frac{(9)(100)}{300}$$
$$= 3 \text{ cms}$$

So basically we used similar triangles to find that for a displacement of 3 cm at a distance of 100 cm, this prism has a power of 3Δ. This is because, by definition, a 3-cm ray displacement at a distance of 100 cm is 3 prism diopters.

If we were to use the equation:

$$\frac{P}{100} = \frac{x}{y}$$

And change the units of measure for the distance from the prism to the screen into meters, then we would have:

$$\frac{P}{1 \text{ meter}} = \frac{x \text{ centimeters}}{y \text{ meters}}$$

or

$$P = \frac{x \text{ centimeters}}{y \text{ meters}}$$

Example 15-7

How much prism power does a prism have if it displaces a ray of light 5 cm from a position it would otherwise strike at a distance of 1 m from the prism?

Solution

If displacement (x) is 5 cm and "screen" distance is 1 m, then:

$$P = \frac{x \text{ centimeters}}{y \text{ meters}}$$
$$P = \frac{5 \text{ centimeters}}{1 \text{ meter}}$$
$$= 5\Delta$$

The answer is 5Δ.

Example 15-8

How much prism power does a prism have if it displaces a ray of light 5 cm from a position it would otherwise strike at a distance of 5 m from the prism?

Solution

The only change in the above problem is the "screen" distance, which increases to 5 m. So if:

$$P = \frac{x \text{ centimeters}}{y \text{ meters}}$$

Then

$$P = \frac{5 \text{ centimeters}}{5 \text{ meters}}$$
$$= 1\Delta$$

Conversion From Degrees of Deviation to Prism Diopters

It is possible to convert back and forth from degrees of deviation to prism diopters using trigonometric functions as described earlier and shown in the equation:

$$\tan d = \frac{P}{100}$$

Example 15-9

How many prism diopters are produced for each degree of deviation?

Solution

For 1 degree of deviation, we begin by finding the tangent of 1 degree.

$$\tan 1 = 0.0175.$$

using:

$$\tan d = \frac{P}{100}$$
$$\tan 1 = 0.0175 = \frac{P}{100}$$

So

$$P = (0.0175)(100)$$
$$= 1.75\Delta$$

So each degree of deviation produces 1.75 prism diopters.

Example 15-10

How many degrees of deviation are produced by 1 prism diopter?

Solution

This time we are going the other way.

$$\tan d = \frac{P}{100}$$
$$\tan d = \frac{1}{100} = 0.01$$

Finding the inverse tan of 0.01 gives a value of:

$$d = 0.573 \text{ degree}$$

So for small amounts of deviation one can simply remember that 1 degree = 1.75Δ, and 1Δ = 0.57 degrees.*

The Prism Centrad (▽)

A seldom-used method of quantifying prism deviation is the centrad (abbreviated ▽). A centrad is similar to a prism diopter in that a ray is displaced 1 cm at a distance of 1 m from the prism. The difference between the two is that a prism diopter is measured on a flat plane 1 m away, whereas the displacement of a centrad is measured

---

*At this point, it should be mentioned that some manufacturing opticians refer to prism diopters by using the term degrees. Although sometimes used in the trade and understood to be the same thing as a prism diopter, this use of the term degrees is technically inaccurate and must not be confused with either degrees of deviation or apical angle as expressed in degrees.

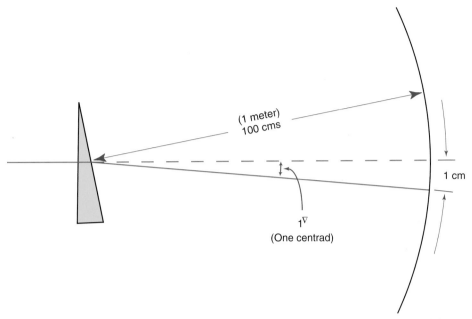

Figure 15-5. One (1) centrad equals one hundredth part of a radian. The one hundredth part is measured on the circular arc. If the radius equals 100 cm, then 1 centrad (∇) is 1 cm measured on the curved arc.

on the arc of a circle having a 1-m radius (Figure 15-5). The centrad is thus a more consistent unit of measurement, but it is not used clinically. For small angles of prism deviation, the centrad and the prism diopter are nearly equal. However, as the amount of prismatic deviation increases, the two become increasingly different.

Image Displacement

If a prism is placed before an eye, the deviated ray enters the eye. The eye itself has no way of knowing that the ray has been deviated. It simply appears to be coming from a different direction. Since this ray comes from a specific object, the object itself appears to be displaced. Since there is no actual displacement, what the eye sees is a displaced image of that object. The phenomenon is referred to as image displacement and is shown in Figure 15-6.

The amount of image displacement is predictable from the power of the prism and can be expressed in prism diopters. This corresponds exactly to the previous definition. As seen in Figure 15-7, if a ray of light is displaced 1 cm at a distance of 1 m from the prism, the image of an object in front of the prism will be correspondingly displaced 1 cm for each meter the object is from the prism.*

---

*For objects closer to the prism than infinity, the divergence of the rays striking the prism causes a ray displacement (and consequently an image displacement as well) that is slightly different than that manifested for an object at infinity. This is called "effective prism power" and is explained later in this same chapter. Rays from an object at infinity strike the prism with neither divergence nor convergence, but are parallel rays.

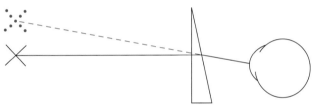

Figure 15-6. When looking through a prism, the image of an object appears to be displaced from its actual location.

Direction of Image Displacement

As previously seen, a single ray of light is deviated in the direction of the prism's base. From the point of view of an observer holding the prism before his or her eye, the prism causes the image of a viewed object to be displaced in the direction of the apex of the prism. To remember this easily, think of the prism as being an arrow with its apex pointing in the direction of the displaced image. *"The eye turns in the direction the prism points."*

Practical Application

Prism is used in a spectacle lens prescription to either cause or allow the eye to turn from the normal straight-ahead viewing direction. If one eye turns upward, a prism may be placed with its base down before that eye. This causes an object to appear as if it is farther up than it actually is. When this is done, the image the eye sees will correspond to the position where the deviant eye is looking so that both eyes may more easily work together as a team. In this simplified example, the direction of

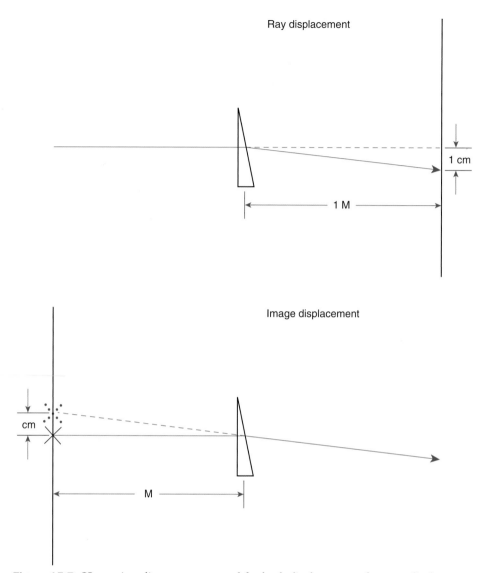

Figure 15-7. How prism diopters correspond for both displacement of rays or displacement of images.

prism orientation would depend on which way the eye tended to point.

How to Specify Prism Base Direction

There is more than one way of specifying prism base direction. Lens prescribers tend to use one method because it fits in more with how they measure the amount of prism needed. The optical surfacing laboratory uses another method because prism can only be ground in a certain manner.

The Prescriber's Method

The person prescribing prism generally uses the wearer's face to reference the prism direction. The top and bottom of the wearer's face and the nose or sides of the head are used to specify base direction. If the prism is "right side up," with the base pointing downward and the apex pointing upward, the prism is said to be a base-down

prism. If it is "upside down," the prism is said to be base up (Figure 15-8).

If the prism is on its side, so to speak, the base of the prism will be oriented either in the direction of the nose or outward away from the nose. Prism oriented with its base toward the nose is said to be base in (Figure 15-9). Prism turned with its base away from the nose is referred to as being base out (Figure 15-10). This is perfectly adequate for those doing the prescribing since vertical and horizontal prism elements are considered separately. If both horizontal and vertical prism corrections are required, then two prism elements are prescribed.

Unfortunately, this is somewhat limiting for the optical surfacing laboratory. First of all, if base-in or base-out prism is prescribed, it depends on which eye is being referenced as to which direction the base of the prism actually faces. For the right eye, base-in prism means that the base goes to the right, but for the left

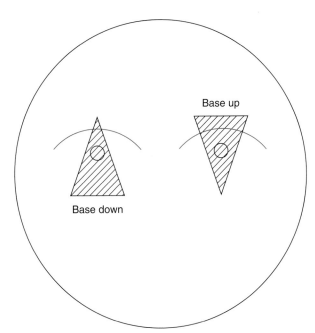

Figure 15-8. It is not necessary to know which eye a prism is on to be certain what "base down" or "base up" means. (However, base down before the right eye has the same effect for the wearer as base up before the left. They are *not* opposite effects.)

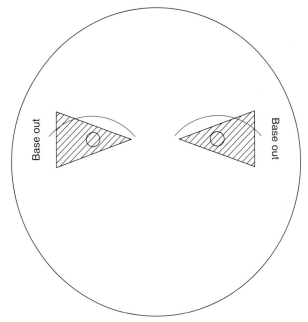

Figure 15-10. Even though the prism bases go in opposite directions, both are classified as "base out." It is not possible to know exactly which way a base-out prism is oriented until a right or left eye is specified.

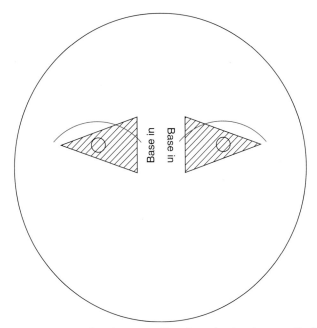

Figure 15-9. When horizontally oriented prism is prescribed for both eyes, it is almost always either base in for both eyes or base out for both eyes. Base-in prisms on both right and left eyes do not cancel each other, but rather augment the desired effect.

eye, a base-in prism means that the base goes to the left.

A 360-Degree Laboratory Reference System
Although the prescriber's method of specifying prism is well suited for those examining eyes and those dispens-

ing eyewear, it is not adequate for the optical laboratory. The optical laboratory uses either a 360-degree system or a 180-degree system of specifying prism base direction.

The 360-degree laboratory reference system uses the standard method of specifying direction in degrees, as shown in Figure 15-11. When a lens is viewed from the front (convex side facing the observer), the base direction is specified as follows: If the base is pointing to the right, it is specified as base 0 degrees. If the base is oriented in an upward direction, it is base 90 degrees. To the left is base 180 degrees, and straight down is base 270 degrees.

The prescriber's method uses a rectangular coordinate system of horizontal and vertical measures. The laboratory method uses a polar coordinate system of degrees.

Converting the Prescriber's Method to the Laboratory System
Suppose a prescription calls for 2 diopters of base-down prism. What is that in the 360-degree laboratory reference system?

Base-down prism is below the 180-degree line. Therefore it must be greater than 180 degrees. Since there are only four directions in the prescriber's method, it must be either 0, 90, 180, or 270 degrees. The 270-degree direction is straight down. Therefore 2 diopters of base-down prism corresponds to base 270.

When there is only one prism element to the prescription lens, there is little difficulty in converting (Figure

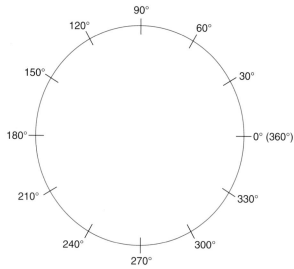

Figure 15-11. The degree system for prism is close to that used for specifying cylinder axis.

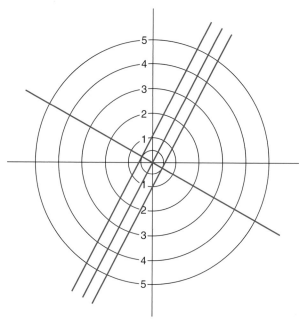

Figure 15-13. When the target is centered in a lensmeter, the optical center of the lens has been located.

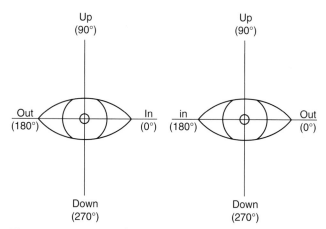

Figure 15-12. Prism base orientation is specified by eye as up, down, in, or out. Base orientations may also be specified in degrees, although prescriptions for an individual's glasses are seldom written as such.

15-12). However, if there are two elements, the conversion may result in any one of the full 360 degrees.

Converting from the Prescriber's Method When Two Prism Elements Are Involved

Sometimes a prescription calls for two amounts of prism in two different directions, both on the same eye. When lenses are ground, it is not possible to work with two prisms. Instead the two prisms are combined into one new prism. Fortunately the end result is the same.

Using one prism instead of two is like taking a short-cut across a field. Instead of walking 2 miles east and 2 miles north, it is possible to walk 2.83 miles northeast and arrive at exactly the same location. (Those familiar with geometry will recognize this as simply the sum of

two vectors.) Therefore instead of grinding 2 diopters of base-out prism for the right eye (prism at 180 degrees) and 2 diopters of base-up prism (prism at base 90 degrees), it is possible to grind 2.83 diopters of prism halfway between (which in this case corresponds to base 135 degrees).

Although this may seem difficult to visualize initially, anyone who is accustomed to using a lensmeter has already been using this system for some time. The lensmeter uses a system of rings inside the instrument to indicate the amount of prism being measured. If the lensmeter is focused, the lines on the target cross at the location of the optical center of the lens. Normally the lens is moved until the target lines are superimposed on the center of the lensmeter reticle, as in Figure 15-13. If the target lines are not centered, the place on the lens where the lensmeter is measuring creates a prismatic effect. The amount of prism is indicated by the location of the intersection of the target lines.

For example, if the target lines intersect on the reticle ring marked "1," the lens shows 1 diopter of prism. If the target lines are on the "1" reticle ring exactly above the center of the reticle, as shown in Figure 15-14, the prism direction is base up. As would be expected, a base-in or base-out effect will be seen to the left or right, depending on which lens is being measured (Figure 15-15).

If a lens is placed in the lensmeter and the intersection of the target lines occurs at a location other than on the vertical or horizontal reticle line, then both vertical and horizontal prism are being manifested. The amount of each is found by drawing imaginary lines from the target center to the horizontal and vertical lines

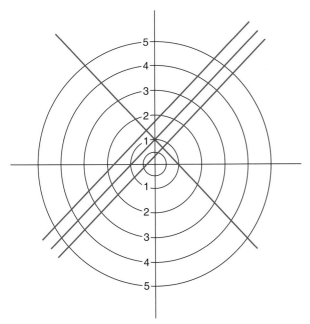

Figure 15-14. If a lens shows this in the lensmeter, there is 1 prism diopter of base-up prism at the point on the lens being looked through. This is true regardless of whether it is a left or a right lens.

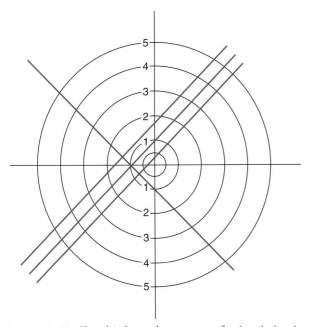

Figure 15-15. For this lens, the amount of prism is 1 prism diopter. However, since we do not know whether the lens is for the left or right eye, we do not know if the prism is base in or base out. If the lens is intended for the right eye, the base direction is base out.

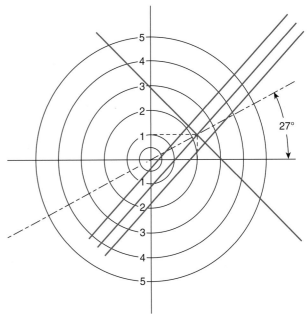

Figure 15-16. Assuming that this lens is for the right eye, the prismatic effect shown is 2Δ base in and 1Δ base up. The base direction of the resultant prism is 27 degrees. It should be noted that the tilt of the triple and single target lines do *not* tell base direction. Within the eyepiece is a hairline that is turned until it crosses the center of the target. This hairline indicates the correct number of degrees. (The interior degree scale is not shown.)

of the reticle. In Figure 15-16, if the lens is a right lens, the amount of prism manifested is 2 prism diopters base in and 1 prism diopter base up. However, the location of the center of the target really shows only one prism. By looking at the figure it can be seen that the amount of

prism is really about 2.25 prism diopters. The base direction is approximately 27 degrees. (Most lensmeters have a degree scale within the reticle that can be used to measure the angle.) We now have a simple system for converting the prescriber's method to the laboratory reference system of recording prism. Since looking into a lensmeter each time is somewhat inconvenient, an alternative is to use a device called a *resultant prism chart*. This chart is shown in Figure 15-17. Such a chart is used in the same manner, but without the lensmeter.

Here are some typical problems for converting the prescriber's method to the laboratory method.

Example **15-11**

If a right lens calls for 1 diopter of base-in prism, what is that in degrees?

Solution

When visualizing prism direction, the lens is always thought of as if the lens (or glasses) has the convex surface facing you (in other words, looking at the glasses as they would appear when being worn by someone else). Therefore for a right lens a base in direction is toward the right. On the prism chart this is in the 0-degree direction. Thus the answer is 1 prism diopter, base 0.

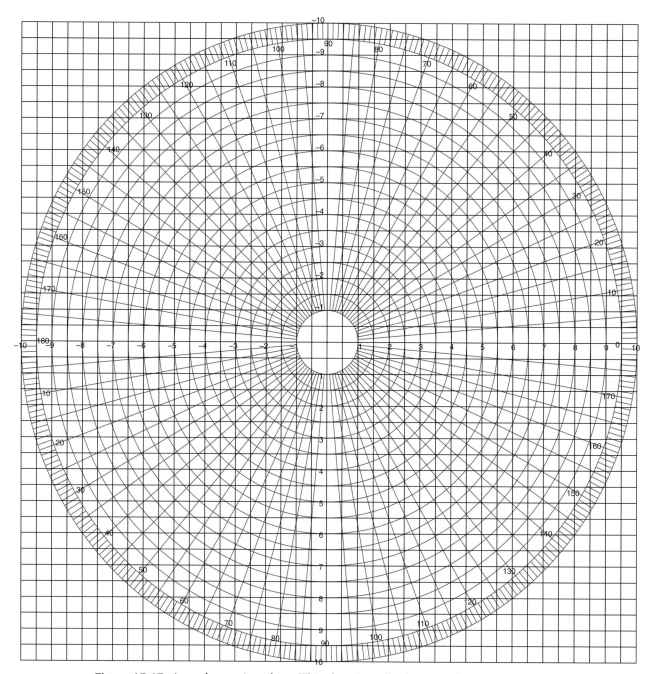

Figure 15-17. A resultant prism chart. This chart is really the same thing as a lensmeter target, but with both a background grid for visualizing the rectangular coordinate system (base in, out, up and down) and the polar coordinate system.

Example **15-12**

What if the prescription for the left eye in Example 15-11 *also* called for 1 diopter of prism base in? Expressed in degrees, what would that base direction be?

Solution

When viewing a left lens from the front, the nose will be to the left. Therefore the base direction is to the left. It can be seen from the prism chart that the base is now in the 180-degree direction.

The answer is 1 prism diopter base 180. So now, even though the prescriber's method indicates base-in prism for both the right and left lenses, the right-eye prism is base 0, and the left-eye prism is base 180.

Example **15-13**

A prescription indicates that the right eye requires 1Δ BI (1 prism diopter base in) and 2Δ BU (base up). Express this in terms of the laboratory reference system.

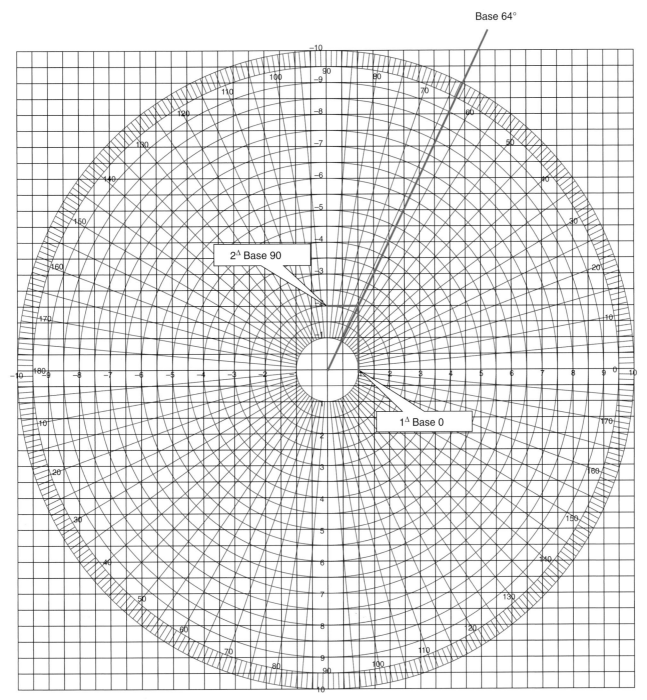

Figure 15-18. Prism chart for Example 15-13.
(Courtesy Coburn Equipment Catalog, Coburn Optical Industries, Muskogee, Okla.)

Solution

Looking at the prism chart in Figure 15-18, we find the location of 1Δ base 0. Next we find the location of 2Δ base 90. If we complete a rectangle using these two points as corners, we find the location of the result as 2.25Δ base 64 degrees.

More practice problems are given at the end of the chapter. Answers are provided at the back of the book.

A Modified (180-Degree) Reference System

Since people in the optical industry are familiar with a 180-degree system when specifying cylinder axis, many prefer to use only 0 to 180 degrees when specifying prism base direction. With cylinder axis there is no difference between axis 90 and axis 270. The cylinder axis is one continuous line. This is not the case, however, with prism base direction. With prism a base 270 direction is exactly opposite a base 90 direction. Thus when using only 0 to 180 degrees, the number must be followed by either "up" or "down." Therefore "base 90" is "base 90 up," and base 270 is "base 90 down."

In practice if the base direction is between 0 and 180 degrees, the word "up" is dropped. But if the base direction corresponds to more than 180 degrees in the 360-degree system, 180 degrees is subtracted from the number, and the word "down" is always added. For example, in the 180-degree reference system, base 270 is (270 − 180), or base 90 DN (down).

Prism Base Direction for Paired Lenses

Prism is normally prescribed to compensate for difficulty the eyes have in working together (i.e., for the purposes of addressing a binocular vision problem). Because eyes work as a team, prism placed in front of one eye affects both eyes. Therefore the full prism correction may be placed before one eye, or the correction may be divided between the two eyes. Dividing the prism may be done as an even split or by placing an unequal portion before one eye and the remainder before the other.

Splitting Horizontal Prism

Very often horizontal prism is split evenly in front of both eyes. Both prisms will be base in, or both will be base out.

It is perfectly legitimate to split prism unevenly. For example, instead of splitting prism as:

R: 2Δ base out
L: 2Δ base out

the prescriber may cause the same effect binocularly with

R: 3Δ base out
L: 1Δ base out

or even

R: 0 prism
L: 4Δ base out

The net effect will be the same. One reason prism may be split unevenly may be because of eye dominance. In other instances, the choice of how to split prism may be made in an effort to either improve the cosmetic appearance of the lenses or equalize lens thicknesses.

Base-out prism in front of the right eye gives the same optical effect as base-out prism in front of the left eye. Base-in prism in front of the right eye gives the same optical effect as base-in prism in front of the left eye.

Splitting Vertical Prism

Vertical prism may also be split evenly or unevenly before the two eyes. An example of prism split evenly would be:

R: 2Δ base up
L: 2Δ base down

For example, the prescriber may cause the same effect binocularly with

R: 3Δ base up
L: 1Δ base down

or

R: 0 prism
L: 4Δ base down

With vertical prism, base up in front of one eye creates the same effect as prism base down in front of the other eye.

This concept is more easily understood by remembering that a prism allows the eye to turn in the direction of the prism apex. Therefore if the right eye turns up, a base-down prism before the right eye will allow the eye to turn upward (in the direction the prism apex points) and should help in preventing eyestrain or double vision.

To summarize:

Right eye		Left eye
Base out		Base out
Base in	is the same as	Base in
Base up		Base down
Base down		Base up

COMPOUNDING AND RESOLVING PRISM

As seen earlier, a prescription may require both horizontal and vertical prism in the same lens. In the manufacturing process, one simple prism may be calculated such that it produces exactly the same effect as the two specified prisms combined would have. When two prisms are combined in power and base orientation to form one prism that is the equivalent of both, the process is known as *compounding prism.*

The reverse of compounding prism is the process of taking a prism whose base orientation is oblique and expressing it as two prisms oriented perpendicularly to one another. The process of expressing a single oblique prism as two perpendicular components is known as *resolving prism.*

When using a lensmeter to analyze a prescription pair of glasses containing both horizontal and vertical components, the two components appear as one compounded prism with the base oriented obliquely. This prism may be resolved into horizontal and vertical components. This may be done easily when the compounding and resolving processes are understood.

Compounding

Compounding of two prisms into one is done by exactly the same process used for obtaining the sum of two vectors (see Chapter 11). The two prisms are drawn to scale as vectors, the unit length of each corresponding to the units of prism power. The arrow points in the direction of prism base orientation.

Example **15-14**

A prescription for the right eye calls for 3Δ base in and 2Δ base up. What compounded prism must be ground onto the lens surface to arrive at the desired prescription?

Solution

The prisms are drawn to scale as shown in Figure 15-19, *A*. A parallelogram is completed (Figure 15-19, *B*), and the resultant prism drawn (Figure 15-19, *C*). This prism is measured and found to be 3.6Δ. The prism base orientation is measured using a protractor and found to be 34 degrees. Therefore the resultant compounded prism is 3.6Δ base at 34 degrees.

This problem may also be solved using geometry and trigonometry. The horizontal prism component is designated *H*, the vertical component *V*, and the resultant prism *R*. The new base orientation of the resultant prism is θ. Because this graphic construction contains a right triangle, the value of the resultant is found using the Pythagorean theorem.

$$R^2 = V^2 + H^2$$
$$R = \sqrt{V^2 + H^2}$$

Since V = 2 and H = 3,

$$R = \sqrt{2^2 + 3^2}$$
$$= \sqrt{13}$$
$$R = 3.61Δ$$

The base orientation is found from

$$\tan\theta = \frac{V}{H}$$

because the side opposite angle θ is the vertical component, and the side adjacent, the horizontal.

By using a calculator, the function inverse tan (tan^{-1}) allows the angle θ to be found as 33.69 degrees.

Therefore the resultant prism is 3.61Δ base at 33.69 degrees.

Resolving

Reversing the previously described process resolves one oblique prism into horizontal and vertical components. First, the oblique prism is drawn to scale as a vector and oriented so that it points in the prescribed base direction. Horizontal and vertical lines are drawn from the tip of the arrow to the 90-degree and 180-degree axis line (*x*- and *y*-axes of the Cartesian coordinate system). The positions of intersection with the *x*- and *y*-axes mark the power of the horizontal and vertical prism resolved from the original prism.

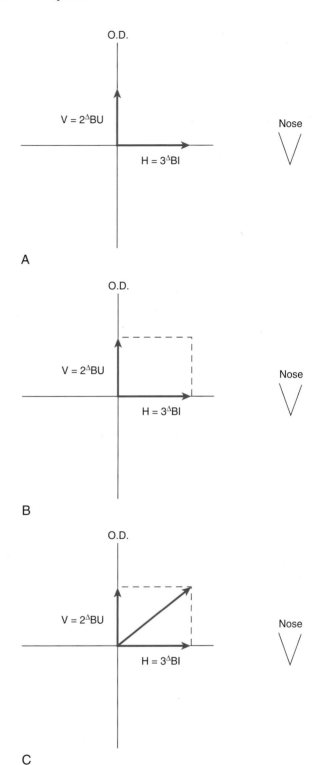

Figure 15-19. A, Compounding two prisms into one using a graphic method begins by entering two vectors on the axes of a Cartesian coordinate system. **B,** From the two prism vector representations, a parallelogram is completed. **C,** The compounded prism that results is the diagonal of the parallelogram, beginning from the origin. (BI = base in; BU = base up.)

Example **15-15**

A wearer's right lens is placed in a lensmeter and prism found. That prism reads 2.00Δ base at 30 degrees. What horizontal and vertical prism values does this prove to be?

Solution

This prism is drawn on a coordinate system as shown in Figure 15-20. Horizontal and vertical lines are dropped from the tip of the vector to the x- and y-axes, and the distance from zero measured. The vertical component measures

1.00Δ base up. The horizontal component measures 1.70Δ base in. (If this were the left lens, the base direction would be away from the nose and would be read as base out.)

In the example given, the target of the lensmeter, representing the spherical and cylindrical powers, will be displaced from its center position to the same degree and in the same direction as the resultant arrow in the graphic method would be (Figure 15-21). By mentally extending lines from the lensmeter target center until they intersect the x- and y-axes, the power of the prisms are determined.

The resolving of prism may also be calculated trigonometrically using equations derived from the geometry of the figure. These are:

$$V = P \sin\theta$$
$$H = P \cos\theta$$

where P is the power of the oblique prism and θ the base orientation. Using the previous problem,

$$V = 2.00 \sin 30$$
$$= 2.00 \times 0.5$$
$$= 1.00$$

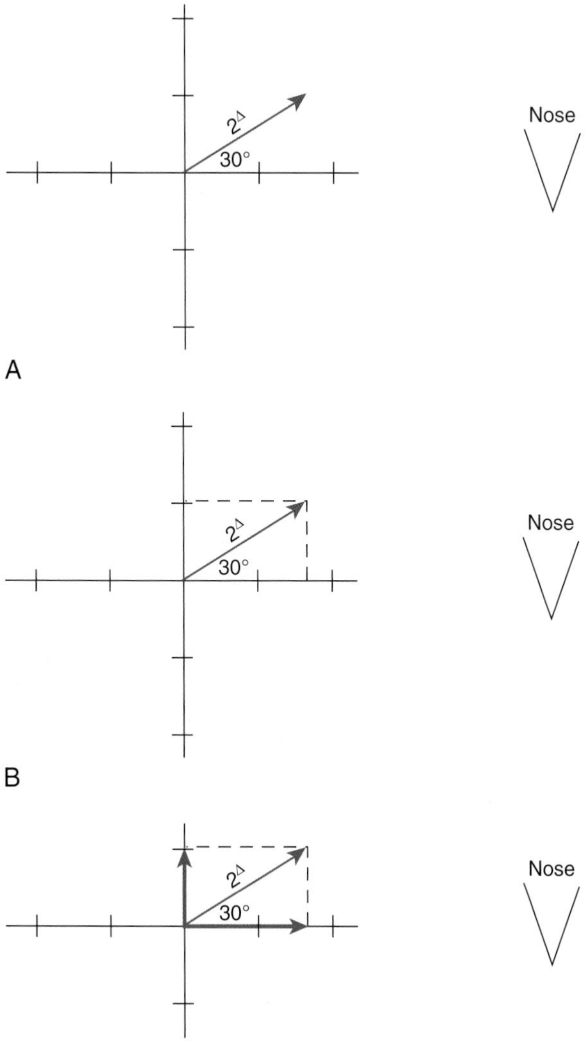

A

B

C

Figure 15-20. A, Resolving a single prism into its equivalent horizontal and vertical components begins by placing a vector on a graph such that it is representative of the prism power in length and represents base orientation in degrees. **B,** Individual component lengths are found by dropping perpendiculars to the x- and y-axes. **C,** In essence by dropping perpendiculars, a parallelogram has been constructed in reverse, using its diagonal. The horizontal land vertical components are easily measured from the lengths of the two sides.

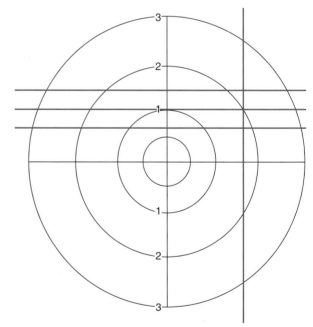

Figure 15-21. The most familiar example of resolving prism occurs daily when using a lensmeter. The intersection of the sphere and cylinder lines gives the location of the prism base. Perpendiculars from this intersection point, down and across to the x-, y-coordinate positions on the inner scale indicate the amounts of the horizontal and vertical prism components. (Because sphere and cylinder target lines may be turned in directions other than 90- or 180-degree positions during verification of a spherocylinder lens, simply following these lines to their intersection with the x- and y-axes will not always give the correct answer as might be initially imagined from the simplified construction of the figure.)

So as before, the vertical component is found to be 1.00Δ.

For the horizontal component

$$H = 2.00 \cos \theta$$
$$= 2.00 \times 0.86603$$
$$= 1.73\Delta$$

The horizontal component has a power of 1.73Δ. Base direction is evident from the orientations of the original prism.

Combining Two Obliquely Crossed Prisms

At first glance, the problem of combining two oblique prisms into one single prism seems difficult. However, there are no new concepts here. In general terms, this can be done as follows:

1. Take each oblique prism and resolve it into its horizontal and vertical components.
2. Add the horizontal components from the two prisms together into one.
3. Add the vertical components from the two prisms together into one.
4. Combine the resultant vertical and horizontal components into a new, single prism.
   Here is an example:

Example **15-16**

Combine these two oblique prisms together into one prism:

2.83Δ base 135
5.00Δ base 037

Solution

Draw these two prisms as vectors to help in visualizing the problem. This is done in Figure 15-22, *A* Take the 2.82Δ base 135 prism and find the horizontal and vertical components. By plotting this out as shown in Figure 15-22, *B1*, we can see that the vertical component is:

$$V = P \sin \theta$$
$$= 2.83 \sin 45$$
$$= (2.83)(6.707)$$
$$V = 2.00\Delta$$

The base direction is 90. The vertical component is 2.00Δ base 90.

Because the triangle is a right triangle with two 45-degree angles, we know the horizontal component will also be 2.00 Δ, and the base direction will be to the left or 180 (i.e., 2.00Δ base 180.

The second oblique prism of 5Δ base 37 is drawn as shown in Figure 15-22, *B2*. The vertical component is:

$$V = P \sin \theta$$
$$= 5 \sin 37$$
$$= 5(0.60)$$
$$= 3.00\Delta$$

The base direction is base up or base 90 (i.e., 3.00Δ base 90). The horizontal component is:

$$H = P \cos \theta$$
$$= 5 \cos 37$$
$$= 5(0.799)$$
$$= 4.00\Delta$$

The base direction is right, or base 0 (i.e., 4.00Δ base 0).

Now we can add the two horizontal and the two vertical components as shown in Figure 15-22, *C*.

$$2.00\Delta Base90 + 3.00\Delta Base90 = 5.00\Delta Base90$$
$$2.00\Delta Base180 + 4.00\Delta Base0 = 2.00\Delta Base0$$

If we only needed horizontal and vertical components, we would be finished. If this was a right eye, the answer would be 5.00Δ base up and 2.00Δ base in. If it was a left eye, it would be 5.00Δ base up and 2.00Δ base out.

However, to complete the problem so that the answer is a single prism, we need to find the vector sum of both prisms. This is shown in Figure 15-22, *D* and calculated as follows:

$$P^2 = V^2 + H^2$$
$$P = \sqrt{5^2 + 2^2}$$
$$= \sqrt{25 + 4}$$
$$= \sqrt{29}$$
$$P = 5.4\Delta$$

The base direction is found this way:

$$\tan \theta = \frac{V}{H}$$
$$\tan \theta = \frac{5}{2} = 2.5$$
$$\theta = 68.2 \text{ degrees}$$

So the final prism amount is 5.4Δ base 68.2. Incidentally, it would have been possible to graph the two prism vectors to scale and find the resultant prism vector of 5.4Δ base 68.2 by measuring it. This is shown in Figure 15-23.

ROTARY PRISMS

There is an application of obliquely crossed prisms that is used on a regular basis in ophthalmic practice. That application is called a *rotary* or *Risley's prism*. A rotary prism is a combination of two prisms. These prisms are placed one on top of the other. Initially, their base directions are exactly identical, but as the prisms are rotated, their bases move by equal extents in opposite directions.

For example, suppose two prisms of 10Δ each are placed on top of one another base-to-base. The total prismatic effect is 20Δ (Figure 15-24, *A*). But if they are placed base-to-apex, then their total prismatic effect is zero (Figure 15-24, *B*).

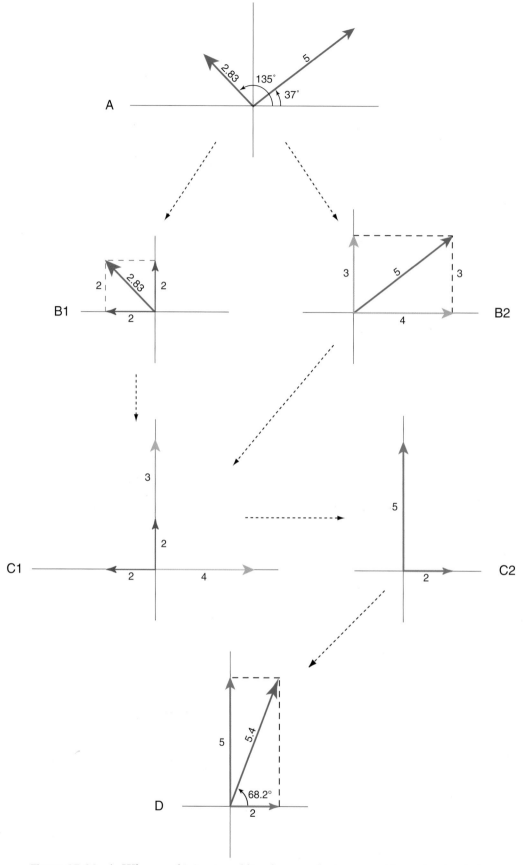

Figure 15-22. A, When combining two obliquely crossed prisms, consider each prism independently and split each prism into horizontal and vertical components. **B1,** A 2.83Δ base 135 prism becomes 2Δ base left or base 180 and 2Δ base up or base 90. **B2,** A 5Δ base 37 prism becomes 4Δ base right (or base 0) and 3Δ base up (or base 90). **C,** When horizontal and vertical components of the two obliquely crossed prisms are added, they become 2Δ base right (or base 0) and 5Δ base up (or base 90). **D,** When 2Δ base right (or base 0) and 5Δ base up (or base 90) are combined, they become 5.4Δ base 68.2.

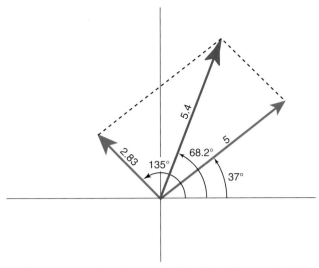

Figure 15-23. When drawn to scale, obliquely crossed prisms can be combined graphically and the resultant prism amount and base direction measured directly without calculating the result using trigonometry, as shown in the previous figures.

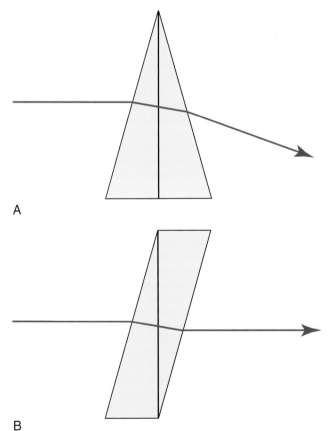

Figure 15-24. A, A Risley's or rotary prism is really two prisms, one on top of the other. When these equally powered prisms are placed base-to-base, their combined prism amount is at a maximum. **B,** When a Risley's or rotary prism has the two prism elements base-to-apex, the resultant amount is zero.

Now suppose we begin with both 10Δ prisms base down. Together they total 20Δ base down. Next we rotate one prism base 37 degrees clockwise and the other base 37 degrees counterclockwise. Now what prismatic effect is being manifested?

We plot each prism in vertical and horizontal components as seen in Figure 15-25. This shows that the horizontal components are equal and opposite. They cancel out. The vertical components are both 8Δ base down, which when added equal 16Δ base down.

As the prisms continue to be rotated in opposite directions, the horizontal components increase equally and continue to cancel out, and the vertical components decrease. This continues until both prisms are fully horizontal-one base left, the other base right. Now there is neither horizontal nor vertical prism. The prismatic effect is zero. If the two prisms continue to be rotated past the horizontal, base-up vertical prism begins to increase and continues to increase until both prisms are fully base up. As these prisms were being rotated, there was never anything but vertical prism being manifested.

The same thing may be done to produce varying amounts of only horizontal prism. To produce only horizontal prism, begin with both prisms base left. Rotate the base of one prism clockwise and the other counterclockwise in equal amounts (Figure 15-26). Now horizontal prism varies, and vertical prism remains at zero.

There are two common forms of the Risley's or rotating prism in ophthalmic practice. One, found on the phoropter, is used to measure phorias and ductions (Figure 15-27). The other is found on some lensmeters and is used to measure large amounts of prism in spectacle lenses (Figure 15-28).

HOW THE EFFECTIVE POWER OF A PRISM CHANGES FOR NEAR OBJECTS

A prism displaces a ray of light consistently. However, it will affect the eye somewhat differently than looking at a near object than it does when looking at a distant object. The eye will turn less when looking through a prism at a near object than it will when looking through that same prism at a distant object. Therefore the *effective* power of the prism, when measured as the angle that light enters the eye, will decrease as an object moves closer to the prism being worn. So although a prism displaces a ray of light consistently, the power of the prism, when measured by the angle that light enters the eye, will be less the closer the viewed object is to the prism.

For an object at infinity, a prism will cause that object to be displaced such that the angle of displacement, (d) equals the angle of rotation of the eye (d_e) (Figure 15-29). In other words, for distance vision, the prism causes the light to deviate or bend by the angle d. This is equal to the actual (effective) turn of the eye d_e.

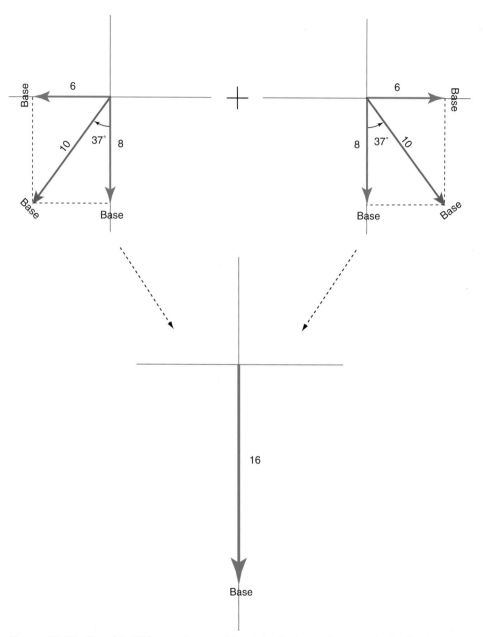

Figure 15-25. For this Risley's prism combination, the base direction for both 10Δ prism elements started out as base down and totalled 20Δ base down. Next they were rotated in opposite directions, one clockwise, the other counterclockwise. This causes their equal and opposite horizontal components to cancel each other out. Their vertical components are additive. Here they add up to 16Δ base down.

Horizontal rotary prism

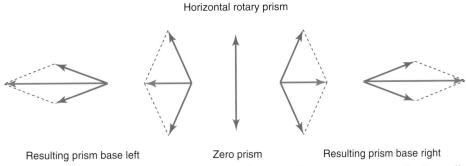

Resulting prism base left   Zero prism   Resulting prism base right

Figure 15-26. Here the combining actions of the two prism components in a horizontally oriented Risley's or rotary prism are shown as vectors.

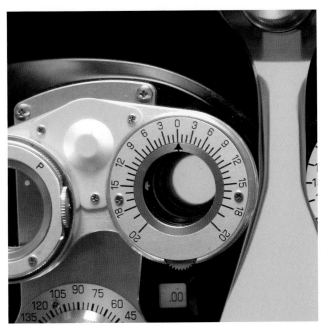

Figure 15-27. The **Von Graefe** prism test used to measure phorias and duction during refraction makes use of a Risley's or rotary prism. Here the rotary prism is set to measure horizontal prism. Turning the small thumb gear at the bottom causes the two linked prisms to rotate in opposite directions.

For near vision, the light is also deviated the same amount by the prism as it is for distance because the prism itself is the same. The amount of deviation of the light by the prism is d, as before. However, for near vision, light is diverging as it enters the prism (Figure 15-30). Though the ray of light is bent the same amount by the prism, the angle at which it enters the eye (d_e) is not as great as it was for distance vision. The effective deviation, d_e, is less than the angular deviation, d.

If we convert the angular measures d and d_e to prism diopters, P prism diopters corresponds to d and P_e prism diopters (effective prism diopters) corresponds to d_e (effective deviation). By the definition of a prism diopter, we are able to say that:

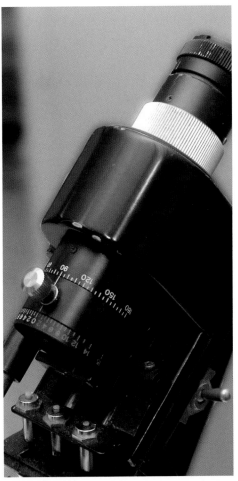

Figure 15-28. The auxiliary prism found on some lensmeters measures high amounts of prism that would normally be beyond the limit of the viewed target area. This auxiliary prism is an example of a Risley's or rotary prism. The red lettering is the amount of prism in one direction, the white lettering on the same ring shows the amount of prism in an opposite base direction. The degree lettering shows the orientation of prism base direction. When the compensating rotary prism axis is on zero, one direction on the prism power scale is Base In and the other Base Out. When the compensating prism axis is on 90 (as shown here), one direction on prism axis scale is Base Up and the other Base Down.

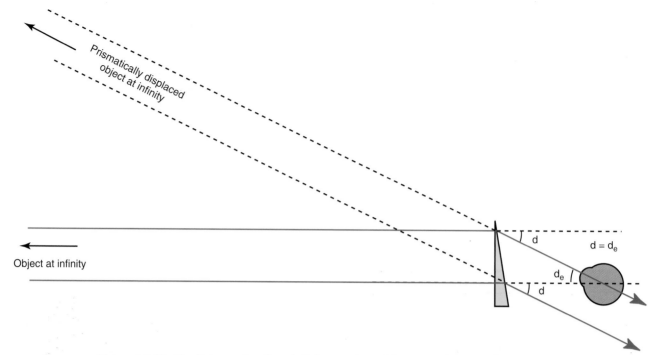

Figure 15-29. For light coming from infinity, a prism with an actual power of P will cause the light from that object to be displaced by the amount of deviation shown in the figure as d. d_e is the amount the eye must turn to see the object. For distance vision, these amounts are equal. When d and d_e are expressed in prism diopters, they are P and P_e, respectively. P_e is the effective power of the prism. Therefore for distance vision, the actual power and effective power of the prism are the same.

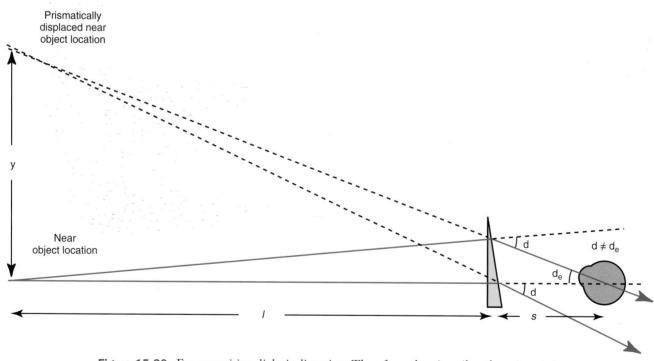

Figure 15-30. For near vision, light is diverging. Therefore when it strikes the prism, it is bent the same amount (check the angle for each of the two rays). However, it enters the eye at a different (and smaller) angle. This causes the effective power of the prism (P_e) to be less than the actual power of the prism (P).

$$\frac{P}{100} = \frac{y}{|l|}$$

The l is written as an absolute value because, by optical sign convention, the lens or prism is at the zero point on a number line. Distance measured from the prism to the right is plus and from the prism to the left is minus.

For the near diagram,

l = the distance from the prism to the near point,
s = the distance from the prism to the center of rotation of the eye
y = the displacement of the image

By the geometry of Figure 15-30

$$\frac{P_e}{100} = \frac{y}{|l| + s}$$

We know that in this instance our l value will be minus. So, in order to maintain sign convention and have the resulting equation work correctly, we write the two previous equations as

$$\frac{P}{100} = \frac{y}{-l}$$

and

$$\frac{P_e}{100} = \frac{y}{-l + s}$$

By transposing the first equation we get

$$y = \frac{P(-l)}{100}$$

And by transposition the second equation becomes

$$y = \frac{P_e(-l + s)}{100}$$

Now we have two values for y that must be equal to one another. Therefore we can combine the two as:

$$\frac{P(-l)}{100} = \frac{P_e(-l + s)}{100}$$

This reduces to

$$p(-l) = p_e(-l + s)$$

and becomes

$$P_e = \frac{P(-l)}{(-l + s)}$$

When transposed the result is what is referred to as the *effective prism power formula*:

$$P_e = \frac{P}{1 - \dfrac{s}{l}}$$

So the effective power of the prism for near objects can be compared mathematically with the actual power of the prism for objects at infinity with the above formula.

If expressed in words, the effective prism power formula reads:

Effective Prism Power =
$$\frac{\text{Actual prism power}}{1 - \dfrac{\text{Distance from prism to center of rotation}}{\text{Distance from prism to near object}}}$$

Example **15-17**

A 5Δ base-in prism is prescribed for distance vision. The prism is worn at a vertex distance of 20 mm. What is the effective power of the prism for objects at 40 cm?

Solution

Before trying to solve by just using the equation, notice that vertex distance was given—not the distance to the center of rotation of the eye. If we use the effective prism power formula, we need to know the distance from the prism to the center of rotation of the eye. The unknown quantity is the distance from the front surface of the cornea to the center of rotation. This distance is usually assumed to be 13.5 mm. If we assume that the distance from the cornea to the center of rotation is 13.5 mm, then the distance from the prism to the center of rotation will be 20 mm + 13.5 mm or 33.5 mm.

Note that because of sign convention, the distance from the lens (prism) to the near object is a negative number (−400 mm). So when putting the numbers into the formula we have:

$$\text{Effective Prism Power} = \frac{5}{1 - \dfrac{33.5}{-400 \text{ mm}}}$$

$$= \frac{5}{1 - (-0.084)} = \frac{5}{1.084}$$

$$= 4.61\Delta$$

The effective power of a 5.00Δ base-in prism, when used to view an object at 40 cm, is 4.61Δ base in.

Example **15-18**

Suppose an object is at a distance of only −10 cm from a base-down prism having a power of 6. If the prism is worn at a distance of 25 mm from the center of rotation of the eye, what is the effective power of that prism?

Solution

Since l = −100 mm, s = 25 mm, and P = 6Δ, then

$$P_e = \frac{P}{1 - \dfrac{s}{l}}$$

$$= \frac{6}{1 - \left(\dfrac{25}{-100}\right)}$$

$$= \frac{6}{1 + 0.25}$$

$$= 4.8\Delta$$

Note: As an object approaches the plane of the prism, the effective power of the prism continues to drop, losing power rapidly until the object finally touches the front of the prism, and the effective power essentially drops to zero.

Proficiency Test

(Answers can be found in the back of the book.)

1. A prism has an apical angle of 4.5 degrees and is made of plastic of index 1.49. What is the angle of deviation of the prism?
   a. 2.2 degrees
   b. 3.0 degrees
   c. 4.5 degrees
   d. 6.7 degrees
   e. none of the above

2. Using the simplified equation for thin prisms, find the angle of deviation for a prism having an apical angle of 5 degrees and an index of refraction of 1.5.
   a. 2.0 degrees
   b. 2.5 degrees
   c. 3.0 degrees
   d. 3.5 degrees
   e. 5.0 degrees

3. A prism with an apical angle of 9 degrees deviates light by 6 degrees. What is the refractive index of the prism material?
   a. 1.49
   b. 1.53
   c. 1.59
   d. 1.67
   e. 1.70

4. A person covers his or her left eye, and a prism is placed before the right eye. The base of the prism is oriented out toward the temporal side of the head. From the point of view of the person looking through the prism, in which direction will the image be displaced?
   a. to the right
   b. to the left
   c. upward
   d. downward
   e. There will be no displacement.

5. A prism deviates light 1.5 degrees. How many diopters of power does this prism have?
   a. 1Δ
   b. 1.5Δ
   c. 2.6Δ
   d. 0.9Δ
   e. none of the above

6. Light entering a prism in air is deviated in the direction of the:
   a. base.
   b. apex.
   c. base or apex, depending on the refractive index of the prism.

7. A prism displaces the image of an object at infinity 6 degrees upward. What is the power of the prism?
   a. 8.75Δ
   b. 99.50Δ
   c. 6Δ
   d. 10.50Δ
   e. none of the above

8. What is the base direction of the prism in the above question?
   a. base up
   b. base down
   c. base in
   d. base out
   e. base at 6 degrees

9. How far will a 3.25Δ prism appear to displace the image of an object 4 m away?
   a. 3.25 cm
   b. 13 cm
   c. 1.3 m
   d. 12.3 cm
   e. none of the above

10. For a 6Δ prism, a point on the wall 6 m away will be made to appear _____ cm away from its actual location.
    a. 36
    b. 1
    c. 6
    d. 60
    e. none of the above

11. An object is displaced 18 cm by a prism of unknown power. If the prism is 4 m from the object, what is the prism power?
    a. 0.22Δ
    b. 7.2Δ
    c. 4.5Δ
    d. 22Δ
    e. none of the above

12. If an image of an object 1.75 m away is displaced 1.75 cm, approximately how strong is the prism?
    a. 1.75Δ
    b. 3.06Δ
    c. 0.10Δ
    d. 3.50Δ
    e. none of the above

13. An object is displaced 4 cm. If the prism is 0.50Δ in power, how far away is the object?
    a. 2 m
    b. 20 cm
    c. 8 m
    d. 8 cm
    e. none of the above

14. One prism has a power of 25Δ, a second prism has a power of 25▽. Which prism is stronger in its ability to deviate light?
    a. the 25Δ prism
    b. the 25▽ prism
    c. The prisms are equal.

15. If a prism has its base direction to the right (the wearer's left):
    a. What base direction is this in reference to the wearer's right eye?
       (1) Base down
       (2) Base up
       (3) Base in
       (4) Base out
    b. What base direction is this in reference to the wearer's left eye?
       (1) Base down
       (2) Base up
       (3) Base in
       (4) Base out

16. A prescription is written with Rx prism of 2.0 prism diopters base in for the right eye. How would this be written in the 360-degree laboratory system?
    a. 2.00 base 0
    b. 2.00 base 180
    c. 2.00 base 90
    d. 2.00 base 270

17. A prescription for Rx prism for the left eye reads:
    4.00 base in
    2.00 base down
    Using the 360-degree laboratory reference system, what is the amount of prism and base direction? What would this be when expressed in the 180-degree reference system?

18. What is prism 3.25 base 287 in the 180-degree reference system?

19. What is prism 1.50 base 1 DN in the 360-degree reference system?

20. A prescription calls for prism in the left lens as follows:
    5.00 base in
    2.00 base up
    What is this when written as one prism? Give amount and base direction.

21. Suppose a prescription calls for Rx prism in the left lens. The amounts are:
    3.00 base in
    1.50 base up
    What is this when written as one prism? Give amount and base direction.

22. a. What are the two other ways of writing 4.00 base 330 for a right lens? (Give the specific base directions and amounts.)
    b. What would the answer be if the lens were a left lens?
    In the following instances of prescribed Rx prism, how much prism in what direction would be surfaced onto the lens? (Give the answer in *both* full 360-degree convention and the method that employs only 180 degrees of reference.)

Two Prism Amounts		Combined Resultant Prism
23. R: 3.00 BO	180	_____
2.50 BU	360	_____
L: 3.00 BO	180	_____
2.50 BU	360	_____
24. R: 1.50 BO	180	_____
2.00 BD	360	_____
L: 1.50 BO	180	_____
2.00 BD	360	_____

Two Prism Amounts		Combined Resultant Prism	Two Prism Amounts		Combined Resultant Prism
25. R: 6.00 BO	180	_____	**37.** R: 1.25 BI	180	_____
5.00 BU	360	_____	0.75 BD	360	_____
L: 6.00 BO	180	_____	L: 1.00 BI	180	_____
5.00 BD	360	_____	1.00 BU	360	_____
26. R: 3.00 BO	180	_____	**38.** R: 3.25 BO	180	_____
4.00 BU	360	_____	0.50 BU	360	_____
L: 3.00 BO	180	_____	L: 3.00 BO	180	_____
4.00 BD	360	_____	1.50 BD	360	_____

27. R: 4.50 BI 180 _____
3.00 BD 360 _____
L: 0.75 BO 180 _____
4.00 BD 360 _____

39.
a. True or false? The prism pair (R: 2 BI, L: No prism) will give the same net prismatic effect binocularly as (R: 1 BI, L: 1 BI).
b. True or false? The prism pair (R: 2 BI, L: No prism) will give the same net prismatic effect binocularly as (R: No prism, L: 2 BO).
c. True or false? The prism pair (R: 2 BU, L: No prism) will give the same net prismatic effect binocularly as (R: No prism, L: 2 BU).

28. R: 5.50 BO 180 _____
1.00 BD 360 _____
L: 2.25 BI 180 _____
4.00 BD 360 _____

29. R: 3.00 BO 180 _____
3.00 BD 360 _____
L: 3.00 BO 180 _____
3.00 BU 360 _____

40. In the lensmeter, a left lens has prism, which reads 2.00 base at 150 degrees. Resolve this prism into vertical and horizontal components (to nearest 1/4 D).
a. 1.00 base up, 1.75 base out
b. 1.00 base up, 1.75 base in
c. 1.75 base up, 1.00 base out
d. 1.75 base up, 1.00 base in
e. none of the above

30. R: 0.75 BI 180 _____
2.50 BD 360 _____
L: 0.75 BI 180 _____
2.50 BU 360 _____

31. R: 2.50 BO 180 _____
4.25 BD 360 _____
L: 2.00 BI 180 _____
4.25 BU 360 _____

41. A 3.00Δ base-up prism is combined with a 4.00Δ base-in prism before the left eye. What is the compounded prism and its base direction that results from this combination?

32. R: 0.50 BI 180 _____
1.75 BU 360 _____
L: 0.50 BI 180 _____
1.75 BD 360 _____

42. Prism base 45 degrees before the right eye is the same as prism base:
a. up and out
b. up and in
c. down and out
d. down and in
e. cannot be determined

33. R: 4.00 BI 180 _____
0.75 BU 360 _____
L: 4.25 BI 180 _____
0.75 BD 360 _____

34. R: 4.25 BI 180 _____
2.00 BU 360 _____
L: 3.75 BI 180 _____
2.00 BD 360 _____

43. What is the prism resulting when each of these sets of two obliquely crossed prisms are combined? Give your answer first in the rectangular coordinate system, then in the polar coordinate system.
a. 5Δ base 37
5Δ base 143
(Right eye)
b. 2.5Δ base 53
2.5Δ base 217
(Left eye)
c. 1.41Δ base 45
5Δ base 323
(Right eye)

35. R: 4.50 BI 180 _____
2.75 BU 360 _____
L: 3.50 BI 180 _____
4.00 BD 360 _____

36. R: 0.75 BO 180 _____
1.00 BD 360 _____
L: 0.25 BO 180 _____
1.25 BD 360 _____

44. A person is wearing 4Δ base down before the right eye and 4Δ base up before the left eye.
   a. What is the effective power of the prisms at 40 cm if the lenses are worn at a vertex distance of 12 mm, and the distance from the cornea to the center of rotation of the eye is 13.5 mm?
   b. This single vision lens wearer works at a very close 15-cm working distance from time to time. What is the effective power of his prism prescription for this working distance?

45. What is the effective power of a 6Δ prism when viewing an object at a 20-cm viewing distance?
   a. 6.99Δ
   b. 6.00Δ
   c. 5.25Δ

CHAPTER 16

Optical Prism: Decentration and Thickness

The relationship between a normal plus or minus spectacle lens and optical prism can sometimes be difficult to understand. For example, when the optical center of a lens is moved away from its expected position in front of the eye, that lens now causes a prismatic effect. The farther the lens is moved or decentered from its original position the greater the amount of resulting prism. This chapter explains how this happens and how prism is related to thickness differences across a lens. Grasping these concepts leads to a much greater understanding of prism and lens prescriptions.

DECENTRATION OF SPHERES

When light goes through the optical center (OC) of the lens, it goes straight through. It is not bent. When light goes through any other point on a lens, the ray of light is bent. The farther from the optical center that a light ray strikes a lens, the more that ray will have to bend to pass through the focal point of the lens. This lens characteristic may be used to advantage when prescribed prism is required in a prescription. However, it will also cause problems if the lens has not been properly centered before the eye.

A Centered Lens

At the exact OC of a lens, front and back lens surfaces are parallel to each other. The line that passes through the OC of a lens is known as the *optical axis*. Light from an object at infinity is focused somewhere on the optical axis. The exact location of the focal point depends on the power of the lens.

If the optic axis of a lens passes through the center of the pupil, the lens is centered in front of the eye. If the lens is moved so that it does *not* coincide with the line of sight of the eye (for our purposes at the center of the pupil), it is said to be *decentered*.

A Decentered Lens

Normally an individual wearing corrective lenses has each lens positioned with its optical center in front of the eye. In this position, when the wearer looks straight ahead there is no displacement of objects from their actual positions (Figure 16-1).

What happens when the lens is moved so that the center of the lens is no longer in front of the center of the eye? To understand what happens, consider the shape of a plus lens. From the side (in cross section), it appears to look much like two prisms placed base to base (Figure 16-2). A minus lens gives the impression of being a combination of two prisms, but this time placed apex to apex (Figure 16-3). When the wearer looks right through the center of the lens, the object is not displaced from its actual location. But when a plus or minus lens is moved off-center in relationship to the location of the eye, the object appears displaced as shown in Figures 16-2 and 16-3. This means that a *decentered* lens causes a *prismatic effect*.

Prentice's Rule

Remember that *prism power* is the amount light is displaced in centimeters at a distance 1 m away from the lens or prism.

The relationship between focal length (f) and decentration (c) is shown in Figure 16-4 using similar triangles. This relationship is the same as the definition of prism power: the displacement in centimeters over the distance in meters.

By similar triangles, as shown in Figure 16-4, B and C, we see that:

$$\frac{c\,(cms)}{f\,(meters)} = \frac{image\ displacement\ in\ cm}{1\ meter}$$

And we know from the definition of a prism diopter that

$$\Delta = \frac{image\ displacement\ in\ cm}{1\ meter}$$

Therefore, we can see that

$$\frac{c}{f} = \Delta$$

So if we know lens decentration in centimeters (c) and lens focal length (f), the prismatic effect caused by the decentration may be calculated.

376

Figure 16-1. When a lens is positioned with its optical center directly in front of the eye, there is no prismatic effect.

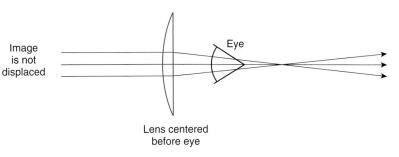

Image is not displaced

Eye

Lens centered before eye

Figure 16-2. Moving the optical center of a plus lens downward will produce a base-down prismatic effect.

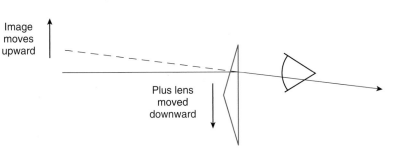

Image moves upward

Plus lens moved downward

Figure 16-3. Moving the optical center of a minus lens downward will produce a base-up prismatic effect.

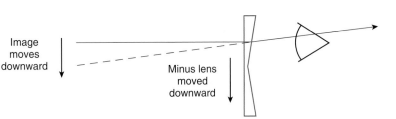

Image moves downward

Minus lens moved downward

Because

$$F = \frac{1}{f}$$

the relationship further simplifies to

$$\Delta = cF$$

The equation $\Delta = cF$ is commonly known as *Prentice's rule.*

Example **16-1**

If a lens having a power of +3.00 D is decentered 5 mm away from the center of the eye, how much prismatic effect will this cause?

Solution

To find the prismatic effect, simply multiply the distance *in centimeters* that the lens has been displaced by the power of the lens. Since 5 mm equals 0.5 cm,

$$\text{Prism diopters} = 0.5 \times 3.00$$
$$\Delta = 1.5$$

Prism Base Direction With Decentration

When a lens is decentered, a prismatic effect is created. With decentration, both prism power and prism base direction are manifested. The power of the prism depends on the amount of lens decentration and the refractive power of the lens being decentered. The prism base orientation depends on the direction of decentration and whether the lens is positive or negative.

As noted before, a plus lens resembles two prisms placed base to base. Both bases are at the center of the lens. Therefore for a plus lens, the base direction created by decentration will correspond to the direction of the decentration. A plus lens decentered down will result in prism with the base down (see Figure 16-2).

A minus lens resembles two prisms placed apex to apex. Both apices are together at the center of the lens. Thus if a minus lens is decentered down, the result will be prism with the base up, opposite to the direction of decentration (see Figure 16-3).

Example **16-2**

If a −4.00 D spherical lens is decentered 5 mm upward, how much of a prismatic effect is induced, and what is the base orientation?

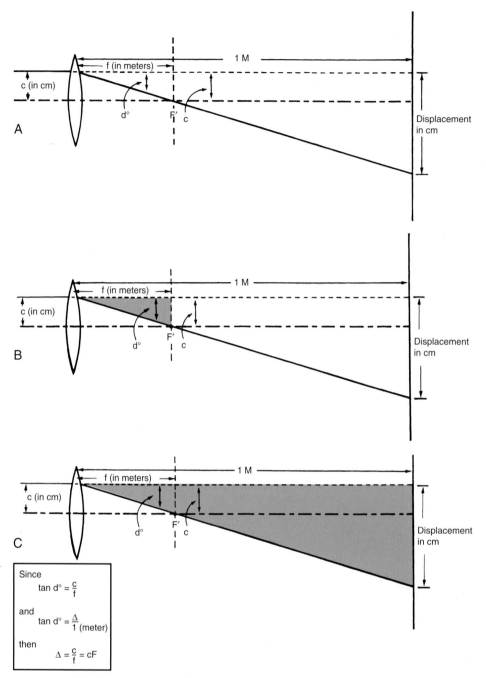

Since
$$\tan d° = \frac{c}{f}$$
and
$$\tan d° = \frac{\Delta}{1 \text{ (meter)}}$$
then
$$\Delta = \frac{c}{f} = cF$$

Figure 16-4. A, When a lens is decentered, the geometry of the displaced ray as it travels through the lens focal point may be illustrated as shown. **B,** Because the deviated ray passes through the focal point, degrees of deviation (d) may be found from the two known parameters (f and c) by using the relationship:

$$\tan d° = \frac{c}{f}$$

C, Once a value for d is known, it can be seen from the figure how prism value expressed in prism diopters may be established. From this relationship, Prentice's rule may be derived as shown in the boxed equation at the bottom left of the figure.

Solution

Prentice's rule is used to find the prismatic effect.

$$\Delta = cF$$

In this instance

$$\Delta = (0.5)(4.00) = 2.00$$

(Normally when using Prentice's rule, the absolute value of the lens power is used. Plus and minus signs are ignored.) The decentration induces 2.00Δ of prism. Since the lens is minus in power, the base direction is opposite to that of the decentration. Therefore the complete answer is 2.00Δ base down.

Example **16-3**

A +6.50 D lens before the right eye is decentered 3 mm nasalward. What amount of prism is induced, and what is the base orientation?

Solution

Prentice's rule is again applied as follows:

$$\Delta = cF$$
$$\Delta = (0.3)(6.50) = 1.95.$$

The lens is plus so the base direction corresponds to the direction of decentration. Since nasalward is inward, the base direction is in. This gives a final answer of 1.95Δ base in.

Example **16-4**

A +4.00 D sphere lens is ordered for the right eye. The prescription also calls for 2Δ of prism base out before the right eye. How should the lens be decentered to obtain the correct amount of prism?

Solution

This time the missing parameters are the amount and direction of decentration. Amount is found by a simple algebraic transformation of Prentice's rule.

$$\Delta = cF$$
$$c = \frac{\Delta}{F}$$
$$c = \frac{2}{4.00}$$
$$= 0.5\,cm$$

Because the lens is plus, decentration must also be outward. The lens must be decentered 5 mm out.

Example **16-5**

The following Rx is ordered:

OD: −5.00 D sphere
OS: −5.00 D sphere
PD = 60 mm

An exceptionally large frame is chosen. The frame is so large that it will not allow the correct interpupillary distance (PD) unless an extra large lens blank is used. Using conventional lens blanks will not allow enough decentration. A gap is created temporally where there is not enough lens material to fill the frame. If the blanks were to be used anyway, the situation would require an incorrect placement of the lenses at a PD of 64 mm. How much prism would be induced and in what direction if this wrong PD is used?

Solution

The problem is shown diagrammatically in Figure 16-5. If the lenses have their OCs 64 mm apart, each lens is erroneously decentered 2 mm outward from the line of sight. It can be seen from the figure that the induced prism is base in (opposite the direction of decentration).
Prentice's rule shows that:

$$\Delta = (0.2)(5.00)$$
$$= 1\Delta$$

The incorrect lens placement was done in order to avoid using large lens blanks. However doing so would cause 1Δ base in of unwanted prism before each of the two eyes.

Horizontal and Vertical Decentration of Spheres

When a sphere lens is decentered both horizontally and vertically, the most straightforward solution for finding the prismatic effect is to consider each component by itself.

Example **16-6**

If a +3.50 D sphere is decentered 4 mm in and 5 mm down, what is the resulting prismatic effect?

Solution

In this situation, the two decentrations may be handled independently.
    The horizontal decentration results in:

$$\Delta = (0.4)(3.50) = 1.40$$
or 1.40Δ base in

The vertical decentration gives:

$$\Delta = (0.5)(3.50) = 1.75$$
or 1.75Δ base down

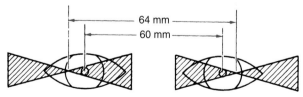

Figure 16-5. For a minus lens, a cross-sectional view suggests two prisms apex to apex. By visualizing the movement of these two prisms before the eyes in decentration, solving for base direction is considerably simplified.

In most cases these results may be left as is. If a single compounded prism is desired, it may be calculated in the manner previously described in Chapter 15 in the section "Compounding and Resolving Prism."

Example **16-7**

A right lens of power −7.00 D sphere is decentered 3 mm out and 4 mm up. What are the resulting horizontal and vertical prismatic effects?

Solution

The horizontal component is:

$$\Delta = (0.3)(7.00) = 2.10$$
$$\text{or } 2.10\Delta \text{ base in}$$

This is shown in Figure 16-6, *A*.
The vertical component is:

$$\Delta = (0.4)(7.00) = 2.80$$
$$\text{or } 2.80\Delta \text{ base down}$$

Which is shown in Figure 16-6, *B*. The combined decentration is shown in Figure 16-6, *C*.

Oblique Decentration of Spheres

When a sphere lens is decentered in an oblique direction, the resulting prismatic effect and base direction will also be along the same meridian of decentration.

Example **16-8**

A right lens of power −7.00 D sphere is decentered 5 mm up and out along the 127-degree meridian. What is the resulting prismatic effect and base direction?

Solution

The prismatic effect for this lens decentration is:

$$\Delta = (0.5)(7.00) = 3.50 \text{ prism diopters}$$

The base direction for a minus lens is exactly opposite the direction of decentration. Therefore the base direction is:

$$(127) + (180) = 307 \text{ degrees}$$

So the resulting prismatic effect and base direction is 3.50Δ base 307 (Figure 16-7). A 307-degree base direction is base down and in for a right eye.

Notice that the previous two examples are really identical. Decentering a lens 3 mm out and 4 mm up is the same thing as decentering that same lens 5 mm up and out along the 127-degree meridian. If we split 3.50Δ base 307 into its vertical and horizontal components, we would find it to be 2.10Δ base in and 2.80Δ base down. This is because a decentration of 3 mm out and 4 mm

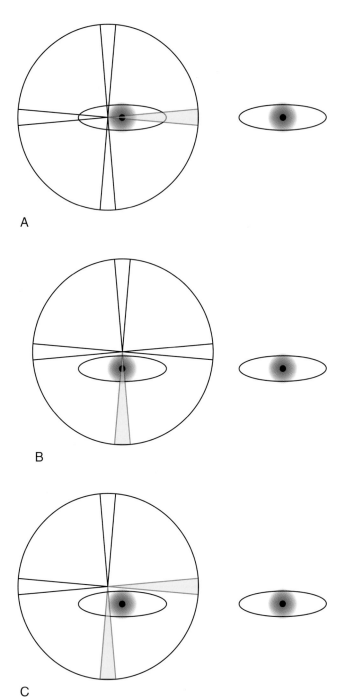

Figure 16-6. A, The −7.00 D sphere lens has been decentered 3 mm out, resulting in base-in prism. **B,** The −7.00 D sphere lens has been decentered 4 mm up, producing a base-down prismatic effect. **C,** The combined up and out movements have produced prism base down and in. It may be expressed as two prismatic effects or these two prismatic effects may be combined into one single prism.

up is the same decentration as 5 mm up and out along the 127-degree meridian.

DECENTRATION OF CYLINDERS

Cylinders produce varying prismatic effects when decentered. These prismatic effects depend not only on the

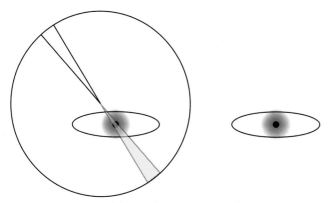

Figure 16-7. An oblique decentration of a sphere lens produces prism in the same meridian as the meridian of decentration.

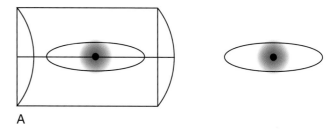

A

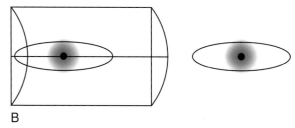

B

Figure 16-8. The cylinder in **(A)** is producing no prismatic effect. **B,** Even though the plus cylinder lens has been decentered to the right, there is still no prismatic effect produced. The eye is still looking through a point on the cylinder axis.

power of the cylinder but also on the orientation of the cylinder axis.

Decentration Along Major Meridians

If the axis of a plano cylinder is oriented in the direction of decentration, there will be no prismatic effect induced regardless of the amount of decentration. This is because there is no power in the axis meridian of a plano cylinder. If, however, the cylinder axis is at right angles to the direction of decentration, the amount of prism induced varies according to Prentice's rule.

Example **16-9**

A plus cylinder lens of power plano +5.00 × 180 is decentered 5 mm to the right. What prismatic effect is produced?

Solution

There is no prismatic effect produced. The decentration is along the axis meridian as shown in Figure 16-8. As long as the eye is looking through any point along the axis of a plano cylinder, there is no prismatic effect.

Example **16-10**

How much prism will be induced and in what direction will the base be oriented by decentering a pl −2.00 × 180 right lens a distance of 3 mm upward?

Solution

Placing the prescription on a power cross reveals that the vertical meridian is −2.00 D in power. Decentering upward causes a base-down prismatic effect for a minus-powered lens. Prism amount is readily determined by:

$$\Delta = cF$$
$$= (0.3)\,(2.00)$$
$$= 0.60$$

The prism induced is 0.60Δ base down.

With plano cylinder lenses, the prism power induced depends only on how far the axis of the cylinder is from the original position. In most cases the original position will be the pupil center. It does *not* necessarily depend on how far the lens was moved.

To illustrate imagine that the cylinder lens in the above example was first decentered 3 mm inward, *then* 3 mm upward (Figure 16-9). The horizontal decentration will have no prismatic effect at all. The second decentration—3 mm upward—still has the same effect of 0.60Δ. The question is somewhat akin to asking how far a straight ruler will be from a certain point on the ground if, while remaining in contact with that point, the straight ruler is slid 3 cm to the right, then lifted 3 cm above the point. Of course, the shortest distance from point to ruler is still 3 cm.

Example **16-11**

A pl +4.00 × 090 cylinder is decentered 5 mm up and 2 mm out. What is the resulting prismatic effect?

Solution

The 5 mm vertical decentration has no prismatic effect at all. This is because the cylinder axis is also up and down (axis 90). However, the horizontal 2 mm out movement is at right angles to the cylinder axis. The horizontal decentration causes this prismatic effect.

$$\Delta = cF$$
$$= (0.2)\,(4.00)$$
$$= 0.80\Delta$$

The lens is plus in power. Therefore the base direction is the same as the direction of decentration. The prismatic effect

Figure 16-10. A, A nondecentered lens having a cylinder component allows the axis of the cylinder to pass through the pupil center. **B,** Decentering a cylinder lens 3 mm outward does not move the axis 3 mm away from the pupil center. (The pupil remains at the origin of the *x*-, *y*-axes.) **C,** To find the power and base orientation of the induced prism, the shortest distance to the cylinder axis is determined.

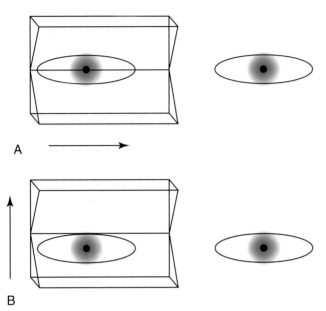

A

B

Figure 16-9. If a minus cylinder axis 180 is moved 3 mm to the right, then 3 mm up, there is no prismatic effect caused by the horizontal movement to the right. When the cylinder is moved at right angles to the cylinder axis, there will be a prismatic effect just as with spheres. **A,** No prismatic effect. The eye is looking through the axis. It will still be looking through the axis even after the lens is moved 3 mm to the right. **B,** The minus-power cylinder lens was moved 3 mm to the right and then moved 3 mm up. The base direction of the prismatic effect produced is down. The base-down prismatic effect is due only to the vertical movement.

caused by both vertical and horizontal decentration is purely horizontal (i.e., 0.80Δ base out).

Decentration of Cylinders Oriented Obliquely

When decentering a plano plus cylinder or a plano minus cylinder, the resulting prismatic effect is always at right angles to the axis of the cylinder. In other words, if a plus cylinder with axis 90 is decentered, the resulting base direction will always be along the 180-degree meridian. It will always be either base 0 or base 180.

Example **16-12**

A cylinder is oriented with its axis at 120. It is then decentered. What are the only two possible resulting base directions?

Solution

There are only two possible answers, regardless of direction of decentration. Both are 90 degrees away from the cylinder

axis. This means that one base direction is 120 + 90, or 210 degrees. The other is 120 − 90, or 30 degrees.

To solve a decentration problem for an oblique cylinder, one of the simplest procedures represents a combination of graphical and algebraic methods. It also helps to understand the concept of what is happening when an oblique cylinder is decentered. And understanding conceptually what is happening is the most important part.

Example **16-13**

A right lens has a cylinder power of +4.00 × 030. What prismatic effects will be caused if the lens is decentered 3 mm outward?

Solution

If such a lens were properly oriented before the eye, it would appear as shown in Figure 16-10, *A.* To solve this problem, a graph is constructed showing the axis position of the lens after the 3-mm decentration has taken place (Figure 16-10, *B*). The power of a cylinder lens is at right angles to the axis. A line is therefore drawn from the point of origin (in this case the eye) to the cylinder axis, meeting the axis line at right angles (Figure 16-10, *C*). When drawn to scale,* this line can be measured and is found to be 1.5 mm long. The distance to this point on the axis is termed the *effective decentration* and abbreviated d_e because the result is the same as if the cylinder lens were decentered to this point.

Because the effective decentration of the cylinder is 1.5 mm away from the point of origin to the axis, the power of the prism may be determined using Prentice's rule.

$$\Delta = (0.15)(4.00) = 0.60$$

The eye is looking through that part of the *plus* cylinder *below* the axis, making the base direction *above* the eye. There are only two possible base directions—120 and 300. (Both are 90 degrees away from the cylinder axis.) And since the base direction is above, or up, the correct base direction is 120.

The induced prism is 0.60Δ base at 120 degrees.[†] This prism could further be resolved into horizontal and vertical

---

*It helps to draw 1 centimeter for each 1 millimeter of decentration. If a drawing is too small, the result cannot be measured accurately enough.

[†]Results may also be obtained purely on the basis of calculations using the formula

$$d_e = y \cos \theta + x \sin \theta$$

where d_e equals the effective decentration, *x* equals horizontal decentration, y equals vertical decentration, and θ equals the angle of the cylinder axis.

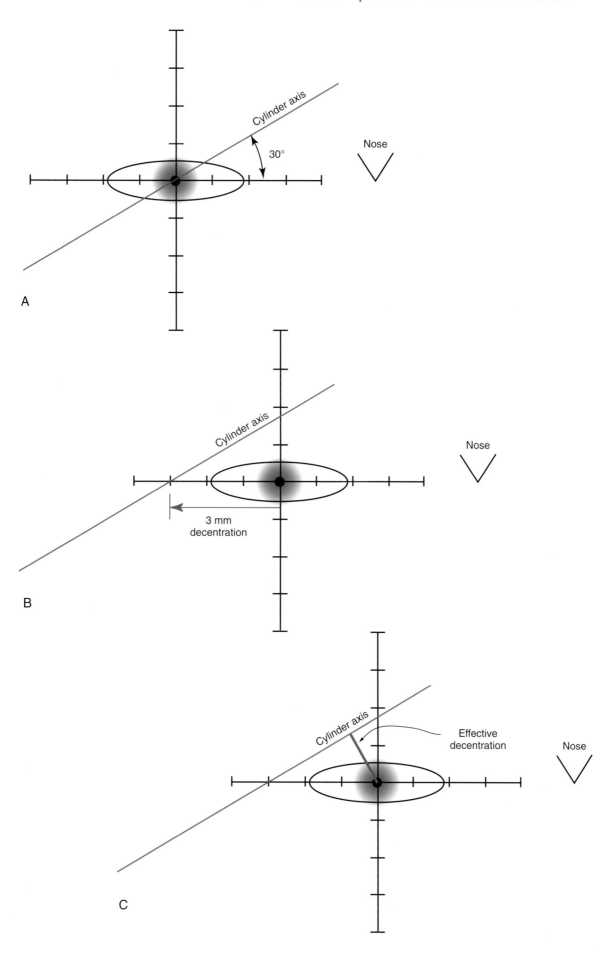

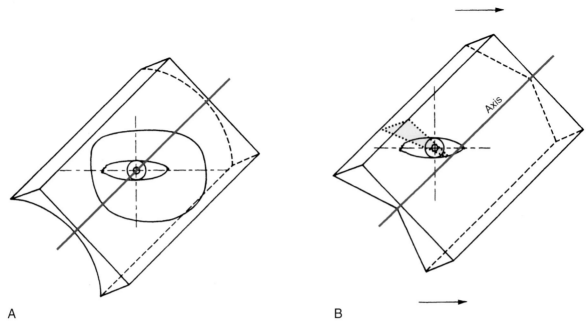

Figure 16-11. A, A minus cylinder lens with an oblique axis appears schematically before the eye as shown here. **B,** If this same oblique cylinder is decentered from its previous location by a purely horizontal movement, it will cause a prismatic effect with an obliquely oriented base direction.

components, as shown previously in Chapter 15. If resolved it would be found that the majority of induced prism would be vertical, even though the decentration was purely horizontal.

Using this formula requires a unique sign convention whereby nasal is positive and temporal is negative. The sign convention is summarized as follows:

- If the point of unknown prismatic effect is nasal to the original position, which we will call the "optical center," (technically a cylinder lens does not have an optical center, but only a cylinder axis), then x is positive.
- If the point of unknown prismatic effect is temporal to the "optical center," then x is negative.
- If the point of unknown prismatic effect is below the "optical center," then y is positive.
- If the point of unknown prismatic effect is above the "optical center," then y is negative.
- If the lens is a right lens, then θ equals the cylinder axis.
- If the lens is a left lens, then θ is 180 degrees minus the cylinder axis.
- When angle θ is acute (less than 90 degrees), then sine is plus, and cosine is plus. (Your calculator will do this for you.)
- When angle is obtuse (greater than 90 degrees), then sine is plus, and cosine is minus. (Your calculator will do this for you.)

Once d_e is found, the prism power is calculated as usual using Prentice's rule.

$$\Delta = d_e F_{cyl}$$

Because the lens is a plano cylinder, the base direction will always be 90 degrees away from the cylinder axis. Base direction will be either upward or downward along this axis.

Example **16-14**

A left lens has a power of *pl* −4.00 × 045. The lens is decentered 4 mm outward from the pupil center. What is the amount and base direction of the prism induced?

Solution

A properly positioned plano cylinder will position the axis across the pupil center, as shown in Figure 16-11, *A*. When the cylinder lens is decentered 4 mm outward, prism is induced. The base direction with either be 135 or 315. The eye is looking above the cylinder axis. Since the cylinder is minus, the prism direction is away from the axis and has an "up" component. Therefore the only possible prism base direction is base 135. Base up and in at 135 degrees is induced (Figure 16-11, *B*).

When drawn to scale, the shortest distance from pupil location to the cylinder axis can be found by direct measurement. The distance in centimeters multiplied by the cylinder power gives the amount of prism. In this case the axis is 2.83 mm from the pupil.

Therefore the power is found by:

$$\Delta = cF$$

which, more specifically, is

$$\Delta = (0.283)(4.00)$$
$$\Delta = 1.13$$

So the answer is 1.13Δ base 135 (Figure 16-12, *A*) The prism found may be resolved into separate horizontal and vertical components, as shown in Figure 16-12, *B*, giving 0.80Δ of base-up prism and 0.80Δ of base-in prism.

Horizontal and Vertical Decentration of Oblique Cylinders

Prism induced by decentration of a cylinder lens both horizontally and vertically is found in exactly the same manner as just described. Once the decentered point is located, an axis line is drawn through it. Thereafter the procedure follows as previously described.

DECENTRATION OF SPHEROCYLINDERS

An accurate solution for prismatic effects induced by a spherocylinder lens may be found in several different ways:

1. Calculate for the sphere and cylinder separately and combine the results.
2. Transpose the prescription to crossed cylinder form. Each cylinder may then be worked independently and the results combined.
3. Use higher mathematical computations.[1]

Perhaps the easiest way is to simply calculate the sphere and cylinder independently. Then results from the sphere decentration and results from the cylinder decentration can be combined for the final answer.

Example **16-15**

A right lens has a power of +3.00 −2.00 × 090. The lens is decentered 7 mm out and 2 mm *up*. What is the prismatic effect induced?

Solution

Considering the sphere first, the horizontal component is:

$$\Delta = cF$$
$$= (0.7)(3.00)$$
$$= 2.1$$

And the base direction is the same as the decentration direction because the sphere is plus. So the horizontal component is 2.1Δ base out.

The vertical component of the sphere is:

$$\Delta = cF$$
$$= (0.2)(3.00)$$
$$= 0.6$$

Since decentration for this plus lens is up, the base direction is up, resulting in 0.6Δ base up.

For the cylinder, the axis is 90, or vertical, so the full amount of the cylinder power is used for the horizontal decentration.

$$\Delta = cF$$
$$= (0.7)(2.00)$$
$$= 1.4$$

The base direction induced by the cylinder is opposite the direction of decentration or base in, resulting in 1.4Δ base in. Because there is no power in the 90-degree meridian for the cylinder, the 2 mm vertical decentration of the cylinder causes no vertical prism.

Now we add the prismatic effects together. The total horizontal prismatic effect is:

$$(2.1\Delta \text{ base out}) + (1.4\Delta \text{ base in}) = 0.7\Delta \text{ base out}$$

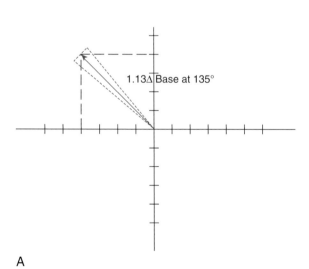

A

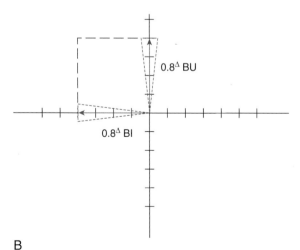

B

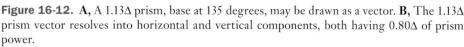

Figure 16-12. A, A 1.13Δ prism, base at 135 degrees, may be drawn as a vector. **B,** The 1.13Δ prism vector resolves into horizontal and vertical components, both having 0.80Δ of prism power.

There is only one vertical component of 0.6Δ base up. These horizontal and vertical components may be left as they are or combined into a single oblique prism.

NOTE: When the direction of decentration is in the same meridian as one of the major meridians of the cylinder, it is actually easier to draw a power cross and consider each meridian. In this example, the horizontal meridian would have a power of +1.00.

$$\Delta = cF$$
$$= (0.7)(1.00)$$
$$= 0.7$$

The vertical meridian remains the same. Although this is easier in this case, it will not work in the case of an oblique cylinder. So next we will consider the case of a spherocylinder with an oblique axis.

Example **16-16**

A right lens has a power of +5.00 −2.00 × 070. What prismatic effect would be found at a point 3 mm up and 5 mm out on this right lens?

IMPORTANT: Notice that the form of the question has changed. Up to this point, the examples were of the lens moving and the eye staying stationary. This time the eye moves and the lens does not.

Solution

Calculate the cylinder component.

Begin by drawing the situation to scale as shown in Figure 16-13. The eye is now 3 mm up and 5 mm out. This is the same as saying the lens was decentered 3 mm down and 5 mm in. Figure 16-13 also shows a perpendicular dropped to the cylinder axis from the point in question (the eye). When measured this effective decentration (d_e) is 5.7 mm long. Since the power of the cylinder is −2.00 D, the prismatic effect induced by the cylinder using Prentice's Rule is:

$$2.00 \times 0.57 = 1.14.$$

The base direction must be either 160 or 340. The cylinder is minus so the base direction is away from the cylinder axis line. The eye is above the axis so the base is upward. The only possible answer is base 160. Therefore the prism

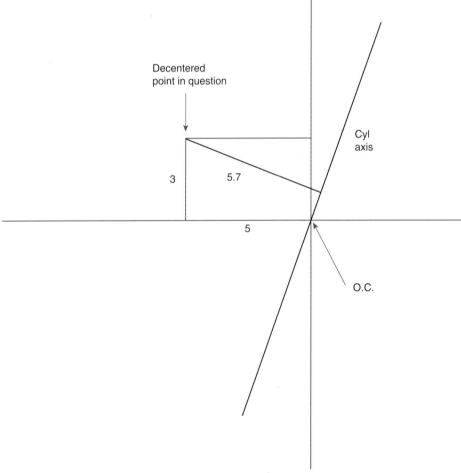

Figure 16-13. The first step in finding prismatic effect produced by decentering an oblique cylinder is to find the effective decentration. When finding the effective decentration, remember that this distance is the shortest distance to the cylinder axis. (*Do not* figure the distance from the point in question to the point marked "OC." This would yield an incorrect answer of 5.83 mm.)

induced by the cylinder portion of the lens is 1.14Δ base 160.

Next we convert 1.14Δ base 160 from the polar to the rectangular coordinate system. To do this we need to make a separate prism diagram as shown in Figure 16-14. Do not try and continue using the previous diagram. Here is how the resulting vertical and horizontal prism components are obtained.

$$\sin 20 = 0.342 = \frac{y}{1.14}$$
$$y = 0.39\Delta\ base\ 90$$
$$\cos 20 = 0.94 = \frac{x}{1.14}$$
$$x = 1.07\Delta\ base\ 180$$

Calculate the sphere component.
The vertical prismatic effect induced by the sphere portion of the lens is:

$$\Delta = 0.3 \times 5$$
$$= 1.50\Delta\ base\ down$$

The horizontal prismatic effect induced by the sphere portion of the lens is:

$$\Delta = 0.5 \times 5$$
$$= 2.50\Delta\ base\ 0$$

Combine sphere and cylinder results.
The combined prism induced by both the cylinder and the sphere are:

$$Vertical = 1.50\Delta\ BD + 0.39\Delta\ BU$$
$$= 1.11\Delta\ BD$$
$$Horizontal = 2.50\Delta\ base\ 0 + 1.07\Delta\ base\ 180$$
$$= 1.43\Delta\ base\ 0\ (base\ in)$$

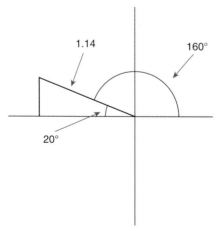

Figure 16-14. Once prismatic effect of the decentered oblique cylinder is found, this prism at an oblique angle is drawn on a different diagram, and the horizontal and vertical components are determined.

Decentration of Spherocylinders Using an Approximation

The optical laboratory needs to be able to move the optical center of a lens away from the boxing center of a frame and over to a location in front of the eye. The laboratory does this by grinding prism into the center of the lens. This moves the optical center to another location. The amount of prism needed for grinding will be the amount that should be found at the boxing center of the lens with the optical center in front of the eye. The laboratory calculates the prism that should be expected at the boxing center of the lens, then grinds that prism amount at the boxing center. The optical center ends up where it is supposed to be.

There is an approximation method for finding decentration prism that was used in the optical laboratory for years. It has now been largely replaced since decentration prism can be found more exactly with the aid of laboratory computers. It is still used in some other instances. The approximation method uses the concept of curvature in an oblique cylinder meridian. This concept was explained in Chapter 13. In that chapter, we found the curvature of a plano cylinder in an oblique meridian (see Figures 13-38 and 13-39).

The curvature of the surface in an oblique meridian was found using the equation:

$$R_\theta = R_{cyl} \sin^2\theta$$

where

R_θ = Curvature in the oblique meridian
R_{cyl} = Curvature in the power meridian
and
θ = the angle between the oblique meridian and the cylinder axis.

From that we derived the equation

$$F_\theta = F_{cyl} \sin^2\theta$$

As noted before, this assumption of power in an oblique meridian is not entirely correct, but can be helpful in certain circumstances.

To find the "power" of a cylinder in an oblique meridian:
1. First find "θ" Theta (θ) is the difference between the meridian in question and the axis of the cylinder.
2. Then apply the sine-squared formula ($F_\theta = F_{cyl} \sin^2\theta$) to the cylinder power.

Example **16-17**

What is the "power" of a pl +3.00 × 030 cylinder in the 180-degree meridian?

Solution

To find theta (θ), take the difference between the cylinder axis and the 180-degree meridian. Here this is 30 degrees. Find the "power" of the cylinder in the 180-degree meridian, using:

$$F_\theta = F_{cyl}\sin^2\theta$$
$$= (+3.00)\sin^2 30$$
$$= (+3.00)(0.25)$$
$$= 0.75\,D$$

The "power" of the cylinder in the 180-degree meridian is +2.25 D.

Using the Sine-Squared Method to Approximate Prism for Decentration

To use the sine-squared method to approximate prism for decentration, the following steps are used[2]:

1. Find the needed decentration.
2. Find the "power" of the cylinder in the 180-degree meridian. This is done by using the formula.
3. Add this reduced cylinder value to the sphere power to find the total power in the 180-degree meridian.
4. Use the total power in the 180-degree meridian to find the prism needed to move the OC. This can be done using Prentice's rule.

$$\Delta = cF$$

where

Δ = prism power
c = decentration in centimenters
F = the power of the lens in the 180 degree meridian

5. Find the base direction of the prism.

Example **16-18**

A left lens has a power of −2.00 −1.50 × 070. What is the "power" of the lens in the 180-degree meridian? How much prism for decentration is needed to move the OC of a lens nasally 3 mm? (Stated another way, how much prism will there be at a point 3 mm temporal to the desired OC location?)

Solution

1. Using the steps listed above, we already know the decentration. It is given as 3 mm.[*]
2. The "power" of the cylinder in the 180-degree meridian is:

---

[*]If it were necessary to figure the decentration amount needed to grind prism for surfacing a lens, we would use the formula

$$\text{decentration per lens} = \frac{A + DBL - PD}{2}.$$

$$F_\theta = F_{cyl}\sin^2\theta$$
$$= (-1.50)\sin^2 70$$
$$= (-1.50)(0.88)$$
$$= -1.32\,D$$

3. Adding the reduced cylinder value of −1.32 in the 180-degree meridian to the sphere power of −2.00, we get a power of −3.32 in the 180-degree meridian.
4. Now we can use the "power" in the 180-degree meridian to find the needed prism using Prentice's rule. This is

$$\Delta = cF$$
$$= (0.3)(3.32)$$
$$= 1.0\Delta$$

5. The lens power in the 180-degree meridian is minus. The point of reference on the finished lens is 3 mm temporal to the OC. Therefore prism base direction is base out. (For the left eye, base out can also be written as base 0.)

Pitfalls of the Sine-Squared Method

For grinding prism for decentration with single-vision lenses in a surfacing laboratory, the sine-squared method works well. There are two pitfalls, however, that prevent it from working every time with every type of lens.

The major pitfall is the failure of this method to take vertical prism into account. Finding a horizontal prism amount by using the "power" in the 180-degree meridian fails to account for the vertical component induced by an oblique cylinder. To see how this works, place a spherocylinder lens in a lensmeter at an oblique axis. Focus the lensmeter and position the lens so that the illuminated target passes through the center of the cross hairs in the lensmeter. Looking through the focused lensmeter, move the lens left and right. Not only will the illuminated target move left and right, but it will also move up and down. The vertical movement is a result of the vertical prism caused by the oblique cylinder. If this vertical prism is not factored into the surfacing process, the OC will be higher or lower on the lens than expected. This can present problems in multifocals.

The second pitfall of the sine-squared method is that the amount of horizontal prism calculated will not exactly duplicate the amount of horizontal prism found using one of the more accurate methods.

Ground-In Prism Versus Prism by Decentration

As we have seen in the previous sections, prism may be created by the decentration of a powered lens. Prism may also be created by grinding the surface of the lens at an angle during the surfacing process.

There is no optical difference between prism created by decentration and prism that has been ground in. Neither is superior nor inferior to the other. It may be that it is possible to create a thinner prismatic lens by surfacing instead of by decentering a finished lens. That is an issue of lens blank thickness rather than prism quality, however.

PRISM THICKNESS

Thickness Differences Between Prism Base and Apex

A prism causes light to change direction. This is because light must pass through two surfaces that are not parallel with one another. Because the surfaces are at an angle to one another, the prism is thin at the top (apex) and thick at the bottom (base). Prismatic power is determined by the angle the front and back surfaces make with one another and by the refractive index of the material. Because lens surfaces of a prism are angled, adding prescribed prism to a lens will cause a change in lens thickness.

Knowing the thickness difference between the base and apex of a prism allows the amount of prism to be found using the formula:

$$P = \frac{100g(n-1)}{d}$$

where

P = the amount of prism
g = the difference in thickness between the apex and the base of the prism
n = the refractive index of the lens material, and
d = the distance between the apex and base of the prism

See Figure 16-15 and be sure to read the caption carefully.

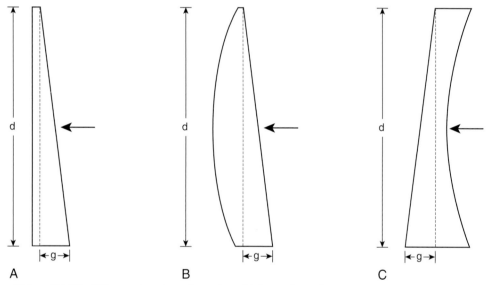

A   B   C

Figure 16-15. When using the prism edge-thickness formula:

$$P = \frac{100g(n-1)}{d}$$

d is the distance between the two measured points, and g is the thickness difference between the points measured. The prismatic effect, P, is for that point halfway between the two points measured. Note that in **(A)** the dimension marked as g does not go the full width of the prism base. The g dimension is the width of the top of the prism subtracted from the width of the bottom of the prism (i.e., the thickness difference). For the plus lens **(B)** the prismatic effect at the halfway point (marked with an arrow) is the same as **(A)** even though the lens has a dioptric power. This is because the thickness difference, g, is the same. **C,** This lens is a minus lens. Even though the lens has minus power, the same thickness difference principle holds. The prismatic effect at the point halfway between the measured points is independent of the refractive power of the lens. In these figures, the measured points were the tops and bottoms of the lenses. They would not have to have been measured at the edges of the lenses, however. Thickness difference will determine the prismatic effect halfway in between the two measured points in the meridian of measurement, regardless of where the points are measured. *To summarize:* In **A** the prism amount is the same across the entire lens, because the prism has only prism power (Δ) and does not have refractive power (D). In **B** and **C** where the lenses have refractive power as well, the prismatic effect is calculated for the halfway point, but will vary at other points across the lens. The amount calculated is for the halfway-between point only.

The thickness difference (g) between the top and bottom of the prism can also be found if the amount of prism is known by simply rearranging the formula to read:

$$g = \frac{dP}{100(n-1)}$$

The prism thickness formula is reliable for all lenses and not just plano prisms. It does not matter if the lens has a plus or minus refractive power. The thickness difference between measured points is still a predictor of prism power halfway between those two points.

Example **16-19**

A lens is made from a material having an index of refraction of 1.5. It is 50 mm in diameter. The top of the lens is 2 mm thick, and the bottom of the lens is 5 mm thick. How much vertical prism is present in the middle of the lens?

Solution

We may use the formula:

$$P = \frac{100g(n-1)}{d}$$

to find the answer.

In this example, the thickness difference (g) between the top and the bottom of the lens is:

$$g = 5 - 2 = 3 \text{ mm}$$

The diameter of the lens is 50 mm, and the index of refraction as 1.5. Therefore we may substitute those values in the prism thickness formula to find:

$$P = \frac{100 \times 3 \times (1.5 - 1)}{50}$$
$$= \frac{300 \times (0.5)}{50}$$
$$= 3\Delta$$

Notice in this particular circumstance, when the index is near 1.5 and the diameter is 50, that the thickness difference is a direct predictor of prism amount.

Example **16-20**

Suppose we have a −6.50 D lens that is made from polycarbonate (index = 1.586). The lens is edged oval for a frame with an A dimension of 48 mm. The nasal edge has a thickness of 4.2 mm, and the temporal edge is 5.8 mm thick. What horizontal prismatic effect is found exactly in the center of the lens?

Solution

To find the answer, we again use the prism thickness formula:

$$P = \frac{100g(n-1)}{d}$$

In this case,

$$g = 5.8 - 4.2 = 1.6 \text{ mm}$$
$$d = 48 \text{ mm, and}$$
$$n = 1.586$$

Substituting these values in the formula, we get

$$P = \frac{100 \times 1.6 \times (1.586 - 1)}{48}$$
$$= \frac{160 \times (0.586)}{48}$$
$$= 1.95\Delta$$

Because the temporal edge is thicker than the nasal edge, the prism base is temporalward, or base out. So the amount of horizontal prism present in the middle of the lens is 1.95Δ base out. (Note that even though the −6.50 D refractive power of the lens was given in the problem, it was not needed to determine prism.)

How Prescribed Prism Affects Lens Thickness

If prism is present in a lens, the lens center thickness will change. Most of the time it is assumed that a lens will be thicker by one half of the prism thickness difference, or ½ g when prism is present, *regardless* of how the prism base direction is oriented. This simplifies the problem, but it is not always true. The base direction determines just how much the Rx (prescribed) prism will change the center or edge thickness. How this works is summarized in Box 16-1 and explained in the following sections.

BOX 16–1

Lens Thickness Changes for Rx Prism

PLUS LENSES
Base in: Center thickness increases by one half of the prism thickness difference.
Base out: Center thickness decreases by up to the full thickness difference, depending upon the amount of decentration present.
Vertical prism with small frame *B*: Center thickness does not change.
Vertical prism with large frame *B*: Center thickness increases by up to one half the thickness difference.

MINUS LENSES
Base in: Center thickness increases slightly (The OC is the thinnest spot on the lens, and it is displaced with Rx prism.)
Base out: Center thickness increases slightly (The OC is the thinnest spot on the lens, and it is displaced with Rx prism.)

Plus Lenses

A plus lens is normally decentered inward because of the wearer's PD. After the lens is in the frame, the thicker portion of the lens edge will be found nasally and the thinner portion temporally (Figure 16-16, *A*). This means that if Rx prism is positioned *base inward*, the thickest portion of the lens will become even thicker (Figure 16-16, *B*). The thinner temporal portion though must retain the same minimum thickness. Therefore the center thickness of the lens will increase by an amount equal to almost half of the difference between base and apex thickness.

This increase in center thickness is necessary because the prescribed prism will be located at what had been the optical center of the lens. With prescribed prism, this location now becomes the major reference point.

Example **16-21**

A plus-powered crown glass lens with a chord diameter of 54 mm is calculated to have a center thickness of 3.4 mm without Rx prism being considered. If the prescription also calls for 2.5 prism diopters of base-in prism, what will the center thickness become?

Solution

To figure the thickness induced by the prism, we begin from the formula:

$$P = \frac{100g(n-1)}{d}$$

and transpose it to:

$$g = \frac{dP}{100(n-1)}$$

The thickness difference between the thick edge and the thin edge is thus:

$$g = \frac{(54)(2.5)}{100(1.523 - 1)}$$
$$= 2.58\,\text{mm}$$

The thickness in the center of the prism will be half of this value, or $\frac{g}{2}$.

$$\text{Increase in center thickness} = \frac{g}{2}$$
$$= \frac{2.58}{2}$$
$$= 1.3\,\text{mm}$$

The new center thickness will be

$$3.4 + 1.3 = 4.7\ \text{mm}$$

Base-Out Rx Prism   If the Rx prism is *base out*, the thicker portion of the prism is turned outward. This corresponds to the thinnest part of an inwardly decentered plus lens. The net effect is a lens that is closer to the same thickness both nasally and temporally. If the lens has sufficient center and nasal edge thickness, it may be *thinned* by an amount up to the full prism thickness difference *g*. Therefore a nasally decentered plus lens with base-out Rx prism can be made thinner than it would be without Rx prism (Figure 16-17).

Base-Up or Base-Down Rx Prism   Small amounts of base-up or base-down Rx prism will not affect the center thickness of the lens if the vertical (*B*) dimension of the frame is small compared with the *A* dimension. However, for prescriptions with larger amounts of prism or for frames with larger *B* dimensions, center thickness will be affected. The amount of center thickness increase

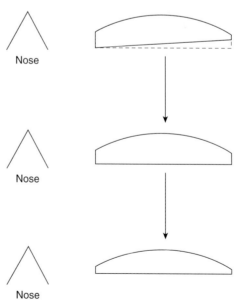

Figure 16-17. When base-out prism is prescribed for a plus-lens wearer, the lens will become thicker temporally. Now because the thinnest edge is thicker, the whole lens may be thinned.

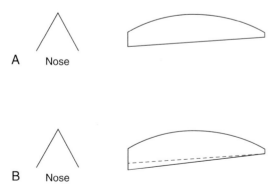

Figure 16-16. **A,** Plus lenses that have been decentered inward to correspond to the wearer's PD are thicker nasally. **B,** If base-in prism is prescribed for the plus-lens wearer, the lens will be thicker still.

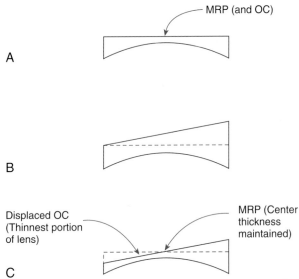

A

B

Displaced OC
(Thinnest portion
of lens)

MRP (Center
thickness
maintained)

C

Figure 16-18. A, Here is a finished but unedged lens with no decentration and no prism. The major reference point (MRP) and optical center (OC) are at the same location. **B,** This minus lens has prism. Simply adding extra thickness to a minus lens by an amount equal to one half the prism's apex-base thickness difference will cause the lens to be unnecessarily thick. **C,** Thinning a minus lens with significant prism back to a normal minimum thickness at the MRP will cause the minus lens to be excessively thin at the now displaced OC. The displaced OC will be at a location other than the MRP.

may then approach one half of the calculated prism thickness difference.

Minus Lenses

With minus lenses the amount of prism affects edge thickness. *Base-out* prism increases the thickness of the temporal edge by an amount equal to the base thickness of the prism.

Center thickness will increase somewhat when *base-out* or *base-in* Rx prism appears in minus lenses. The thinnest point on the lens moves from the major reference point to the location of the displaced optical center, as shown in Figure 16-18.

REFERENCES

1. Long WF: Decentration of spherocylindric lenses, Optom Weekly 66:878-880, 1975.
2. Brooks C: Understanding lens surfacing, Newton, Mass, 1992, Butterworth/Heinemann.

Proficiency Test

(Answers can be found in the back of the book.)

1. A +4.00 D lens is decentered 3 mm inward from the center of the pupil. What prismatic effect is induced, and what is its base direction?

2. A lens is decentered up 3 mm and creates a 2.10Δ base-down prismatic effect. What is the power of the lens?

3. A minus lens has its optical center displaced too far temporally. What kind of prismatic effect will be produced?
   a. base in
   b. base out
   c. cannot tell from information given

4. A person wearing an Rx with O.D. −1.25 +0.25 × 180 requires 1.00Δ base-up prism. The frame is rectangular with a vertical dimension of 40 mm. How much decentration is required to create this amount of prism?
   a. 8 mm up
   b. 8 mm down
   c. 10 mm up
   d. 10 mm down
   e. none of the above

5. When looking through a point on a spherical lens 7 mm to the right of the OC, it is noted that the image of an object 6 m away is displaced 42 cm to the right. What is the power of the lens?
   a. +7.00 D
   b. −7.00 D
   c. +10.00 D
   d. −10.00 D
   e. none of the above

6. In verifying a pair of glasses, it is known that the wearer has a PD of 60. The distance between the centers of the lenses is 68, and the lenses both are −4.00 D. How much prism (to the nearest 0.25Δ), in what base direction, is being worn for both eyes together?
   a. 2.50Δ BI
   b. 1.50Δ BO
   c. 1.50Δ BI
   d. 3.25Δ BO
   e. 3.25Δ BI

7. A wearer has a PD of 70 mm. The distance between the OC of a pair of −6.25 D lenses is 63 mm. There is no prism indicated in the Rx. How much prism is included and in what direction? (Do not round off.)

8. Wearer's binocular PD is 66. The eyes are symmetrically placed, and the Rx is:
   O.D. −5.00 D sph.
   O.S. −8.00 D sph.
   The OCs were erroneously placed at 62 mm. What is the prismatic effect induced?

9. A pair of glasses read as follows on the lensmeter:
   R +2.75 −1.00 × 180
   L +2.75 −1.00 × 180
   Distance between OCs is 56 mm. The wearer's PD is actually 66 mm. How much prism, and in what direction, is this person wearing? (Putting the Rx on a power cross may help in working the problem.)

10. A pair of glasses reads as follows on the lensmeter:
    O.D. −2.00 −1.00 × 180
    O.S. −3.00 −1.00 × 090
    (Watch the cylinder axis.) Distance between OCs is 76 mm. (Both dots are equal distances from the center of the glasses.) The wearer's PD is 66 mm. How much total prism, and in what direction, is being worn? (Assume the eyes to be symmetrically placed in the head [i.e., monocular PDs are equal].)

11. An Rx is:
    O.D. −3.50 −1.00 × 090
    O.S. −5.50 −1.50 × 090
    The PD is 64 mm. To keep from using oversized blanks, the laboratory "pushed the PD" so that the OCs are 2 mm too far out per lens giving a binocular PD of 68 mm. How much total prismatic effect is induced?

12. The following Rx is ordered:
    −1.00 −1.75 × 090
    −1.50 −1.75 × 090

Wearer's PD is 59. The frame chosen has a large eye size. When the Rx is returned from the laboratory, in dotting the lenses the OCs are found to be 63 mm apart. Using prevailing prism tolerance standards of 0.67Δ prism error for both eyes combined, is the 63 PD acceptable?
   a. yes
   b. no
   c. insufficient information present

13. A right lens of a pair of spectacles is examined through the lensmeter. The lens is positioned so that initially the lensmeter stop is positioned on the horizontal midline of the lens and temporal to the lens geometric center. As the lens is moved to the operator's left, the target is observed to move from the lower half of the field (prism base-down effect) to the upper half. What may be said about the lens?
   a. It contains prism.
   b. It contains base-down prism.
   c. It contains an oblique cylinder, with the axis of the minus cylinder between 90 and 180.
   d. It contains an oblique cylinder with the minus cylinder between 0 and 90.
   e. It is not possible to make any of the above statements with the information given.

14. A right lens of power pl −3.00 × 045 is decentered out. What is the resulting prismatic effect?
   a. Base up and out
   b. Base down and in
   c. Base down and out
   d. Base up and in
   e. Base in

15. (This is a concept problem. You should not be doing any calculating.)

    The right lens shown below has already been surfaced. The OC has been moved nasally. The lens is facing you, convex side up. There are several possible lens prescriptions listed. For each lens prescription, there will be prism present at the location of the blank geometric center. Tell what base direction(s) you would expect for the prism at this location. (If you are using the rectangular coordinate system and both horizontal and vertical prism are present, there will be more than one base direction.)

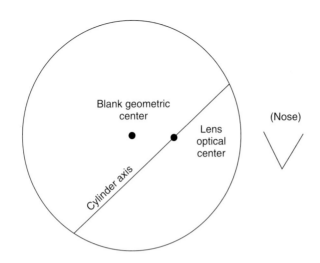

a. +4.00 D sphere (Ignore the cylinder axis drawn on the lens.)
   (1) Base in
   (2) Base out
   (3) Base up
   (4) Base down
b. pl −3.00 × 040
   (1) Base in
   (2) Base out
   (3) Base up
   (4) Base down
c. Expressed in the polar coordinate system, what is the base direction for the prism at the blank geometric center for the lens in "b" above?
d. +4.00 +1.00 × 040 (*Note: The lens is a plus cylinder lens.*)
   (1) Base in
   (2) Base out
   (3) Base up
   (4) Base down
e. +4.00 −1.00 × 040 (*Now the lens is a minus cylinder lens.*)
   (1) Base in
   (2) Base out
   (3) Base up
   (4) Base down

16. A right lens has an Rx of −6.00 +1.00 × 090 with 3.00Δ of prism base in. How far nasalward or temporalward from the MRP is the OC?
    a. 6 mm temporalward
    b. 5 mm temporalward
    c. 5 mm nasalward
    d. 6 mm nasalward
    e. none of the above

17. The following Rx is ordered:
    pl −2.75 × 015
    pl −2.75 × 165
    PD 63

The Rx is verified and found to have a PD of 67. Assuming the wearer's eyes are symmetrically placed, how much combined vertical and horizontal prism results O.U.?

18. A right lens having a power of pl +3.50 × 075 is decentered 5 mm out. How much prism, expressed as vertical and horizontal components, is induced?

19. A −4.00 −2.00 × 055 right lens is decentered 3 mm out. How much prism, expressed in vertical and horizontal components, is created before the eye?

20. A −3.50 −2.75 × 030 left lens is decentered 3 mm out. How much prism, expressed in vertical and horizontal components, is created before the eye?

21. An Rx reads as follows:
    O.D. −4.00 −2.00 × 055
    O.S. −3.50 −2.75 × 030
    If this Rx were ground with OCs separated by 65 mm, what would the total net prismatic effect be if worn by someone having a 59-mm PD?

22. Find the "power" in the 180-degree meridian for each of the following lenses using the "sine-squared θ" method:
    a. pl −2.00 × 180
    b. pl −2.00 × 090
    c. pl −2.00 × 020
    d. pl −2.00 × 070
    e. −1.00 −2.00 × 090
    f. −1.00 −2.00 × 150

23. A right lens has a power of −3.00 −2.50 × 120. Using the shortcut sine-squared method, answer the following questions.
    a. What is the "power" of the lens in the 180-degree meridian?
    b. How much horizontal prism for decentration is needed to move the OC of a lens nasally 4 mm? (Stated another way, how much prism will there be at a point 4 mm temporal to the desired OC location?)

24. A right lens has a power of +4.00 −1.50 × 020. Using the shortcut sine-squared method, respond to the following questions.
    a. What is the "power" of the lens in the 180-degree meridian?
    b. How much horizontal prism for decentration is needed to move the OC of a lens nasally 2 mm? (Stated another way, how much prism will there be at a point 2 mm temporal to the desired OC location?)

25. A 1.80-index lens, edged oval, has a temporal edge thickness of 4.2 mm and a nasal edge thickness of 3.2 mm. The lens has an A dimension of 54 mm. What is the prismatic effect at the geometric center of the edged lens?

26. A right lens with a power of +4.75 D sphere has an index of refraction of 1.66. It is edged and in the frame. You dot the MRP of the lens. You measure the thickness of the lens at a point 20 mm nasal to the MRP and again at a second point 20 mm temporal to the MRP. The thickness of the lens 20 mm temporal to the MRP is 7.8 mm. The thickness 20 mm nasal to the MRP is 5.4 mm. What is the prismatic effect and base direction at the MRP?

CHAPTER 17

Fresnel Prisms and Lenses

Normal lenses and prisms vary in thickness depending upon the power of the lens or prism and upon the size of the lens or prism. This is not the case with Fresnel lenses and prisms, since they are constructed differently. Though not a replacement for normal lenses, Fresnel lenses and prisms are highly versatile and are very useful in certain specific circumstances.

WHAT IS A FRESNEL PRISM?

A traditional prism has two flat, nonparallel surfaces. Parallel light entering the prism is bent toward the base of the prism and leaves the back surface at an angle. A prism is thicker at the base than at the apex. The larger the prism, the thicker the base of the prism will be.

A *Fresnel prism* attempts to circumvent thickness by building a "tower" of small, wide prisms. To understand how a Fresnel prism works, imagine cutting off the tops of a large number of equally powered prisms and gluing them, one above the other, onto a thin piece of plastic (Figure 17-1). Although a Fresnel prism is molded into one flexible piece, its construction duplicates this imaginary example (Figure 17-2). A Fresnel prism is only 1 mm thick.

What Are the Advantages of a Fresnel Prism?

There are several advantages of a Fresnel prism. First, it is very *thin and extremely lightweight*. It is *flexible* and can be applied to an existing spectacle lens, making it *possible to apply the lens in-house*, without an in-house optical laboratory.

Because the lens is made from a soft, flexible material, it *can be cut to any shape* with scissors or a razor blade. This means that it can be cut and applied to one sector of a lens. (Practical applications are explained later.)

Because conventional prisms have a large increase in thickness from apex to base, a high-powered prism is troubled by magnification differences and changes in power across the lens. Although Fresnel lenses do not eliminate this problem, they do *reduce magnification differences* considerably.

What Are the Disadvantages of a Fresnel Prism?

Fresnel prisms *look different* than conventional lenses. They are different enough that they may be noticed by others. Because Fresnels have a number of small ledges, they are *harder to clean* than conventional lenses.

High-powered prisms will cause a slight decrease in visual acuity. Most of this is due to the chromatic aberration and distortion associated with prisms. This decreased acuity occurs in both conventional and Fresnel prisms. Fresnel prisms also cause a *slight loss of visual acuity caused by reflections* at the prism facets, especially under certain sources of illumination. The minimal acuity decrease through Fresnel prisms may be slightly less than a line on a Snellen chart at a 90% contrast level compared with acuity through conventional prisms.[1]

WHEN ARE FRESNEL PRISMS USED?

There are a variety of clinical applications for Fresnel prism. The following six sections discuss major applications.

High Amounts of Prism

Because of its thickness advantage, Fresnel prism is especially useful for high amounts of prism.

Use and Reuse

Fresnel prism lenses are easy to apply and remove. They may be used and reused. This is helpful when determining how a given prism amount will work long term or for use during visual training.

Sectorial Application

A partially paralyzed extraocular muscle may result in a different amount of prism needed for different directions of gaze. A Fresnel lens can be cut to fit that particular lens area. Prism is present only where it is needed.

For Vertical Imbalance Correction

When a person may require a correction for vertical imbalance, Fresnel prism can be applied to existing lenses to see if a vertical imbalance correction of a certain amount will be helpful before it is actually ordered.

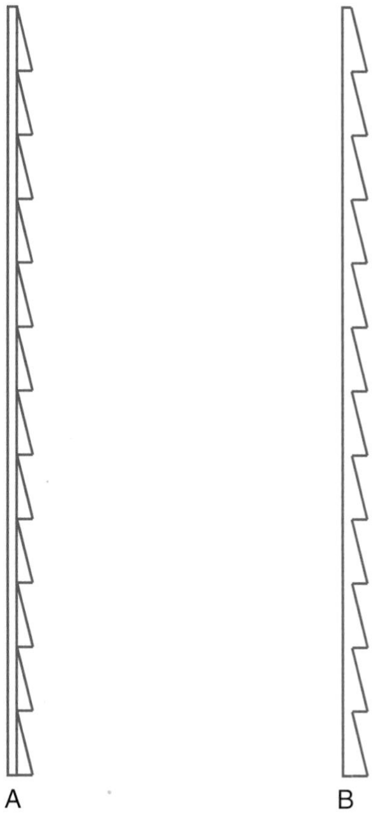

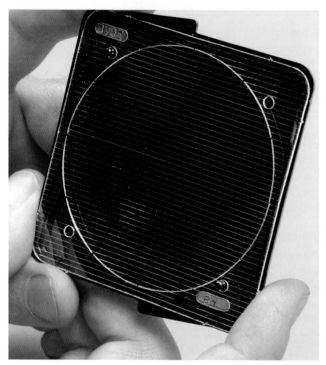

Figure 17-1. A, Fresnel prism is thin because it is really a series of prisms stacked one on top of the other. The concept of individual prisms attached to a thin piece of plastic is shown. **B,** In actuality, the Fresnel prism in molded from one piece of material.

Figure 17-2. A Fresnel lens has a series of slightly visible lines on the surface. These lines are really ledges that indicate the location of the base of the prism. The base direction is at right angles to the direction of the visible lines.

(For more on vertical imbalance correction, see Chapter 21.)

For Horizontal Prism at Near

For a prescription with horizontal prism for near only, it is feasible to use Fresnel prism applied to the lower portion of the lenses only. (For more on horizontal prism at near, see Chapter 19.)

Visual Field Defects

With visual field defects, prism may be applied in one section of the lens with the base direction in the direction of the defect and the edge of the prism close to the central visual area. This way the eye travels only a short distance before it picks up the image through the prism. The image appears closer to the center and can be seen without moving the head.

A person may have a visual field defect where the right half of the visual field is blind for both right and left eyes. The defect is call homonymous hemianopia. Fresnel lenses can be applied to the right side of both lenses. In this instance, prism base direction would be base right. With prism in place, the wearer looks to the right, but does not have to turn the eyes as far to see an object in the right-hand field of view.

If the defect is a constricted visual field down to 5 to 15 degrees of viewing area, prism from 20 to 30 prism diopters could be placed base out on the temporal sides of the lenses and base in on the nasal sides.[2]

Homonymous Hemianopia Application

To measure for correct placement of a prism on one half of the spectacle lens in the case of homonymous hemianopia, the spectacles, properly adjusted, should be on the subject's face. The subject looks into the viewing eye of the practitioner. The eye with the visual field loss nasally is occluded, usually with a cover paddle. A near-point card or other straight edge is brought in from the temporal, nonseeing side. When the subject first reports seeing the card, the location of the card is marked on the lens with a vertical line (Figure 17-3, A). The edge of the prism is placed 3 to 5 mm temporalward from this position (Figure 17-3, B).[3] The amount of prism may vary. Though others have used Fresnel prism, Lee and Perez used 12 prism diopters of sectorial prism,* but not Fresnel prism, maintaining that Fresnel prism reduced acuity too much.

In the past sectorially applied prism for homonymous hemianopia has been placed on each eye in the blind area. Many practitioners are using only a single sectorially applied prism on the eye with the temporal field defect.

---

*Slab-off prism may be ground vertically instead of horizontally as is normally done for the correction of vertical imbalance. There are other types of low-vision prism options available.

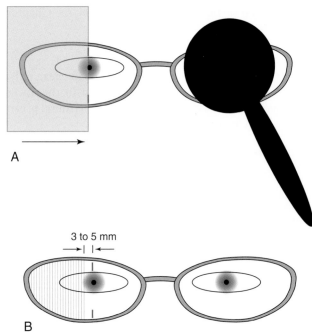

A

B

3 to 5 mm

Figure 17-3. A, To position a Fresnel prism for homonymous hemianopia, occlude the eye with the nasal field loss. On the eye with the temporal field loss, move the card from the temporal side until the person first sees the card. Mark the position of the card. (Marks are shown in red.) **B,** Measure back 3 to 5 mm from this point to find the location of the apical edge of the prism and apply the prism to the temporal portion of the lens.

Eli Peli's High-Powered Prism Segment

Another method of sectorial application of prism for helping the person with homonymous hemianopia places high-powered (30 to 40 Δ) prism in certain segment areas of the lens.[4] Two prism segment areas, with their base-apex axis in the horizontal position, are placed on the lens prescribed for the eye with the visual field loss. The upper one is placed above the pupil in alignment with the upper limbus and the lower one below the pupil in alignment with the lower limbus (Figure 17-4). These prisms are placed base out and create diplopia in that eye. Objects seen through the segment areas are shifted from the nonseeing to the seeing part of the visual field. With adaptation the individual is able to visualize the parts of the objects viewed through the prism in the areas where they would normally be located, expanding the visual field area by up to 20 degrees.

Such prisms may be constructed as a prism segment within the carrier spectacle lenses. The first trials are done with Fresnel prisms cut to the expected dimensions of the finished prism segment areas.

Cosmetics of Nonseeing Eyes

In Chapter 21 of this text, the use of prism to improve the appearance of a blind or prosthetic eye is discussed. Fresnel prisms can be used in such instances.

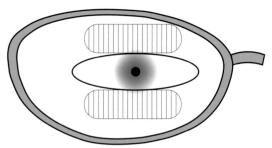

Figure 17-4. These temporary 30 to 40 Δ base out Fresnel prism segment areas are used to create peripheral diplopia for those who have homonymous hemianopia visual field loss. They will later be replaced with prism segments constructed within the carrier spectacle lens.

Slowing of Nystagmus

Nystagmus is a condition characterized by a constant back and forth movement of the eyes. Such movement is involuntary and reduces vision. In some cases nystagmus may slow when the person looks to one side or the other. For example, if the examiner sees that movement slows when the person looks to the right, equal amounts of prism may be applied to both lenses. The correct base direction would be base left. Because the eyes turn toward the apex, prism base left will keep the head pointed straight while the eyes turn to the right. Since the eyes are turned to the right, nystagmus slows. For a summary of Fresnel prism uses, see Table 17-1.

WHAT IS A FRESNEL LENS?

Chapter 12 explained how a lens works. Figure 12-20 presented the concept of how a plus lens is like a series of prisms, each more powerful than the one before. The front and back surfaces at the optical center (OC) of a lens are flat. But as the distance from the OC increases, the lens surface becomes more angled.

A Fresnel lens is similar to a series of concentric prisms, each with a slightly higher prismatic effect (Figure 17-5). When the concentric surfaces are angled correctly, a plus or minus sphere of any desired power may be created. Advantages and disadvantages of Fresnel lenses parallel those of Fresnel prisms.

When Are Fresnel Lenses Used?

Nonspectacle Uses

Fresnel lenses are not just used for spectacles. A common application may be found when looking through the writing surface of an overhead projector. (Adjust the focus to be slightly off and see the concentric rings of the lens projected on the screen.)

Large minus Fresnel lenses are sometimes applied to a window to create a wider field of view, or are used for the warning beams of seaside lighthouses so that the illumination projected from the source within the building is increased.

TABLE 17-1
Clinical Applications for Fresnel Prisms

Use	Comments
High prism amounts	Keeps lens thin
Temporary prism	The practitioner can get an idea of how the prism will work before ordering
	It is possible to change prism amount without remaking glasses
Sectorial application of prism for palsied muscle	Can apply to half the lens or to any portion of the lens
Visual field defects such as homonymous hemianopia	Place the sectorially applied prism in the blind area
	Orient the prism base toward the blind area
Prism in bifocal portion only	Can be horizontal and/or vertical prism
Cosmetic improvement of blind, turning eye	Use inverse prism (e.g., if the eye turns out, give base out prism)
Treatment of nystagmus	Used yoked prism to reduce eye movement (e.g., both base left or both base right)
For those who cannot sit up in bed	Use yoked base-down prism of 15–30Δ
	(Note: There are also "recumbent spectacles" that are specially made for these purposes)
Use as a partial occluder	Place prescribed prism over the nonamblyopic eye as Fresnel prism to slightly decrease acuity

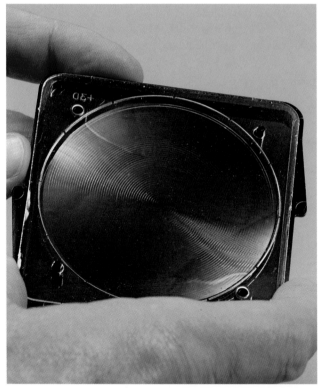

Figure 17-5. The Fresnel lens shown here is in the original container, but has been turned around so that the rings will be more readily apparent. When worn, the rings will be much less visible than their appearance in the photograph because they will be on the back surface of the Fresnel lens, and the Fresnel lens will be on the back surface of the carrier spectacle lens.

Short-Term Wear

Clinically, Fresnel lenses are useful on a temporary basis, such as during vision training or frequent changes in refraction that may result from unstabilized diabetes or certain postsurgical situations.

Creating Adds

Fresnel lenses can also be applied to one portion of the spectacle lens. High add powers can be created for low-vision or occupational purposes.

Fresnel lenses are available as precut flat-top bifocal segments in powers ranging from +1.00 D to +6.00 D. These segments will also work well in the dispensary to give a realistic simulation of bifocal heights (see Chapter 5, Figure 5-22).

Fresnel lenses or lens segments can be used to create special occupational lenses. For example, if a person has a need for a double D occupational lens, the current bifocal or progressive add lens can be converted to an occupational lens using an upside-down Fresnel bifocal segment at the top. If Fresnel segments are placed on a pair of single-vision sunglasses, it changes them into prescription bifocals.

For a summary of Fresnel lens uses, see Table 17-2.

How to Apply a Fresnel Lens or Prism to a Spectacle Lens

Fresnel prisms and lenses are applied using the following steps:

1. For lenses, mark the desired position of the lens OC on the *front* of the carrier lens. (The carrier lens is the spectacle lens already in the eyeglass frame.)

   For prisms determine correct base direction. (In the presence of horizontal and vertical prism, determine what single prism amount and base

---

TABLE 17-2

Clinical Applications for Fresnel Lenses

Use	Comments
To create a thin lens	Fresnel lenses are always thin, regardless of lens power
Temporary lenses	Fresnel lenses can be especially handy during visual training or for unstabilized diabetes when lens powers may need to be changed frequently
Underwater diving masks, swimming goggles, etc.	Application to optical surfaces is easy
Sectorial applications	Plus lenses of normal or high powers can be used as a multifocal add; this add can be used temporarily or permanently for certain unusual occupational needs or for low-vision needs
Trial bifocals	Available in powers from +1.00 to +6.00 D
	Used for accurate determination of bifocal height, for temporary wear, or for making prescription sunglasses into multifocals

---

direction will result from the combination of the two prisms.)

2. Take the carrier lens out of the spectacle frame.
3. Place the Fresnel lens or prism on the *back* of the carrier lens with its smooth side against the carrier. Be sure the OC or base direction is properly oriented.
4. With a razor blade, trim the Fresnel lens or prism flush with the beveled edge of the carrier lens. (It is also possible to use sharp, high-quality scissors.)
5. Remove the Fresnel lens or prism and reinsert the carrier lens into the frame.
6. Wash both carrier and Fresnel lens with a weak solution of lotion-free, liquid detergent.
7. In a bowl of warm water, or under a stream of warm water, apply the smooth side of the Fresnel to the carrier. Work out any air bubbles that may be trapped between the two surfaces.
8. Give the lenses to the wearer, but instruct the wearer to handle with care for 24 hours until drying is complete.

It is possible to substitute rubbing alcohol for water when applying Fresnel lenses and prisms. The lens is said to adhere faster, the bubbles slide out easier, evaporation is faster, and the lens can be dispensed sooner without fear that the Fresnel prism will slide out of place.[5]

How to Clean Fresnel Lenses or Prisms

The manufacturer's recommended method of cleaning these lenses is to rinse under warm running water. If the lenses have dirt in the grooves, use a soft brush. Blot dry with a soft, lint-free cloth. Hard contact lens cleaning solutions have also been used to clean Fresnel optics.

REFERENCES

1. Flom MC, Adams AJ: Fresnel optics. In Duane TD, editor: Clinical ophthalmology, vol 1, Philadelphia, 1995, Lippincott-Raven.
2. Tallman KB, Haskes D, Perlin RR: A case study of choroideremia highlighting differential diagnosis and management with Fresnel prism therapy, J Am Optom Assoc 67:421-429, 1996.
3. Lee AG, Perez AM: Improving awareness of peripheral visual field using sectorial prism, J Am Optom Assoc 70(10):624-628, 1999.
4. Peli E: Field expansion of homonymous hemianopia by optically induced peripheral exotropia, Optom Vis Sci 77(9):453-464, 2000.
5. Rubin A: Fitting tip: applying Fresnel prisms, Opt Dispensing News (215): 2005.

Proficiency Test

(Answers can be found in the back of the book.)

1. If a Fresnel prism is to be placed base out, will the visible lines on the lens be horizontally or vertically oriented?
   a. horizontally
   b. vertically

2. True or false? Visual acuity is better with Fresnel prisms than with conventional prisms.

3. True or false? Fresnel lenses and prisms are not reusable.

4. Fresnel prisms and lenses are applied:
   a. to the back of the spectacle lens with the smooth side out.
   b. to the front of the spectacle lens with the smooth side out.
   c. to the back of the spectacle lens with the smooth side in.
   d. to the front of the spectacle lens with the smooth side in.

5. Prism is to be used to slow nystagmus. If the nystagmus slows when the individual turns the head to the left while still looking straight ahead, the prism should be applied:
   a. base to wearer's right for the left eye and base to the wearer's left for the right eye.
   b. base to the wearer's left for the left eye and base to the wearer's right for the right eye.
   c. base to the wearer's right for both right and left eyes.
   d. base to the wearer's left for both right and left eyes.
   e. This type of prism use for slowing nystagmus is not valid.

6. For those with homonymous field defects, an "increase" in field (or at least an increase in the ability to quickly view more of the blind field area) is achieved by placing Fresnel prism (or slab-off prism) on the spectacles in the defect area. If this is done, the base direction should be:
   a. base toward the side or direction of the defect.
   b. base away from the side or direction of the defect.

CHAPTER 18

Lens Design

A well-designed lens has excellent optics both through the center and the periphery of the lens. In addition, the lens should be as attractive as possible and easy to wear. This chapter attempts to bring understanding in what to look for in a lens and how to make an appropriate choice of lens design.

A SHORT HISTORY OF LENS DEVELOPMENT

Lenses have gone through several stages of development. To quickly summarize, here are some general categories and time lines.[1] These describe not the theoretical development of the lens, but when these lenses were introduced and available.

1. *"Flat" lenses* (1200 to 1800): Actually the word "flat" is deceiving, since neither side of the lens was flat. Instead the lens was bean shaped, like a lentil—the bean that resembles the shape of a lens. The lenses worked well for central vision, but vision was poor through the edges.
2. *Periscopic lenses* (1800s): An improvement in peripheral vision occurred when a −1.25 D back surface was used.
3. *Six-base meniscus lenses* (Beginning in the 1890s): These lenses improved vision in several ways. The quality of peripheral vision increased markedly. The lenses could also be fit closer to the eye because the vault of the lens cleared the lashes. Six-base lenses were still used up until the 1960s. During the 1950s and 1960s, the use of six-base lenses moved almost entirely to places that were known for low-end pricing. Eventually, companies simply stopped producing these types of lenses.[2]
4. *Corrected curve lenses* (early 1900s): In 1908 the Carl Zeiss Company introduced Punktal lenses that corrected for oblique astigmatism found in the lens periphery. These lenses required a very large number of base curves and became available in the United States in 1913. In 1919 American Optical introduced a corrected curve series of lenses that also corrected for oblique astigmatism, but, unlike the earlier Punktal lenses with a large number of required base curves, the AO lenses were designed with base curves that changed in 1 or 2 diopter

intervals. This made stocking semifinished lenses much more practical. In the 1960s there was a transition time while single vision lenses were being converted from plus cylinder form (with the toric surface on the front) to minus cylinder form to match the back surface torics that were already being used for multifocals.
5. *Aspherics*: Aspherics have been available for very high plus "cataract" style corrections beginning in the early part of the twentieth century. They have been available in lower powered plus and minus single vision lens form during the latter part of the twentieth century, but only began to enjoy more widespread use as higher index plastic lens materials became available.
6. *Atorics*: Atorics are rapidly replacing aspheric lens series for new lines of single vision finished lenses. However, atorics are generally not available in multifocal lenses. The exceptions to this are those progressive lenses that are individually designed and custom produced by free-form generating techniques.

LENS ABERRATIONS

To understand the developments and characteristics of these lens designs, it is necessary to understand what problems the designer is attempting to prevent. Such problems, which cause lenses to deliver less than a perfect image, are known as *aberrations*.

When light from a point source goes through a correctly powered spectacle lens yet fails to create a perfect image, the cause is lens aberration. There are several types of lens aberrations that can contribute to an imperfect image. These aberrations can be grouped into two major types: *chromatic aberration* and *monochromatic aberration*.

Chromatic aberration is color related. It causes an image to have a colored fringe. Monochromatic aberration occurs when the light source contains only one wavelength (one color).

Chromatic Aberration

There are two manifestations of chromatic aberration. One is called *longitudinal chromatic aberration*.

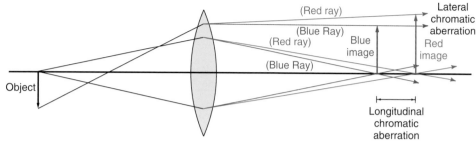

Figure 18-1. Chromatic aberration has two aspects. One is longitudinal chromatic aberration. This means that light of different wavelengths will focus at different focal distances from the lens. The other aspect is lateral chromatic aberration. Lateral chromatic aberration is shown here and in Figure 18-2.

Longitudinal chromatic aberration occurs when a point light source that is composed of several wavelengths (e.g., white light) forms a series of point images along the optical axis. Each of these images is of a different color, and each has a slightly different focal length.

The second manifestation of chromatic aberration is called *lateral chromatic aberration*. This type of chromatic aberration will produce images of slightly different sizes at the focal length of the lens, depending on the color of the light.

Longitudinal (Axial) Chromatic Aberration

Since each color or wavelength undergoes a slightly different degree of refraction at the same surface curvature, longitudinal chromatic aberration results in a series of foci spread out along the optic axis (Figure 18-1). Thus longitudinal chromatic aberration can be expressed as the dioptric difference between two extremes—blue light (F_F) and red light (F_C). Written as a formula, longitudinal chromatic aberration is:

$$\text{longitudinal chromatic aberration} = F_F - F_C$$

Longitudinal chromatic aberration is not directly related to prismatic effect. Therefore plano prisms do not have longitudinal chromatic aberration.

Normally, we think of glass or plastic lens material as having one specific index of refraction (n). In actuality lens material has a slightly different index of refraction for each wavelength. The index of refraction we memorize for a given lens material is really the index of refraction for yellow light. Lens materials that are relatively free of chromatic aberration have indices of refraction that are nearly the same for each wavelength. Materials that have a lot of chromatic aberration, such as the glass for crystal chandeliers, have indices of refraction that span a larger range.

Longitudinal chromatic aberration can be written another way. To find out how, we start with the Lensmaker's formula:

$$F = (n - 1)R$$

Where
F = the power of the lens,
n = the refractive index of the lens (for yellow light), and
R = the curvature of the lens.
(NOTE: $R = R_1 - R_2$, where R_1 = the curvature of the first lens surface and R_2 = the curvature of the second lens surface.)

This means that since:

$$\text{longitudinal chromatic aberration} = F_F - F_C$$

longitudinal chromatic aberration can also be expressed as:

$$\begin{aligned}
\text{longitudinal chromatic aberration} \\
= (n_F - 1)R - (n_C - 1)R \\
= (n_F - 1 - n_C + 1)R \\
= (n_F - n_C)R
\end{aligned}$$

The quantity ($n_F - n_C$) helps to define the chromatic nature of the material and is called the *mean dispersion*.

Since lens power is specified in terms of yellow light, F can also be more specifically written as F_D.

If

$$F = (n - 1)R$$

then

$$F_D = (n_D - 1)R$$

which can be transposed and written as

$$R = \frac{F_D}{n_D - 1}$$

And because

$$\text{longitudinal chromatic aberration} = (n_F - n_C)R$$

it can also be written as

$$\text{longitudinal chromatic aberration} = (n_F - n_C)\frac{F_D}{n_D - 1}$$

or even as

$$\text{longitudinal chromatic aberration} = \frac{n_F - n_C}{n_D - 1}F_D$$

The quantity

$$\frac{n_F - n_C}{n_D - 1}$$

is useful for quantifying chromatic aberration of a given material. It is called the *dispersive power*. Dispersive power is abbreviated as the Greek letter omega, or ω. This means that longitudinal chromatic aberration can be written as:

$$\text{longitudinal chromatic aberration} = \omega F_D$$

The Abbé Value
Because the value for dispersive power ends up as a decimal value, working with it can be unwieldy. It is easier to work with its reciprocal value. The reciprocal of dispersive power comes out as a whole number. The reciprocal of ω (dispersive power) is symbolized by the Greek letter nu, or ν. In other words,

$$\frac{1}{\omega} = \nu$$

The value has three different names. It is called the *nu value*, the *constringence*, or the *Abbé number* or *value*.

The *Abbé value* is the most commonly used number for identifying the amount of chromatic aberration for a given lens material. The higher the Abbé value, the less chromatic aberration present in the lens. The lower the Abbé value, the more likely it will be that color fringes will be seen through the lens and that visual acuity will be reduced in the periphery of high-powered lenses. Table 18-1 shows the Abbé values and refractive indices for some representative ophthalmic materials.

Using the Abbé value means that longitudinal chromatic aberration can even be written as

$$\text{longitudinal chromatic aberration} = \frac{F}{\nu}$$

Example **18-1**

We are interested in knowing how longitudinal chromatic aberration compares between two +6.00 D lenses when one is made from polycarbonate and the other crown glass. Find

TABLE 18-1
Abbé Values for Some Representative Lens Materials

Lens Material	Refractive Index	Abbé Value
Crown Glass	1.523	58
CR–39 Plastic	1.498	58
Corning Photogray Extra (Glass)	1.523	57
Trivex (plastic)	1.532	43-45
Spectralite (plastic)	1.537	47
Corning 1.6 index PGX (glass)	1.600	42
Essilor Thin-n-Lite (plastic)	1.74	33
Essilor Stylis (plastic)	1.67	32
Schott High-Lite Glass	1.701	31
Polycarbonate	1.586	30

the longitudinal chromatic aberration for this lens in both crown glass and polycarbonate.

Solution

Longitudinal chromatic aberration can be found by dividing the power of the lens by the Abbé value of the material from which the lens is made. Polycarbonate has an Abbé value of 30 and crown glass an Abbé value of 58. Beginning with polycarbonate we find:

$$\text{Longitudinal Chromatic Aberration}_{(polycarb)} = \frac{F}{\nu}$$
$$= \frac{6}{30}$$
$$= 0.20 D$$

Glass has a longitudinal chromatic aberration of:

$$\text{Longitudinal Chromatic Aberration}_{(crown\ glass)} = \frac{F}{\nu}$$
$$= \frac{6}{58}$$
$$= 0.10 D$$

Lateral (or Transverse) Chromatic Aberration and "Chromatic Power"
Lateral chromatic aberration is expressed either as differences in image magnification or differences in prismatic effect.

Magnification Differences With refractive lenses, lateral chromatic aberration is thought of in terms of *magnification differences*. A magnification difference is the difference in size between the images formed by two different wavelengths, such as red and blue (see Figure 18-1).

Differences in Prismatic Effect When quantified by prismatic effect, the lateral chromatic aberration of a prism is the difference in prismatic effect for light of two different wavelengths (Figure 18-2). As a formula this would be expressed:

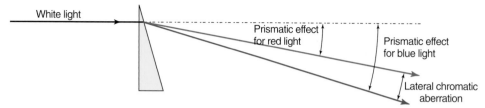

Figure 18-2. Lateral chromatic aberration occurs when a prism bends light of two different wavelengths by different amounts.

lateral chromatic aberration = (prismatic effect for blue light) – (prismatic effect for red light)

or

lateral chromatic aberration = $\Delta_{blue} - \Delta_{red}$

Lenses have prismatic effects as well, but for a lens, the prismatic effect will depend on the distance from the optical center (OC) of the lens. We know that prismatic effect increases as we look farther away from the center of the lens. Prismatic effect for a given point on a lens is determined by Prentice's rule. Prentice's rule states:

$$\Delta = cF$$

where c is the distance from the OC in centimeters, and F is the dioptric power of the lens. Sometimes the letter d (for distance) is used instead of c (for centimeters). This is the case when working with lateral chromatic aberration. Therefore since

$$\Delta_{blue} = dF_F \text{ and } \Delta_{red} = dF_C$$

and

lateral chromatic aberration = $\Delta_{blue} - \Delta_{red}$

then

lateral chromatic aberration = $dF_F - dF_C$
$$= d(F_F - F_C)$$

For longitudinal chromatic aberration, both the formulas:

longitudinal chromatic aberration = $F_F - F_C$

and

longitudinal chromatic aberration = $\dfrac{F}{v}$

are useable and equal to one another. Therefore we know that:

$$F_F - F_C = \frac{F}{v}$$

If both sides of the equation are multiplied by d (decentration), we see that:

$$d(F_F - F_C) = d\frac{F}{v}$$

Looking at the left-hand term in the equation, we recognize the formula for lateral chromatic aberration. This means that lateral chromatic aberration can also be written as:

$$\text{lateral chromatic aberration} = \frac{dF}{v}$$
$$= \frac{\text{Prismatic Effect}}{v}$$
$$= \frac{\Delta}{v}$$

Since v is the Abbé value, it is now possible to find lateral chromatic aberration quickly if the Abbé value of a lens is known.

When lateral chromatic aberration refers to differences in prismatic effect, as shown previously, it is sometimes called *chromatic power*.

The concept of chromatic power allows us to see that as prismatic effect increases, the effects of chromatic aberration become more powerful and hence more disturbing to vision.

Example **18-2**

In the previous example, we found the longitudinal chromatic for a +6.00 D lens. Lateral chromatic aberration is a function of prismatic effect. We can find the lateral chromatic aberration for a prism of a certain material. But we cannot simply ask "What is the lateral chromatic aberration for a +6.00 D lens of a certain material." However, we can ask (and are asking) this question. What is the lateral chromatic aberration for a point 8 mm away from the optical center of a +6.00 D lens when it is, (A) made from polycarbonate material, and (B) made from crown glass?

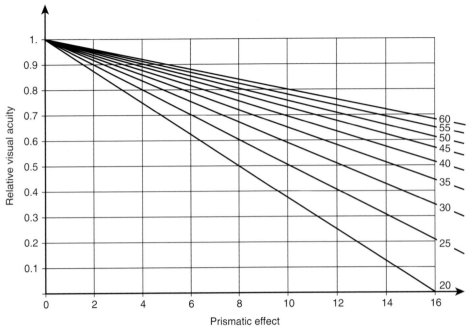

Figure 18-3. Chromatic aberration can be measured as an Abbé value. In the graph, the Abbé value is shown on the right. Prismatic effect increases toward the periphery of a strongly powered lens. The graph shows what happens to visual acuity as prismatic effect increases. The more chromatic aberration present in a lens, the faster visual acuity will be affected. (From Meslin D, Obrecht G: Effect of chromatic dispersion of a lens on visual acuity, Am J of Optom Physiol Opt 65:25–28, 1988. Figure 2, The American Academy of Optometry, 1988.)

Solution

For a prism, lateral chromatic aberration is the prism amount (Δ) divided by the Abbé value (v).

$$\text{lateral chromatic aberration} = \frac{\Delta}{v}$$

For a certain point on a lens, to find the lateral chromatic aberration, we need to know the prismatic effect at that particular point. For a lens with power, the prismatic effect is the power of the lens times the distance of the decentered point from the optical center, or $\Delta = dF$. This makes the lateral chromatic aberration equal to:

$$\text{lateral chromatic aberration} = \frac{dF}{v}$$

For a point 8 mm from the center of a polycarbonate lens, the lateral chromatic aberration is:

$$\text{lateral chromatic aberration}_{(polycarb)} = \frac{(0.8)(6)}{30}$$
$$= 0.16\Delta$$

For the same point on a crown glass lens, the lateral chromatic aberration is:

$$\text{lateral chromatic aberration}_{(crown\ glass)} = \frac{(0.8)(6)}{58}$$
$$= 0.08\Delta$$

When Does Chromatic Aberration Reduce Visual Acuity? Suppose a person is wearing a pair of prescription spectacle lenses and is looking at an object directly through the OCs. When the wearer looks through the OCs, there is no prismatic effect and thus no chromatic power.

As the wearer looks to the right or left, the prismatic effect of the lenses increases. So does the chromatic power. The more the chromatic power (lateral chromatic aberration) increases, the more the image blurs. There is more prismatic effect in the periphery of a high-powered lens than in the periphery of a low-powered one. So peripheral visual acuity drops off faster for high-powered lenses than it does for low-powered ones.

The higher the chromatic aberration, the lower the Abbé value. The lower the Abbé value, the faster the reduction in relative visual acuity peripherally. (This is shown in Figure 18-3.)[3]

Fortunately the peripheral areas of a lens are seldom used for intensive viewing during normal spectacle lens wear. Instead if something needs to be seen clearly, the head is turned. Otherwise, lens materials with low Abbé values would not be as well tolerated as they are.

To reduce the possibility of chromatic aberration becoming troublesome, the dispensing factors shown in Box 18-1 should be considered.

Important Dispensing Factors for Lenses With Low Abbé Values (Polycarbonate and Some High-Index Materials)

1. Use monocular interpupillary distances.
2. Measure major reference point heights, considering pantoscopic angle (see Chapter 5).
3. Use shorter vertex distances.
4. Have sufficient pantoscopic angle, but not more than 10 degrees for high lens powers.
5. Give attention to comparative edge thicknesses (OCs that are too high above the horizontal midline of the edged lens will cause large differences in top and bottom edge thicknesses).

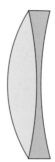

Figure 18-4. An achromatic lens is constructed from two different materials, each with a different refractive index chosen to counteract the effects of chromatic aberration. Achromatic lenses are not used in normal spectacle lenses.

Example **18-3**

What is the expected visual acuity when looking through a point 12 mm temporal to the distance optical center of a −7.00 D CR-39 lens with an Abbé value of 58? How would this compare with a polycarbonate lens when looking through this same point?

Solution

To find the answer to this question, we will use Prentice's rule to find prismatic effect and to look up relative visual acuity in Figure 18-3. Prismatic effect is:

$$\Delta = cF$$
$$= (1.2)(7)$$
$$= 8.4$$

Looking up a prismatic effect of 8.4Δ for a 58 Abbé-value material shows a relative visual acuity of 0.82. To find this in Snellen acuity equivalent:

$$\text{Relative visual acuity} = \frac{\text{measured visual acuity}}{\text{maximum visual acuity}}$$

$$0.82 = \frac{20/x}{20/20} = \frac{20}{x}$$

$$x = \frac{20}{0.82} = 24$$

$$\text{measured visual acuity} = \frac{20}{24}$$

So for the CR-39 lens, the Snellen visual acuity is $\frac{20}{24}$.

Looking up the same 8.4Δ point for a polycarbonate lens and calculating acuity will yield a Snellen acuity of $\frac{20}{29}$.

Achromatic Lenses

A lens would be considered totally without chromatic aberration if all of the wavelengths across the visible spectrum focused at one point. This does not happen with ophthalmic lens materials. To create a lens that is considered achromatic, a plus lens of one material is used in combination with a minus lens of another material.

The two lens powers must add up to the needed lens power and light from the F (blue) and C (red) spectral lines must focus at the focal point of the lens. Such a lens is called an *achromatic lens* or a *doublet* (Figure 18-4). Acromatic doublets are not used for ordinary spectacle lens wear.

To create an achromatic lens, this is what must happen:

1. The longitudinal chromatic aberrations of the two lenses must neutralize each other. That is

$$\frac{F_1}{v_1} = -\frac{F_2}{v_2}$$

2. And the two lenses must equal the desired power, so that the needed power is

$$F = F_1 + F_2$$

3. Combining these two equations give this equation for the first lens in the doublet.

$$F_1 = \frac{Fv_1}{v_1 - v_2}$$

4. Once F_1 is found, then the second lens (F_2) can be found from

$$F_2 = F - F_1$$

Example **18-4**

What would the two needed lens powers of an achromatic doublet be for a lens having a needed power of +6.00 D? Use these two lens materials to make the lens:

Index 1.523 with an Abbé value of 58

Index 1.701 with an Abbé value of 31

Solution

To find the first component of the lens, use the equation

$$F_1 = \frac{Fv_1}{v_1 - v_2}$$
$$= \frac{(6)(58)}{58 - 31}$$
$$= \frac{348}{27}$$
$$= +12.89D$$

The second component is:

$$F_2 = F - F_1$$
$$= 6 - 12.89$$
$$= -6.89\ D$$

The Monochromatic Aberrations

Aberrations can occur in a lens even when the light entering the lens is only one color. These aberrations, called *monochromatic aberrations* may be more troublesome for cameras or optical systems than for prescription ophthalmic lenses, but are still of definite concern when designing a spectacle lens and evaluating visual performance.

Seidel Aberrations

When rays of light pass through a lens, we expect them to focus at one predictable location. When those rays are paraxial (or central) rays, we can predict the location of focus using the fundamental paraxial equation:*

$$F = L' - L$$

which, written another way is:

$$L' = L + F$$

The fundamental paraxial equation is derived from Snell's law on the basis of an assumption. The assumption is that for small angles (measured in radians instead of degrees) $\sin\theta = \theta$. However, a still more accurate approximation for $\sin\theta$ is a polynomial series expansion given as:

$$\sin\theta = \theta - \frac{\theta^3}{3!} + \frac{\theta^5}{5!} - \frac{\theta^7}{7!} + \dots$$

The first term represents the paraxial approximation $\sin\theta = \theta$. If we use both the 1st and 2nd terms of this equation we are using third order terms for $\sin\theta$. In other words, instead of saying $\sin\theta = \theta$, we say that $\sin\theta = \theta - \frac{\theta^3}{3!}$ (again measured in radians instead of degrees). This substitution gives us the next higher order

of approximation. This third order approximation is used as a basis of comparison when determining the quality of how well a given wave front of light is able to come to a proper focus after passing through a lens, a lens surface or a lens system. In the process of passing through a lens, the wave front may lose some of its spherical shape. This reveals aberration and a resulting imperfect focus.

Using third order terms, Seidel classified aberrations into 5 categories. The 5 are interrelated. Making a lens change to reduce the amount of one aberration can affect the magnitude of other aberrations. These 5 aberrations have become known as the *Seidel or 3rd order aberrations*. (There are other aberrations that will occur when using higher order approximations such as 5th or 7th order.) The 5 Seidel aberrations are *spherical aberration, coma, oblique (radial or marginal) astigmatism, curvature of field (power error)*, and *distortion*. These will be described shortly.

One of the drawbacks of expressing aberration as Seidel aberrations is that all lens surfaces are assumed to be spherical. To better describe aberration for surfaces that may not be spherical, such as the refracting surfaces of the eye, a different system works better.

Classifying Aberrations Using Zernike Polynomials

There are other systems for classifying how a given wave front deviates from a perfect sphere when leaving a refracting surface, a lens, or a refracting system. One system that describes aberrations of the human eye uses Zernike polynomials. The use of Zernike polynomials is a more complete representation of the aberrations that could be present in a lens or eye. Furthermore it does not assume spherical surfaces, which Seidel aberrations do. The Zernike system has gained visibility because of an ever increasing interest in aberrations within the human eye. This interest is driven by several factors, including:

1. A desire to see into the eye clearly to detect disease-driven changes. The aberrations of the eye degrade the view of retinal elements within the eye. Correcting these aberrations will allow earlier diagnosis of ocular disease.
2. The challenge of refractive surgery. Unfortunately aberrations of the eye are often increased because of refractive surgery. Ideally one would want to not only correct sphere and cylinder refractive errors, but also reduce other aberrations so as to enhance visual performance.
3. A desire to measure ocular aberrations so that they might be corrected. If ocular aberrations can be measured, the next logical step is to figure out a way to correct them. Options will include not only refractive surgery, but also contact lenses or other methods.

As stated earlier, the use of Zernike polynomials has become a popular system to describe and measure ocular monochromatic aberrations. Zernike polynomials use a

---

*See the section in Chapter 14 called "Reduced Thickness and Refractive Index."

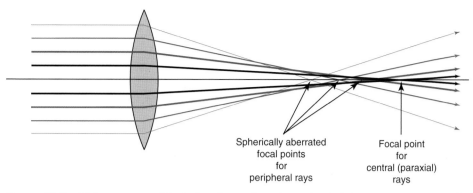

Spherically aberrated
focal points
for
peripheral rays

Focal point
for
central (paraxial)
rays

Figure 18-5. This exaggerated depiction shows that when spherical aberration is present, the closer to the edge of the lens the rays are, the shorter their focal length will be. The peripheral rays have an increasingly shorter focal length than the central (paraxial) rays. (This particular form of spherical aberration is positive spherical aberration. There is a form of spherical aberration called negative spherical aberration where the peripheral rays have a longer focal length than the central rays.)

numbered term that describes a geometric shape for the aberration. These terms are grouped into orders. (These orders are not the same as those described in the previous section on Seidel aberrations, although some Zernike terms are similar to certain Seidel terms.) Here are how the Zernike orders describe some of the commonly known aberrations related to the eye.[10]

Order	Aberration
1st	Prism
2nd	Defocus and astigmatism
	(Defocus includes spherical refractive error such as myopia and hyperopia)
3rd	Coma and trefoil
4th	Spherical aberration and other modes
5th to 10th	Higher order irregular aberrations

According to the orders within this classification, second order aberrations are errors which are corrected by the written ophthalmic eyeglass prescription. These "aberrations" of the human eye are corrected using sphere and cylinder lenses. Those aberrations classified as 3rd order and up are referred to as *higher order aberrations*.

The Five Seidel Aberrations

Spherical Aberration

Spherical aberration is a Seidel aberration that occurs when parallel light from an object enters a large area of a spherical lens surface (Figure 18-5). When spherical aberration is present, peripheral rays focus at different points on the optic axis than do paraxial rays. (Peripheral rays are those that enter the lens nearer the edge than the center. Paraxial rays are those that pass through the central area of the lens.)

Spherical aberration occurs when the object point is on the optical axis of the system. All of the other Seidel aberrations occur when the object point is off the optic axis.

Because the pupil of the eye limits the number of rays entering the eye for any given direction of gaze, spherical aberration is not a large problem in ophthalmic lenses.

Coma

The second Seidel aberration is coma. When the object point is off the axis of the lens, there is a difference in magnification for rays passing through different zones of the lens. (Zones could be considered to be imaginary doughnut-shaped rings on the lens, each having a longer radius.) The focal areas of the peripheral "zones" lie in a different location than those of the more central rays. Instead of forming a single point image off the optic axis, the image appears comet or ice cream cone shaped. The point of the cone points toward the optic axis. This aberration is known as coma (Figure 18-6).

Oblique Astigmatism

Oblique astigmatism is another Seidel aberration that occurs when rays from an off-axis point pass through the spectacle lens. When a small bundle of light strikes the spherical surface of a lens from an angle, oblique astigmatism causes the light to focus as two line images, known as the tangential and sagittal images, instead of a single point (Figure 18-7). It is as if the light were passing through an astigmatic lens, rather than a spherical lens.

The distance between the two line foci that occurs in oblique astigmatism is called the *astigmatic difference*. When expressed in diopters, this difference is called the *oblique astigmatic error*. Oblique astigmatic error is a measure of oblique astigmatism.

Oblique astigmatism is troublesome for the spectacle lens wearer and must be taken into consideration when designing spectacle lenses. Oblique astigmatism may be reduced by finding the optimum base curve for a given lens power. There is a graph that shows the best lens form(s) for eliminating oblique astigmatism at a particular off-axis viewing angle. This graph is in the shape of an ellipse and is called *Tscherning's ellipse* (Figure 18-8). The size of the ellipse may vary, depending on the

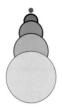

Figure 18-6. Coma is an aberration that causes light from peripheral areas of the lens to be focused farther from the true image point than it should be. Because light farther in the periphery is displaced increasingly farther from the point focus, the image is distorted in cometlike fashion as shown. The drawing is simplified to show the way the image is created. In actuality there are unlimited "circles" of blur that blend together in a flared appearance like the tail of a comet.

viewing distance and angle the lens designer uses when trying to reduce oblique astigmatism.

There are two synonyms for oblique astigmatism. These are *radial astigmatism* and *marginal astigmatism*.

The Effects of Tilting Lenses

Oblique astigmatism is also manifested when lenses are tilted in front of the eye. This happens because the optic axis of the lens tilts with the lens. The object of regard, which used to be on the optic axis of the lens, now becomes an off-axis object or point. Because the lens is angled in reference to the object of regard, oblique astigmatism will affect the image of that point. Before the tilt, the object, located on the optic axis, formed a single-point image based on the actual spherical power of the lens. With tilt the image is now formed as if it were refracted through a new sphere and cylinder.

The new sphere and cylinder powers manifested through the "old" tilted lens can be determined by first finding the effective powers in the sagittal and tangential meridians of the lens.[4] It turns out that the sagittal

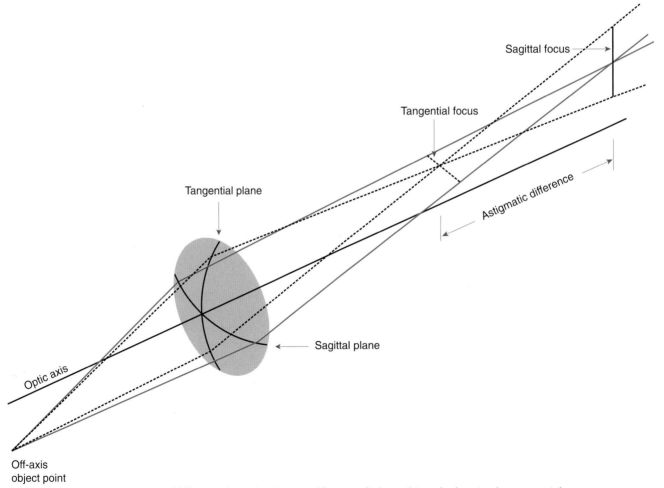

Figure 18-7. Oblique astigmatism is caused because light striking the lens in the tangential plane focuses at one line focus, whereas light striking the lens in the sagittal plane focuses at another line focus. (The tangential plane of the lens is the plane that intersects the optic axis and the off-axis object point. The sagittal plane is 90 degrees away from the tangential plane.)

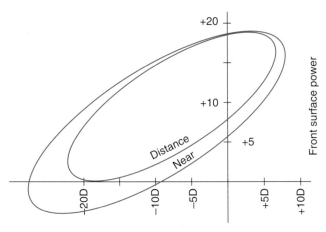

Figure 18-8. A Tscherning's ellipse graphically shows the base curves needed to correct for oblique astigmatism. There is a different ellipse for each viewing distance. (From Keating MP: Geometric, physical and visual optics. Boston, 1988, Butterworth-Heinemann.)

meridian coincides with the axis of lens tilt. For a pantoscopic tilt, the axis of tilt is along the horizontal or 180-degree meridian, and so the horizontal meridian is the sagittal meridian. For a face-form tilt, the axis of tilt is along the vertical or 90-degree meridian, and so the vertical meridian is the sagittal meridian. (The tangential meridian is perpendicular to the sagittal meridian, as shown in Figure 18-7.)

The effective power in the sagittal meridian is:

$$F_s = F\left(1 + \frac{\sin^2\theta}{2n}\right)$$

Where

F_s = the power in the sagittal meridian
F = the power of the lens being tilted (i.e., the "old" lens)
θ = the angle of tilt and
n = the refractive index of the lens.

The power in the tangential meridian is:

$$F_T = F\left(\frac{2n + \sin^2\theta}{2n\cos^2\theta}\right)$$

The difference between sagittal and tangential powers is the amount of astigmatism induced. In other words, the cylinder power induced is:

$$\text{induced cylinder} = F_T - F_S$$

For a spherical lens, the equation for tangential power is sometimes skipped, and the induced cylinder is directly approximated by:

$$\text{induced cylinder} \approx F\tan^2\theta$$

where

F = the power of the lens being tilted (i.e., the "old" lens) and
θ = the angle of tilt.

The sign (+ or −) of the induced cylinder is the same as the sign of the tilted lens. The axis of the induced cylinder is the same as the axis of tilt. Finding the induced cylinder with this equation is not as accurate as finding the difference between tangential and sagittal powers.

Wrap-Around Prescription Lenses Wrap-around prescription eyewear presents unique optical problems that can require compensating power changes in lens powers to keep the optical effect of the prescription as intended. Here are some examples of what can happen optically to a prescription placed in a wrap-around frame.

Example **18-5**

A person orders wrap-around sunglasses with a drop-in prescription front. The prescription lenses are made from 1.50 index plastic and have a power of −5.75 D sphere. The wrap-around design of the front causes the drop-in front and lenses to be angled 9 degrees. In the drop-in front there is no decentration. In other words, the wearer's interpupillary distance equals the A + DBL of the front. What is the effective power induced by the wrap around?

Solution

If there is no decentration, no face form is required (see Chapter 5). Yet the lenses are tilted 9 degrees. Since the lens tilt is from wrap around, the angle of tilt is in the 90-degree meridian.

We begin by finding the sagittal power. This will become the new effective sphere power. Using the formula previously given, the sagittal power equals

$$F_s = -5.75\left(1 + \frac{\sin^2 9}{2(1.5)}\right)$$
$$= -5.75\left(1 + \frac{0.02447}{3}\right)$$
$$= -5.75(1.008)$$
$$= -5.80\,\text{D}$$

To find the effective cylinder power, we will use the alternate equation, which gives an approximate answer and is:

$$\text{induced cylinder} \approx F\tan^2\theta$$
$$\approx -5.75\,(\tan^2 9)$$
$$\approx -5.75\,(0.025)$$
$$\approx -0.14\,\text{D}$$

The axis of the induced cylinder is the same as the axis of tilt, 90 degrees. Therefore the lens effectively becomes:

$$-5.80 - 0.14 \times 90$$

In this example, the effect of tilting the lens is relatively small. A larger lens power or an increased lens tilt will produce a greater amount of change.

Example 18-6

Now suppose that this same −5.75 D lens is made from polycarbonate material of index 1.586 and is placed in a "wrap" frame having tilt around the 90-degree axis of 25 degrees. (Some wrap frames can approach 30 degrees in their tilt.[5]) Again, there is no decentration required since the wearer's PD equals the (A + DBL) of the frame front. What will the effective power of this tilted lens be, when placed in this frame?

Solution

Repeating the same computations as before, we find the sagittal power that will become the new effective sphere power.

$$
\begin{aligned}
F_s &= -5.75\left(1 + \frac{\sin^2 25}{2(1.586)}\right) \\
&= -5.75\left(1 + \frac{0.1786}{3.172}\right) \\
&= -5.75(1.0563) \\
&= -6.07\,\text{D}
\end{aligned}
$$

This time we will find the tangential power in the other meridian, allowing a more exact cylinder power.

$$
\begin{aligned}
F_T &= F\left(\frac{2n + \sin^2 \theta}{2n\cos^2 \theta}\right) \\
&= -5.75\left(\frac{2(1.586) + \sin^2 25}{2(1.586)\cos^2 25}\right) \\
&= -5.75\left(\frac{3.172 + 0.179}{(3.172)(0.821)}\right) \\
&= -5.75\left(\frac{3.351}{2.605}\right) \\
&= -7.40\,\text{D}
\end{aligned}
$$

Taking the difference between sagittal and tangential meridians, we find the effective cylinder power to be:

$$
\begin{aligned}
\text{induced cylinder} &= F_T - F_S \\
&= -7.40 - (-6.07) \\
&= -1.33\ \text{D}
\end{aligned}
$$

The lens effectively becomes:

$$
-6.07 - 1.33 \times 90
$$

It is evident that the effect of tilting the lens can become large and will be problematic unless the effect of tilt is considered and the power of the lens changed to compensate for the induced change in sphere and cylinder. Some prescriptions will be significantly affected by lens tilt when placed in a frame with a large amount of wrap around.

Example 18-7

What powered lens of 1.586 index of refraction would be needed to produce a −5.75 D sphere after the frame has been given a face-form wrap around that tilts the lens 25 degrees?

Solution

This is essentially asking how we must compensate a −5.75 D sphere prescription so that it comes out right in a frame with a 25-degree tilt for each lens. To figure this out, we need to work backwards. In other words, using the formula:

$$
F_s = F\left(1 + \frac{\sin^2 \theta}{2n}\right)
$$

We need to end up with F_s equal to −5.75 D. We need to find the value of F for the meridian of tilt. In this case the meridian of tilt is the 90-degree meridian.

$$
\begin{aligned}
F_s &= F\left(1 + \frac{\sin^2 \theta}{2n}\right) \\
-5.75 &= F\left(1 + \frac{\sin^2 25}{2(1.586)}\right) \\
-5.75 &= F\left(1 + \frac{0.179}{3.172}\right) \\
-5.75 &= F(1.056) \\
F &= \frac{-5.75}{1.056} \\
F &= -5.45\,\text{D}
\end{aligned}
$$

So the needed power in the 90-degree meridian is −5.45 D.

Since the lens is a sphere we also need to end up with a power of −5.75 D in the tangential (180-degree) meridian. Here we also work backwards using the formula:

$$
F_T = F\left(\frac{2n + \sin^2 \theta}{2n\cos^2 \theta}\right)
$$

We want a power of −5.75 for F_T when we are finished. Therefore:

$$
\begin{aligned}
F_T &= F\left(\frac{2n + \sin^2 \theta}{2n\cos^2 \theta}\right) \\
-5.75 &= F\left(\frac{2(1.586) + \sin^2 25}{2(1.586)\cos^2 25}\right) \\
-5.75 &= F\left(\frac{3.172 + 0.179}{(3.172)(0.821)}\right) \\
-5.75 &= F\left(\frac{3.351}{2.605}\right) \\
-5.75 &= F(1.286) \\
F &= \frac{-5.75}{1.286} \\
F &= -4.47\,\text{D in the 180}
\end{aligned}
$$

If we have −5.45 D in the 90 and −4.47 D in the 180, the theoretical lens needed is −4.47 −0.98 × 180. The lens used would be −4.50 −1.00 × 180.

Tilting of Spherocylinders When tilted, a spherocylindrical lens also has induced power changes. For either pantoscopic or face-form tilt of a spherocylinder lens with axis 90 or 180, the tilted spherocylindrical lens acts similar to a spherocylinder with a new sphere power and a new cylinder power. The principal meridians of the "old" (or untilted) lens are horizontal and vertical. The lens power chosen to calculate the effective sagittal power (F_S) is the power of the spherocylinder in the sagittal meridian. The lens power chosen to calculate the effective tangential power (F_T) is the power of the spherocylinder in the tangential meridian.

After calculating the new powers, one can then put them on a horizontal and vertical power cross and from it determine the new (or effective) spherocylindrical parameters (sphere, cylinder, *and* axis) in the usual manner.

For pantoscopic or face-form tilt of a spherocylindrical lens with an oblique axis, there is an effective change in cylinder axis and an effective change in the sphere and cylinder powers. Here the computations are more complicated and require resultant calculations combining obliquely crossed cylinders. It is also feasible to work backwards as we did above to find what prescription must be placed in a wrap-around frame to prevent unwanted power changes. For an explanation of how this may be done, see Keating MP: Geometric, Physical, and Visual Optics.[4]

Induced Prism with Wrap-Around Eyewear There are also induced prismatic effects associated with tilting lenses. To see how this works, take a lens prescription and center the optics in a lensmeter with the prescription correctly neutralized. Then tilt the prescription to simulate a wrap-around effect. The prism that appears is a result of that lens tilt.

This prismatic effect depends on the angle of tilt, the steepness of the base curve, the index of the material, and the thickness of the lens. It is predictable using the equation[6]

$$\Delta = 100 \tan\theta \frac{t}{n} F_1$$

Where

Δ = the prism induced
θ = the angle of tilt
t = the thickness of the lens at the reference point in meters
n = lens refractive index
F_1 = the front curve of the lens

Notice that the refractive power of the lens does not enter into this equation for prismatic effect, only front curve lens power.

The base direction of the prism induced is determined by the angle at which the light enters the lens. If

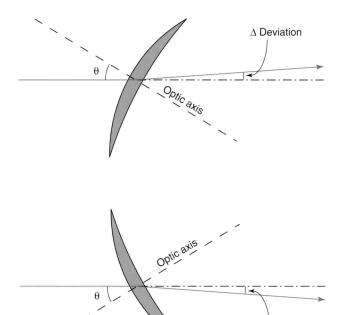

Figure 18-9. Lens tilt will cause a slight amount of prismatic effect. The amount of prism deviation is equal to

$$\Delta = 100 \tan\theta \frac{t}{n} F_1.$$

In this figure θ is the angle between the optic axis and the incoming central ray.

the light enters the lens from above the optic axis, the orientation of the prism will be base down. If the light enters the lens from the left of the lens, then the base of the induced prism is to the right.

For lenses with pantoscopic tilt, the bottom of the lens is tilted in toward the face. Light coming from straight ahead strikes the lens as if it were entering from above. Therefore the prism induced is base down. Since the induced prism is base down for both right and left lenses, there is a net prismatic effect of zero. Both lenses cause the image to move up by basically the same amount so no compensation would be required.

For wrap-around lenses, the right lens is tilted such that light coming into the lens from in front of the wearer is striking the lens as if it were coming from the left (Figure 18-9). Therefore the prism base direction is base right. For the right eye, base right is the same as base out. For the left eye, the base direction will be base left, which is also base out. With both eyes having base out prism, the eyes must turn slightly inward to retain a single image of the object viewed. To compensate for induced base out prism, base-in prism would need to be used. This is true even for wrap-around lenses that have no power when made with a curved lens. However, if the front of the lens is flat, then the prismatic effect drops to zero.

Example **18-8**

A prescription is to be placed into a pair of wrap-around frames with a wrap angle of 25 degrees for each lens. It is ground onto a +8.00 D base curve polycarbonate lens with a 2.0-mm center thickness. What would be the amount of prism induced and in what base direction? If compensatory prism is placed in the glasses to counteract the induced prism, what base direction would be used?

Solution

Using the formula for prism induced by tilt, the prism amount is:

$$\Delta = 100 \tan\theta \frac{t}{n} F_1$$
$$= 100 \tan 25 \left(\frac{0.002}{1.586}\right) 8$$
$$= 0.47$$

The amount of prism is 0.47Δ. Since the light enters the lens at an angle on the nasal side, the prism base direction is on the other side, which is base out. The induced prism is 0.47Δ base out per eye. The prism needed to compensate for induced base out is base in.

For orders with significant wrap around and a moderate to high-powered prescription, use a laboratory that is experienced with making any necessary compensatory changes in refractive power and prism caused by lens tilt.

Intentionally Tilting a Lens to Prevent Problems

Earlier lens tilt examples present situations where the wearer's interpupillary distance and the frame A + DBL dimensions are the same. In other words, there is no necessity for decentration. Yet most prescriptions do require at least a small amount of decentration inward since the wearer's PD is generally smaller than the frame's A + DBL measurements.

If a prescription *does* require some decentration inward, then the frame front *should* have a certain amount of face form. A lens with decentration inward and no face form will end up having tilt at the optical center. This is explained in more detail in Chapter 5. (Note especially Figures 5-2, 5-3, and 5-4.) Decentration that is compensated for with a certain amount of face form will actually *prevent* the decentered lens from being tilted at the OC. However, adding more face form than the needed amount will end up causing those unintended sphere and cylinder power errors that have been just described.

Curvature of Field (Power Error)

If a designer makes a lens that is completely free of oblique astigmatism, there will still be another aberration the wearer encounters when looking through the periphery of the lens. This fourth of Seidel's five aberrations is called *curvature of field* or *power error*. Power

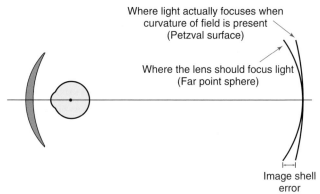

Figure 18-10. The aberration curvature of field occurs when light entering the peripheral areas of the lens does not focus where it should; namely, on the far point sphere. (The far point sphere is curved because the eye turns to see objects toward the periphery of the lens.) Instead it focuses on the Petzval surface. The Petzval surface is formed when oblique astigmatism is corrected. Another name for the Petzval surface is the image sphere.

error is the most descriptive term because this aberration causes the spherical component of the lens to have the effect of being off-power in the periphery when worn (Figure 18-10). (The dioptric difference between the place where the image actually focuses and where it should focus is called the *image shell error.*)

It is important to use the manufacturer's recommended base curve for each given lens power. The optimum base curve will ensure that oblique astigmatism and power error are held to a minimum. When using the wrong base curve, the wearer will not be able to see as well through the periphery of the lens.

Distortion

The last of the five Seidel aberrations is distortion. *Distortion* occurs because there is a different magnification at different areas of the periphery of the lens in proportion to the distance of those areas from the OC of the lens. For plus lenses, magnification increases proportionately toward the periphery, whereas in minus lenses, the magnification decreases proportionately. When looking at the center of a square window through a high plus lens, the corners of the window are farther away from the center of the lens than the middle of the sides (or the middle of the top and bottom). This means the corners will be magnified more, making the window look like a pincushion (Figure 18-11). This is known as *pincushion distortion.*

For minus lenses, the corners would receive less magnification than the middle of the sides, causing *barrel distortion.*

Spectacle Lens Design

As noted previously, some aberrations are more important than others when designing spectacle lenses. To summarize:

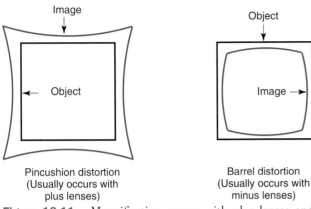

Figure 18-11. Magnification occurs with plus lenses and minification with minus lenses. However, the magnification is not even across the lens. This results in the types of distortion of the magnified or minified images shown here.

- Chromatic aberration is important when considering possible high-index materials to use for spectacle lenses or when choosing the fused multifocal segment of a glass spectacle lens.
- Because of pupil size, the Seidel aberrations of spherical aberration and coma are less problematic.
- The three Seidel aberrations proving to be most troublesome in ophthalmic lenses are oblique astigmatism, power error, and distortion.

Looking at design possibilities simplistically, there are three possibilities:

1. A lens designer can correct the oblique astigmatism completely, leaving the power error uncorrected. A lens designed in this fashion is referred to as a *point focal lens.*
2. A designer can concentrate on eliminating power error, but choose to leave residual astigmatism uncorrected. This type of lens is referred to as a *Percival form lens.*
3. A designer can design a lens referred to as a *minimum tangential error form* that is a compromise between the first two choices. At this point in time, designing a lens that is strictly a "point focal" or a "Percival" form lens is not likely. A lens which compromises between the two forms is common practice.

It should be noted that all three of the above choices are referred to either as *corrected curve* or *best form* lenses.

Four Variables of Lens Design

There are four variables the designer can use to arrive at the best form for an individual lens of a specific power. These four are:

1. Vertex distance
2. Lens thickness
3. Refractive index
4. Front and back lens surface powers

For a single vision series of lenses, the first three variables must be decided for the whole series. Therefore the only practical variables left to work with are front and back surface powers.

The Importance of Using the Correct Base Curve for Surfaced Lenses

When a laboratory receives a single vision series of finished lenses, the base curve of the lens is set. When the lens is removed from the package, the only choices left are related to lens edging. When a lens has to be surfaced, however, the laboratory looks at the desired lens power and chooses a lens blank with a front (base) curve appropriate for that particular power. Lens designers have already recommended certain base curves for specific lens powers so the laboratory usually tries to remain within those guidelines.

Failure to select the correct base curve for a given lens power will not affect the quality of vision a person has through the center of the lens. It will reduce the quality of vision through the periphery of the lens, however.

By using the correct base curve, the most troublesome monochromatic aberrations can be reduced. By looking at Tscherning's ellipse (see Figure 18-8), we see that it is possible to completely correct for oblique astigmatism* for sphere powers ranging from approximately +7.00 D to −23.00 D. For powers outside of this range, there is no spherical base curve that will eliminate oblique astigmatism. There is another option, however. That option is to use an aspheric lens.

The Tscherning's ellipse also shows that there are really two base curves that correct for oblique astigmatism. The lower half of the ellipse corresponds to the lenses that are customarily used today.

APPROPRIATE BASE CURVES

It is possible to create the same power using an almost infinite variety of lens forms. A lens with a front curve of +2.00 D and a back curve of −6.00 D will produce virtually the same power that a lens with a +3.00 D front curve and a −7.00 D back curve will produce. If many lens forms produce the same power, is there a particular front curve that should be chosen for a given lens power?

Although there is a range of possible lens forms that will prove acceptable, there are limits beyond which the overall results will be poor. If an incorrect base curve is selected, the quality of vision is acceptable while looking straight ahead. But vision will be degraded when turning the eyes to view an object off to the side. This effect is due to lens aberrations brought about by an incorrect lens form.

---

*The phrase "completely correct for oblique astigmatism" means that for one viewing distance at one oblique viewing angle, oblique astigmatism can be eliminated. At other viewing angles and distances, oblique astigmatism will be considerably reduced, but not entirely eliminated.

Manufacturers' Recommendations

Lens manufacturers recommend specific base curves for each lens power. These recommendations list the range of powers and tell which base should be used for those powers.

A General Guideline

The power of a lens determines its shape.

- Plano lens powers usually have back surface curves close to −6.00 D.
- As lens power becomes more minus, the back surface steepens, and the front surface flattens.
- As plus lens power increases, the back surface becomes progressively flatter, while the front curve becomes steeper.

From the front, minus lenses look flatter, and plus lenses look steeper.

Base Curve Formulas

One method for estimating the range in which an appropriate base curve might be found is to use a simplified formula derived from precalculated base curves. Such a formula is not a replacement for manufacturers' recommendations. One such formula is *Vogel's formula*,[7] which states that, for plus lenses, the base curve of the lens equals the spherical equivalent of the lens power plus 6 diopters. Written as a formula this is:

$$\text{Base curve}_{(plus\ lenses)} = \text{spherical equivalent} + 6.00\ D$$

(The *spherical equivalent* of a lens is the sphere power plus half of the cylinder power.) For minus lenses, Vogel's formula for base curve begins with the spherical equivalent of the lens, divides the spherical equivalent by 2, then adds 6 diopters. Written as a formula this is:

$$\text{Base curve}_{(minus\ lenses)} = \frac{\text{spherical equivalent}}{2} + 6.00\ D$$

These formulas are summarized in Box 18-2.

(Remember that this formula is to help in determining approximately what base curve might be expected for a given lens power. Actual base curves for lenses will vary. Plus lenses will be somewhat flatter than calculated and lenses of higher index of refraction may be considerably flatter.)

Example **18-9**

Using Vogel's formula, find an approximate base curve for a lens having a power of +2.00 D sphere.

Solution

For spheres there is no need to calculate a spherical equivalent. So for this lens, the base curve is:

$$\text{Base curve}_{(plus\ lenses)} = +\ 2.00\ D + 6.00\ D$$
$$= 8.00\ D$$

> ### BOX 18-2
>
> **Vogel's Formula for Base Curves***
>
> Plus lenses:
>
> $$\text{Base curve} = \text{spherical equivalent} + 6.00\ D$$
>
> Minus lenses:
>
> $$\text{Base curve} = \frac{\text{spherical equivalent}}{2} + 6.00\ D$$
>
> Where
>
> $$\text{Spherical equivalent} = \text{sphere} + \frac{cyl}{2}$$

*Note: These base curves are estimates for glass and low index plastic lenses and will estimate a somewhat higher base curve for plus lenses. They are for general reference purposes and should not be used for actual lens production.

Example **18-10**

Suppose a lens has a prescription of +5.50 −1.00 × 70. Using Vogel's formula, what is the base curve?

Solution

Since this lens has cylinder, we begin by finding the spherical equivalent of the lens.

$$\text{Spherical equivalent} = +5.50 + \frac{(-1.00)}{2}$$
$$= +5.00\ D$$

The approximate base curve is:

$$\text{Base curve}_{(plus\ lenses)} = +5.00\ D + 6.00\ D$$
$$= +11.00\ D$$

Example **18-11**

A minus lens has a power of −6.50 −1.50 × 170. Using Vogel's formula, what is the approximate base curve?

Solution

The spherical equivalent of −6.50 −1.50 × 170 is:

$$\text{Spherical equivalent} = -6.50 + \frac{-1.50}{2}$$
$$= -7.25\ D$$

The base curve formula for minus lenses is different than that for plus lenses; therefore the approximate base curve is:

$$\text{Base curve}_{(minus\ lenses)} = \frac{-7.25}{2} + 6.00\ D$$
$$= -3.62\ D + 6.00\ D$$
$$= +2.38\ D$$

Rounded to the nearest $1/2$ D, this is +2.50 D. (In practice this would be rounded to the nearest base curve in the series stocked by the laboratory.)

Considering Right and Left Lenses As a Pair

Up to this point, we have only been choosing the base curve on the basis of the power of one individual lens. This works fine as long as both left and right lenses have exactly the same power. But if the powers are different in the left and right eyes, one lens might call for one base curve, whereas the other lens requires a different curve. This could be problematic in certain instances.

Consider for instance, the situation where one lens in a pair has a power that is only 0.50 D stronger than that of the other. Yet when looking at manufacturer's recommendations for each lens, the right and left base curve powers straddle two available base curves. (Lens blanks come in power jumps, such as 2, 4, 6, etc.) One lens calls for a +6.00 base, whereas the other calls for a +8.00. If the lenses were chosen with two different base curves, there would be both a visible difference in the appearance of the two lenses and a difference in magnification created between the images seen by the right and left eyes. Therefore a decision needs to be made to modify the base curve(s).

Because an error in base curve selection is worse for high-powered lenses than for lenses closer to zero power, from an *optical* standpoint, the higher powered lens would drive the choice.

This would mean that:

1. In instances *where both lenses are plus*, the steeper base curve (higher numerical base curve) of the two would be the correct optical choice. From a cosmetic standpoint, this choice may not always be followed.
2. If *both lenses are minus*, the flatter base curve of the two should be chosen.
3. If *one lens is plus and one lens is minus*, again, from an optical standpoint the base curve for the lens with the highest numerical value should be chosen.

It is usually advisable to maintain individual lens base curve choices when the difference between the right and left base curves is greater than 2 diopters. A correctly chosen base curve will produce clear vision, regardless of whether the wearer is looking through the center or off toward the edges. If the recommended base curve is changed too much, vision in the periphery of the lens will be poor. (Aniseikonia considerations may also influence base curve choice. For more on Aniseikonia and base curve, see Chapter 21.)

Other Factors That Modify Base Curve Choice

Most *metal frame* eyewires are curved to best accept a lens with a six-base curve since this is the most common base curve. For this reason, prescriptions that would normally have steeper base curves may have those curves flattened somewhat so that the lenses will stay in the frame better. (Instead of flattening the lens, a better choice would be to use an aspheric lens. Aspherics can be made on a flatter base curve without degrading optical quality.)

Plastic frame styles that have a poor lens retention record may retain their lenses better if the lenses have flatter base curves.

Prescriptions with *large amounts of prism* end up being thicker. Lens thickness increases lens magnification and makes the eye look larger. This is especially true for plus lenses. Much of this magnification comes from a steep front curve. This means that magnification may be reduced by using a flatter base curve. As an added benefit, large prisms are easier to work with when produced on a somewhat lower base curve.

ASPHERICS

What Is an Aspheric Lens?

The term *aspheric* means "not spherical." The degree of curvature of a spheric lens is continuously uniform with a consistent radius of curvature throughout its entire surface, like that of a ball or sphere. An aspheric lens surface changes shape. It does not have the same radius of curvature over the entire surface. Aspherics are, generally speaking, based on a surface curvature that comes from a conic section. A conic section is a slice through a cone. There are 4 basic types of conic sections (Figure 18-12). These are:

1. *A circle:* A circle is the shape formed by a horizontal plane, or slice through an upright cone.
2. *An ellipse:* An ellipse is a shape formed by an angled plane through a cone that does not intersect the base of the cone.
3. *A parabola:* A parabola is a curve that is formed by the intersection of a cone with a plane having one side parallel to the side of the cone.
4. *A hyperbola:* A hyperbola is a shape formed when a cone is intersected by a plane that makes a greater angle with the base of the cone than the side of the cone makes with its base.

When these shapes are used as the shape for the front of a lens, they compare as shown in Figure 18-13.

The type of asphericity used on a lens surface is often classified by "*p*-values." *P*-values refer to the value p in the equation[8]:

$$y^2 = 2r_0x - px^2$$

This equation describes the conic sections referred to previously. The r_o value is the radius of curvature at the vertex of the conic section. Knowing the p value will differentiate the conic sections from each other, as shown in Box 18-3.

These were shown in Figure 18-13. Thus knowing the "p-value" of an aspheric surface helps to understand which type of asphericity is being used and how far the surface departs from a circular or spherical shape. For example, a surface having a p-value of −3.0 is a hyperbolic surface. This surface departs further from a spherical shape than one having a value of +0.5.

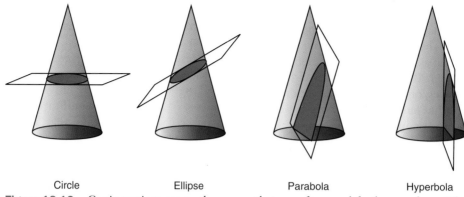

Circle   Ellipse   Parabola   Hyperbola

Figure 18-12. Conic sections create the curves that are often used for lens surfaces. The circle is used for spherically based lenses. The ellipse, parabola, and hyperbola are used for aspheric surfaces.

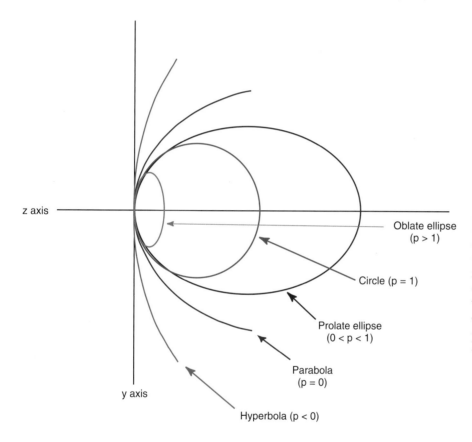

z axis

Oblate ellipse
(p > 1)

Circle (p = 1)

Prolate ellipse
(0 < p < 1)

Parabola
(p = 0)

y axis

Hyperbola (p < 0)

Figure 18-13. This figure shows how geometric conic sections could be used on front or back lens surfaces to produce different types of asphericity. The type of asphericity used on a surface may be classified by "*p*-values." *P*-values refer to the value p in the equation and describe the varying shaped conic sections referred to in Figure 18–12. Using a different approach it is also possible to classify asphericity by "Q-values," with Q being a measure of conicoid asphericity. Using Q-values, a circle has a value of zero compared with this system in which a circle is classified with a p-value of 1. (From Jalie M: Ophthalmic lenses & dispensing, ed 2, Boston, 2003, Butterworth-Heinemann.)

BOX 18-3

p-Values for Aspheric Surface Shapes

If the p-value is:		Then the type of aspheric surface will be:
p > 1	(p is greater than 1)	Oblate ellipse (The long axis of the ellipse is vertical)
p = 1	(p is equal to 1)	Circle
0 < p < 1	(p is between 0 and 1)	Prolate ellipse (The long axis of the ellipse is horizontal)
p = 0	(p is equal to 0)	Parabola
p < 0	(p is less than 0)	Hyperbola

One having a p-value of +0.50 is a prolate elliptical surface.

Aspheric surfaces have a changing radius of curvature and thus a varying amount of surface astigmatism everywhere except at the center of the lens surface. This means that it is possible to select a specific type of aspheric surface that will neutralize unwanted oblique astigmatism. For example, suppose we want to use a lens that has a considerably flatter base curve than normal. Just flattening the base curve on a spherically based lens will mean increased oblique astigmatism resulting in poor peripheral optics. Yet this flatter base can be used successfully if a type of aspheric surface that has a matching

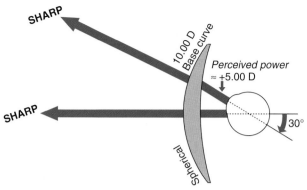

Figure 18-14. The normal base curve for a plano lens is +6.00 D. The +10.00 D front surface of this +5.00 D lens looks considerably steeper and causes more magnification. However, this spherical corrected curve lens will give sharp vision both centrally and peripherally. (From Meslin D: Varilux practice report no. 6: asphericity: what a confusing word!, Oldsmar, Fla, November, 1993, Varilux Press. Figure 1A. Courtesy Varilux Corp.)

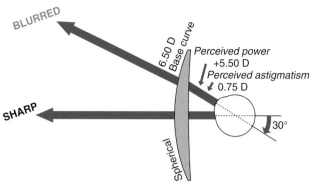

Figure 18-15. Flattening a +5.00 D lens from a +10.00 D spherical base curve lens back to a +6.50 makes it look more like a low-powered plus lens. With this flat curve, it is no longer optically sound. Even though the center may produce 20/20 vision, the periphery suffers from both power error and oblique astigmatism. (From Meslin D: Varilux practice report no. 6: asphericity: what a confusing word!, Oldsmar, Fla, November, 1993, Varilux Press. Figure 1B. Courtesy Varilux Corp.)

but counterbalancing amount of surface astigmatism is chosen.

Purposes for Using an Aspheric Design

There are at least five good reasons for producing a lens that has an aspheric surface.

1. The first reason is to be able to optically correct lens aberrations.
2. The second reason is to allow the lens to be made flatter, thereby reducing magnification and making it more attractive.
3. The third reason is to produce a thinner, lighter-weight lens.
4. A fourth reason may be to ensure a good, tight fit in the frame.
5. The fifth reason is to make a lens with progressive optics.

Asphericity for Optical Purposes

As stated earlier, for most powers, it is possible to produce a lens that is optically sound using regular, spherical surfaces. Once lens powers go beyond the +7.00 D to −23.00 D range, however, it is necessary to use an aspheric design.

In the middle, an aspheric lens surface starts out as any other spherical surface. Then at a certain distance from the OC, the lens surface gradually changes its curvature at a rate calculated to offset peripheral aberrations. (This concept will be discussed in greater depth in the section on high plus lenses later in the chapter.)

Asphericity for Flattening Purposes

For lenses with spherical base curves, higher plus power always results in steeper base curves (Figure 18-14). Unfortunately, for high plus lenses the steeper the base curve, the worse the lenses look. Choosing a flatter base

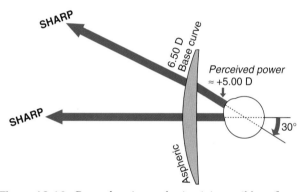

Figure 18-16. Properly using asphercs, it is possible to flatten a lens and still overcome peripheral aberrations. Here, this +5.00 D lens has been flattened to have a +6.50 front curve, yet because the front curve is aspheric, vision remains clear in the periphery. (From Meslin D: Varilux practice report no. 6: asphericity: what a confusing word! Oldsmar, Fla, November 1993, Varilux Press. Figure 1C. Courtesy Varilux Corp.)

curve will make the lens look less bulbous and also reduce magnification. Cosmetically the lens looks much better. It even looks considerably thinner than before, although in reality it is only slightly thinner. Because flat base curves reduce magnification, the wearer's eyes do not look as big.

Unfortunately, just flattening a regular lens results in bad optics. In the periphery, the sphere power will be off (because of power error), and there will be unwanted cylinder (because of oblique astigmatism) (Figure 18-15).

If the flattened lens surface is aspheric, it is possible to get both good cosmetics and good optics (Figure 18-16). Such a lens may even change the degree of asphericity when approaching the edge of the lens to further flatten the lens.

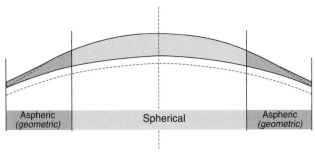

Figure 18-17. When using asphericity for the purpose of thinning a plus lens, the front surface is flattened to give the edge more thickness. For a plus lens, center thickness is limited by edge thickness. If edge thickness can be added with asphericity, then the whole lens can be thinned, and center thickness will be reduced. (Dotted lines show the shape of the unthinned, spherical lens.) (From Meslin D: Varilux practice report no. 6: asphericity: what a confusing word! Oldsmar, Fla, November 1993, Varilux Press. Figure 2A. Courtesy Varilux Corp.)

Another Reason for Flatter Base Curves

The steeper the base curve, the easier it is to dislodge the lens from a metal frame. So it is not unusual for a laboratory to flatten a base curve to make it fit more securely in the frame. Yet rather than flattening a regular lens, a better option is to use a flatter, aspherically designed lens.

Asphericity for Thinning Purposes (Geometric Asphericity)

Asphericity can be engineered with the express purpose of making the lens thinner. To do this for plus lenses, the lens front and back surface are flattened quite a bit toward the edge. Flattening the periphery makes it possible to grind the whole lens thinner (Figure 18-17). Of course there are several aspects for thinning lenses, often combined with one another. Figure 18-18 shows how lens thickness responds to a decrease in lens diameter, an increase in lens index, and a change to an aspheric design.

To thin minus lenses, either the peripheral portion of the lens front surface is steepened, or the peripheral portion of the back surface is flattened toward the periphery, or both. This reduces edge thickness (Figure 18-19).

To Ensure a Good, Tight Fit in the Frame

Most frames are made to best hold a lens with around a 6 D base curve. Using ordinary methods for edging lenses, the steeper the base curve is, the harder it is to keep the lens tight in the frame. Since a lens can be made closer to a 6 D base curve in an aspheric design without compromising peripheral vision, an aspheric design will help in ensuring that the lens stays in the frame.

Asphericity for Producing Progressive Power Changes

By definition, any lens surface that is not spheric is aspheric. Progressive addition lenses achieve their add

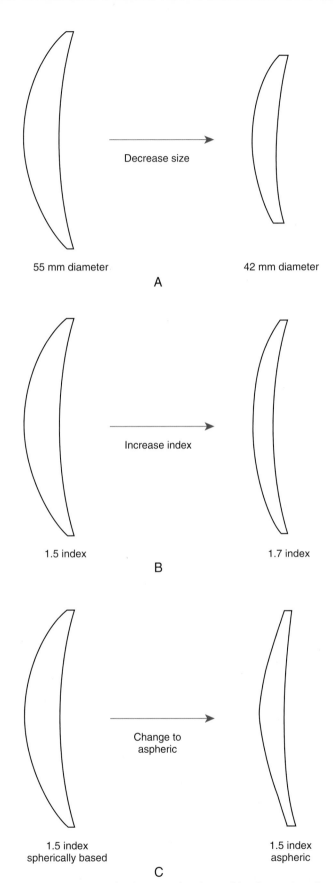

Figure 18-18. A plus lens may be thinned by decreasing the overall diameter of the lens (**A**), increasing the refractive index of the lens (**B**), and changing from a spherical surface to an aspheric surface (**C**).

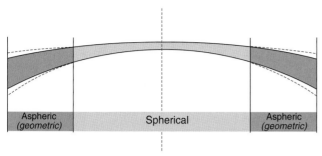

Figure 18-19. Asphericity can be used to thin the edge of a high minus lens. This is done by steepening the periphery of the front and/or flattening the periphery of the back curve. (From Meslin D: Varilux practice report no. 6: asphericity: what a confusing word! Oldsmar, Fla, November 1993, Varilux Press. Figure 2B. Courtesy Varilux Corp.)

power gain from a progressively steepening surface curvature. So progressive addition lenses are also aspheric lenses.

Most progressive addition lens designs continue to follow the same rules as spheric base curve lens designs. In other words, their distance portion will have the same base curve as one would expect for spherically based corrected curve lenses.

A progressive lens can also be made with a flatter base curve for the distance portion. To prevent unwanted aberrations, the front surface should be aspherically compensated as in any other nonprogressive aspheric lens. (As would be expected, the combined asphericities will become considerably more complex to design.)

ATORIC LENSES

A spherically based lens using a properly chosen base curve to create a corrected curve design can do a very good job of minimizing peripheral lens aberrations. So can an aspheric lens. In fact an aspheric lens is able to create a lens that has a flatter base curve and is often thinner and lighter while still maintaining corrected curve quality for reduction of aberrations.

Yet like the spherically based lens, the base curve and/or asphericity combination of an aspheric lens is designed for one specific lens power. The problem is when a lens corrects for astigmatism and introduces a cylinder component into the prescription, the lens has two powers. A lens with two curves on the same surface is called a *toric* lens. Which power will be used to determine the correct amount of asphericity? Choosing to correct one power means that correction for peripheral aberrations for the other power will be less than ideal. Usually a compromise power somewhere in between the two is chosen, with neither being optimum.

An aspheric lens changes the curvature of the surface in all directions equally. With two lens powers, the rate of change in surface curvature would have to be different for each power meridian. Changing the curvature at

different rates for each of the two meridians means that each rate of change can be optimized for the power in that meridian. When each meridian is optimized on a toric lens, the design is called an *atoric* lens. For a lens having cylinder power, an atoric design is able to expand the peripheral range of clearer vision beyond what is found for either a well-designed (best form) spherically based lens or an aspheric lens (Figure 18-20).

Atoric lenses should be recommended for all cylinder powers above 2.00 D, even when the spherical component of the prescription is low. They may also prove advantageous for anyone with cylinder power beyond 1.25 D. Fortunately, many of the newer high-index single vision series of lenses being marketed are now being made as an atoric series and not just aspheric.

Comparing the Construction of Spherically Based Lenses, Asphercis, and Atorics

Here is a quick and general comparison of the way single vision lenses are constructed for spherically based, aspheric, and atoric lenses.

Spherically based lenses
- For simple spheres (no cylinder), the front surface is spherical, and the back surface is also spherical.
- For spherocylinders, the front surface is spherical, and the back surface is toric.

Aspheric lenses
- In most cases, for simple spheres (no cylinder), the front surface is aspheric, and the back surface is spherical.
- For spherocylinders, the front surface is aspheric. The back is toric. It is not possible to correct both of the major meridians of a cylinder lens for aberrations when a lens is designed this way.

Atoric lenses
- There are both spheres and spherocylinders in a given lens series that use an atoric design. This means that in the case of spheres, the lens is really an aspheric. Technically it cannot be an atoric because it has no cylinder power.
- There are several ways atoric lenses can be made. It can be anticipated that the number of these possibilities will expand.
  1. A finished single vision lens with the front surface spherical and the back surface atoric.
  2. A semi-finished single vision lens with the front surface having the gradual changes in power associated with the lens atoricity. The back surface is the normal toric surface correcting for cylinder power. So the back surface takes care of the refractive power of the cylinder, whereas the front surface makes atoric changes for peripheral aberrations.
  3. A third category is an atoric design in conjunction with a progressive addition lens.

In the past, atorics had only been available in single vision lenses. Atorics had been out of the question with

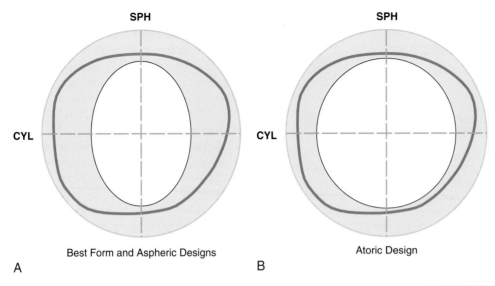

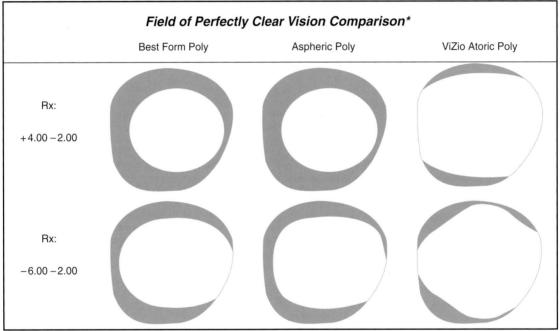

Figure 18-20. A, This is conceptual drawing showing the zone of optimum vision for a best form spheric or an aspheric spherocylinder lens when the design is optimized for the sphere power meridian. The cylinder power represented in this drawing is fairly high. Here the wider area produced by the sphere meridian happens to fall in the narrower vertical meridian because of cylinder axis orientation. **B,** In B an atoric lens allows the design to be optimized for both sphere and cylinder power meridians, resulting is a larger area of better vision. (Illustrations **A** and **B** courtesy of Darryl Meister, Carl Zeiss Vision.) **C,** Here is a comparison of the size of sharp, clear vision for three polycarbonate lenses in best form, aspheric, and atoric forms for two specific spherocylinder lens powers. There is little difference in peripheral lens clarity between the best form (corrected curve) spherically based lens and the aspheric design, assuming that both lenses are fit correctly. Because an atoric lens can correct peripheral aberrations for both astigmatic meridians independently, the atoric design is able to widen the peripheral area of sharp, clear vision. (From Meister D: ViZio the next generation of aspheric lenses, Sola optical publication #000–0139–10460, 10/98.)

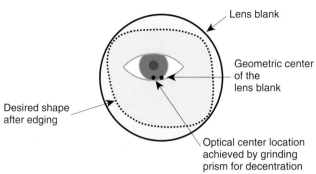

Lens blank

Geometric center
of the
lens blank

Desired shape
after edging

Optical center location
achieved by grinding
prism for decentration

Figure 18-21. When the unsurfaced, unedged lens blank is small or the frame is large, it may be necessary for the laboratory to move the OC away from the center of the lens blank. This is done by grinding prism in the center of the lens blank so that the OC will be properly placed after the lens has been edged.

multifocals and progressives. The segment or progressive zone of the lenses requires that the lenses be surfaced to prescription to correctly place the cylinder axis direction. The segment or progressive zone is already on the front of the lens. Since there was no practical way to grind and polish atoric optics onto the back side of the lens, atorics were only made in single vision lenses. Now "free-form" generating and polishing is making atorics available for an increasing number of newer custom progressive lens designs.

WORKING WITH ASPHERICS AND ATORICS

An Aspheric Design Prohibits Grinding Prism for Decentration

When a conventional (nonaspheric) single vision lens is surfaced, the laboratory can move the OC to any location on the lens. This is done by grinding prism for decentration and is especially helpful when using large frames. Grinding prism for decentration moves the OC away from the center of the lens blank. On a spherically based lens, the OC may be moved without creating any new optical problems (Figure 18-21). Decentration prism is helpful when the lens blank would otherwise be too small for the frame size.

But what will happen if the OC is moved away from the geometric center of an *aspheric* lens blank? If the OC of an aspheric lens is moved, the asphericity will be misplaced relative to the position of the eye (Figure 18-22). When the eye looks one way, it reaches the aspheric portion too soon. When it looks the other way, the aspheric area is not reached soon enough. In short the OC of an aspheric lens must remain locked to one position on the lens blank.

Rx Prism Still Works With Aspherics
Just because aspherics do not allow prism for decentration does not mean that aspherics cannot be used for prism prescriptions. They can be used with Rx prism. The prism must be ground in prism done in the surfac-

ing laboratory so that the correct amount of prism will be found at the center of the aspheric zone. A finished single vision lens cannot simply be decentered to create a prismatic effect as is done with normal spherically based lenses. Decentering a stock aspheric lens to create prism will mean that the wearer will no longer be looking through the middle of the aspheric zone.

Identifying a Lens As an Aspheric or Atoric Lens

When someone comes into the office already wearing glasses, it is helpful to know if the lenses being worn are aspheric lenses. It is not always easy to tell. Here are some possibilities for identifying an aspheric lens.

- *Use a lens clock:* By placing the three pins of a lens clock on the front surface of a lens and moving the lens clock sideways, it may be possible to identify some aspherics. If front surface lens power changes, the lens is aspheric. However, if the lens is edged and in the frame, it is not possible to move the lens clock very far. Therefore many, if not most aspherics may be missed.
- *Use a grid pattern:* View a grid pattern through a higher plus lens. Not seeing distortion of the grid may identify certain types of aspherics, but not all types.
- *Notice lens curvature:* Notice the flatness of the front (and back) curve compared with other lenses of equal powers. Of these first three suggestions for identifying the possibility of having an aspheric lens, this may be the best.
- *Look for identifying markings:* Fortunately, some manufacturers are putting identifying markings on the front surface of their lenses. This will allow the identification of a lens as being a specific brand of aspheric, much like the system used for identifying progressive addition lenses. Remember, however, that whereas progressive lens marks will appear along the 180-degree line, aspheric lens markings may appear in any lens meridian because of the lens being rotated during edging.

Why Dispensing Rules Take on Special Importance for Aspherics

A well-designed aspheric lens can produce excellent optical and cosmetic results. There is one thing that must be kept in mind, however. Aspheric lenses are not as forgiving of dispensing errors as regular lenses. If a regular lens is fit without adhering to all the proper fitting rules, vision may still be acceptable enough to produce a happy wearer. But if an aspheric lens is fit improperly, the lens can end up being optically worse than a regular spheric-based lens would have been.

Fitting Guidelines for Aspherics
Fitting rules for aspherics are really no different than careful fitting rules for any other lens. Remember to

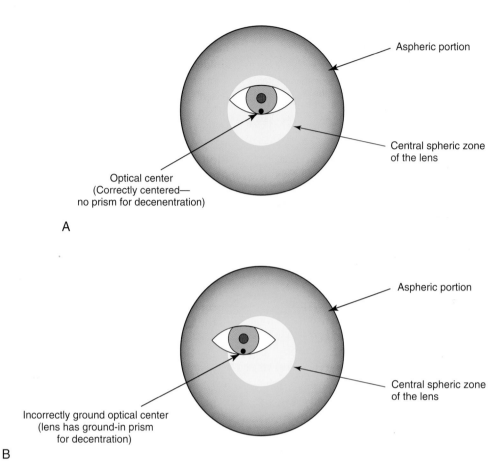

Aspheric portion

Central spheric zone
of the lens

Optical center
(Correctly centered—
no prism for decenentration)

A

Aspheric portion

Central spheric zone
of the lens

Incorrectly ground optical center
(lens has ground-in prism
for decentration)

B

Figure 18-22. A, An aspheric lens should always have the OC in the middle of the central, spheric portion of the lens. This way as the eye looks left and right, the lens is used as intended. If an aspheric lens is ground with prism for decentration as shown in **B,** the eye will run into aspheric changes too quickly in one direction and not quick enough in the other direction. (The eye is slightly above the OC to allow for pantoscopic tilt and reading.) NOTE: Do not confuse prism for decentration with prescribed (Rx) prism. Prism ground onto an aspheric lens as Rx prism is always acceptable.

always use monocular PDs, measure for MRP height, and use the correct amount of pantoscopic tilt.

Use Monocular Interpupillary Distances
The eye must be horizontally centered in the "concentric aspheric rings" of the lens. Taking monocular interpupillary distances will ensure that this happens.

Measure Major Reference Point Heights and Compensate for Pantoscopic Angle
First, measure MRP heights in the conventional manner (see Chapter 5). Then use the rule of thumb for tilt compensation (i.e., subtract 1 mm of MRP height for each 2 degrees of pantoscopic tilt). Aspheric areas concentrically surround the lens OC. Therefore do not move the MRP more than 5 mm below the pupil, even if the rule of thumb for tilt calls for more than 5 mm. Moving the MRP too far downward can cause the peripheral aspheric area to interfere with normal distance vision. Because the MRP should not be dropped more than 5 mm below the pupil, it is not advisable to

use more than 10 degrees of pantoscopic tilt with high-powered aspheric prescriptions.

Alternative Method for Determining Major Reference Point Height: Tilt the Head and Measure An alternative method for finding MRP height is to first tilt the wearer's head back until the frame front is perpendicular to the floor. Next measure MRP height with the subject's head tilted back. (If the frame has a large amount of pantoscopic tilt, remeasure height without tilting the head. The difference in measurement should not exceed 5 mm.) This head-tilt method should give the same results as compensating for pantoscopic tilt and is certainly easier. (See Chapter 5 for more details regarding MRP height.)

Caution: Some laboratories assume that the MRP height specified on the order form places the MRP in front of the eye. Since this is incorrect in the presence of pantoscopic tilt, some laboratories drop the MRP below the ordered amount to compensate for tilt. You will need to know how your laboratory is treating so-called MRP heights.

BOX 18-4

Fitting Guidelines for Aspherics

1. Use monocular interpupillary distances.
2. Measure major reference point heights in the conventional manner. Then subtract 1 mm for each 2 degrees of pantoscopic tilt. (The OC should not be more than 5 mm below the pupil.)
   Alternative method for finding major reference point height: First tilt the wearer's head back until the frame front is perpendicular to the floor. Next measure the major reference point height in this position. This alternative method should give the same results as compensating for pantoscopic tilt will give.
3. Remember that the laboratory cannot grind prism for decentration with aspheric lenses. Moving the OC away from the center of the aspheric zone will destroy any aspheric optical advantage.

The guidelines for fitting aspherics are summarized in Box 18-4.

Full Versus Nonfull Aspherics

When thinking of aspherics, we generally think of the lens surface radius of curvature changes as beginning nearly at the optical center of the lens. The changes start gradually and increase more rapidly as distance increases from the center of the lens. This type of aspheric lens is referred to as a *full aspheric* lens. Because changes start almost centrally, it is important to follow recommended fitting guidelines. If the eye in not correctly located in the aspheric configuration, this poor fitting can produce results worse than would be experienced if spherically based lenses were poorly fit.

To help reduce poor fitting problems, some aspheric lenses are designed with a spherical central area or *cap* that may vary in size depending upon who makes the lens. In this central area, the lens behaves like a spherically based lens. If the eye is not properly centered, the consequences are not supposed to be as noticeable. Such a lens is referred to as a *nonfull aspheric*.[9] Another advantage is that the lens may be able to be decentered for smaller amounts of prism without having as many adverse affects.

When to Recommend Aspherics and Atorics

For Plus Lens Wearers

For plus lenses, an aspheric may easily be recommended when the power goes above +3.00 D. However, opinions vary on when to recommend aspherics with beginning points ranging from +2.00 D to +4.00 D or even lower. Remember that as frame size increases, the amount of plus power needed before recommending an aspheric lens decreases. The larger the lens, the lower the power will be when aspheric lenses are recommended.

For Minus Lens Wearers

For a minus lens wearer, an aspheric may be recommended for powers above −3.00 D. The "minimum" lens power that is recommended continues to drop. Again differences as to what the lowest power is for recommending a minus aspheric will differ, depending upon frame size and wearer concerns. (Note: If a high-index aspheric is being used primarily to thin the lens, it is counterproductive to place such a lens in a frame with a small eye size and narrow vertical dimension if that frame is a nylon-cord frame. Nylon-cord frames need a minimum edge thickness to allow for grooving the edge. Such high-index lenses may have to be made thicker because of the frame.)

Aspherics Are Recommended for Anisometropia

When a person has a difference in power between the left and right eyes that is greater than 2.00 D, there will also be differences in magnification. Aspherics are normally flatter, thinner, and closer to the eyes and reduce magnification differences.

Other Possibilities for Using Aspherics

Aspherics can also be recommended for

- Children who are sensitive about how their glasses look;
- Contact lens wearers so they will not overwear their contacts to avoid wearing thick, ugly spectacle lenses; and
- Older wearers to decrease lens weight.

Adapting to Aspherics and Atorics

Changing base curve and lessening the amount of distortion a person experiences when switching from a spherically based lens to an aspheric or atoric would seem like a good thing. And it is. However, the person who has been wearing lenses that cause straight lines to appear curved has already made some adaptations. They have mentally been able to correct the distortions caused by the lens. Their mind straightens the optically distorted (curved) line and sees it as straight. Now when a new correcting lens no longer curves straight lines, the mind tries to compensate as before, and the world takes on an unfamiliar appearance. Until readaptation takes place, nothing looks right. Those being changed from conventional spherically based lenses into aspheric or atoric lenses should be warned about the adaptation time that will be necessary. Once a person is used to wearing aspherics and atorics, they find them much to their liking. (This is assuming that the lens has been carefully measured and fit.)

HIGH PLUS LENS DESIGNS

Before the advent of intraocular lens implants following cataract surgery, high plus lenses were common, and a number of high plus spectacle lens options were

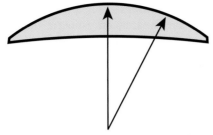

Figure 18-23. This lens has the same radius of curvature over the entire front surface of the lens. A "full-field" lens is one that is optically useable over the entire viewing area. There-fore technically, even this regular spherically based lens could be called a full-field lens.

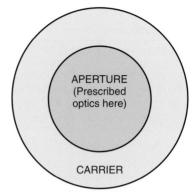

Figure 18-24. When a lenticular lens is viewed from the front, the optically useable central aperture is seen in the center of the outer carrier portion.

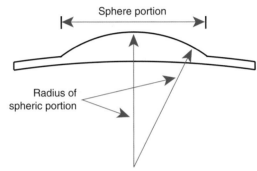

Figure 18-25. The cross section of a spheric lenticular lens shows that the optically useable central portion has the same radius of curvature across its entire surface. The outer carrier portion is considerably flatter.

developed. Many of these options are still available. Because high plus options are often thought of simply as "cataract lenses," they may not be used to full advantage. People who need a high plus correction and have never had cataract surgery are still candidates for these special lens designs.

Regular Spheric Lenses

It is possible to use a regular, spherically based lens for a high plus wearer, even though the optics are not as good. Sometimes these lenses are called "full-field lenses" to make them sound better. Actually, any lens that has the prescribed lens power over the whole viewing surface could be described as a full-field lens (Figure 18-23).

High-Index Aspheric

Whenever possible, it is best to use a high-index aspheric lens for high plus lens wearers. High index aspherics may not be available in some of the very highest plus powers.

Unfortunately, many of the specialty high plus lenses described in the next sections are only available in regular 1.498-index CR-39 lens material because these lenses were designed when CR-39 was the preponderant material.

Lenticulars

A lenticular lens is one that has a central area with the prescribed lens power surrounded by an outside area of little or no power. The central area is called the *aperture*, and the outer area is called the carrier (Figure 18-24). The lenticular style was developed for the purpose of thinning the lens. It is like a small, plus lens that is attached to a thin plano lens (Figure 18-25).

Lenticular lenses are available as either spheric or aspheric lenticulars. *Spheric lenticulars* look just like the lens shown in Figure 18-25. *Aspheric lenticulars* have an aspheric aperture. An aspheric lenticular can be thought of as a small, aspherically designed plus lens that has been placed on a near-plano carrier (Figure 18-26). Of the two lenticular designs, the aspheric lenticular is the better choice.

Advantages of a Lenticular Design
The main advantages of the lenticular design are weight reduction, thickness reduction, and, for aspheric lenticulars, good optics.

Disadvantages of a Lenticular Design
The main drawback to the lenticular design is looks. Even for small eye sizes, the edge of the aperture is usually visible. If the frame eye size is too large, the lens looks like the yolk of a fried egg.

The Development of High Plus Multidrop Lenses
The *Welsh 4-Drop* lens was developed in an effort to overcome the cosmetic negatives of the lenticular design while maintaining a thin lens. The Welsh 4-Drop had a back surface curve that was almost flat. The front surface of the lens had a 24-mm spherically based central area. Outside of that central area, the lens surface became aspheric and dropped in power, 1 diopter at a time, for a total of 4 diopters (Figure 18-27). For example, if the lens had a central base curve of +14.00, there were four outer concentric areas with powers of +13.00 D, +12.00 D, +11.00 D and +10.00 D. Each area blended into the other so that the changes in power were not visible.

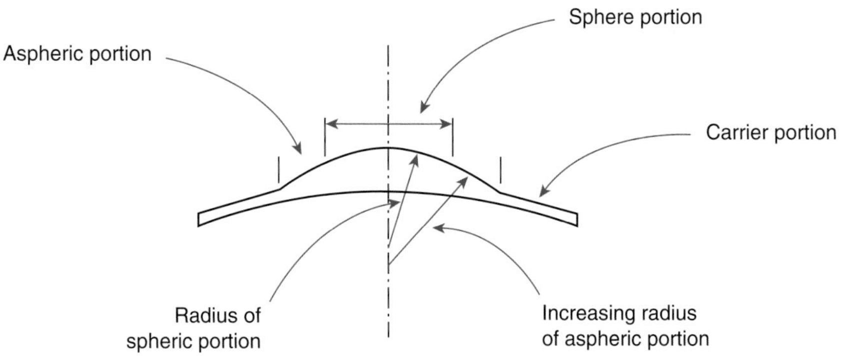

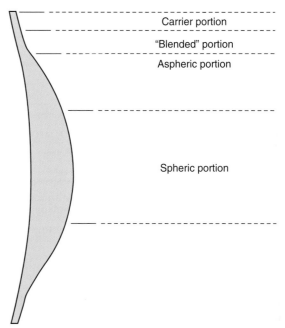

Figure 18-26. The cross section on an aspheric lenticular has a varying radius of curvature across the aperture. There is still an abrupt, visible demarcation between the central aperture and the carrier.

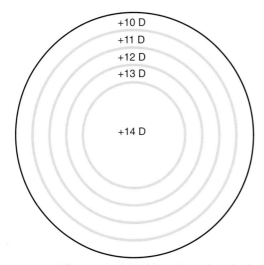

Figure 18-27. The original Welsh 4-Drop lens had a front surface that dropped 4 D from center to edge.

Figure 18-28. A multidrop lens can incorporate the advantages of optically sound aspherics for near-peripheral viewing, plus a fast-changing aspheric drop toward the edge resulting in what could almost be considered a blended aspheric lenticular.

The Welsh 4-Drop was a radical change over previous plus lens designs. The optics were less than ideal, but the lens was thin and better looking. The concept was picked up by competing lens companies and modified.

In the competing products, the concentric areas no longer changed as abruptly. The amount of aspheric drop was no longer limited to 4 D, regardless of base curve. The general category of lenses that emerged became known as *multidrop* lenses.

In the early stages of multidrop development, the issue of using aspherics to correct for aberrations instead of just for cosmetic and weight purposes had not yet been substantially addressed. Eventually, multidrop lenses were developed that more effectively took into account both peripheral aberrations and cosmetics. The central portion of the newer multidrop lens has an area that resembles the optics of an aspheric lenticular. Once outside of this more traditionally designed central area, the front surface suddenly flattens. The outer zone of the lens functions more like a carrier. In essence the lens resembles a large, blended aspheric lenticular (Figure 18-28).

HIGH MINUS LENS DESIGNS

Perhaps the greatest lens problem facing the high minus wearer is thick edges. This can be substantially addressed through appropriate frame selection. (For a review of frame selection for high minus wearers, see Chapter 4.)

Many of the options for high minus lenses discussed in the following sections may not be needed if the dispenser first applies traditional dispensing principles, such as small effective diameter sizes, high-index lenses, roll and polish, and antireflection coating. Yet if lens power is high enough, these measures may still prove insufficient. If this happens, a special high minus lens design is in order.

Lenticular Minus Designs

A lenticular design for a high minus lens uses the same idea as the lenticular design for high plus lenses. The

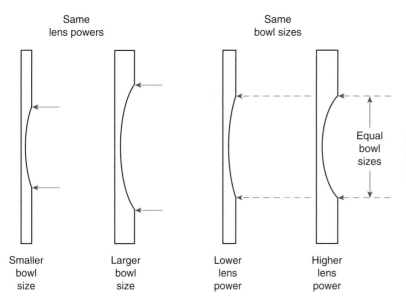

Same lens powers Same bowl sizes

Equal bowl sizes

Smaller bowl size | Larger bowl size | Lower lens power | Higher lens power

Figure 18-29. For a myodisc lens (having a plano carrier), edge thickness increases with both lens power and bowl size.

central area of the lens contains the prescribed refractive power of the lens. The peripheral (carrier) area serves only to extend the physical size of the lens without increasing its thickness.

Lenticular minus lenses can be found in several forms; one of which is the myodisc. It is important to remember that minus lenticular lens designs are not limited to one type of lens material and can be made of higher index material.

The Myodisc

According to the traditional definition, the myodisc design has a front surface that is either flat or almost flat. The front usually contains the cylinder component of the prescription. A myodisc also has a plano back carrier area. There is a high minus "bowl" in the middle of the back surface. (Originally, these lenses, made from glass, had a small 20- or 30-mm bowl size. Myodisc was a trade name.)

In a myodisc type of lens, the carrier is near plano. Therefore the thickness of the carrier portion is constant. The larger the bowl area is, the thicker the carrier will be. For lenses with the same-sized bowl areas, increases in lens power will mean an increase in carrier thickness (Figure 18-29).

Because the myodisc carrier is plano, as bowl size and/or lens power increases, edge thickness can become significant. It is conceivable to reduce edge thickness by using a different form of a minus lenticular design.

Minus Lenticular

A high minus lens with a lenticular design can be made so that the carrier is not plano. Several examples of minus lenticular lenses are shown in Figure 18-30.

If the back side of the carrier is made positive, as shown in Figure 18-31, B and D, the outer edge will thin down considerably. Often the laboratory makes this type

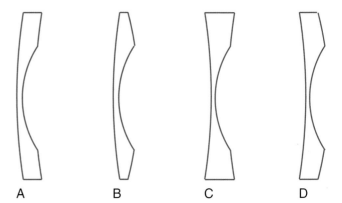

A   B   C   D

Figure 18-30. Minus lenticular lenses may be made in a variety of forms. Here are some examples. All have a high minus power in the central bowl area. The numbers are for illustration purposes only. **A,** A minus lenticular with a –2.00 D back carrier curve and a +2.00 D front curve. **B,** A minus lenticular with a +6.00 D back carrier curve and a +2.00 D front curve. The plus 6 back carrier helps to thin the lens edge. **C,** A minus lenticular with a –2.00 D back carrier curve and a –2.00 D front curve. The minus front curve increases the total minus power without having to make the back bowl curve even more concave. **D,** A minus lenticular with a +6.00 D back carrier curve and a –6.00 D front curve. Again the plus back carrier helps to thin the lens edge. It would be possible to put a higher plus carrier curve on the back of the lens to obtain more edge thinning.

of lens by beginning with a semifinished lens that has a plus six or greater front curve. The minus bowl is ground into the "front" of the semifinished lens. This will become the back of the minus lenticular lens. The cylinder and remaining power is ground onto what will become the front of the lens.

REFERENCES

1. Bruneni JL: The fine art of aspherics, Eyecare Business 56-62, 2000.

2. Bruneni JL: The evolution continues: a review of current aspheric technology, LabTalk, 27, 1999.
3. Meslin D, Obrecht G: Effect of chromatic dispersion of a lens on visual acuity, Am J Optom Physiol Opt 65:27, 1988.
4. Keating MP: Geometric, physical and visual optics, ed 2, Boston, 1988, Butterworth-Heinemann.
5. Yoho A: Curve control, Eyecare Business 28, 2005.
6. Meister D, Sheedy JE: Introduction to ophthalmic optics, Petaluma, Calif, 2002, Sola Optical.
7. Borover WA: Opticianry: the practice and the art in the science of opticianry, vol 2, Chula Vista, Calif, 1982, Gracie Enterprises.
8. Jalie M: Ophthalmic lenses & dispensing, ed 2, Boston, 2003 Butterworth-Heinemann.
9. Bruneni J: The evolution continues: a review of current aspheric technology, LabTalk 24-27, September 1999.
10. Liang J, Williams DR, Aberrations and retinal image quality of the normal human eye, J. Opt. Soc. Am. Vol. 14, No. 11, November 1997, p. 2879.

Proficiency Test

(Answers can be found in the back of the book.)

1. One of the factors that causes chromatic aberration to become a problem is:
   a. the additional monochromatic aberrations that are brought on by poor fitting techniques.
   b. the presence of oblique cylinder in the prescription.
   c. antireflection coating a lens that has a low Abbé value.

2. True or false? Chromatic aberration may be irritating, but it does not reduce the visual acuity when the wearer looks through the periphery of the lens, regardless of lens power.

3. Which other aberration has a resemblance to spherical aberration, but is manifested when the object is in an off-axis position?

4. You read about a new lens. The lens has an Abbé number of 22. What does this tell you?
   a. The lens will be lighter in weight than most.
   b. The lens will have more chromatic aberration than most.
   c. The lens will be heavier than most.
   d. The lens will have less chromatic aberration than most.
   e. The Abbé number has nothing to do with either weight or chromatic aberration.

5. Tscherning's Ellipse shows lens design possibilities for:
   a. choosing the overall best lens design when working with spherical lenses.
   b. choosing a Percival form lens.
   c. choosing a Point Focal lens.
   d. choosing a corrected curve lens.
   e. none of the above.

6. What two parameters are plotted by Tscherning's Ellipse?

7. A Tscherning's ellipse:
   a. is the same size, regardless of working distance.
   b. shows that oblique astigmatism can be brought to zero for distance viewing by using specific sphere curves between the approximate powers of +7.00 and −23.00 D.
   c. shows the one lens form per given lens power, which corrects oblique astigmatism.

8. A corrected curve lens is:
   a. one which corrects for oblique astigmatism.
   b. one which corrects for curvature of field.
   c. one which attempts to reduce both oblique astigmatism and curvature of field.
   d. All of the above are correct responses.
   e. None of the above are correct responses.

9. Of the following base curves, which is the best choice to create −10.00 D sphere?
   a. +6.00 D
   b. plano
   c. +8.00 D
   d. +4.00 D

10. When lens base curves are properly selected, the further from plano the lens power goes in the plus direction, the _____ the *back* curve of the lens becomes.
    a. steeper (more concave).
    b. flatter (less concave).

    For each of the following lens powers (Questions 11 to 18), use Vogel's formula to find the approximate base curve. (Do not round off your answers.)

11. +3.00 D sph

12. +4.50 −1.50 × 025

13. +2.00 −0.50 × 175

14. −4.00 D sph

15. −1.00 −1.00 × 090

16. −2.75 −0.75 × 075

17. −2.75 −2.75 × 160

18. −5.25 −1.50 × 015

19. True or false? High plus aspheric lenses with flat-top bifocal segments have a fixed seg drop and inset that the prescriber cannot change.

20. What are the possible reasons for using an aspheric lens design for a wearer whose distance Rx is +3.75 D? (There may be more than one correct response.)
    a. to produce a thinner lens
    b. to produce a lighter weight lens
    c. to produce a flatter base curve
    d. to produce a lens that results in a better visual acuity through the center of the lens than a spherically based lens of the same power

21. For a myodisc, the thickness of the carrier portion increases with:
    a. a decrease in bowl diameter.
    b. an increase in bowl diameter.
    c. an increase in minus lens power when there is no change in bowl size.
    d. a decrease in minus lens power when there is no change in bowl size.

22. The outermost area of a lenticular lens is called the:
    a. aperture.
    b. closure.
    c. carrier.
    d. cortex.
    e. none of the above

23. Compared with a spheric design, which lens design may result in a thinner lens?
    a. a lenticular design
    b. an aspheric design
    c. neither a lenticular nor an aspheric design
    d. both a lenticular and an aspheric design

24. True or false? All lenticular lenses have an aspheric central portion.

25. True or false? The center thickness of a lenticular lens will vary according to the effective diameter and decentration of the lens.

CHAPTER **19**

Segmented Multifocal Lenses

Most spectacle lenses correct for just one distance. These are called *single vision lenses*. Yet a person's visual needs may require different lens powers for different distances. These needs can be met by changing the power in one or more areas of a lens.

MULTIFOCAL LENSES

Multifocal lenses meet the wearer's needs for focusing light at more than one, or *multi*ple distances. Originally all multifocal lenses had visible segments. There were no progressive addition lenses with gradually changing powers hidden from view. To help distinguish multifocal lenses with progressive optics from multifocal lenses with distinctly different powers in sharply demarcated areas of the lens, the lenses with visible segments may be referred to as *segmented multifocals*.

The Concept of a Near Addition

The crystalline lens within the eye becomes nonelastic as a result of the aging process. This condition is called *presbyopia*. Because of presbyopia, a person becomes unable to see clearly at close range, regardless of how well vision is corrected for distance. To see clearly at near, the wearer needs additional plus lens power.

Suppose a person has no need for correction of distance vision. If no distance correction is required, the only factor to be considered is the necessary plus lens power to see clearly at near. The amount of plus power needed for near vision is +2.00 D. This can be given in the form of a regular, single vision lens having the same +2.00 D power over the whole lens. It can also be given as a lens with no power in the main portion of the lens, but with a small area of plus power in the lower portion of the lens, as shown in Figure 19-1. This is the concept of a bifocal lens.

However, if the wearer does have a correction for distance, the extra required power for near must be "added on" to the power found in the distance prescription already being worn; hence the term *near addition*. The near addition is the same as a small plus lens placed in the lower portion of the lens. For that reason, it is often referred to as the *near segment* or, in abbreviated form, the *seg*. The net power resulting from the combination of the distance power and the add power is termed the *near power*, or *near Rx*.

An example of how the power of the near addition is written in prescription form is:

> O.D. +3.25 D sph
> O.S. +3.25 D sph
> Add +2.00 D

By this it is understood that both lenses are to contain a near segment whose power of +2.00 D adds that much more plus power to that part of the lens.

In the above example, since an addition is made to the distance power, the measured power through the distance portion of the right lens is +3.25 D sphere, and the measured power through the near portion is +5.25 D sphere (Figure 19-2). In simplified terms, if the near object is at the focal point of the near addition "lens," the add allows incoming light to enter the distance lens as if it were coming from a distant object. This way light focuses at the same point as it does for distance vision (Figure 19-3).

To go one step further, consider an example of a lens that has both sphere and cylinder power. If a lens has a distance power of +2.00 −0.75 × 180 with a +2.00 D add, then the actual measured power through the near portion will be +4.00 −0.75 × 180. This may be explained with two power crosses, as shown in Figure 19-4. When both meridians are added together, the total near power still contains the same cylinder power. Regardless of whether the distance portion is plus or minus in power, the near portion is still the algebraic sum of distance power and near add.

Example **19-1**

The distance portion of a lens is a −2.50 D sphere. The near add power is +2.50 D. What is the near power through the segment portion?

Solution

Since the total near power is calculated as:

(distance power) + (near addition) = (near power)

431

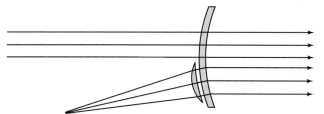

Figure 19-1. A bifocal segment is a small plus lens positioned on a lens that normally corrects for distance vision. Here the bifocal is placed on a lens that has no power in the distance portion.

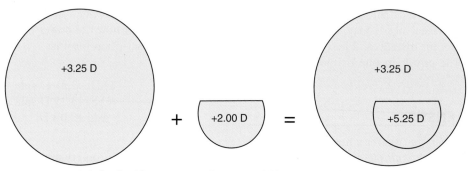

Figure 19-2. A bifocal addition is just that—an addition to the distance power. Here the distance power of +3.25 D is supplemented with a +2.00 D add for near viewing. The total power at near is +5.25 D. The +5.25 D power is the power that would be used in a pair of single vision lenses intended to be used only for reading.

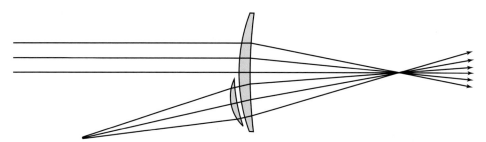

Figure 19-3. A plus lens with a bifocal near addition.

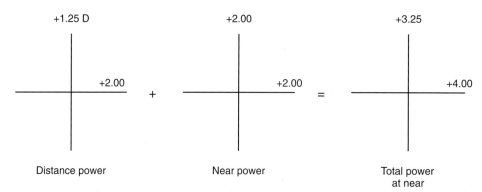

Figure 19-4. The near portion of a lens having an add of +2.00 D does not necessarily manifest a +2.00 D power, but rather will be the sum of the distance power and near addition combined.

then

$$(-2.50) + (+2.50) = 0.00$$

The total power through the bifocal will be zero. Looking at the near power this way for people with lower minus-powered distance prescriptions makes it easier to understand why they are not enthusiastic about going into multifocals. They can do very well just removing their glasses.

The Trifocal Intermediate

Some lenses have an intermediate area between distance and near portions. This area is used for viewing objects that are not at the normal reading distance. Yet what is being looked at is close enough to make clear vision through the distance portion impossible. The solution for these situations when using segmented multifocal lenses is a *trifocal* (Figure 19-5).

In trifocals the power of the intermediate portion is normally one half that of the prescribed near add. It is expressed as a percent. Normally the intermediate portion will be 50% of the near add. Lenses for special intermediate viewing distances may also be obtained having intermediate powers of 61% of the near addition.

To calculate the expected power through the intermediate portion of a trifocal lens, first the prescribed trifocal percent of the near add is found. For example, a lens having a +2.50 D add has an intermediate power that is +1.25 D greater than the distance power. Since +1.25 D is half of +2.50, the lens has an intermediate power of 50%. This +1.25 D intermediate add value is added to the distance power to find the expected total intermediate power as measured in the lensmeter.

When to Use a Trifocal

Eyes that still have a limited ability to focus and only require additions of +1.50 D or less will have clear vision in all areas of viewing. When looking through the upper (distance) part of the lens, the eye can focus on objects at an intermediate distance by using its own focusing ability. This eliminates the need for an intermediate trifocal area. For this reason, most trifocals are not available in add powers below +1.50.

After the add power increases above +1.50, there will be intermediate areas of vision that are not clear through either the distance portion or the near portion of a normal bifocal. To see these areas clearly, the wearer will either have to look through the upper part of the lens and back away from the object, or look through the lower bifocal part of the lens and move closer. A trifocal intermediate will furnish clear vision at this previously blurred in-between distance. (A progressive addition lens will solve this problem as well. For more information on progressive addition lenses, see Chapter 20.)

Terminology

Bifocals are available in a wide variety of segment shapes and sizes from small, round segs to segs that occupy the entire lower half of the spectacle lens. Their size and locations are quantified by means of a few standardized terms.

The size of a seg horizontally, or *seg width*, is measured across the widest section of the segment area (Figure 19-6). If part of the segment area has been cut away in edging the lens for the frame, the dimension is still considered to be the widest portion that the segment had before edging.

The longest vertical dimension of the seg is the *seg depth*. *Seg height* is dependent on the frame for which the

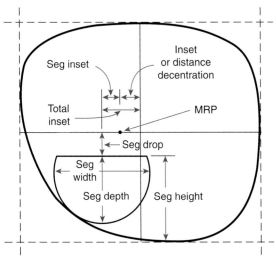

Figure 19-6. The *major reference point (MRP)* of a lens is positioned in the same vertical plane as the pupil and a few millimeters below it. If no prescribed prism is present in the prescription, the MRP and the optical center of the lens are one and the same point. (When prescribed prism is present in the distance portion, the optical center is no longer in the same location as the MRP.) The amount the MRP is moved laterally from the geometric center of the lens is the *inset* or *outset* (also referred to as *distance decentration*). The additional amount the center of the near segment is moved inward from the MRP is the *seg inset*. The inset plus the seg inset is known as *total inset* (or *total seg inset*).

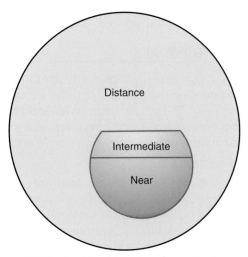

Figure 19-5. A trifocal lens has three viewing areas.

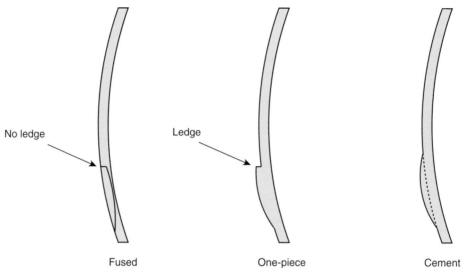

No ledge   Ledge

Fused   One-piece   Cement

Figure 19-7. A fused segment lens as shown on the left is made using glass that has a higher index of refraction in the segment than in the main part of the lens. One-piece lenses have a ledge that can be felt and may be made from almost any lens material. Cement segs are made by gluing a single vision distance lens and a small, segment-sized lens together.

lenses have been edged and is measured vertically from the lowest point on the lens to the level of the top of the seg (see Chapter 5). *Seg drop* is the vertical distance between the major reference point (MRP) of the lens and the top of the seg.

The distance portion of the lens must be decentered from the geometric center of the lens opening of the frame to correspond to the wearer's interpupillary distance (PD). This is referred to as *inset* or *outset*. The segment must be further decentered to correspond to the near PD. This seg decentration is referred to as *seg inset*.

Inset (or outset) + seg inset = *total inset*

(Outset would be written as a negative number.)

How Multifocals Are Constructed

Bifocals and trifocals are usually constructed in three main ways: fused, one piece, and cemented (shown in cross section in Figure 19-7).
1. *Fused*—Fused multifocals are available only in glass. The segment of the lens is made from glass having a higher refractive index than that of the distance "carrier" lens.* A fused glass bifocal has no ledge or change of curvature on the front. The segment cannot be felt because it is fused into the distance portion.
2. *One piece*—One-piece multifocals are made from one lens material. Any change in power in the segment portion of the lens is due to a change in the surface curvature of the lens. One-piece multifocals can be

identified by feeling the segment border. If either a ledge or a change in curvature is felt, the lens is not fused and is most likely a one-piece design.

One-piece multifocals may be made from any lens material. All plastic lenses are made as one-piece multifocals. One-piece glass multifocals are usually either the full-segment Franklin-style lens with the near portion occupying the entire lower portion of the lens, or they are large round-segment lenses.
3. *Cement lenses*—Cement lenses are custom-made lenses that have a small segment glued onto the distance lens. Used only for specialized custom purposes, such lenses are usually in the form of small, round segments.

Another occasionally used segmented lens is one that is actually two lens sections glued together. The upper half is a distance lens, and the lower half is a near lens. Both are cut in half, and half of each is used. The most common application for such lenses is for creating horizontal prism in the near portion only.

TYPES OF BIFOCALS

There are a few major groupings of bifocal segment styles, but many variations within those styles (Figure 19-8 and Table 19-1). The basic styles include round segments, flat-top segments, curve-top and panoptik segments, and Franklin- or Executive-style segments.

Round Segments

Round segments vary in size from a small lens of 22 mm up to the largest, 40 mm. The most common size is 22 mm. For large, round seg sizes, 38 mm may be occasionally used. Logically the optical center (OC) of a round segment is always at the center of the segment. The round segment lens is a versatile lens because the

---

*The distance lens is denoted the "carrier" lens because it is the portion to which the multifocal segment is attached. The segment is carried by the distance portion.

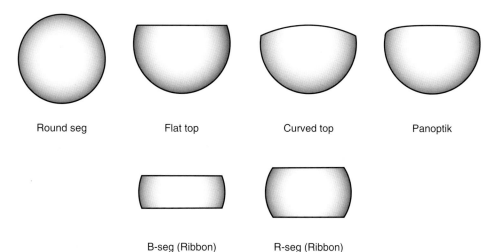

Round seg   Flat top   Curved top   Panoptik

B-seg (Ribbon)   R-seg (Ribbon)

Figure 19-8. A sampling of available bifocal segment types.

round segment can be rotated and still not look tilted. It can also be positioned at odd locations on the lens, such as in the upper temporal corner of a golfer's right lens. (Assuming, of course, that the golfer is right-handed.) This keeps the segment out of the golfer's way and still allows access to a near add for score card marking and reading.

Blended bifocals are round-segment bifocals with the border smoothed out to keep the segment from being seen.

Flat-Top Segments

Flat-top segments are basically round segments with the top cut off. The top is generally "cut off" 4.5 to 5.0 mm above the center of the segment. Stated another way, the segment OC is about 5 mm below the seg line. This allows the lens segment to have maximum reading width where a person will be reading. Very wide flat tops have the segment OC on the line. Flat tops are also known as *D segs*.

Flat tops are the mainstay of lined multifocal lenses. Segment sizes range from 22 up to 45 mm. Most flat tops used now are 28 mm or greater.

Curve-Top and Panoptik Segments

Curve-top segments look similar to flat tops, except that the upper line is arched, rather than flat. There is a distinct point on either corner. The top of panoptik segments are curved as well, but the corners are rounded.

Ribbon Segments

Ribbon segments are basically round segments with the top *and* bottom cut off. There are two types: a B and an R segment. The B is only 9 mm deep and is good for someone who must be able to have distance vision below the bifocal area. Some remember the letter and function by identifying "B" with *bricklayer*. Bricklayers often work in high places and can appreciate the ability to look below the segment and have clear distance vision.

The R segment has a 14 mm depth. It is seldom used as a regular bifocal lens. The R-segment bifocal is the same lens that is modified to create the "compensated 'R'" segment pairs that may occasionally be used for the correction of vertical imbalance.

Both B and R segments have their segment optical centers in the middle of the segment. Ribbon segments are available only in glass.

Franklin-Style (Executive) Segments

Franklin-style lenses are more commonly known by the trade name, *Executive*. It is a one-piece lens with the segment extending the full width of the lens. The lens has the advantage of a very wide near-viewing area.

There are some disadvantages to this lens. As the add power increases, the segment ledge gets bigger and more unsightly. Because the thickness of the lens is dependent on the near power rather than the distance power, the whole lens is thicker than a flat top would be. Thickness also increases with each increase in add power, making the lens progressively heavier. (It is possible to thin the lens by using yoked base-down prism. This principle is used for progressive addition lenses and is explained in Chapter 20.)

The Franklin-style bifocal has the segment OC on the segment line. For this reason, some have referred to these lenses as "monocentric" bifocals. However, a monocentric bifocal is one where the distance and segment OCs occupy exactly the same spot on the lens. It *is* possible for an Executive lens to be monocentric, but only if the lens is surfaced so that the distance OC is on the bifocal line at the same location where the segment optical center is found. This would not be expected to happen using today's surfacing practices.

If Executive lenses are used, it is important to avoid large eye sizes and large effective diameters. A better alternative to the Franklin-style lens for someone desiring a large bifocal reading area is a large flat-top lens,

TABLE **19-1**
Bifocal Lenses

General Style	Segment Name	Segment Width (mm)	Location of Seg OC (mm)	Comments
Flat-top	FT, straight-top (ST), or D style segment	22 25 28 35 40 45	5 below 5 below 5 below 4.5 below On line On line	The flat top is the most commonly used bifocal style.
Curve-top	CT	22 25 28 40	4.5 below	This lens is basically the same design as a flat-top segment, except that the upper seg line is curved.
Panoptik	P style	24 28	4.5 below	Panoptiks are a further variation of the curved-top segments, except that the top is flatter and the corners are rounded.
Ribbon	B-seg	22 or 25 wide 9 deep	4.5 below	A ribbon seg is similar to a flat-top segment, except both top and bottom are flat.
	R-seg	22 or 25 wide 14 deep	7 below Seg OCs are centered.	
Franklin	Executive E-Line Full Seg	Full lens width	On line	The top of the segment is a straight line that transverses the whole lens. The segment occupies the whole bottom half of the lens.
Round	Round seg	22 24 25	Seg OCs are centered.	A 22-mm round segment is often called a "Kryptok." In actuality, a Kryptok applies only to an inexpensive fused glass segment.
	A style	38		Large round segments are one-piece designs in either glass or plastic. A 38-mm A-style seg is semicircular because the blank is cut through the center of the seg. This means the maximum height of the seg can only be 19 mm.
	AA or AL R-40 style	38 40		The AA, AL, or R-40 segs are not semicircles, but almost a full circle. For this reason, they can be used if a round segment with a higher seg height is needed. One-piece round-segment glass or plastic lenses are sometimes called "Ultex" lenses. Ultex is a trade name for one-piece round segment multifocals.
	Blended bifocals (Invisible segs)	22 25 28	Seg OCs are centered.	A blended segment is a one-piece round segment with the line smoothed away.
	Rede-Rite (Minus Add Upcurve)	38	Seg OC is centered.	A semicircular upcurve design with the near power located in the main lens and the distance power in the "add," which is located at the top of the lens. It is often called a "minus add" lens. The entire lower area is for near work.

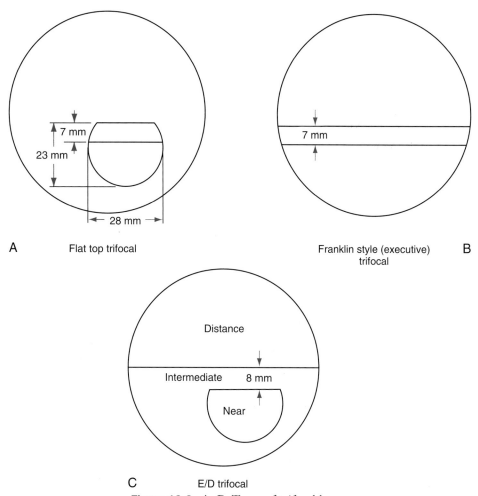

<table>
</table>

A Flat top trifocal

Franklin style (executive) trifocal **B**

C E/D trifocal

Figure 19-9. A-C, Types of trifocal lenses.

TABLE **19-2**
Trifocal Lenses

General Style	Segment Name	Segment Dimensions (mm)	Comments
Flat-top		7 × 25 7 × 28 7 × 35	The first number in the segment designation refers to the depth of the intermediate; the second number refers to the width of the segment. Lenses with segments having especially deep intermediate areas are more like occupational lenses and are found listed as occupational lenses.
Franklin	(Executive)	7-mm intermediate	
E over D	E/D Trifocal	Full width intermediate, D 25 style near.	The intermediate is 8 mm deep and extends around the near "D" seg, which is 25 mm wide.

such as a flat-top 35. A large flat top will reduce weight and thickness, but still allow as wide a near field of view.

TYPES OF TRIFOCAL LENSES

Most bifocal styles are also available in a corresponding trifocal style. Trifocals offer the convenience of intermediate vision in a moderately large field of view (Figure 19-9 and Table 19-2).

Flat-Top Trifocals

Flat-top trifocals come with intermediate sections that vary in width from 22 mm to 35 mm and in depth from 6 mm to 14 mm (see Figure 19-9, *A*).

Any trifocal that has a depth of more than 8 mm should not be considered an all time–wear lens. Such lenses are better for occupational situations requiring a large intermediate working area. Trifocals are also available with intermediate powers other than the standard 50% intermediate.

Franklin (Executive) Trifocals

The Executive, or Franklin-style, lens is a full-width segment lens with a 7-mm full-width intermediate (see Figure 19-9, *B*). It suffers from the same problems as the Franklin-style bifocal lens and because of the very visible twin ledges, loudly announces the wearer's need for an age-related lens correction.

The E/D Trifocal

The E/D trifocal combines the characteristics of the Executive-type lens with a 25-mm *D* (flat-top) segment (see Figure 19-9, *C*). It is constructed with a full, wide line across the lens dividing the distance portion from the intermediate portion and looks just like an Executive lens trifocal line. A flat-top segment is also placed in this lower, intermediate-powered portion. This is the segment needed for the near-working distance.

The lens is an excellent segmented lens for working at a desk. Intermediate viewing is available not only in the area 8 mm above the near seg, but also on either side of the near segment. This gives clear vision for wide, arm's-length working areas in every direction.

OCCUPATIONAL MULTIFOCALS

Any lens that is chosen by careful forethought and positioned for a specialized viewing situation may be classified as an occupational lens. However, there are certain lens styles that are specifically designed with certain work circumstances in mind. These lenses are called *occupational multifocals* (Figure 19-10 and Table 19-3). The following three sections discuss those available at the time of this writing.

Double-Segment Lenses

Some people require intermediate or near viewing while looking upward, including plumbers, pharmacists, librarians, electricians, auto mechanics, and many others in specialized working situations. Double-segment lenses were developed with these types of individuals in mind. Double-segment lenses have a segment in the normal position and a second segment at the top of the lens (see Figure 19-10, *A*). The two segments are normally separated by a 13-mm or 14-mm vertical distance (see Table 19-3 for more detailed information).

Double-segment lenses are underused. There are a great many people who would benefit from being able to see at close range just by looking up through an upper segment area. Instead they are required to tilt their head back in a very uncomfortable position for long periods of time because no one has told them that there is a lens that could solve their neck problems.

The upper segment comes in a variety of power possibilities. These include:

1. An upper segment that is identical in power to the lower segment.
2. An upper segment with a power that is ½ D less than the lower segment power.
3. An upper segment that is a given percentage of the lower segment, such as 50% or 60%, much like a trifocal.

The right way to decide which segment is most appropriate is to recreate the wearer's working situation, measure the working distances, and determine what the upper power should be. Once that has been done, choose the lens that fulfills the prescribed power needs. (For information on how to measure segment heights for double-segment lenses, see Chapter 5.)

Double-segment lenses are most commonly seen as flat tops, such as the double D.

The *quadrafocal* lens is a double-segment lens with a flat-top trifocal on the bottom and an upside-down flat-

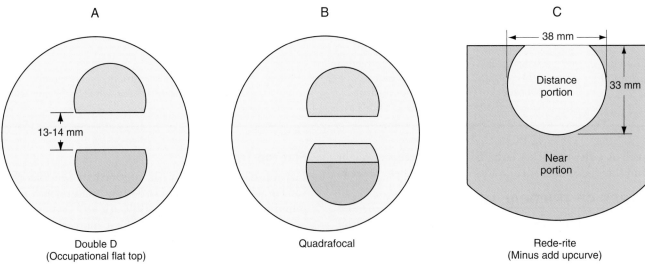

A	B	C
13-14 mm		38 mm / Distance portion / 33 mm / Near portion
Double D (Occupational flat top)	Quadrafocal	Rede-rite (Minus add upcurve)

Figure 19-10. Three types of occupational multifocals.

TABLE **19-3**
Occupational Lenses

General Style	Segment Name	Segment Dimensions (mm)	Comments
Double Segment	Occupational flat top or "double D"	22/22 25/25 28/28 28/25 35/35	Lower segment same as flat top. Upper segment same as upside-down flat top. Segments are normally 13-14 mm apart but may range from 12-15 mm for special orders in glass. The upper segment add power may be a. The full value of the add, like the lower seg. b. One-half diopter less than the lower seg add power. c. A percentage of the full add power such as 60% or 50%.
	Double round	22/22 25/25	Segments are normally 13 or 14 mm apart. For glass, factory orders can be made for seg separations of from 11 to 20 mm apart.
	Double executive	Full segment	
	Quadrafocal	7 × 22 (22 upper) 7 × 25 (25 upper) 7 × 28 (28 upper)	Has a flat-top trifocal below and an upside-down flat-top bifocal above. Available only in glass. Segment separation: 10 mm and 13 mm. With special orders with segment separation varying from 9 mm to 20 mm are available.
Occupational Trifocals	Flat top	8 × 35 9 × 35 10 × 35 8 × 34 10 × 35 12 × 35	These wide-intermediate trifocals have 50% intermediate powers. These trifocal lenses have deep intermediate segment areas combined with 61% intermediate powers.
Round bifocal segs	Custom segment sizes	7-25	It is possible to get custom sizes in glass. Round segments, from 7 mm up to 25 mm are available on special order
Progressive Add Lenses			For occupational progressive lenses, see Chapter 20.

top segment on the top (see Figure 19-10, *B*). It is appropriate for those who have need of both a trifocal and a double-segment lens. Since "quad" means four, the lens takes its name from the four distinct viewing areas. This lens is only available in glass.

The Minus Add "Rede-Rite" Bifocal

The *Rede-Rite* bifocal is a lens with a long history. It is a so-called upcurve bifocal because it has a large round segment at the top (see Figure 19-10, *C*), most of which is cut off after edging. This leaves the upper edge of the lower portion in the form of a circle that curves upward; hence, the term *upcurve*. It is a minus add, which means that the segment at the top has more minus power than the rest of the lens. In reality the lens is a bifocal with a huge add area at the bottom and a small distance-viewing area at the top. It is a lens for people who want a segmented lens and need a full, near-working area. But they still want to see clearly in the distance without taking their glasses off.

More versatile alternatives are progressive add lenses that have wide near portions but also give clear, wide vision in the intermediate. Two such lenses are the AO Technica and the Hoya Tact. The Technica has a small distance portion located in the same place as that of the

Rede-Rite. (For more information on these occupational progressives, see Chapter 20.)

ORDERING THE CORRECT LENS POWER FOR READING GLASSES

When a spectacle lens prescription is written with an add power, it is often written before a decision is made on what type of lenses are to be used. This means that the prescription may have to be written in a different form when ordered so that the same optical effect is maintained. For example, if an individual wants reading glasses only, the order form will not be written with an add, but will be written for single vision lenses.

Example **19-2**

A prescription is written as follows:

$$+0.25 \ -0.50 \times 180$$
$$+0.25 \ -0.50 \times 180$$
$$\text{Add: } +1.50$$

The wearer decides they do not want anything but single vision reading glasses. What power would be ordered?

Solution

The power ordered for reading must be the same as would be found through the bifocal segment. Earlier in this chapter, we stated that:

(distance power) + (near addition) = (near power)

Since reading glasses must be made for the near power, in this example, the near power is figured by adding the add power to the sphere power of the distance prescription.

$$\begin{array}{r} +0.25 -0.50 \times 180 \\ +1.50 \\ \hline +1.75 -0.50 \times 180 \end{array}$$

A common mistake is to simply order +1.50 D sphere for reading. The needed near power is really +1.50 D sphere *in addition* to the distance prescription. The add power is *added to* the distance sphere power *and* the cylinder contained in the distance prescription to create the correct power for reading glasses. Astigmatism is still present in the eye regardless of whether distant or near objects are viewed. This requires that the cylinder power be included.

Ordering the Correct Lens Power for Intermediate and Near Only

Certain individuals work in circumstances in which they need to see at intermediate and near-viewing distances only. A distance correction is not needed. It is as if they need only the intermediate and near-viewing powers of a trifocal (Figure 19-11).

Example **19-3**

A prescription reads as follows:

R: +0.25 −0.25 × 170
L: +0.25 −0.25 × 010
Add: +2.50

The wearer has half-eye frames, is satisfied with them, and is not interested in a distance prescription. The wearer needs to see at intermediate distances. The decision is made to place a bifocal lens in the half-eye frame. What power lens should be ordered?

Solution

To find the new "distance" power, we need to know what the power of the lenses through the intermediate area of a regular trifocal in this prescription would be. To do this, we must first know the "intermediate add."

A normal intermediate power is 50% of the near addition. Fifty percent, or half of the +2.50 near addition, is:

$$\frac{+2.50}{2} = +1.25$$

Therefore the top of the new half-eye bifocal must be the wearer's distance Rx plus the addition in the intermediate, or +1.25 D. For the right eye this is:

$$\begin{array}{r} +0.25 -0.25 \times 170 \\ +1.25 \\ \hline +1.50 -0.25 \times 170 \end{array}$$

and for the left eye:

$$\begin{array}{r} +0.25 -0.25 \times 010 \\ +1.25 \\ \hline +1.50 -0.25 \times 010 \end{array}$$

These are the powers of the new "distance" portions of the lenses.

The near portion of the half-eye bifocal must read the same in the lensmeter as a regular bifocal lens would have read if it had been made in the original prescription. In the original prescription, the near power for the right eye is:

$$\begin{array}{c} \text{(distance power)} \\ +\text{(near addition)} \\ \hline \text{(near power)} \end{array}$$

or

$$\begin{array}{r} +0.25 -0.25 \times 170 \\ +2.50 \\ \hline +2.75 -0.25 \times 170 \end{array}$$

So through the lensmeter, the near power must read: +2.75 −0.25 × 170.

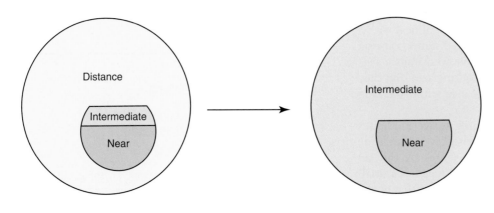

Figure 19-11. If a segmented multifocal lens is to be used for intermediate and near viewing only, the intermediate power goes where the distance power would normally have been found. This will affect how the lens must be ordered, with even the add power changing to remain correct.

If

$$(distance\ power) + (near\ addition) = (near\ power)$$

then we know by transformation

$$(near\ addition) = (near\ power) - (distance\ power)$$

This can be written as:

$$\begin{array}{r} (near\ power) \\ -(distance\ power) \\ \hline (near\ addition) \end{array}$$

So the add power is:

$$\begin{array}{r} (+2.75-0.25\times170) \\ -(+1.50-0.25\times170) \\ \hline +1.25\ add \end{array}$$

Therefore the half-eye bifocal must be ordered as:

$$+1.50-0.25\times170$$
$$+1.50-0.25\times010$$
$$Add:\ +1.25$$

When ordered like this, the lens powers come out the same as they would have in the original prescription.

Example **19-4**

After wearing a new pair of trifocals for awhile, the individual returns, saying the trifocals are acceptable, but do not have enough reading area through the intermediate area. Instead they want a pair of bifocals just to wear at work. The strength through the top of a new bifocal lens should be the same as the existing trifocal intermediate. They do like the size and strength of the near portion and want it left as is. Their current prescription reads:

$$-2.50-1.25\times160$$
$$-2.50-1.25\times015$$
$$Add:\ +2.25$$

Another pair of frames is chosen, and bifocal heights are measured. What powers should be ordered for the new lenses?

Solution

First, determine the power through the present trifocal intermediate area. This could be done with a lensmeter, but is better accomplished by looking at the written prescription. Assuming that the intermediate is 50%, or half of the add power, the "intermediate add" will be:

$$\frac{+2.25}{2} = +1.12$$

The power of the new "distance" portion will be the power through the old intermediate. Power through the old intermediate for the right eye is the wearer's distance Rx plus the intermediate addition.

$$\begin{array}{r} -2.50-1.25\times160 \\ +1.12 \\ \hline -1.37-1.25\times160 \end{array}$$

and for the left eye:

$$\begin{array}{r} -2.50-1.25\times015 \\ +1.12 \\ \hline -1.37-1.25-015 \end{array}$$

To stay with the nearest quarter diopter, we must change the −1.37 sphere power to either −1.50 or −1.25. We choose to round up so that the new "distance" prescription for the right eye will be −1.50 −1.25 × 160.

Next we need to know the near power of the prescription so that we can determine the add power for the new glasses. In the original prescription, the near power for the right eye is:

$$\begin{array}{r} (distance\ power) \\ +(near\ addition) \\ \hline (near\ addition) \end{array}$$

or

$$\begin{array}{r} -2.50-1.25\times160 \\ +2.25 \\ \hline -0.25-1.25\times160 \end{array}$$

So through the lensmeter, the near power must read: −0.25 − 1.25 × 160.

Since

$$\begin{array}{r} (near\ power) \\ -(distance\ power) \\ \hline (near\ addition) \end{array}$$

the new add power is

$$\begin{array}{r} (-0.25-1.25\times60) \\ -(-1.50-1.25\times60) \\ \hline +1.25\ add \end{array}$$

Therefore the half-eye bifocal must be ordered as:

$$R:\ -1.50-1.25\times160$$
$$L:\ -1.50-1.25\times015$$
$$Add:\ +1.25$$

(NOTE: If we had chosen −1.25 −125 × 160 for the "distance" power when we rounded, the add power would have been +1.00 D.)

As demonstrated in the above examples, to maintain the intent of the prescription, it is sometimes necessary to change the powers of the lenses. Using these examples

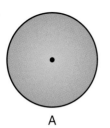
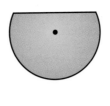
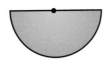

A   B   C

Figure 19-12. A-C, The distance from the top of the seg to the seg optical center varies with seg style. Three different seg styles, all set at the same height, can have very different locations for their segment optical centers.

as a beginning, it is possible to see how specialized eye-glasses can be designed to suit specific needs while maintaining the intent of the original prescription.

IMAGE JUMP

The segment portion of a bifocal lens is like a minilens. It has the same characteristics as a normal single vision lens, except it is smaller. The bifocal section is really a smaller lens on a larger lens. When the segment is round, the segment's OC will be exactly in the middle of the seg (Figure 19-12, *A*). For example, if the segment is 22 mm round, the seg OC will be 11 mm from the top of the seg.

However, not all segs are round. Some are shaped with the upper section cut off so that the upper dividing line is closer to the OC of the seg (Figure 19-12, *B*). It is also possible to have a segment constructed such that the OC is exactly on the upper line (Figure 19-12, *C*). The style of segment chosen depends on the wearer's occupational visual requirement.

One noticeable side effect of segment shape happens as a result of the position of the segment OC compared with the location of the upper edge of the segment. The farther from the OC the eye looks, the greater will be the prismatic effect.

When wearers drop their eyes while wearing single vision lenses, prismatic effect increases as the eyes travel downward. If the lens is a bifocal, the segment also contains a prismatic effect. The value of the prismatic effect in the segment is dependent on the location of the segment optical center. When crossing the border of the seg, the prism induced by the distance portion is suddenly changed by the amount of prism that is being induced by the segment portion. This abrupt change in prismatic effect causes objects to be suddenly displaced.

This sudden displacement of the image as the bifocal line is crossed is known as *image jump*. The amount of image jump for a given style of bifocal is independent of the power in the distance portion. It can be calculated using Prentice's rule.

Example **19-5**

How much image jump does a bifocal with a 22-mm round segment have if the add is +2.00 D?

Solution

Since the segment is round with the seg OC in the middle, the upper bifocal border is 11 mm above that center. When looking through a point 11 mm away from the OC of a +2.00 D lens, a prismatic effect is created equal to:

$$\Delta = cF = (1.1)(2.00) = 2.20$$

Therefore a 22-mm round seg of +2.00 D add power has an image jump of 2.20Δ.

Example **19-6**

How much jump does a flat-top segment, such as the one shown in Figure 19-12, *B*, have? The segment dimensions are as follows:

seg width = 25 mm
seg depth = 17.5 mm
Add power = +1.50 D

Solution

A flat-top style seg is essentially a small round lens with the top cut off. Therefore to find the distance from the seg line to the seg optical center, subtract one half of the seg width from the seg depth.

$$17.5 \text{ mm} - 12.5 \text{ mm} = 5 \text{ mm}$$

Image jump is determined by finding the prismatic effect of the segment at the point on the upper seg line. In this case since the distance from the seg OC is 5 mm we use:

$$\Delta = cF = (0.5)(1.50) = 0.75$$

giving an image jump of 0.75Δ.

ACCOMMODATION AND EFFECTIVITY

There are several mysteries when it comes to comparing plus and minus lens wearers. Here are a few of them:

- Why do hyperopic spectacle lens wearers seem to need bifocals or progressives before myopic lens wearers?
- Why do middle-aged myopes sometimes have trouble with reading when switching into contact lenses, but middle-aged hyperopes do not? In fact the hyperopes going into contact lenses seem to postpone the need for a reading correction.

- Why do some previous spectacle lens–wearing myopes have trouble with reading after undergoing refractive surgery?

All of these questions stem back to the effect that spectacle lenses have on what is called accommodative demand. In this section, we will be showing how accommodative demand is affected by spectacle lenses, compared with contact lenses and no lenses at all.

Who Needs Bifocals or Progressives First, the Hyperope or the Myope?

The amount of accommodation required for an individual to see clearly at near is determined by three things:
1. The near-viewing distance
2. The power of the distance spectacle lens prescription being worn
3. The distance from the lens to the principal planes of the eye

The primary and secondary principal planes of the eye are those planes perpendicular to the optic axis at which refraction of incident and emergent light is considered to take place. The distance from the spectacle lenses to the principal planes of the eye can be considered as being the vertex distance plus 1.5 mm.* Therefore this distance is the vertex distance plus 1.5 mm.

To tell who will need a bifocal first, consider the situation of an emmetrope[†] who wears no lenses at all. Suppose an emmetrope is wearing an empty frame at a 12.5-mm vertex distance. No accommodation is required for viewing objects in the distance. This is because light entering the eye from infinity is parallel, having a zero vergence.[‡] At the normal reading or near working distance, the emmetrope looks at an object that is 40 cm from the spectacle plane. This means that light first travels 40 cm from the near object to the frame, then 12.5 mm from the spectacle plane to the cornea, and finally 1.5 mm from the cornea to the principal planes of the eye. In other words, the near object is −41.40 cm or −0.4140 m away from the principal planes. The amount of accommodation required to focus the near object through the "glasses" is the difference between the vergence of light coming from a distant object and the vergence of light coming from a near object. That is to say,

$$\text{Ocular Accommodation} = L_d - L_n$$

where L_d is the vergence of light reaching the principal planes of the eye from a distant object (infinity), and L_n

is the vergence of light reaching the principle planes of the eye from a near object.

For the emmetrope, ocular accommodation is:

$$
\begin{aligned}
\text{Ocular Accommodation} &= L_d - L_a \\
&= \frac{1}{\infty} - \frac{1}{-0.414} \\
&= 0 - (-2.42) \\
&= +2.42 D
\end{aligned}
$$

The question is, does this required ocular accommodation of 2.42 D remain the same for a hyperopic spectacle lens wearer? To find out, solve Example 19-7.

Example **19-7**

How much must a wearer of +7.00 D single vision spectacle lenses have to accommodate to clearly see an object that is 40 cm away from the spectacle plane? (Assume a 12.5-mm vertex distance.)

Solution

Remember, ocular accommodation is the difference between distance and near vergence at the principal planes of the eye. Finding the vergence of light at the principal planes of the eye after being refracted through a lens is basically the same as working an effective power problem (see Chapter 14). Written as a formula, effective power is:

$$L_d = \frac{1}{\dfrac{1}{F_v'} - d}$$

where
L_d is the vergence of light at the corneal plane from infinity,
F_v' is the power of the lens, and
d is the distance in meters from the reference position of the lens to the new reference position.

This time, however, instead of using vertex distance as was used in working effective power problems in Chapter 14, use principal plane distance (i.e., vertex distance plus 1.5 mm) (Figure 19-13). This will make L_d equal to the vergence of light at the principle planes of the eye. Therefore for the +7.00 D hyperope,

$$
\begin{aligned}
L_d &= \frac{1}{\dfrac{1}{+7} - 0.014} \\
&= +7.76\,D
\end{aligned}
$$

For a near object at 40 cm, the vergence of light striking the lens is 1/−0.40, which is the same as −2.50 D (Figure 19-14). This vergence must be added to the power of the lens to find the vergence of light leaving the lens. The vergence of light leaving the lens is:

$$\left(\frac{1}{-0.40}\right) + F_v'$$

---

*According to Gullstrand's schematic eye, the principle planes of the eye are 1.47 mm and 1.75 mm behind the cornea.
[†]An emmetrope is neither nearsighted (myopic) nor farsighted (hyperopic).
[‡]In this case, the vergence of light is found by taking the reciprocal of the distance in meters from the eye to the source.

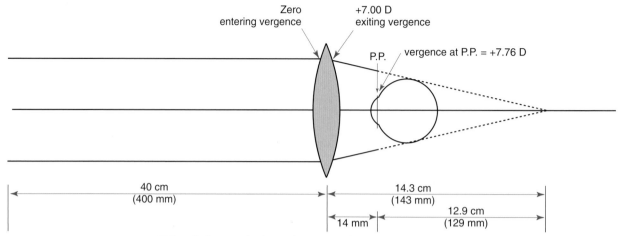

Figure 19-13. When light travels through a spectacle lens, the vergence of light reaching the eye is different from the vergence of light that left the back surface of the lens.

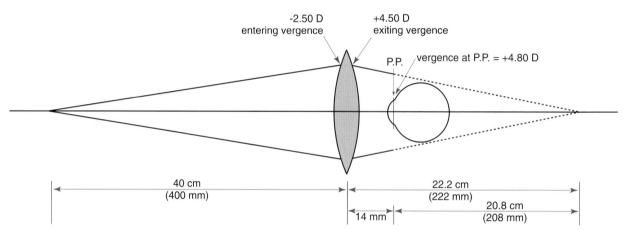

Figure 19-14. The amount of ocular accommodation required is the difference between distance and near vergence at the eye. In this case the amount of ocular accommodation required is +7.76 − 4.80 = +2.96. This is more than the approximately +2.50 D of accommodation expected for an object viewed at 40 cm.

This means that the vergence of light for the near object at the principal planes of the eye would be:

$$L_n = \cfrac{1}{\left(\cfrac{1}{\left(\cfrac{1}{-0.40}\right)+F'_v}\right) - d_v}$$

$$= \cfrac{1}{\left(\cfrac{1}{-2.50+F'_v}\right) - d_v}$$

$$= \cfrac{1}{\left(\cfrac{1}{-2.50+7.00}\right) - 0.014}$$

$$= \cfrac{1}{\left(\cfrac{1}{4.5}\right) - 0.014}$$

$$= \cfrac{1}{0.208}$$

$$= +4.80\,D$$

If, then for a +7.00 D hyperope, the amount of accommodation required to clearly see an object at 40 cm would be +7.76 −4.80 = 2.96 D. This amounts to approximately ½ D more accommodation required than for an emmetrope.

If the same calculations were done for a −7.00 D myope, the ocular accommodation would be found to be only +2.00 D. This is less than would normally be expected. In other words, a +7.00 D hyperope wearing single vision lenses must accommodate almost a full diopter more to clearly see an object at 40 cm than a −7.00 D myope. *This means that a spectacle-wearing hyperope will require a near addition to their glasses before a myope will.*

How Contact Lenses Affect Required Accommodation

In spite of differences in required accommodation for spectacle lens–wearing myopes and hyperopes, a contact lens–wearing hyperope will not need bifocals any sooner than a contact lens–wearing myope. This is because the spectacle lenses are the factor causing the difference in accommodation required. Contact lenses rest directly on the eye. This will return high plus and high minus lens wearers to a situation that closely resembles the emmetrope, equalizing accommodative differences.

What Happens as Add Power Increases

Interestingly, once a spectacle-lens wearer goes into bifocals, as the add power increases, differences in the amount of accommodation required for hyperopes and myopes decrease. When full presbyopia is reached, the +7.00 D hyperope does not need the nearly +3.00 D add that might be expected. This is because light from 40 cm diverges to −2.50 D at the spectacle plane, but the +2.50 add in the spectacle plane changes the diverging light back to parallel. Thus light rays leaving the add enter the distance lens parallel and are able to be focused on the retina just as if they were coming from a distant object.

Determining Occupational Add Powers for New Working Distances

When someone needs a second pair of glasses for a specific occupational need, the working distance may not be the same as it is for normal wear. Usually the near prescription has been determined for a 40-cm working distance. At the new working distance, the wearer needs to be accommodating the same amount as they did for their regular working distance. This ensures that the near prescription will be neither too strong nor too weak. Therefore there must be a change in the add power. The prescriber can test at this new working distance and find the correct add power, or if the prescription is already written, it is possible to calculate the new add power using the optical principles previously described.*

Why Some Nonpresbyopes Need a Different Cylinder Correction for Near

Occasionally a nonpresbyope with an occupation requiring intense near work complains of eye fatigue with near viewing. In spite of all efforts on the part of the examiner to uncover the source of the problem by checking and rechecking the refraction, the solution remains illusive. When the prescription contains a high cylinder power, there may be an optical answer that is not immediately obvious.

As shown previously, the power of a spectacle lens will affect the amount of accommodation required for near viewing. A spectacle lens containing a large cylinder component has a considerable difference in refractive power between its two major meridians. This means that a single vision lens wearer may require a different amount of accommodation for one meridian of the lens than for the other when comparing the effectiveness of that lens at distance and near. If the distance sphere power is also large, this effect can be even more significant. The net effect of these differences results in a new astigmatism at near that is different from the value found for distance vision. This new amount of astigmatism is not fully corrected at the near reading distance.

The initial response may be to calculate a new cylinder correction for near. Yet rather than try and calculate a new cylinder correction to remedy the near problem, the best solution is to test for cylinder power and axis for near vision. Retesting with a near target during refraction is better than recalculating because there can sometimes be a slight amount of cyclorotation† of the eyes on convergence. A slight cyclorotation will change the cylinder axis. Therefore in cases like this it is best to test for both cylinder power and axis at near.

If there both a difference in distance cylinder values and near cylinder values that is combined with an axis change, a second single vision pair of glasses may be adviseable for near work. Differences in accommodative demand between the two meridians diminish when presbyopia advances and add power increases.

CREATING HORIZONTAL PRISM AT NEAR ONLY

Occasionally a prescription will call for horizontal prism, but only for near viewing. Why might someone need prism only at near? Although the situation does not happen often, there are times when it can be an advantage to create base-in or base-out horizontal prism for

---

*It is possible to find an occupational add power that is equivalent to the regular add power using a formula. That formula is based on the difference in the vergence of light at the principal planes of the eye coming from an object at the distance for which the add was prescribed (usually 40 cm), compared to the vergence of light at the eye coming from the new "occupational" distance. The difference represents a change in the amount of accommodation required at the new working distance. This change in accommodation is then added to the original add power to find the occupational add. The formula is as follows:

New add power = (current add power) + (change in ocular accommodation at the principal planes of the eye.)

$$\text{New add power} = \text{(current add power)} + \left(\begin{array}{c}\text{vergence of light at the principal planes for}\\ \text{normal 40-cm working distance}\end{array}\right) - \left(\begin{array}{c}\text{vergence of light at the principal planes for}\\ \text{new occupational working distance.}\end{array}\right)$$

$$\text{New add power} = \text{(current add power)} + \cfrac{1}{\cfrac{1}{\left(\cfrac{1}{-d_{(1)}}\right) + F_v' + F_a} - (d_{pp})} - \cfrac{1}{\cfrac{1}{\left(\cfrac{1}{-d_{(2)}}\right) + F_v' + F_a} - (d_{pp})}$$

where F_v' is the power of the distance lens, F_a is the power of the current add, $d_{(1)}$ is the distance for which the add is prescribed, $d_{(2)}$ is the occupational working distance, and d_{pp} is the distance from the lens to the principal planes (i.e., vertex distance plus 1.5 mm).

†Cyclorotation is a clockwise or counterclockwise turning of the eye around an imaginary axis corresponding to the line of sight.

near only. It could also happen that there is already horizontal prism in the distance portion of the lens, but a different amount is needed in the near viewing area. Here are some examples of situations where this might occur:

1. *The AC/A ratio is either high or low.* Some individuals have an abnormally high or low AC/A ratio. The *AC/A ratio* is "the ratio of accommodative convergence (AC) to accommodation (A), usually expressed as the quotient of accommodative convergence in prism diopters divided by the accommodative response in diopters."[1] People with this problem do not lose binocular vision. Both eyes still accurately point at the object being viewed. However, the fusion required to keep from seeing double makes concentrated viewing at near a strain.

2. *There is a periodic strabismus (tropia) at near only.* Strabismus is an eye condition where one eye looks at the object being viewed, but the other eye does not. (Such an individual is often referred to as being "cross-eyed" or "walleyed.") Sometimes a tropia exists during near viewing only. When this is the case, prescribed base-in or base-out prism for near viewing may enable the individual to see with both eyes simultaneously.

3. *Nonconcomitant strabismus is present.* With *nonconcomitant strabismus*, the angle of deviation varies. The eye turns at a different angle when the person looks at distant objects compared with when he or she looks at near objects. Using one amount of prism for both distance and near may solve the problem for distance, but not for near. For such cases, creating a different amount of prism at near could provide the answer.

If horizontal prism is ordered for near only (or a different amount at near than at distance), then there are several ways to address the issue:

1. *Use two pairs of glasses*—With two pair of glasses, the distance prescription is given without prism. A second pair for near viewing is given and includes both horizontal prism and the near add power.

2. *Use Fresnel press-on prism for near only*—Although Fresnel prism fulfills the intent of the prescription, it does not offer a permanent solution.

3. *Use larger-segment flat-top lenses and decenter the segments*—Base-in or base-out prism is created by having the laboratory move the segments in or out, relative to their traditional near PD location.

4. *Use a split lens*—Each lens in the pair is formed from two separate lenses as described for a Franklin bifocal. The upper half of a distance-powered lens is cemented to the lower half of a near-point powered lens containing the desired prism. This is described in greater detail on pages 448 and 449.

5. *Use a cement seg construction*— Some laboratories are able to use a single vision lens for the distance prescription and glue a specially constructed segment lens onto the single vision lens. The segment must have a back curve equal to the front curve of the distance lens. The segment can be made with prism only or with prism and an add power.

Horizontal Prism at Near by Segment Decentration

The least expensive method for correcting horizontal prism at near with a multifocal lens is to use larger flat-top segments. These segments are decentered more or less than they normally would be for the near PD (Figure 19-15). The amount of segment decentration required

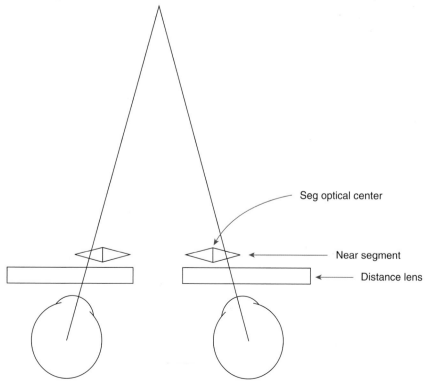

Seg optical center

Near segment

Distance lens

Figure 19-15. Bifocal segments are really small plus lenses. This means that if the segment OCs are moved nasalward, they will cause a base-in prismatic effect. This prismatic effect occurs only in the near position.

depends on the power of the near addition. There are some restrictions:

- If too much decentration is required, it will not be possible to move the segment far enough. The lens size will not allow it.
- If the segment is too small, the edge of the segment will be too close to the line of sight, and there will not be enough reading area.

Thus the practitioner must know how far the segments must be decentered and what the minimum size of those segments must be so that there is still enough segment reading area remaining (Figure 19-16).

Steps in Finding Seg Decentration and Size for Prism at Near

The following steps outline how the amount of segment decentration is determined and reveal how large the segment must be so that sufficient segment area remains for reading. (These steps are summarized in Box 19-1.)

1. Find the customary seg inset.

$$\text{Seg inset} = \frac{\text{distance PD} - \text{near PD}}{2}$$

2. Find the additional seg inset needed to produce the prism prescribed for near using a transposed form of Prentice's rule.

Now for some examples on how this is done.

Example **19-8**

A prescription reads:

+2.00 −1.00 × 180	1.25Δ base in at near only
+2.00 −1.00 × 180	1.25Δ base in at near only
Add +2.25	
PD = 64/60	

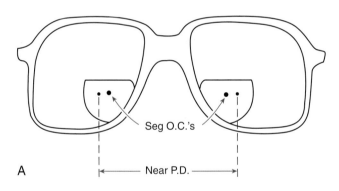

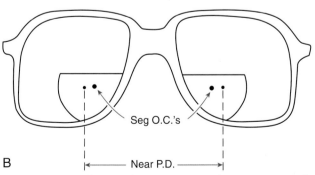

Figure 19-16. The eyes do not remain at the near interpupillary points when close work is done, but scan back and forth. The production of lateral prism at near through segment decentration requires that attention be given to seg width. **A,** There will be insufficient outer seg area to permit normal eye movement. **B,** If a larger seg is chosen, the problem is alleviated.

BOX 19-1

Finding Seg Decentration and Size for Prescribed Prism at Near Only

1. Find the customary seg inset.

$$\text{Seg inset} = \frac{\text{distance PD} - \text{near PD}}{2}$$

2. Find the additional seg inset needed to produce the prism prescribed.

$$c_a = \frac{\text{near prism}}{F_a}$$

where c_a = additional seg inset, and F_a = the add power.

3. Determine if the additional seg inset is inward or outward. Because the segment is really a small plus lens, if the prescribed near prism is base in, the additional seg inset will be inward. If the prescribed near prism is base out, the additional seg inset is outward.

4. Find the net seg inset.

$$\text{Net seg inset} = \text{seg inset} + \text{additional seg inset}$$

5. Find the minimum segment size needed to give the wearer enough area to read with.

$$\text{Seg size} = 2(10 + \text{additional seg inset})$$

Could this amount of prism correction be achieved using decentered flat-top segments? If so, how large should the segs be so that they give at least a 10-mm distance from the reading center to the edge of the segment? The reading center is at the location of the near PD.

Solution

To find the answers to these questions, proceed through the steps outlined in the preceding section.
1. For this prescription, the customary seg inset is:

$$\text{Seg inset} = \frac{\text{distance PD} - \text{near PD}}{2}$$
$$= \frac{64 - 60}{2}$$
$$= 2\,\text{mm}$$

2. Find the additional amount of decentration needed beyond what would normally be required for the near PD. To do this, use the formula:

$$c_a = \frac{\text{near prism}}{F_a}$$

In this case

$$c_a = \frac{1.25\Delta}{2.25D}$$
$$= 0.55\,\text{cms}$$
$$= 5.5\,\text{mm}$$

3. Because the horizontal prism at near is base in, the additional seg inset is also inward.
4. Therefore the net seg inset is:

$$\text{net seg inset} = \text{seg inset} + \text{additional seg inset}$$
$$= 2 + 5.5$$
$$= 7.5\,\text{mm}$$

5. The minimum segment size needed will be:

$$\text{Seg size} = 2(10 + \text{additional seg inset})$$

Additional seg inset was the c_a value found in step 2. So in this case

$$\text{Seg size} = 2(10 + 5.5)$$
$$= 2(15.5)$$
$$= 31\,\text{mm}$$

Since flat-top segs do not come in 31-mm sizes, the next largest segment is chosen. That size is a 35-mm segment. To summarize, use flat-top 35-mm segments and decenter these segments 7.5 mm inward for each eye.

Example **19-9**

Suppose we want to specify the position of the seg in the previous example in terms of "near PD" on the order form instead of net seg inset. What would the "near PD" be for this prescription? (In this case the "near PD" is really the

horizontal segment center separation and does not at all correspond to the wearer's PD at near.)

Solution

If net seg inset is 7.5 mm per lens, then the distance between the near segs will be closer together than the distance PD by an amount equal to twice the net seg inset. This means that the distance between the near segs is (2) × (7.5) or 15 mm less than the distance PD. The distance between seg centers for this prescription is:

$$\text{"near PD"} = 64 - (2)(7.5)$$
$$= 64 - 15$$
$$= 49\,\text{mm}$$

The amount of prism at near will be achieved when the far PD equals 64 mm, and the distance between the near PD seg centers is 49 mm. Written on the order form, this would read 64/49. (When writing something like this on the order form, there should be some explanation, or it will be taken as an error.)

Additional Comments on Prism at Near

If a frame with a large eye size is chosen, the decentered lens blank may not be large enough. When it appears that blank size may become an issue, it is advisable to check for minimum blank size (see Chapter 5).

If the segment requires a significant amount of outward decentration to achieve base-out prism at near, a blank size problem can often be solved by having the laboratory swap lens blanks: left for right and right for left. In other words, use a left lens blank to grind the right lens and a right lens blank to grind the left lens.

Ordering Horizontal Prism at Near

As stated previously, the least expensive option for producing prism at near only is that of decentered near segments. By figuring the decentration needed, making certain the lenses will cut out, and specifying the prism as "distance PD/near PD" as in Example 19-9, costs are kept lower.

Aside from cost issues, however, the practitioner should be able to determine ahead of time if decentering segments to create near prism will work before placing an impossible order. The method just outlined makes this feasible.

A Split Lens for Prism at Near

When the amount of prism prescribed for near is different from the distance prism correction, it is possible to use a split lens. Each of the lenses in the pair begins as two lenses—one nonprism distance lens and another lens for near that includes the prescribed prism, along with the add power. In fact the prism can be in any base direction since there are really two lenses. The lenses are both cut in half. The upper half of the distance-powered lens and the lower half of the near-powered lens are glued together.

The laboratory does this by making both lenses with the same base curve. The laboratory will try to match the center thicknesses of the two lenses. Once the two lenses are made, the lens to be used as the upper half is spotted, and a "seg line" is marked on this distance lens so that the distance optical center will be 3 or 4 above the seg line. The lens will be cut along the seg line. Another "seg line" is marked on the near lens. For this lens, the part below the "seg line" will be used. The lenses are cut, and the cut edges are smoothed. Then the two halves are glued together and allowed to dry. Now the newly created lens is spotted, blocked, and edged for the frame.

The person receiving a split lens should be told that this lens is not as impact resistant as other lenses and should be asked to sign a disclaimer for impact resistance. Although it may be possible to make a cement seg lens from a single vision lens that could be more impact resistant, such a lens may not be as suitable.

REFERENCES

1. Hofstetter HW, Griffin JR, Berman MS et al: The dictionary of visual science, ed 5, Boston, 2000, Butterworth-Heinemann.

Proficiency Test

(Answers can be found in the back of the book.)

Segmented Multifocal Lenses

1. Which of the following is correct?
   a. (distance power) + (near power) = (near Rx)
   b. (near power) - (distance power) = (near addition)
   c. (near addition) = (distance power) - (near power)
   d. (near power) - (distance power) = (near Rx)
   e. None of the above is correct.

2. Which of the following statements is correct?
   a. Seg height is always equal to seg depth.
   b. Seg depth is always greater than or equal to seg height.
   c. Seg height is always greater than or equal to seg depth.
   d. Seg height is always greater than seg depth.
   e. None of the above is correct.

3. If a right lens has an outset of 1 mm and a seg inset of 2.5 mm, what is the total inset?
   a. 1.0 mm
   b. 1.5 mm
   c. 2.5 mm
   d. 3.5 mm
   e. None of the above is correct.

4. The lensmeter reads:
   $-1.00 -1.00 \times 180$ in the distance portion
   $+0.50 -1.00 \times 180$ in the intermediate portion
   $+1.50 -1.00 \times 180$ in the near portion
   What is the near add?
   a. +1.50 D
   b. +1.75 D
   c. +2.00 D
   d. +2.25 D
   e. +2.50 D

5. In Question 4, what percent is the intermediate seg power?
   a. 40%
   b. 50%
   c. 60%
   d. 70%
   e. None of the above is correct.

6. If you could not see a lens and were only able to feel the surfaces, which of the following multifocals could not be distinguished from a single vision lens?
   a. a fused glass multifocal lens
   b. a one-piece construction multifocal lens
   c. a cement segment multifocal lens
   d. All could be distinguished from a single vision lens.
   e. None could be distinguished from a single vision lens.

7. An Executive lens is an example of which type of construction?
   a. fused
   b. one piece
   c. cement segment

8. Which of the following multifocal construction methods are used only with glass?
   a. fused
   b. one piece
   c. cement segment

9. True or false? One-piece multifocal construction is used only with plastic lenses, not with glass.

10. Match the bifocal lens segment with how far the segment OC is below the top of the segment. (It may be possible to use an answer more than one time.)

    a. 22-mm round segment   1. 4.5 or 5 mm below
    b. flat-top 28 segment   2. 19 mm below
    c. Franklin-style segment   3. 11 mm below
    d. 38-mm round segment   4. 0 mm below
    e. curved-top segment   5. 3 mm below
        6. 7 mm below

11. Which of the following bifocal lenses are always monocentric?

    a. 22-mm round segment
    b. flat-top 45 segment
    c. Franklin-style segment
    d. curved-top 25
    e. None of the above is always monocentric.

12. A lens that could be substituted for a Rede-Rite bifocal and probably do the job better would be

    a. an ED trifocal
    b. a regular progressive addition lens
    c. an upside-down Executive lens
    d. an occupational progressive such as the Hoya Tact or AO Technica
    e. There is no lens that would serve as a suitable replacement.

13. A trifocal lens that looks similar to a combination of a Franklin-style lens and a flat-top bifocal is called:

    a. a quadrafocal.
    b. an ED.
    c. a DBL.
    d. a Rede-Rite.

14. A lens that looks similar to a flat-top trifocal with an upside-down flat-top bifocal in the upper half is called:

    a. a quadrafocal.
    b. an ED.
    c. a DBL.
    d. a Rede-Rite.

15. This lens has what appears to be a large round segment at the top of the lens and no segment at the bottom. The round segment area at the top is the distance prescription, and the rest of the lens contains the near add. It is called:

    a. a quadrafocal.
    b. an ED.
    c. a DBL.
    d. a Rede-Rite.

16. True or false? Double-segment occupational lenses are available with Franklin-style segments.

17. A lens has the following dimensions:
    Shape: rectangular
    Depth of lens (the "B" dimension) = 36 mm
    Width of the lens (the "A" dimension) = 50 mm
    Rx: O.D. +2.50 −1.50 × 090
         O.S. +2.50 −1.50 × 090
         Add: +1.75 O.U.
    Seg dimensions: seg width = 28 mm
                   seg depth = 19 mm
                   seg height = 15 mm
                   seg inset = 2 mm
    What is the seg drop?

    a. 6 mm
    b. 5 mm
    c. 4 mm
    d. 3 mm
    e. None of the above is correct.

Image Jump

18. For the lens in Question 17, what is the image jump?

    a. 0.525Δ
    b. 0.70Δ
    c. 0.875Δ
    d. 1.05Δ
    e. None of the above is correct.

19. What is the "jump" in a 20-mm round bifocal with a distance Rx of +2.00 D sphere, seg 3 mm below distance center, and power of add + 2.00 D?

    a. 0.60Δ
    b. 2.00Δ
    c. 1.40Δ
    d. There is no jump with this lens.
    e. None of the above is correct.

20. Calculate the "jump" for the following bifocal lens: +3.00 − 1.00 × 080; add of +2.50 D
    Seg top is 3 mm below distance OC. Seg style is a straight-top 25 with the segment OC 5 mm below the dividing line.

    a. 1.25Δ
    b. 1.75Δ
    c. 2.25Δ
    d. 2.75Δ
    e. None of the above is correct.

21. For the lens described above, what would the jump be if the seg top were 5 mm below the distance OC?

    a. 1.25Δ
    b. 1.75Δ
    c. 2.25Δ
    d. 2.75Δ
    e. None of the above is correct.

22. Give the image jump for the following Rx:
O.D. +3.00 −1.00 × 180
O.S. +3.50 −1.25 × 180
Add: 2.25 D
Seg height = 15 mm
Seg style is an Ultex A.
Lens is in a 48-mm round frame with no distance decentration and a seg inset of 2.5 mm.
a. 6.75Δ
b. 2.025Δ
c. 8.55Δ
d. 3.375Δ
e. None of the above is correct.

Ordering for Reading and Intermediate Distances

23. A prescription reads as follows:
−0.50 −0.25 × 180
−0.50 −0.25 × 180
Add: +2.00
The wearer wants a pair for distance and a pair for reading. What powers would be ordered for the reading glasses?
a. +2.00 D sph
+2.00 D sph
b. +2.00 −0.25 × 180
+2.00 −0.25 × 180
c. +2.50 −0.25 × 180
+2.50 −0.25 × 180
d. +1.50 D sph
+1.50 D sph
e. +1.50 −0.25 × 180
+1.50 −0.25 × 180

24. A trifocal wearer has the following Rx:
O.D. −1.25 −0.50 × 005
O.S. −1.75 −0.25 × 175
Add: +2.50 D
Trifocal with 50% intermediate portion
The wearer finds the intermediate power exactly correct for the computer console at which she must work, and the near is just right for paperwork. She never uses the distance portion. What Rx would serve the purpose?
a. pl -0.50 × 005
−0.50 −0.25 × 175
Bifocal add: +2.50
b. -0.62 −0.50 × 005
−1.12 −0.25 × 175
Bifocal add: +1.75
c. -2.25 −0.50 × 005
−2.75 −0.25 × 175
Bifocal add: +1.25
d. pl −0.50 × 005
−0.50 −0.25 × 175
Bifocal add: +1.25
e. None of the above is correct.

25. An Rx is:
+2.00 −1.00 × 090
+2.00 −1.00 × 090
Add +2.50 D
Trifocal with 70% intermediate portion
What power will be read through the intermediate portion using a lensmeter?
a. +3.15 −1.00 × 090
b. +3.75 −1.00 × 090
c. +2.45 D
d. +3.25 -1.00 × 090
e. None of the above is correct.

Accommodation and Effectivity

26. A 41-year-old individual is just beginning to have some problems working at near distances for prolonged periods of time. Interest is expressed in the possibility of changing from spectacles to contact lenses. The distance prescription is:
R: +6.75 −0.75 × 180
L: +6.75 −0.75 × 180
Which of the following is true?
a. This individual will have even more difficulty with fatigue at near in contact lenses than in spectacle lenses.
b. This individual will have less difficulty with fatigue at near in contact lenses than in spectacle lenses.
c. This individual will not experience much difference in contact lenses versus spectacle lenses regarding fatigue at near.

27. Of the following spectacle lens prescriptions, which wearer may have more difficulty with eye fatigue at near?
a. +2.00 −1.00 × 180
+2.00 −1.00 × 180
b. +3.00 −2.50 × 180
+3.00 −2.50 × 180
c. +5.50 −3.50 × 180
+5.50 −3.50 × 180
d. +6.00 −3.75 × 180
+6.00 −3.75 × 180
add: +2.25

28. A 50-year-old −6.00 D myope with a +1.00 add power decides to have refractive surgery. What would you expect after refractive surgery, assuming that after surgery both eyes have a zero distance refractive error?

a. This person will probably still need a +1.00 D add, even after refractive surgery.

b. This person will need a slightly lower add power than he or she had before surgery.

c. It is doubtful that this person will even need an add following refractive surgery, regardless of the type of intraocular lens implant used by the surgeon.

d. This person will need an add power greater than +1.00 D following refractive surgery.

29. An individual is wearing a +6.00 D spectacle lens prescription at a 13-mm vertex distance. How much ocular accommodation is required to clearly view an object at 25 cm from the spectacle plane?

Horizontal Prism at Near Only

30. A prescription calls for 0.75Δ of base-in prism per lens in the segment only. To produce this amount by seg decentration, how much additional seg inset is required beyond the amount that has been determined by near PD measurement or calculation? (The power of the add in question is +2.00 D.)

a. 1.5 mm additional seg inset per lens

b. 2.7 mm additional seg inset per lens

c. 3.8 mm additional seg inset per lens

d. 1.5 mm counterbalancing seg outset per lens

e. none of the above

31. A prescription reads:

+0.50 −0.75 × 005   1.50Δ base in at near only
+0.50 −0.75 × 175   1.50Δ base in at near only
add: +2.00
PD = 66/62

a. How much net seg inset is required to achieve the correct amount of prism at near only using flat-top segments?

b. How large should the segs be so that they give at least a 10-mm distance from the reading center at the near PD to the edge of the segment? Give your answer first as theoretical segment size. Next indicate the size you would use from those flat-top segment sizes that are currently available.

32. A prescription has distance powers of pl −1.00 × 180 with a +2.00 add power. The prescription also calls for 1.5Δ of prism base in per eye at near only. If you were to use decentered flat-top 35s to create prism at near, which direction would you decenter the segments?

a. inward

b. outward

33. For Question 32, how far would you decenter the segments from their normal location at the near PD to create the needed prismatic effect at near only?

a. 1.3 mm

b. 3.0 mm

c. 7.5 mm

d. 13.0 mm

e. There is not enough information given to answer the question.

The following applies to Questions 34 and 35.

A prescription reads:

+1.00 −0.50 × 180   2.00 base in near only
+1.00 −0.50 × 180   2.00 base in near only
Add: +2.25
The wearer's PD is 65/62.
The prism at near is to be created by decentering the segs horizontally.

34. To the nearest millimeter, what should the distance between segment optical centers be for the wearer's glasses if measured with a PD ruler in the usual manner?

a. 40 mm

b. 44 mm

c. 47 mm

d. 80 mm

35. To the nearest millimeter, what would the minimum theoretical lens segment size be to permit near work? (The answer does not have to correspond to an available lens multifocal segment.)

a. 28 mm

b. 31 mm

c. 35 mm

d. 38 mm

e. 45 mm

36. A prescription reads:

−2.00 −0.50 × 090   2.50 base out near only
−2.00 −0.50 × 090   2.50 base out near only
Add: +2.00
The wearer's PD is 64/61.
The prism at near is to be created by decentering the segs horizontally. To the nearest millimeter, what would the TOTAL seg inset or outset need to be for each segment?

a. 6.5 mm outset

b. 8 mm outset

c. 11 mm outset

d. 12.5 mm outset

e. 14 mm

37. For the prescription in Question 36, what is the minimum segment size that would be required so the reading area will be sufficiently large?
    a. 28 mm
    b. 35 mm
    c. 40 mm
    d. 45 mm
    e. None of these segments are large enough.

38. This is a difficult question. Think it through carefully. A spectacle-lens wearer has a distance prescription of −2.50 D sphere and an add power of +2.50. If the segment is decentered either nasally or temporally, will there be any change in horizontal prismatic effects in the segment viewing area?
    a. yes
    b. no

CHAPTER 20

Progressive Addition Lenses

Progressive addition lenses are sometimes referred to as invisible bifocals. However, invisible bifocals have round segments where the demarcation line between the distance portion and the bifocal segment has been polished out, causing the two areas to appear as if blended together. Invisible bifocals are really blended bifocals, not progressive addition lenses. (For more information on blended bifocals, see Chapter 5.)

SECTION 1
Measurement and Dispensing of Progressive Lenses

Progressive addition lenses are made with the help of specially designed front surface curves. These changing surface curves cause the lens to gradually increase in plus power, beginning in the distance portion and ending in the near portion. These variable-powered progressive addition lenses should, according to design, permit clear vision at any given viewing distance merely by positioning the head and eyes.

PROGRESSIVE LENS CONSTRUCTION

Like a segmented multifocal, a progressive addition lens, or *PAL*, has certain distinct areas to the lens. But those areas in a progressive lens are not visible. If we were able to see them, they would look like the lens in Figure 20-1.

The upper portion of the lens is basically the distance portion. The near portion of the lens, where the full near addition power is found, is down and inward. In between the distance and near portions is a *progressive corridor* where the power of the lens is gradually changing.

SELECTING THE FRAME

When choosing a frame for someone wearing a progressive addition lens, there must be enough room for the progressive zone and near portion. Because these areas are not visible like a bifocal segment is, they may be unintentionally cut off. This was a problem when progressive lenses were first introduced in the United States. At that particular time, many frames had narrow vertical dimensions. When progressive lenses were dispensed in

these frames, much of the near portion was cut off. Since people could not see very well up close, dispensers falsely concluded that the lenses were no good. So frame selection is an important part of fitting progressives. Here are some important points to keep in mind:

1. The frame must have sufficient vertical depth. Each lens type has a manufacturer-recommended minimum fitting height. The recommendations of the lens manufacturer should be followed. Standard minimum progressive addition lens fitting heights will vary, going down to a low of about 18 mm. If there is not enough vertical depth to allow the minimum fitting height, then either a different frame must be chosen, or a special short corridor lens that is designed for frames with a narrow vertical dimension should be used. Otherwise there will not be enough reading area left.

2. The frame must have sufficient lens area in the lower nasal portion where the near progressive optics are found. Sometime the frame has a large enough "B" dimension, but the shape is cut away nasally. Aviator shapes are an example of this type of frame.

3. The frame should have a short vertex distance. The closer the frame is to the eyes, the wider the field of view will be for both reading and distance vision.

4. The frame must be able to be adjusted for pantoscopic angle when facial structure will allow. A 10- to 12-degree angle is recommended. The intermediate and near fields of view are effectively wider when the progressive and near zones are closer to the eyes.

5. The frame must have sufficient face form. This also allows a wider viewing area through the progressive corridor.

Frame selection criteria for progressive lenses are discussed in greater detail in Chapter 4. The reader is encouraged to review this section, noting especially Figure 4-14.

CHOOSING THE RIGHT TYPE OF PROGRESSIVE

Most progressive lenses are made for general purpose wear since the majority of wearers only have one pair of

Basic areas of a
progressive addition lens

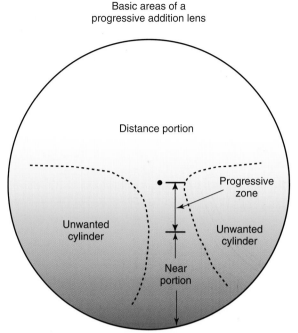

Figure 20-1. The basic construction of a progressive addition lens consists of a distance portion in the upper lens area, a near portion in the lower central area (slightly displaced nasally), and a progressive corridor between the distance and near areas where power gradually increases. On both sides of the progressive and near zones are areas containing a certain amount of unwanted cylinder. New designs are able to control the optics in these peripheral areas better, making them considerably more useful than might be anticipated.

glasses. Although general purpose progressives work for most people, here are some additional considerations:

1. What type of general purpose progressive is appropriate? It is possible to choose a certain type of general purpose progressive to fit the needs of the wearer. This is discussed in more detail in Section 2 of this chapter under General Purpose Progressives.
2. Does the wearer have a significant amount of cylinder power in the prescription? If so consider using a lens design that is atoric. (See the sections found on pages 474 and 475, beginning with "Designs Using Aspheric and/or Atoric Surfacing Methods.") Using such a design will reduce the amount of unwanted distortion that will otherwise be present in the periphery of the lens.
3. If the vertical "B" dimension of the frame is small, choose a short corridor progressive lens. A short corridor lens is still used for general purposes, but is meant for this type of frame. For more on this topic, see Section 3, Specialty Progressives.
4. Does this person use a computer a lot? Do they work in a small office environment where intermediate vision is important? If so they may need a near variable focus occupational progressive

lens. This type of lens is made for closer viewing distances through the top of the lens and has both a wider intermediate progressive corridor and a wider near-viewing area. An occupational progressive lens should not be used as a person's only pair of glasses, unless this person does not need a distance prescription and would otherwise only be wearing reading glasses. These lenses should be considered for a second pair of glasses. For more on this topic, see Section 3, Specialty Progressives.

MEASURING FOR AND ORDERING THE PROGRESSIVE

A progressive addition lens has a rather narrow progressive corridor linking the distance and near portions of the lens. It is through this corridor that intermediate vision takes place. Unless the eye tracks down the exact center of this corridor, the lenses do not work very well. Therefore PD measurements must be taken for each eye individually and an exact vertical height specified for each eye.

To help make sure the progressive corridor is where it should be, the manufacture uses a *fitting cross*. The fitting cross is usually 4 mm above the start of the progressive corridor and is intended to be placed exactly in front of the wearer's pupil center.

Standard Method for Taking Progressive Lens Fitting Measurements

The following measurement techniques are applicable to all manufacturers or designs of progressive lenses, provided the centration chart of the specific manufacturer is used for the lenses being measured. An example of such a chart is shown in Figure 20-2.

1. Measure monocular distance PDs. The recommended method is to use a pupillometer. (The use of a pupillometer is explained in Chapter 3.)
2. Fit and fully adjust the actual frame to be worn. This includes pantoscopic tilt, frame height, vertex distance, face form, and nosepad alignment. Make certain the frame is straight on the face. If the temples are not adjusted, hold the frame in place while measuring so that it will not slip down the nose.
3. If the frame does not contain clear plastic lenses or the wearer's old lenses, place clear (nonfrosted), transparent tape across the eyewire of the empty frame.
4. The dispenser is positioned with his or her eyes at the wearer's eye level. With the wearer looking at the bridge of the fitter's nose, the dispenser draws a horizontal line on the lens or tape. The line should go through the center of the pupil. This is done for both right and left eyes.
5. Place the frame on the manufacturer's centration chart and move it left or right until the bridge is

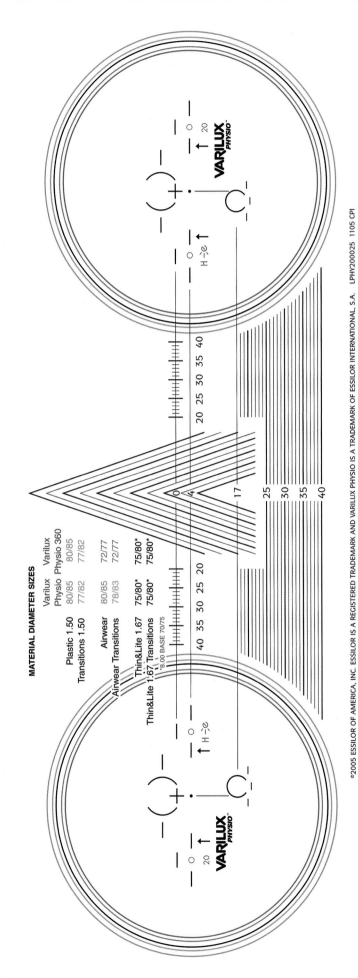

Figure 20-2. The manufacturer's centration chart allows for easy reading of the fitting cross height. When monocular interpupillary distances have not been previously measured with a pupillometer but were marked on the lenses, their distances may be easily determined with the help of the horizontal scale on the chart. (The circles are for determining minimum blank size.) (Courtesy of Essilor of America, Dallas, TX)

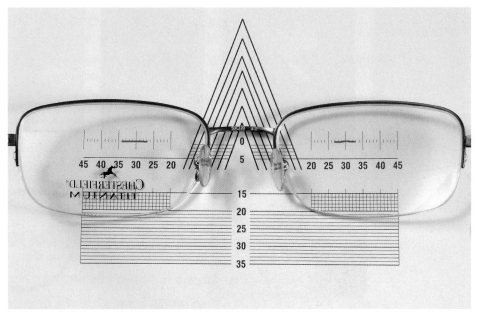

Figure 20-3. For this pair of glasses, the fitting cross heights are marked. The frame bridge is centered on the arrowhead lines. The fitting cross lines are positioned on the horizontal line, and their heights read as the lowest level of the lens on the lower, horizontal line scale.

centered on the diagonally converging central alignment pattern. Then move the frame up or down until the marked horizontal pupil center lines are on the chart's horizontal axis (Figure 20-3). Mark the previously measured PD for each eye as a vertical line that crosses the horizontal one (Figure 20-4).

6. For first one lens, then the other, read the fitting cross heights from the chart. (Fitting cross height is the vertical distance from the fitting cross to the level of the inside bevel of the lower eyewire of the frame.) Record these fitting cross heights and the monocular PDs on the order form and in the wearer's record. (Note: Fitting cross heights are usually erroneously referred to as major reference point (MRP) heights, which they really are not.)

7. Check the size and shape of the frame on the lens picture portion of the centration chart. Do this by placing the frame on the lens blank circles of the centration chart so that the cross on the glazed lens overlaps the fitting cross on the picture (Figure 20-5). The circle should completely enclose the frame's lens shape.

8. Send the frame to the laboratory with the marks still on the lenses or tape.

Fitting Cross Heights for Children

Progressive addition lenses are sometimes used for children. If they are, it is recommended that the lenses be fitted 4 mm higher than normal.[1] An example of when progressives might be used for children is in the case of accommodative esotropia.

The only time a child would not be fitted 4 mm higher than pupil center would be if the child has no accommodation, as after cataract surgery. In this case the fitting cross is positioned normally.

A fitting cross height 4 mm higher than the pupil center helps to ensure that the child is actually looking through the near zone for reading. This is consistent with the recommendation for children's bifocal fitting height. For children bifocals are normally fit with the segment line at the center of the pupil.

Children adapt well to a 4-mm fitting cross raise and use the near portion for their near work. Kowalski et al[2] compared the adaptability of 235 myopic children wearing progressive addition lenses with 234 myopic children wearing single vision lenses. The progressive addition lens wearers were fit with the fitting cross 4 mm above the pupil center. The study concluded that "most children with mild to moderate myopia are able to successfully adapt to PALs with a modified fitting protocol 4 mm higher than the adult standard protocol. This higher fitting protocol will help ensure that children are getting the full benefit of the near addition. Just like with adults, it is important to demonstrate and reinforce the proper use of PALs to children, including possible changes in head posture, head movements, and eye movements, as well as providing information about possible initial adaptation symptoms. These results indicate that PALs do not interfere with children's visual demands

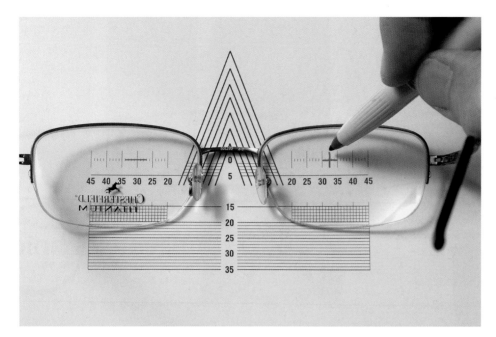

Figure 20-4. In preparation for checking whether a lens blank will be large enough for the frame chosen, the wearer's previously measured monocular interpupillary distances are marked on the lens.

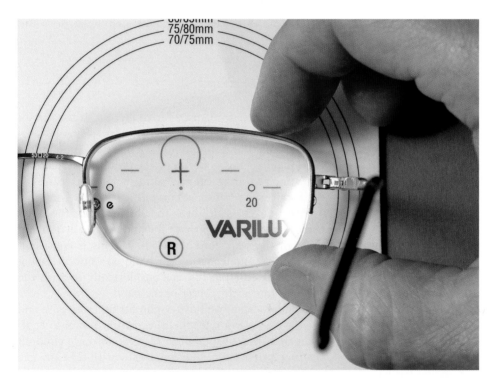

Figure 20-5. To see if the lens blank will be large enough for the frame, the fitting cross that has been drawn on the glazed lenses is placed over the fitting cross in the picture of the lens blank. The smallest lens size that completely encircles the edged lens or lens opening is the minimum blank size needed. If the largest pictured lens blank size fails to encircle the edged lens or lens opening, the frame is too large, and another frame must be selected.

in the classroom, using the computer, or for physical activities such as playing sports.[2]"

Even though the study only used mild-to-moderately myopic children, it would be logical to assume that similar results would be found with children having other refractive errors.

Alternative Methods for Taking Progressive Lens Fitting Measurements

Marking a Cross on Glazed Lenses or Tape
Sometimes a pupillometer is not available for measuring monocular PDs. If this is the case, here is a method

that uses only an overhead transparency pen and the frame:
1. Fully adjust the frame to fit the wearer correctly.
2. Position yourself at the same level as the wearer and approximately 40 cm away.
3. Close your right eye and instruct the wearer to look at your open left eye.
4. Use an overhead transparency marking pen to mark a cross on the right lens. If there is no lens in the frame, place clear tape across the lens opening and mark the tape instead. Draw the cross directly over the center of the wearer's right pupil (see Chapter 3, Figure 3-5).

5. Next close your left eye, open your right eye, and instruct the subject to look at your open eye. Then mark a cross on the lens or tape directly over the left pupil center.

6. Because of the movement involved in marking pupil centers and the ease with which unintentional head movement can occur, it is important that these markings be carefully rechecked. If the wearer turns the head slightly to one side, an error in monocular PDs will occur. It may be hard to catch this error since both monocular PDs may be slightly off, but still add up to what would otherwise be a correct binocular PD.

7. When you are confident that pupil centers are accurately marked, remove the frames. Measure and record the distances from the center of the bridge to the center of each cross using the progressive lens manufacturer's centration chart.

For those who prefer to use corneal reflections instead of the geometric center of the pupil, a penlight positioned directly below the dispenser's open eye will provide the source for the needed reflection (see Chapter 3).

Using the Red Dot Procedure to Subjectively Verify Fitting Cross Positions

To subjectively verify the position of the fitting cross, use the preceding method, but either substitute a red dot for the cross, or draw a red dot in the center of the cross. When measurements are complete, ask the wearer to look straight ahead and view a distant object. The object should appear pink if the wearer is correctly viewing through the red dots. First one eye and then the other is covered. If the wearer must move the head to see pink with either or both eyes, the lenses need to be remarked.[3]

VERIFYING A PROGRESSIVE LENS

Major Points or Areas

When the Rx is returned from the laboratory, it contains removable markings, such as a distance power arc, the fitting cross, horizontal dashes, and a prism reference point (PRP) dot. It may also contain a near-point power circle (Figure 20-6). The distance power arc indicates the recommended position of the lens through which the distance power should be read on the lensmeter.

- The distance reference point (DRP) is at the center of the arc.
- The fitting cross will normally be centered in the pupil.
- The two horizontal dashes to the left and right sides of the lens help to tell if the lens is level or tilted.
- The centrally located PRP dot is used to verify prism power. This is the same as the MRP.

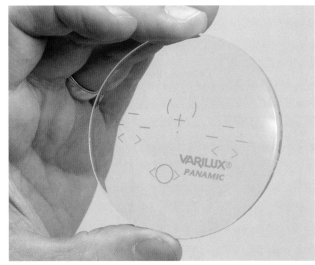

Figure 20-6. A progressive addition lens usually arrives with visible markings or a decal. These markings are used for verification and fitting purposes and are shown in the photograph. The upper semicircle or parentheses area is where the lens is verified for distance power. The fitting cross should fall directly in front of the pupil. The dot directly below the fitting cross is the location of the prism reference point (major reference point) and is where prismatic effect is verified. The lower circle is where near power is verified. The left and right sets of dashes denote the location of hidden marks used for remarking the lens once the visible markings shown here have been removed. The left and right sets of carets <> bracket the locations of the hidden identifying trademark and the marking for the add power. A hidden trademark, whether denoted by an oval or not, is on all progressive lenses and is important in identifying the brand of an unknown progressive lens.

- The circle in the lower part of the lens locates the near reference point (NRP) and is used to verify near power (Figure 20-7).

It is preferable that these markings on the surface of the progressive lens be left on the lens until the finished prescription is both verified and fitted on the patient. This enables the dispenser to verify the powers at far and near and to more easily judge the accuracy of the positioning of the lenses on the wearer's face when the frame is finally adjusted. When the temporary markings are gone, they can be reconstructed using hidden surface engravings.

Verifying Distance Power, Prism Amount, and Add Power

The distance power of a progressive lens should be measured with that portion of the lens that is marked by the distant power arc or circle positioned in front of the lensmeter aperture (Figure 20-8). The place where distance power should be measured is set by the manufacturer and is known as the DRP.

Prism, however, is measured at the specified location of the PRP (Figure 20-9), even though the target may

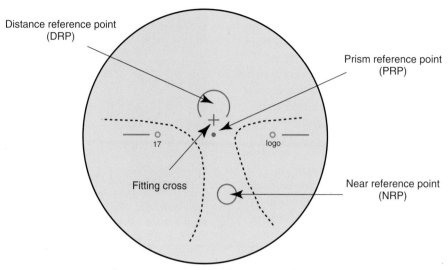

Progressive lens
fitting and verification points

Distance reference point
(DRP)

Prism reference point
(PRP)

Fitting cross

Near reference point
(NRP)

Figure 20-7. In verifying a progressive addition lens, the distance power is verified higher on the lens than it would be on any other type of lens. The manufacturer determines where it should be verified, calls it the distance reference point (DRP), and marks its location with a semicircle.

Prism is verified at the prism reference point (PRP), which is the same thing as the major reference point (MRP). (Note that the fitting cross where the pupil center is located is *not* the same as the MRP. Nevertheless, many dispensers erroneously use the terms "fitting cross height" and "MRP height" interchangeably.) The add power is verified at the location set by the manufacturer, marked with a circle, and called the near reference point (NRP). No verification is done at the fitting cross.

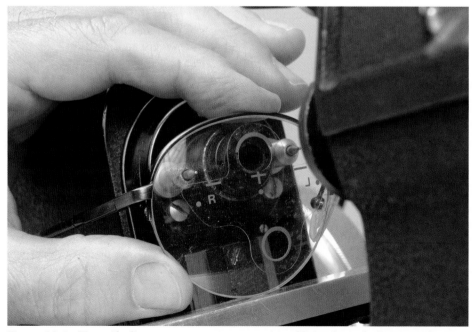

Figure 20-8. To verify distance power on a progressive addition lens, the lens must be positioned with the arc around the lensmeter aperture as shown. This ensures that the power reading will not be affected by the changing power in the progressive zone.

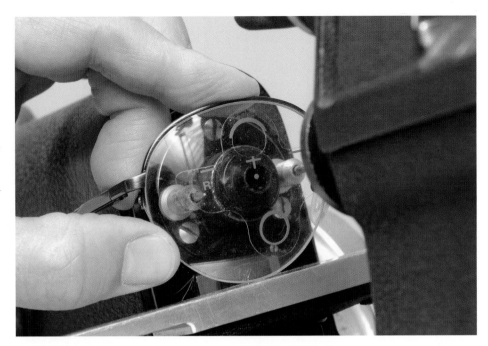

Figure 20-9. To verify prismatic effect, the lens is verified at the prism reference point (PRP) located by the central dot directly below the fitting cross.

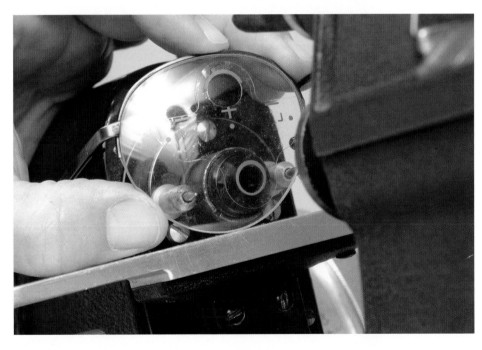

Figure 20-10. When both distance and near powers are low, the near power may be verified using the back vertex power as shown in the figure. In any case the near power must be read through the near circle. The correct method, however, is to find the near add using front vertex powers. This is shown in Figure 20-11.

be slightly blurred. The target may be blurred in the lower half of the viewing field because the progressive corridor begins at the PRP.

As can be expected in all types of multifocals, the near portion of progressive lenses will demonstrate power in an amount dependent on the power of the distance portion and add. It should be read through the circular marking that identifies the center of the near power area (Figure 20-10). This point is set by the manufacturer and is referred to as the NRP.

Although Figure 20-10 shows the near addition being measured as back vertex power, as with standard multifocals, to determine the add most accurately, distance and near powers should be read with the lenses in a reversed position and the add power calculated (Figure 20-11). In practice back vertex power measurements will work for low-powered lenses with low-powered adds, but front vertex powers will give more accurate readings with either or both increasing distance and add powers. (For more information, see Chapter 6.)

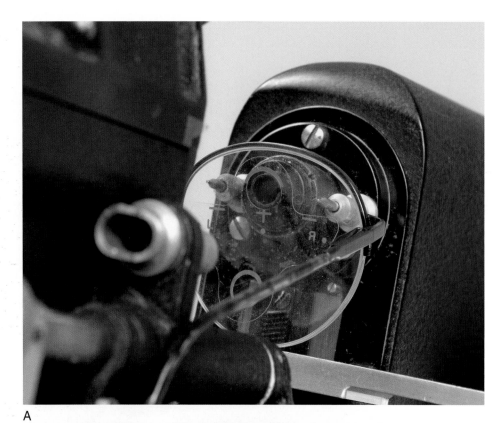

A

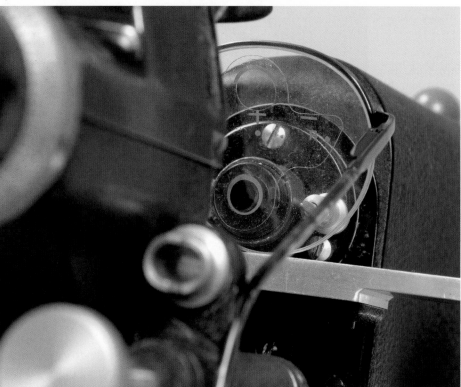

B

Figure 20-11. If the power of the distance and/or add powers are high, the add power (not the distance power) is measured using front vertex powers. This is no different from any other multifocal lens. **A,** The front vertex power is measured through the distance portion as the first step in obtaining an accurate add power. **B,** The second step in accurately measuring the add power is to measure front vertex power through the near portion. This difference between distance and near front vertex powers is the power of the near addition.

In practice the power of the near addition is seldom measured for progressive lenses. This is because the near addition power amount appears as a hidden number on the front surface of the lens. Instead of using the lensmeter for near power, verifying this hidden number is common practice.

Verifying Fitting Cross Height and Monocular Interpillary Distances

Fitting cross height and monocular PDs can be checked by centering the bridge of the glasses on the diagonally converging central alignment pattern of the manufacturer's centration chart. The horizontal lines on the lens must be on (or parallel to) the horizontal axis of the centration chart with the fitting cross height at the "zero" level. From this position, the monocular PDs and fitting cross heights can be verified.

It is important to verify the location of the hidden engravings on the lens as well (Figure 20-12). This will ensure that the lens is indeed properly marked. It is not unusual for the laboratory to have to reapply the visible markings if they were removed during processing. If the visible markings appear correct but the hidden engravings do not coincide with them, the lens is not correct.

Locating the Hidden Engravings on a Progressive Lens

All progressive lenses have fairly similar markings or engravings on their surfaces. These markings are directly used to identify design, manufacturer, and add power. They are used indirectly to reconstruct the temporary markings that allow distance power, PRP, and near power to be found. The engravings that allow reconstruction of temporary markings are found in the forms of circles, squares, triangles, or trademarks at lateral positions on either side of the lens.

On most brands, the power of the add is engraved 4 mm below the temporal symbol, although it may be above that symbol on some. On many brands, but not all, a mark identifying the design or the manufacturer is engraved 4 mm below the nasal symbol.

The hidden engravings can sometimes be hard to see. The following three sections discuss methods that may help dispensers locate them.

Use a Black Background
Using a black background, hold the lens so that there is plenty of light on it. It is often helpful to locate the light source on the other side of the lens, off to the side or above it. Tilt the lens to inspect the front surface from different angles until the markings become visible.

Use a Fluorescent Bulb
It may be possible to find the hidden markings on a lens by using a fluorescent light source behind the lens. To use this method, hold the lens up with a fluorescent ceiling light in the background and view the lens surface.

Use a Hidden Circle Finding Instrument
The Essilor instrument for finding hidden circles consists of a magnifier and an area for the lens that is illuminated with a bulb. This facilitates lens identification in a controlled manner (Figure 20-13). Markings are considerably easier to see because they are clearer and also appear larger. Figure 20-14 shows a view of what the hidden markings look like through this instrument.

Identifying an Unknown Progressive Lens
When someone is wearing a progressive lens and the lens manufacturer, lens design, or lens material of the progressive are unknown, the hidden markings will reveal the needed information. Remember that normally a hidden marking identifying the design is engraved 4 mm below the nasal hidden circle or symbol. To "decode" these markings, look in the Optical Laboratory

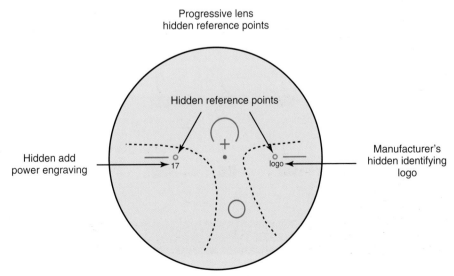

Figure 20-12. Manufacturers place hidden marks on the front surface of a progressive lens for four reasons: (1) to identify their product so that the dispenser is certain the product is the brand ordered, (2) to identify unknown lenses already being worn, (3) to indicate power, and (4) to provide reference points to allow the reapplication of visible markings for verification purposes. In this illustration, the number 17 indicates a +1.75 D add power.

Progressive lens
hidden reference points

Hidden reference points

Hidden add
power engraving

17

logo

Manufacturer's
hidden identifying
logo

Association's (OLA) *Progressive Identifier* (Figure 22-15). This publication shows pictures of each type of progressive lens with all their hidden markings. In the front is an index by symbol. Find the symbol in the index and look up the lens on the appropriate page. The *Progressive Identifier* gives information on lens type, material, fitting cross location, and minimum recommended fitting height. It is available through wholesale optical laboratories or direct from the OLA.

Remarking a Lens Using Hidden Engravings

To remark a lens, the two hidden engraved circles (or marks) can be emphasized by dotting their centers on the front side with a thin felt-tip or fiber-point pen. These dots are then placed on the respective manufacturer's centration or verification chart. The other markings for the power control circles, fitting cross, and optical center (OC) can be traced from the chart. Alter-

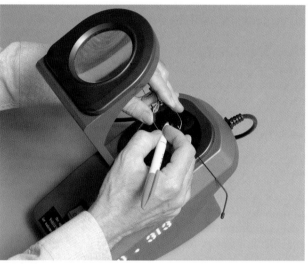

Figure 20-13. This Essilor instrument allows the hidden markings on a progressive addition lens to be seen much more easily than with the naked eye. The open placement of the lens on the instrument means that the markings can be dotted with a marking pen while looking through the instrument.

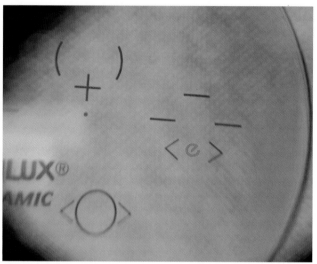

Figure 20-14. This photo shows the permanent, hidden marking on a progressive addition lens using the Essilor instrument. The permanent lens identification logo is found between the nonpermanent, caret marks. (The photographic view through the instrument as seen in this figure has been retouched for clarity.)

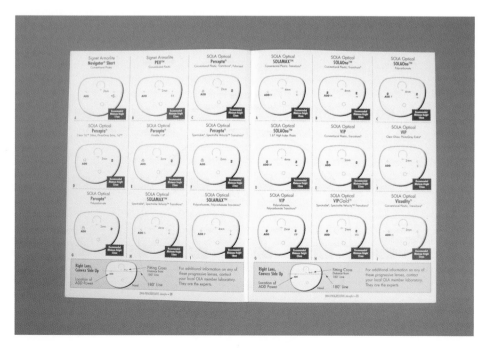

Figure 20-15. This is a page from the Optical Laboratory Association's (OLA) *Progressive Identifier* used to find information about progressive addition lenses.

natively a set of plastic dispensing decals may be used, if available. The decals form a set of two, one for each eye, with the near circle decentered nasally on each.

DISPENSING PROGRESSIVES

Validation on the Patient

Once the prescription has proved to be correct, it is adjusted to fit the wearer. Normal frame fitting rules apply. In addition, to provide the maximum possible field of view, adjust the frame for:

1. A small vertex distance
2. Adequate face form
3. A maximum pantoscopic tilt that still looks appropriate for the wearer

With the visible markings still on the lenses, also check the following:

1. The fitting crosses should be in front of each pupil center. (Ensurance of the placement of the fitting crosses is especially important when the two eyes are not at an equal vertical height.)
2. The horizontal dashes on the lenses should be exactly horizontal and not tilted.

Removing the Visible Markings

The visible marks that are on a progressive addition lens when it comes back from the laboratory are nonwater soluble. To remove them, use alcohol or an alcohol swab. Sometimes these marks can be stubborn. Some say that stubborn markings will come off easier if the lens is first heated in the hot air frame warmer. The alcohol may work better on the heated mark.

Instructing the Wearer at Dispensing

Adapting to progressive lenses can be made easier for a new wearer if the characteristics of the lenses are demonstrated at the time they are dispensed.

To demonstrate the full range of progressive lens versatility, hold a near-point chart at eye level at an intermediate distance. Instruct the wearer to look directly at the near-point card through the distance portion. Next ask the patient to tilt his or her head back until the letters on the card are clear. Gradually, bring the card closer to the eyes as the head is tilted still farther back, demonstrating the full range of viewing available.

More head movement is required with progressive lenses. Therefore some fitters recommend instructing the wearer to first point his or her nose at the object to be seen, then to move the head somewhat up or down until things clear.

Attention should also be called to any distortion present during peripheral gaze so the wearer understands that this is to be expected. While the wearer holds the head still, demonstrate areas where vision is not as clear by moving the near-point card to the left and right in the reading area while the wearer follows the card with the eyes. As observed in some studies, adjustment to distortion and increased head movement are adaptations that depend on steady wear of the lenses. In other words, wearing the lenses at all times will speed the adaptation process. Emphasize this point to the new wearer.

Once again remember that it is better to point out any areas of distortion, rather than having the wearer "discover" them and report back with a problem. If this lens characteristic is pointed out ahead of time, the dispenser is considered to be knowledgeable when it occurs. If the wearer discovers the problem and points it out, the dispenser is in the awkward position of having to explain after the fact.

TROUBLESHOOTING PROGRESSIVE PROBLEMS

Most problems encountered by progressive lens wearers are a direct result of basic fitting principles being ignored. Here are a few typical errors that should never occur, but do.

- One monocular PD is correct; the other is wrong. This happens when the monocular PDs are done with a ruler or by marking the PD measurements on the lenses, and the fitter uses only one eye to measure both lenses.
- The PD is given as a binocular PD, rather than as two monocular PDs.
- Fitting cross height is measured for one eye, and the same measurement is written down for both eyes. Fitting cross heights must be individually measured for both eyes.

When a wearer does come back with a complaint, the most straightforward way to check for possible problems is to *first* put the progressive markings back on the lenses and see if they are correct in relation to where they should be when the prescription is worn. Often the problem will be obvious.

If the solution is not immediately apparent, Table 20-1 gives some common complaints with reasons they may occur and possible solutions.

Using the Near PD Method When Near PD Proves Incorrect

Sometimes it becomes necessary to troubleshoot a problem of insufficient near-viewing area. There are numerous possible reasons for this happening. These are listed in Table 20-1. When none of the other solutions are applicable, it may be that monocular distance PDs are correct, but the monocular near PDs are either too large or too small. Here is one way to solve the problem.

For many progressive add lenses, the near-viewing area is inset from 2.0 mm to 2.5 mm per lens. Most manufacturers use 2.5 mm per lens. (Newer progressives

TABLE 20-1

Troubleshooting Progressive Addition Lens Problems

Complaint	Possible Cause	Possible Solution
The wearer has to lower the head to drive or see well in the distance.	1. The fitting cross is too high. The wearer is looking through the beginning of the progressive zone.	A. Adjust the frame to lower the fitting cross. B. Re-measure fitting height and reorder the lenses.
Central distance vision is blurry.	1. The fitting cross is too high. The wearer is looking through the beginning of the progressive zone.	A. Adjust the frame to lower the fitting cross. B. Re-measure fitting height and reorder the lenses.
	2. The distance refraction is off.	A. Recheck the refractive prescription.
Distance vision is clear in the center but blurry on either side (in the periphery).	1. The lens is a soft design and the vertex distance is too great.	A. Adjust the frame to decrease the vertex distance.
	2. The wearer has little or no distance prescription and the lens has a soft design with some distortion in the distance periphery.	A. Change to a harder design with less peripheral distortion in the distance.
	3. The lens has been made on the wrong base curve.	A. Check to see if the base curve is what is recommended for the distance power of the lens.
Near viewing area is too small and/or near vision is poor.	1. The lens-to-eye (vertex) distance is too great.	A. Adjust the frame to decrease the vertex distance so the frame fits closer to the face. B. Increase the pantoscopic angle to bring the lower (near viewing area) of the frame closer to the face.
	2. The wearer has not been instructed on how the lens is to be used.	A. Instruct the wearer on how to use the lenses and see if he or she recognizes the appropriate area of the lens to use for near viewing.
	3. One or both of the monocular PDs are incorrect. The eyes are not in the center of the reading portion, narrowing the useable reading area.	A. Re-measure for monocular PDs and remake lenses.
	4. The lens or frame is fit too low.	A. Adjust the frame to move it higher on the face. B. Re-measure and re-make the lens.
	5. The vertical dimension of the frame is too small for the progressive lens and too much near viewing area is being cut off.	A. Use a frame with deeper vertical dimension. B. Use a short-corridor lens design appropriate for frames with narrower vertical depths. C. DO NOT increase the add power in an attempt to avoid or correct this problem!
	6. The add power is incorrect.	A. If the add power is too high, the correct power will not be found in the normal near viewing area. Re-check the refraction and reorder the lenses if necessary.
	7. The lens design has insufficient width for the near viewing needs of the wearer.	A. Choose a lens design with a wider near area. B. Suggest a second pair of occupational lenses for a small office environment.
	8. The monocular *distance* PDs are correct, but the monocular *near* PDs are either too large or too small.	A. Re-measure the monocular PDs as monocular *near* PDs. Add the manufacturer's segment inset to the monocular near PDs and order these values for monocular distance PDs.

TABLE **20-1**
Troubleshooting Progressive Addition Lens Problems—cont'd

Complaint	Possible Cause	Possible Solution
The wearer has to hold the reading material to one side in order to read.	1. The monocular PDs are probably off.	A. Re-measure and remake the lenses to the correct monocular PDs.
The wearer has to tilt the head back in order to read	1. The lenses are fit too low.	A. Adjust the frame so that is sits higher on the face. B. Re-measure and remake the lenses.
	2. The progressive corridor is too long for the wearer.	A. Go with a shorter corridor progressive lens.
There is not enough width for intermediate viewing distances	1. The lenses are fit too far away from the eyes (vertex distance is too long). 2. The monocular distance PDs are incorrect. 3. The fitting cross heights are incorrect.	A. Adjust the frame so that the lenses are closer to the face. A. Re-measure for monocular PDs and remake the lenses. A. Adjust the frame for the correct fitting height. B. Re-measure the fitting cross heights and remake the lenses.
	4. The lens design is too hard. 5. The wearer's needs for intermediate viewing are too great for a general-purpose progressive lens	A. Use a lens with a softer design. A. Suggest a second pair using an occupational progressive lens.
Objects in the periphery seem to move or "swim" when the wearer is moving around.	1. The lenses are not fit close enough to the wearer's eyes.	A. Adjust the frame for a closer vertex distance. B. Increase the face form of the frame.
To see objects clearly for intermediate and near distances, the wearer needs to move the head more than would be expected.	1. The lenses are not fit close enough to the wearer's eyes. 2. The add power is too high.	A. Adjust the frame for a closer vertex distance. B. Increase the face form of the frame. A. Recheck the near add power and remake the lenses for a lower add power.

Data from Enhancing patient satisfaction with Varilux Comfort, video #306-922043, 0399-CP, Essilor of America, St. Petersburg, Fla; Brown WL: Progress in progressive addition lenses, 2001 Ellerbrock memorial continuing education program, Philadelphia, PA, 12/6/2001, pp 303-306; Reference Guide 2002, LPAN200009 05/02CP, Essilor of America.

will vary the near inset based on distance power.*) For some wearers, this "seg" inset per lens may not agree with their pupillometer-measured near-point PD. Too much inset may displace the channel position too far nasally and limit the near-point field, resulting in some nonadaptable situations.[4]

For individuals with small distance PDs, less inset is required than is present for a standard progressive addition lens. This can happen with children who are being fitted for progressive lenses.

Here is how to base a progressive lens order on near PD measurements:

1. Measure the monocular near PDs using a pupillometer.

2. Add the manufacturer's seg inset value to the measured right and left monocular near PDs.
3. Order the lenses according to the new, calculated distance PDs.

There is a way to know if an incorrect near PD might be a problem ahead of time. This procedure is explained in Box 20-1. This same method may also be used to check near PD placement and to evaluate the problem of a new progressive lens wearer complaining about the width of the near-viewing field.

Example **20-1**

A new progressive lens wearer returns complaining that the lenses do not allow sufficient reading area. You remark the lenses and find that the fitting crosses are located correctly. Tilting the wearer's head back and having the wearer look at the bridge of your nose, you discover that the wearer's eyes are not looking through the near circles. The circles are inset too far nasally. Currently the monocular distance PDs are R: 28.5, L: 29.0. How would you reorder for a successful fit?

---

*Those with high minus distance prescriptions may also require less "seg" inset because of the base-in prism induced by viewing nasally through the lenses during convergence. (See Chapter 3 on how to predict the near PD based on distance PD and distance lens powers.)

Checking for the Near Viewing Area

If a person has an especially small PD, or *if you are concerned that the near viewing area may not come out right*, it is possible to check ahead of time using the following steps:

1. Measure for monocular distance PDs and fitting cross height.
2. Mark the sample lenses that are in the frame with these measurements.
3. Use the lens manufacturer's centration chart to locate the proposed location of the near lens power. This area is identified with a circle on the chart.
4. Use a marking pen to trace the circle on the lenses.
5. Close one eye, position a penlight directly under the open eye, and point the penlight at the wearer's eyes. (You should be at the wearer's normal near working distance, which is usually 40 cm, or 16 in.)
6. Instruct the wearer to look at your open eye. Place your fingers under the wearer's chin and tilt the chin back until the eyes can be seen through the drawn circles.
7. If the circles are not centered, you will need to adjust the PD so that the circles will be centered.

To evaluate *the problem of a new progressive lens wearer complaining about a small near viewing area*, find the hidden circles on the lens. Trace the fitting crosses and near circles back on the lenses. (This is explained in more detail in this chapter in the section Remarking a Lens Using Hidden Engravings.) Follow steps 5 though 7 above.

Solution

Set the pupillometer for a near-working distance of 40 cm. Measure the monocular near PDs. They are:

R: 27.5 mm
L: 28.0 mm

Lens manufacturer's information indicates that the progressive lens you are using has a seg inset value of 2.5 mm per lens.* To have the near PD come out correctly, the distance PD needs to be set 2.5 mm wider than the measured near PD for both right and left lenses. Therefore the monocular distance PDs will be

R: 27.5 + 2.5 = 30.0
L: 28.0 + 2.5 = 30.5

The distance PDs should be ordered as

R: 30.0 mm
L: 30.5 mm

---

*If not indicated elsewhere, this inset distance may be found by measuring the horizontal distance from the fitting cross to the center of the near reference circle on the manufacturer's lens centration chart.

When the distance lens powers are low, this method of near PD method of measurement works well. With high-powered distance PDs, however, incorrect distance PDs may induce too much prismatic effect.

SECTION 2
General Purpose Progressives

OPTICAL CHARACTERISTICS OF GENERAL PURPOSE PROGRESSIVES

The first successful progressive addition lenses were designed to maintain some of the characteristics of a bifocal. One criterion considered to be important was maintaining traditional lens optics in the upper half of the lens. If this is done, the power from the midline upward corresponds exactly to the prescribed distance power. At the midpoint of the lens and downward following the expected path of the eyes, plus power begins to increase. Once the full add power is reached, lens power does not vary. The progressive zone connects distance and near lens areas. These types of lenses are said to have *spherical upper halves* because the front surface of the upper half of the lens is spherical, rather than aspheric.

The first really successful progressive lens was the original 1959 Varilux lens.[5] The 1959 Varilux lens used this design philosophy.

Unwanted Cylinder

Unwanted cylinder is the greatest problem inherent in progressive addition lenses. Although the progressive zone gives clear vision when properly fitted and dispensed, the area to either side of this zone will have some unwanted cylinder power. This cylinder varies in amount and orientation, depending on design and add power. It will be noticeable if the eye moves far enough laterally from within the progressive zone.

A Sandbox Analogy

There are certain design characteristics that change the amount of unwanted cylinder in the periphery of the lens. To help understand how this works, we will use an oversimplified example of a sandbox. Think about a round sandbox with the surface of the sand smoothed to a spherical shape to resemble the front surface of a regular, single vision lens. Suppose we want to change the surface curvature of one area of the sand. The object is to give the surface a new "power" so that it will resemble the near portion of a progressive addition lens.

We can do this by starting at the center and gradually increasing the curvature of the surface in a certain area corresponding to the progressive portion of a lens. In other words, we start shaving the surface of the sand, removing sand from that area. But one of the first sandbox rules is, "You are not allowed to throw sand out of the sandbox."* So where do we put the sand? If we wanted to keep the upper half of the lens at exactly the distance power, it could not go there. So sand would have to be piled on either side of the progressive zone and then smoothed out. This changes the curve of the surface and causes unwanted cylinder.

Interrelating Progressive Design Factors

Here are some general design factors that may influence unwanted cylinder power and other lens parameters.[†]

1. *Add power*—as add power increases, so will the amount of unwanted peripheral cylinder.
2. *Rate of progressive power change*—progressive power can change from distance to near zones in either a rapid or slow fashion, making the progressive corridor either short or long. A rapid change means that the progressive zone surface curvature changes over a very short distance resulting in a short corridor lens.
   When the power changes rapidly
   - The intermediate zone width will generally be smaller.
   - The near zone is generally wider and larger.[6]
   If the progressive zone is longer, the plus power changes more slowly. A longer progressive zone means less unwanted cylinder; a shorter progressive zone means more unwanted cylinder.
3. *Intermediate zone width*—a larger minimum zone width is associated with lower amounts of unwanted cylinder.[6] The smaller the intermediate zone width and area, the greater the unwanted cylinder will be. However, there is not as direct a relationship between the amount of unwanted astigmatism and near-viewing zone size.
4. *Zone widths*—distance and intermediate and near zone widths influence each other. When one zone is made larger or wider, the other two zones will become narrower and smaller.[6]

The Use of Contour Plots to Evaluate Progressive Lenses

In 1982 a standard format was initiated for representing the surface characteristics of progressive addition lenses. This took the form of connecting points having equal powers. The concept is similar to that of topographic maps that show mountainous heights. These line diagrams are known as contour plots.

One form of contour plot maps the amounts of unwanted cylinder power, showing how fast cylinder power increases over the lens surface. Areas of equal cylinder power are plotted with a connecting line. These lines are called *isocylinder lines* (Figure 20-16, *B*). Another type of contour plot maps areas having equal spherical equivalent powers (Figure 20-16, *A*). With these it is possible to see:

1. How fast the power increases in the progressive corridor
2. What kind of power changes take place in the upper and lower lens peripheries

Being able to read contour plots allows for a greater understanding of the features common to all progressive lenses and the individual characteristics that may differentiate one lens design from another. It should be understood, however, that contour plots in themselves may not precisely convey a given lens' actual performance when being worn. Clinical choices made by progressive addition lens wearers may not agree with predictions anticipated from contour plots.

Contour plots do demonstrate relative progressive zone width, the presence of a hard or soft optical design, and the anticipated amount of unwanted cylinder in the upper half of the lens. They may also be helpful in matching a certain style of progressive addition lens to the optical needs of the wearer.

HOW PROGRESSIVE LENS DESIGNS HAVE CHANGED

We would not expect today's progressive addition lenses to be the same as they were when first successfully used. Progressive lens designs come forth as a result of professional judgments as to what lens characteristics are most important when worn. These judgments do not always agree. In addition, one philosophy may be correct for one wearing situation, but not for another. Here are some of the contrasting ways lenses have been designed.

Spherical and Aspherical Distance Portions

Originally, progressive lenses were designed to maintain an upper half just like a regular single vision lens. The upper half had a spherical front surface (Figure 20-17). In 1974 Varilux introduced a design that attempted to reduce the intensity of unwanted cylinder by spreading it out over a larger area.* It soon became evident that small amounts of induced astigmatism could be tolerated in the periphery of the distance portion. Lenses designed in this manner are aspherical[†] in the upper *and* lower portions of the lens surface instead of just in the lower section containing the progressive corridor (Figures 20-18 and 20-19). Returning to the oversimplified sandbox

---

*Keep in mind that this is an analogy only and is not what really happens with progressive lenses. It is only meant to characterize the problems faced by lens designers.
[†]Much of the information found in this section is taken from Sheedy JE: Correlation analysis of the optics of progressive addition lenses, *Optometry and Vision Science* 81(5):350–361, May 2004.

---

*This lens was called the Varilux 2 or Varilux Plus.
[†]An aspherical surface is one that does not maintain a constant spherical curve, but changes in curvature over a given area. Aspherical means nonspherical.

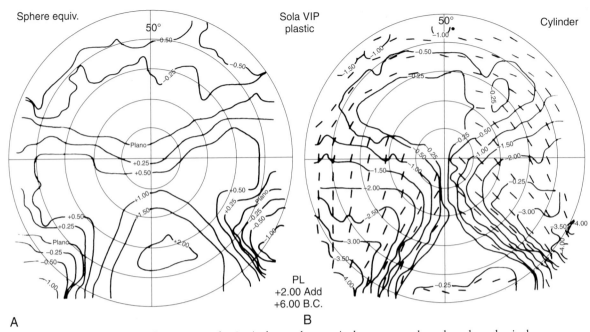

Figure 20-16. The contour plot in **A** shows changes in lens power plotted as the spherical equivalent.

$$\text{Spherical equivalent} = \text{sphere} + \frac{\text{cylinder power}}{2}$$

The contour plot shown in **B** is plotted as unwanted cylinder alone. Both plots are of the same lens having a plano distance power and a +2.00 add power. (From Sheedy JE, Buri M, Bailey IL et al: Optics of progressive addition lenses, Am J Optom Physiol Optics 64:90-99 1988, Figure 1.)

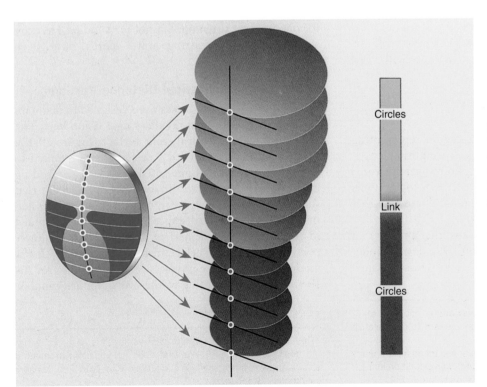

Figure 20-17. The original Varilux lens was designed to maintain a spherical surface in the upper half of the lens. It had two large and spherical distance and near vision zones linked together.

(From Progressive addition lenses, Ophthalmic Optics File, p. 28, Figure 25, Esselor International, Paris France, undated publication.)

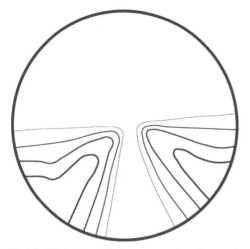

Figure 20-18. This simplified contour plot shows a lens with a spherical upper front surface. The concentric lines represent the areas of increasing astigmatism. (This contour plot is theoretical only and is not a representation of any existing lens.)

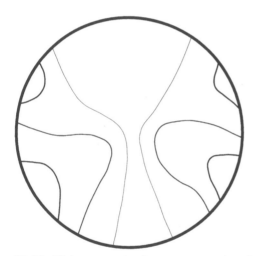

Figure 20-19. This progressive lens representation shows a lens with an aspheric upper front surface. Asphericity is allowed to continue into the upper half of the lens, with small amounts of astigmatism being evident in the periphery of the top half of the lens. (This contour plot is theoretical only and is not a representation of any existing lens.)

analogy, we can see that in allowing the displaced "sand" to be spread over a larger area the amount of unwanted cylinder in any given area will be reduced. Usually a lens with a spherical upper half resembles a "hard" design and one with an aspherical upper half, a "soft" design. These terms will be explained shortly.

Hard Versus Soft Designs

When an individual wearing a progressive addition lens is using the near-viewing area of the lens and slowly looks to one side, the eyes begin to leave the region of the near zone. Outside of this near zone, the power begins to change, and unwanted cylinder power increases.

Hard Designs

With a bifocal lens, there is a distinct, lined border between the near-viewing area and the rest of the lens. There is no question as to where the near portion ends. With some types of progressive addition lenses, the change in power and increase in astigmatism is more demarcated than in others. For example, the unwanted cylinder may rapidly increase from nothing up to 0.50 D, then move quickly to 1.00 D, and on up to 1.50 D in the space of only a few millimeters. Because of the rapid change along the border between viewing areas, this type of design is known as a hard design (Figure 20-20).

Hard designs generally offer larger and more delineated areas of unvarying optical power for distance and near viewing. Often in hard designs, the power in the progressive channel increases rapidly. When a person looks down, the eyes reach the level of full add power sooner.

The disadvantages of hard designs are linked with the rapid increase in cylinder power and the areas in which that unwanted cylinder is concentrated. Distortions caused by more rapid power change may mean a slightly longer period of adaptation. Straight lines may appear more curved when viewed through the lower half of the lens than they do with other designs. (It should be noted that all progressive add lens designs cause this effect to some extent, at least during initial adaptation. Even the near portion of a bifocal lens can cause a straight line to appear curved.) The intermediate viewing area of the lens may be more limited both vertically and horizontally, requiring the wearer to zero in more consciously to view intermediate objects with clarity.

Soft Designs

A soft design is one in which the change from the near zone to the peripheral area is gradual when compared with a hard design (Figure 20-21). As the wearer's eye begins to leave the near zone laterally, the amount of unwanted cylinder increases, but more gradually. From the wearer's point of view, it is not easy to determine where the near zone ends. A soft design has a slower vertical change in power as the wearer looks from distance to near. In other words, the progressive channel is longer and usually wider. This means that the wearer has to drop the eyes farther down into the lower areas of the lens before reaching the full near power.

The advantages of a soft design are easier, more rapid adaptation times; less distortion of peripherally viewed objects; and less "swim" of objects with head movement. Soft designs typically start with a smaller near zone and allow aberrations to spread over a larger area, including parts of the upper half of the lens. This means that the

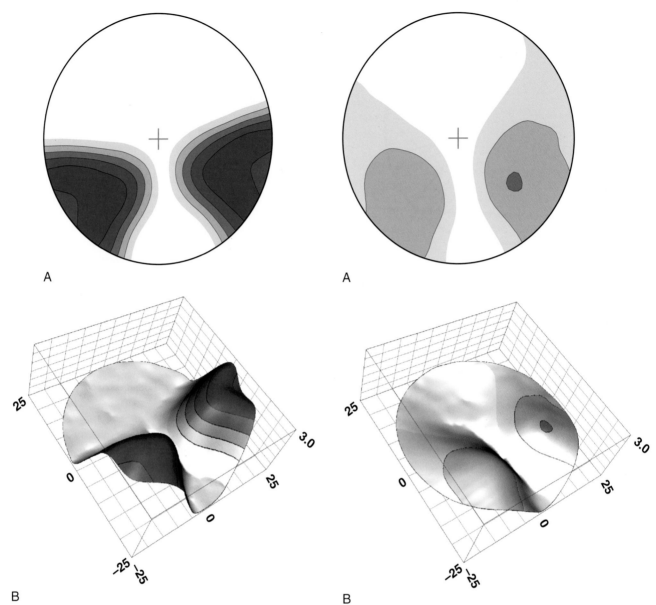

A

A

B

B

Figure 20-20. This is an example of a lens that has a somewhat hard progressive addition design. **A,** The contours of increasing astigmatism start at the border of the corridor and near zone. Each contoured area farther from the zone shows darker in on the diagram and represents a change in measured cylinder power. The near portion is fairly wide, and the contour lines are closely spaced at the border of the progressive and near zones. This indicates a more rapidly changing cylinder power. **B,** This 3-dimensional rendition of the same lens shows increasing cylinder as seen by increasing elevation. The lens is a 50 mm round lens.

(Illustrations courtesy of Darryl Meister, Carl Zeiss Vision.)

Figure 20-21. A, Here is an example of a very wearable soft progressive lens design. The near zone appears narrow, but the intervals of astigmatic increase are farther apart, indicating a more gradual increase in cylinder power. **B,** This 3-dimensional perspective of the same lens shows how a softer design usually results in a smaller dioptric maximum amount of cylinder power spread over a wider area of the lens.

(Illustrations courtesy of Darryl Meister, Carl Zeiss Vision.)

Differences Between Hard and Soft Progressive Add Lens Designs

Hard Designs	Soft Designs
Wider areas of stable optics in both distance and near	Longer distance down to the near viewing area
Narrower intermediate	Wider intermediate
Longer adaptation	Shorter adaptation
Some apparent curving of straight lines	Less apparent curving of straight lines
Highest dioptric value of peripheral distortion larger than soft designs	A soft design's highest dioptric value of peripheral distortion is generally less than for hard designs
Shorter distance down to near viewing	

dioptric power of the unwanted cylinder will not be as large.

The disadvantages of soft designs include the possibility of a slight reduction in visual clarity in the upper peripheral areas of the distance lens, the necessity of dropping the eyes farther to reach the full add power* and a "smaller" near zone. It should be noted, however, that wearers do not always find the near zone to be functionally as small as it may appear on an astigmatic contour plot. Because the amount of unwanted cylinder increases so gradually as the eyes leave the near zone laterally, the wearer may be able to use the outer limits of the near area anyway, even though these areas contain a certain amount of unwanted cylinder power. For a summary comparing hard and soft designs, see Box 20-2.

Monodesigns Lead to Multidesigns

As can be imagined, there are a multitude of ways to design a progressive addition lens. It is the job of the designer to try and anticipate the needs of the wearer. Initially, all progressives had a single design for all powers. This was later called a "monodesign." A monodesign is limited in its effectiveness.

When a person first enters the age of presbyopia, the power of the needed near addition is low. This means that a new presbyope still has a considerable amount of accommodation left. For example, an individual with a +1.00 D add power really does not need a special correction for intermediate distances. If presbyopes with a

---

*To counter this problem, the designer may increase power progression so that most of the add power is reached earlier. For example, a Varilux Comfort lens reaches 85% of add power 12 mm below the fitting cross.

+1.00 D add needed a special correction for intermediate viewing, there would be people wearing trifocals with a +1.00 D add. Yet trifocals are not made for add powers below +1.50 D.

With this in mind, designers began to ask whether or not consideration should be given to using more than one design for the same progressive lens, depending on the power of the near addition for that lens.

If changing add power is a major factor that alters the design needs for a progressive add lens, it would be logical to design a different lens for each add power. This is the basis for the *multidesign* lens, which varies to allow for changing needs with changing add powers.

Progressives Should Be Uniquely Right and Left Specific

From a historical perspective, when progressives were first emerging, it was not unusual for both left and right lens blanks to be identical. There was no difference between a right and left lens blank. Since the eyes turn inward for reading, the progressive corridor must tilt inward. Each lens was rotated so that the channels tilted nasalward.

This was not the best design, because when the lenses are rotated, prismatic effects are different for left and right eyes in certain directions of gaze. If both eyes looked into the lower right areas of their respective lenses, those two locations were not the same in power and prismatic effect.

Right- and left-specific lenses should be designed to work as a pair so that peripheral power, cylinder, and vertical prism are matched for binocular viewing.

NEW MANUFACTURING METHODS ALLOW NEW LENS DESIGNS

Recently there have been some major changes in the way lenses can be manufactured. These changes employ a method of generating the lens surface that differs from what is normally done. It is now possible to individually shape a lens surface to a unique form with a varying surface curvature and then polish that surface to optical quality. This type of manufacturing has commonly been referred to as *free-form generating*, although Shamir has trademarked that term, and a general term to replace it has not yet emerged.

Here are some examples of what these changes in manufacturing mean in terms of possibilities for progressive lenses. Some possibilities may be used by one design, some by another. Not all will be used for the same lens.

- The back surface of the progressive can be made as an aspheric or an atoric surface. Atoric curves can reduce the peripheral aberration called oblique astigmatism. (See Chapter 18.) This is especially important for progressive addition lens wearers with cylinder. When uncorrected oblique astigmatism is present, it combines with the peripheral distortion inherent in progressive addition lenses and can further degrade peripheral vision. An atoric design can improve peripheral vision.

- Progressive lenses are normally made as semifinished lenses with certain fixed base curves. These semifinished lenses are then surfaced in the laboratory. With free-form generating, the front surface can be custom surfaced to any base curve and the progressive optics included during surfacing. Then the back surface is generated at the completion of the front surface. This way the base curve can be more closely matched to the power of the lens.
- If a frame is fit with a specific vertex distance, the prescribed power of the lens can be altered for the vertex distance of the frame. These power changes are not limited to quarter diopter increments. The smoothing (fining) and polishing process no longer uses power-specific tools to bring the surface to optical quality.
- When a lens is tilted, there is a change in the sphere power, and a cylinder is induced whose axis is in the meridian of rotation. (See Chapter 18.) This power change can be compensated for on an individual basis, whether the tilt is pantoscopic tilt or face form. Again the compensation may be done more exactly because it is not limited to quarter diopter increments.
- With this type of generating, it is possible to make a progressive lens to order with the progressive power on the front of the lens, the back of the lens, or on both the front and the back of the lens. (The Definity lens is made this way with the progressive add split between the front and back surfaces.)
- This type of generating allows for the progressive portion of the lens to be made at different widths, depending upon the needs of the wearer.
- The progressive zone of a lens can be shortened or lengthened to custom fit the vertical depth of the frame and the vertical height of the wearer's eyes.

DESIGNS USING ASPHERIC/ATORIC SURFACING METHODS

Lens quality is limited by how well lens aberrations can be corrected. In Chapter 18, the basics of spectacle lens design were explained. One of the limiting factors has been the ability to correct oblique astigmatism for lenses with cylinder power. Oblique astigmatism could be corrected for spherical lenses by using a specific base curve or by using an aspheric surface. But if the lens had two different powers, as it does when prescribed cylinder power is present, then oblique astigmatism could only be corrected for both meridians at once if an atoric lens design was used. Atorics are easier to make for single vision lenses because they can be molded at the factory. But atorics could not be made for a segmented multifocal

or progressive lens because these lenses were surfaced for the correct power in the optical laboratory. The laboratory could only surface a spherical or a toric surface, not an atoric surface.

It is now possible to custom grind and polish an aspheric or atoric surface (although the equipment required is quite expensive). This makes it possible to correct more of the oblique astigmatism present in any spectacle lens, not just progressive lenses.

Progressive lenses have unwanted cylinder in the periphery of the lens simply because they are progressives. Oblique astigmatism caused by lens aberrations will combine with this cylinder and degrade peripheral vision even more. If this oblique astigmatism can be reduced, peripheral vision will improve.

One of the first types of progressives to include aspheric/atoric surfacing methods was the so-called *position-of-wear* or *as-worn* progressive lens design.

POSITION-OF-WEAR OR AS-WORN LENS DESIGNS

A major change in progressive lenses that took place because of free-form generating resulted in lenses sometimes referred to as *position-of-wear* or *as-worn* designs. A primary example of this is the Rodenstock Multigressiv 2 lens. This lens includes all the following factors in the design of the lens on an individual basis:

- Pantoscopic tilt
- Vertex distance
- An aspheric or atoric surface to optimize correction of lens aberrations

The practitioner specifies the sphere, cylinder and axis measures, along with vertex distance and pantoscopic tilt. When the prescription is received, an optimum base curve is chosen for the front surface of the lenses, and the prescription is modified to allow for tilt and vertex distance (Figures 20-22 and 20-23.) Then the amount of asphericity needed in each major meridian back surface is calculated. When the lenses are returned, the accompanying order information will include the sphere, cylinder, axis, and add power as originally ordered. It will also include new sphere, cylinder, axis, and add powers based on the calculated changes. For example, a lens may be ordered with powers of

$$-4.00 \;\; -0.25 \times 45$$
$$+2.00 \text{ add}$$

The order may be returned with powers listed as

$$-3.96 \;\; -0.27 \times 36$$
$$+1.82 \text{ add}$$

The second set of powers is what the lens actually will be. This second set of numbers is used for verification purposes.

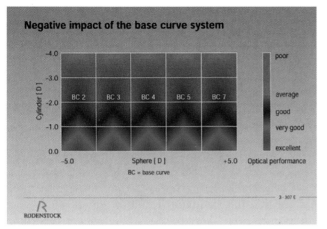

Figure 20-22. When a lens is made from semifinished blanks that come in certain finite intervals, the optical quality varies, depending upon how close that base curve comes to the ideal. However, even the ideal base curve does not deliver ideal optics when the lens has a high amount of cylinder. This figure shows conceptually how an ideal base curve, made with spherically curved surfaces, cannot be ideal for two different powers at the same time. It is not meant to show actual measures of vision or visual acuity.

(From Baumbach P: Rodenstock Multigressiv—a technical prospective, Rodenstock, RM98052, p. 3, Figure 4.)

Even if vertex distance and pantoscopic tilt were not specified for these types of lenses, the lenses still have great advantages because base curves can be optimized by varying the amount of asphericity on the surface of the lens.

ATORIC PROGRESSIVES

A progressive lens does not have to be a position-of-wear lens to incorporate atoric optics into the lens. Lenses dispensed in the United States are less likely to be measured for vertex distance and pantoscopic tilt. However, using atoric optics can be a large advantage, particularly for lenses with prescribed cylinder. Each lens may still be more exactly corrected for aberrations and individualized for prescription powers. However, the lenses must be custom surfaced using free-form generating techniques. At the time of this writing, such lenses are, with limited exceptions, only available through major manufacturers.

Examples of these lenses are Shamir Autograph, Zeiss Gradal Individual and Zeiss Short i,* and the Varilux Physio 360.

The Varilux Physio is a lens that is designed using wave front technology, but is surfaced in the traditional manner. It is not atoric. The Varilux Physio 360 uses the

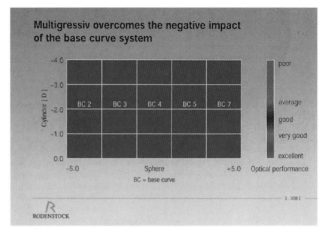

Figure 20-23. This figure shows conceptually what can happen to optical quality when optics can be corrected for base curve in both meridians of a lens surface at once when a prescription has cylinder power. This is done using an atoric surface custom cut for the prescription. The illustration is not meant to show any actual measures of vision or visual acuity.

(From Baumbach P: Rodenstock Multigressiv—a technical prospective, Rodenstock, RM98052, p. 7, Figure 15.)

same basic design as the Varilux Physio, but also uses generating procedures necessary to make the lens atoric, optimizing optics for all meridians of the lens.

PERSONALIZED PROGRESSIVES

Because of the ability to generate any surface on demand, the next logical step in progressives is to produce a lens with the progressive optics tailored to the distinct, individual needs and habits of the wearer. The Varilux Ipseo lens takes a major step into this area. The Ipseo lens is designed to match the unique head and eye movement habits of the wearer. Some individuals turn their eyes much more than they turn their head to see an object. Others are head turners, moving their head more than others do. The Varilux Ipseo uses an instrument called the VisionPrint System to measure head and eye movement (Figure 20-24). The lens is designed so that the near-viewing area will better match the personal viewing habits of the wearer.

In addition, the Ipseo lens design program takes the prescription and frame characteristics into consideration. When the lens returns from the laboratory the ordered prescription powers will have been altered because of surface asphericity and should be verified using the modified parameters. For example, a lens of power

$$+2.25 -1.25 \times 27, \text{ add } +2.25$$

may need to be verified as

$$+2.21 -1.22 \times 25, \text{ add } +2.07$$

---

*The Zeiss Short i is designed for frames with a small vertical dimension.

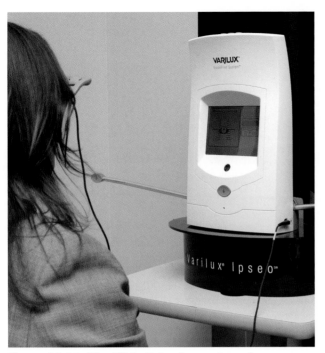

Figure 20-24. The VisionPrint System is used to measure head and eye movements. Results determine how the Varilux Ipseo personalized progressive lens will be custom designed for the head and eye movement requirements of the wearer.

It would be expected that other lens manufacturers may develop lenses that have alternate designs based on other personal characteristics, visual habits, and occupational needs of the wearer.

SECTION 3
Specialty Progressives

For years bifocal and trifocal lenses were worn by the majority of presbyopic spectacle lens wearers. Yet they were not able to satisfy all the visual needs for every wearing situation. As a result, a number of segmented specialty lenses developed.

Even though progressive lenses are clearly overtaking segmented multifocals, it is also unrealistic to think that general purpose progressives are able to fulfill everyone's specialized needs any more than segmented lenses could. If a progressive lens is truly for specialized tasks and will not be used for full-time wear, the lens may be called an *occupational progressive lens* and may be abbreviated *OPL*. Progressive addition lenses as a general category are often abbreviated as *PALs*.

SHORT CORRIDOR PROGRESSIVE LENSES

The *short corridor* category of specialty progressives is really a subcategory of general purpose progressives. The thing that makes this lens unique is that it is designed to allow a progressive addition lens to be worn in a frame with a small vertical dimension. Regular progressive lens corridors are too long. Too much of the near portion of a regular progressive lens is cut off when the lens is edged for frames with narrow B dimensions.

The short corridor progressive has a faster transition between the distance and near portions of the lens. This means that the wearer is quickly into the near portion when looking downward. Because the transition is short, near vision is suitable. Yet it is only logical that there will be some sacrifice of the otherwise larger intermediate portion.

When choosing a short corridor progressive, be certain that the minimum fitting height is suitable for the frame. Even short corridor progressives can come up short on near viewing if the frame is exceedingly narrow.

Some examples of short corridor progressives are shown in Box 20-3.

Short corridor progressives are fitted in the same manner as regular progressive lenses. Monocular PDs are needed, and the fitting cross is placed in the center of the pupil.

NEAR VARIABLE FOCUS LENSES

Near variable focus lenses started out as a replacement for single vision reading glasses. This lens also goes by other names, including, *small room environment progressives*, *reader replacements*, or simply *OPLs*. Over time the lens has become the lens of choice for someone working in a small office where intermediate and near vision are the primary viewing needs.

To get an idea of how the lenses are constructed, take the example of a prescription that has no power in the distance and a +2.00 D add. The normal progressive addition lens would have powers as shown in Figure 20-25 with no power in the upper (distance) portion. Power gradually increases until it reaches the prescribed +2.00 D add power in the lower near portion.

BOX 20-3	
Examples of Short Corridor Progressive Lenses*	
	Minimum Fitting Height
Hoya Summit CD (Compressed Design)	14 mm
Varilux Ellipse	14 mm minimum to 18 mm maximum
Shamir Piccolo	16 mm
Rodenstock Progressiv Life XS	16 mm
Zeiss's Gradal Brevity	16 mm
Kodak Concise	17 mm

*These are only a small number of the short corridor progressive addition lenses available. It is not meant to be an inclusive list. Nor will it necessarily be a current list. Short corridor lens designs, like other progressives, will continue to change.

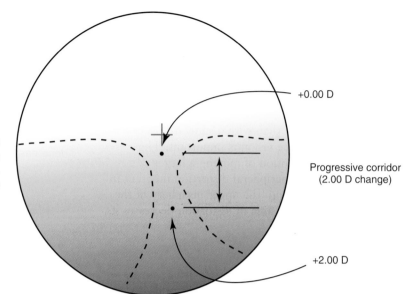

Figure 20-25. This is a simplified drawing of the structure of a progressive addition lens with a plano distance prescription and a +2.00 D add. The "power range" of this lens is a full two diopters.

Standard progressive

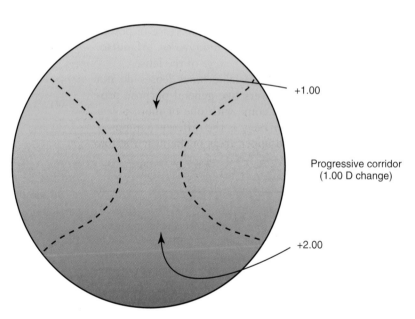

Figure 20-26. When a prescription with plano distance power and a +2.00 D add is placed in near a variable focus lens having a 1.00 D power range, the power difference between upper and lower portions is less. The progressive zone is also lengthened. This makes the progressive zone wider and reduces the intensity of peripheral distortion. This simplified drawing of the lens structure, based on the same prescription, can be compared with the standard progressive in Figure 20-25.

Intermediate/Near specialty progressive

This is usually not the case with most near variable focus lenses. The farthest distance that people who work in small office environments need to see clearly might be the distance of someone sitting across the desk from them. They also need a clear view of a computer monitor placed at an intermediate viewing distance and at the normal 40-cm near-working distance for reading. With this in mind, our example lens could be designed with a moderate amount of plus power in the distance.

If we use +1.00 D of power in the upper portion of the lens, we can gradually increase plus power until a total of +2.00 D is achieved for near. This would appear as shown in Figure 20-26. Note that the progressive zone for this type of lens is longer and wider than the normal progressive corridor found in a general wear progressive lens. This works well, and for this type of working environment, these OPLs give excellent intermediate and near vision with less peripheral distortion. Here is why:

- A longer progressive zone will result in less peripheral distortion.
- In a near variable focus lens, the difference between the powers in the upper and lower halves of the lens

are usually smaller. In the example, instead of having a difference of +2.00 D, this lens has a difference of only +1.00 D. In reality this is a +1.00 D add instead of a +2.00 D add. The smaller the add power, the smaller will the unwanted cylinder be.

- When wearing a near variable focus lens, more visual work will be done with midlevel and downward viewing than with a standard progressive where clear distance vision is important. The designer has the option of moving a larger proportion of the peripheral distortion inherent in progressive lenses into the upper periphery of the lens.[7] Increasing the area of distortion decreases its intensity.

Power Ranges

With regular progressives we think of beginning with the distance power in the upper portion and increasing plus power as we go downward. With near variable focus lenses, we begin with the near power. The reference power is the near power instead of the distance power. We start with the near power in the lower portion and decrease plus power moving up to the distance portion. This is no longer an addition, but a decrease in power. This decrease in power is called a *degression*.[7] Manufacturers often call this the *power range* of the lens.

This means that near variable focus lenses do not come in regular add powers like general purpose progressives. They instead come with one or more power ranges. Again the *power range* is the difference in power between the lower and upper areas of the near variable focus lens.

Example **20-2**

Suppose a variable focus lens made by a certain manufacturer comes in only one power range and that power range is 1.00 D. This means that there will always be 1.00 D difference (degression) between the lower and upper portions of the lens. If a person has a prescription of

$$\text{R: plano}$$
$$\text{L: } +0.25 -0.50 \times 180$$
$$\text{Add: } +2.25$$

what powers would be found in the lower and upper areas of the lenses when using this manufacturer's near variable focus lenses?

Solution

When trying to anticipate the powers in a variable focus lens, begin with the total near power. Total near power is the sum of the distance power and the near add.

For the right lens this power is

$$\frac{\begin{array}{r}\text{(distance power)} \\ +\text{(add power)}\end{array}}{=\text{(total near power)}}$$

or

$$\frac{\begin{array}{r}0.00 \\ +2.25\end{array}}{=+2.25}$$

Since the lens has a power range, or degression of 1.00 D, the upper area of the lens will have 1.00 D less plus power than the lower area of the lens. So the upper area of the lens has a power of

$$\frac{\begin{array}{r}\text{(total near power)} \\ -\text{(degression)}\end{array}}{=\text{(upper power of the lens)}}$$

or

$$\frac{\begin{array}{r}+2.25 \\ -1.00\end{array}}{=+1.25}$$

In a lensmeter, the upper portion of the lens reads +1.25 D, and the near portion reads +2.25 D.
For the left lens, the total near power is

$$\frac{\begin{array}{r}\text{(distance power)} \\ +\text{(add power)}\end{array}}{=\text{(total near power)}}$$

or

$$\frac{\begin{array}{r}+0.25 -0.50 \times 180 \\ +2.25\end{array}}{=+2.50 -0.50 \times 180}$$

So the upper area of the lens has a power of

$$\frac{\begin{array}{r}+2.50 -0.50 \times 180 \\ -1.00\end{array}}{=+1.50 -0.50 \times 180}$$

Near Variable Focus Lenses Differ

Near variable focus lenses are made by a number of different manufacturers. They are not all the same. Each has its own characteristic power ranges and should not be expected to perform in the same way. Table 20-2 shows some examples for several variable focus lenses.

Example **20-3**

A wearer has a normally written prescription for distance and near of

$$+0.75 -0.75 \times 175$$
$$+0.75 -0.75 \times 005$$
$$\text{Add } +2.50$$

However, the wearer works in a small office environment and uses a computer a fair amount of the time. If a near variable

TABLE **20-2**
Examples of Near Variable Focus Lenses*

Near Variable Focus Lens Type	Power Ranges (Degressions)	Manufacturer's Range Recommendations
Essilor Interview	0.80 D	All add powers
Sola Continuum	1.00 D	All add powers
Sola Access	0.75 D and 1.25 D	0.75 D range for adds of +1.50 and below. 1.25 D range for adds of +1.75 and above.
Zeiss Business	1.00 D and 1.50 D	1.00 D range for adds of +1.75 D and below. (This lens is said to be suitable for use in half-eye frames as well.) 1.50 D range for adds of +2.00 and above.
Rodenstock Cosmolit Office	1.00 D and 1.75 D	1.00 D range for adds from +1.00 up to and including +1.75 1.75 D range for add powers of +2.00 and above.
Zeiss Gradal RD (Room Distance)	Power ranges are always 0.50 D less than the wearer's regular add power	Each add has a lens with a power range of 0.50 D less than the add. For example, a +2.00 D add uses a lens with a +1.50 D power range.

*These are examples of some lenses available at the time of this writing. They are intended as examples only. New lens designs will continue to appear and availability will change rapidly.

focus lens with a power range (degression) of 1.50 D is chosen, what powers will be found in the lower portion and upper portion of the right lens?

Solution

With a near variable focus lens, it is easiest to begin with the near power first, then find the power in the top part of the lens. The near power will be found by adding the near addition to the prescribed distance power.

$$
\begin{array}{r}
+0.75 -0.75 \times 175 \\
+2.50 \\
\hline
= +3.25 -0.75 \times 175
\end{array}
$$

A lens with a degression of 1.50 D shows a plus power decrease from the near power by the amount of the degression. The power in the upper portion of the lens is found by subtracting 1.50 D of power from the near power.

$$
\begin{array}{r}
\text{(total near power)} \\
-\text{(degression)} \\
\hline
= \text{(upper power of the lens)}
\end{array}
$$

or

$$
\begin{array}{r}
+3.25 -0.75 \times 175 \\
-1.50 \\
\hline
= +1.75 -0.75 \times 175
\end{array}
$$

The power in the upper portion of the lens will be +1.75 −0.75 × 175.

Power Changes in the Vertical Meridian

As may be seen from Table 20-2, power degressions among lenses will vary considerably. The greater the power degression, the more the contour plot of the lens will resemble that of a general purpose progressive. Figure 20-27 shows a simplified representation of a lens with a small degression compared with a lens with a larger degression. Higher degressions result in narrower progressive zones and greater amounts of unwanted peripheral astigmatism. (Yet even with higher degressions, the OPL zone will be considerably wider than that of the standard progressive lens because of its increased length.)

Customizing the Near Variable Focus Lens to the Needs of the Wearer

When someone has two specific distances at which they do most of their work, the examiner may decide to prescribe for those distances. In this case the type of lens should be chosen with a power range appropriate for the prescription. Here is how it is done.

Example **20-4**

Suppose a person has a regular prescription of

R: +1.25 −0.50 × 090
L: +1.25 −0.50 × 090
+2.25 add

This person does most of her near work at the conventional 40-cm working distance, but uses a computer screen situated at an intermediate distance. The examiner tests for the best refractive correction for this computer screen distance.

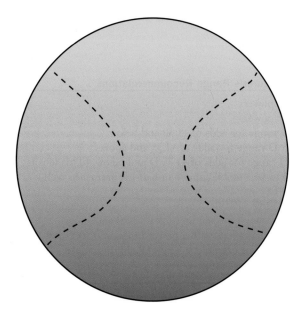
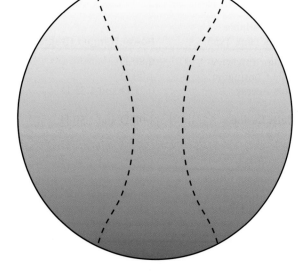

OPL with a smaller
power range

OPL with a larger
power range

Figure 20-27. When a near variable focus lens has a small degression (power range), the zone of optimal vision will be larger. Here are two simplified drawings comparing how a lens with a small degression might compare with another with a larger degression. Which of the two would be the most appropriate lens will depend upon the intermediate and/or near tasks for which the lenses are intended.

This distance is found to have an intermediate add power of +1.25. If a near variable focus lens is to be used:

A. What would the prescription read in the lensmeter through the upper and lower portions of the appropriate near variable focus lens? (Assume that the power of the upper portion and mid portion of the lens will be the same.)

B. What would the correct power range be?

C. When choosing from the lens types found in Table 20-2, which lenses would have this power in the upper portion of the lens?

Solution

A. Through a lensmeter the lower portion of this lens would have the regular near power of the prescription. This would be

$$\frac{+1.25 -0.50 \times 090}{+2.25\ \text{add}}$$
$$= +3.50 -0.50 \times 090$$

In the top part of the lens, we want to have the prescribed intermediate power. This will be the sum of the distance power plus the intermediate add, which is

$$\frac{+1.25 -0.50 \times 090}{+1.25\ \text{add}}$$
$$= +2.50 -0.50 \times 090$$

B. The power range, or degression, is the power decrease between lower and upper parts of the lens—in other words, the power difference between intermediate and near powers.

This can be found by taking the difference between +2.50 −0.50 × 090 and +3.50 −0.50 × 090, which is

$$\frac{(+3.50 -0.50 \times 090)}{-(+2.50 -0.50 \times 090)}$$
$$= 1.00$$

Power range or degression may also be found by taking the difference between the intermediate and near *add* powers, which would be

$$\frac{(+2.25)}{-(+1.25)}$$
$$= 1.00$$

Both methods result in a power range of 1.00 D.

C. In looking through the possibilities in Table 20-2, there are several possible choices with a 1.00 D power range. These include the Sola Continuum, Zeiss Business, and Rodenstock Cosmolit Office. It is likely that there are also other near variable focus lenses with this same power range that are not specifically listed in this example table.

The example just given assumes that the occupational progressive lens is to be used with maximum viewing distance being the distance from the eyes to the computer screen. If the viewing distance is to go beyond the computer viewing distance, then a larger power degression might be chosen.

Fitting the Near Variable Focus Lens

Near variable focus lens fitting recommendations vary widely, depending upon the lens style. For example, the Access lens only requires a binocular near PD and does not require any measured fitting height. It is fit just like a single vision prescription for reading glasses. The reason it is possible to use a binocular PD instead of monocular PDs is because the progressive zone of the lens is much wider than in a standard progressive lens. So if the eyes do not track down the exact center of the zones, there are not the same problems encountered.

In contrast the Rodenstock Office lens is fit like a standard progressive lens using monocular distance PDs and fitting cross heights measured to the center of the pupil. The distance prescription and standard near addition would be specified. If no power range is specifically requested, the laboratory will use the recommended range for the add power of the prescription.

OCCUPATIONAL PROGRESSIVES THAT INCLUDE DISTANCE POWERS

There are occupational progressive lenses that are used for small office environments and computer viewing, but still include a small distance portion located at the very top of the lens. This requires that the wearer drop the chin and look through the upper portion to see in the distance. Yet since the lens is entirely an occupational lens, this is not necessarily a disadvantage and may be considered an expected trade-off for intermediate viewing enhancement.

The intermediate area of the lens is positioned in front of the eye, as if looking through a trifocal segment straight ahead (Figure 20-28). Because the progressive zone is longer, going almost from the top to the bottom of the edged spectacle lens, the intermediate and near zones will still be considerably wider than standard progressives, though not as wide as near variable focus lenses with smaller degressions.

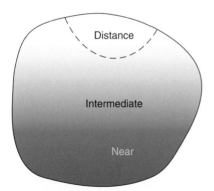

Figure 20-28. The Technica lens shows a large functional intermediate zone area with a small distance area in the upper portion of the lens.

These lenses are fit like regular progressives, but require enough vertical depth to the frame to keep from cutting off the needed top and bottom areas of the lens. They are certainly not feasible for frames with narrow B dimensions.

Two examples of these lenses are the AO Technica and the Hoya Tact. Neither of these lenses should be used as a replacement for regular, full-time-wear progressive addition lenses.

SECTION 4
Prism and Progressive Lenses

PRISM THINNING

One slight drawback to progressive addition lenses in certain power ranges is thickness. Increased thickness is especially evident when the distance powers are either plus or low minus. Progressive lenses in plus or low minus power ranges will be thicker than a flat-top multifocal lens of equal power. This increased thickness is a result of the steepening front curve in the lower half of the lens. (This same problem also occurs in "Executive" multifocals and can be solved in the same way.) As the lower progressive portion of the lens increases in plus power, the surface curvature steepens. This thins the bottom edge. To keep the lower lens edge from becoming too thin, the whole lens must be thickened.

To overcome the problem, the lower edge must somehow be thickened without thickening the upper edge. This can be done by adding base-down prism to the whole lens. When this is done properly, overall lens thickness will actually decrease. The technique, known as yoked base-down prism, is illustrated in Figure 20-29. Naturally, both right and left lenses must receive the same amount of base-down prism, otherwise the wearer will experience double vision as a result of unwanted vertical prism differences.

The exact amount of prism needed to thin the lens effectively varies according to the strength of the addition, the size and shape of the lens after edging, and the design of the lens. As a rule of thumb, Varilux suggests adding prism power amounting to approximately two thirds of the power of the add. (The use of yoked base-down prism for Varilux lenses has been referred to by the name Equithin.)

Most wholesale optical laboratories now use prism thinning routinely without consulting the account. Prism thinning has a very positive effect on reducing lens thickness and weight for lenses in the appropriate power range and should be used.* According to a study by Sheedy and Parsons,[9] small amounts of yoked

---

*Darryl Meister points out that in some cases high minus lenses may be prism thinned using base-up prism. This would occur if the fitting cross of a minus lens were located high enough in the lens to result in a thicker bottom edge.[8]

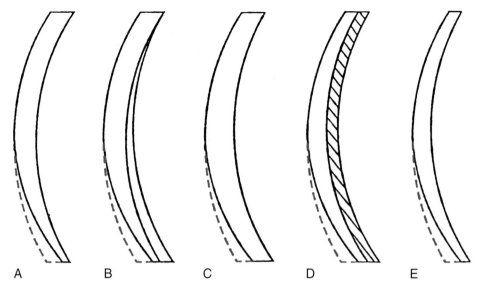

Figure 20-29. This figure shows the use of base-down prism to thin a progressive addition lens. **A,** The progressive addition lens as ground without prism thinning. The dotted lines indicate how the lens would be curved if it were a single vision lens instead of a progressive lens. **B,** Adding base-down prism thickens the bottom of the lens only. **C,** The line between prism and original lens has been removed. It is now possible to see how this lens with newly added base-down prism could be further thinned because both top and bottom are thick. **D,** The hatched area shows how much lens thickness may be removed now that both edges are equally thick. **E,** Excess lens thickness has been removed and progressive lens prism thinning achieved.

base-down prism are not disturbing to the wearer. Those tested could not differentiate between the absence of prism and 2Δ base down in both eyes. However, when prism was increased to 4Δ base down, there were significant postural changes by the wearer.

Prism Thinning Causes Prism at the PRP

It should be mentioned that base-down prism used to thin the lens will show up at the PRP of the lens. This is particularly important to note when only one lens is to be replaced since both right and left lenses must have the same amount of vertical prism. Thus vertical prism found at the PRP of the lens is acceptable when both left and right lenses have the same amount of vertical prism.

THE EFFECT OF PRESCRIBED PRISM ON PROGRESSIVE LENS FITTING

Success in fitting progressive addition lenses depends on accurate horizontal placement of the monocular PDs. If monocular PDs are incorrect, the eyes do not track down the progressive corridor. This reduces intermediate vision. Incorrect PDs also displace the reading zone, reducing its usable size.

Success in fitting progressive addition lenses is also influenced by the accuracy of fitting cross heights. An inaccurate fitting cross height will cause one eye to track down the corridor ahead of the other. This means that the add power is not increasing equally for the two eyes. The eye farther down one corridor is looking through more plus power than the partner eye following a few steps behind. An inaccurate fitting cross height also causes the eye to track down the progressive corridor off-center, narrowing the effective width of the intermediate viewing.[10]

When prism is placed before the eye, it causes the image of an object to be displaced in the direction of the prism apex. The eye must turn toward the apex to view the displaced image. For example, if base-down prism is placed before one eye, that eye turns upward toward the apex to fixate the displaced image. (This concept was explained in Chapter 5 and is shown in Figure 5-29.)

Vertical Rx Prism Changes Fitting Cross (and Bifocal) Heights*

When vertical prism is present in a prescription, it causes one of the wearer's eyes to turn slightly up or down. But when fitting cross height measurements are taken, the prism is not present. When the wearer is able to keep the eyes working together without the prism the eyes are looking straight ahead. One eye will not likely be turned upward or downward in relationship to the other.

---

*Much of the information presented in this section is taken from Brooks CW, Riley HD: Effect of prescribed prism on monocular interpupillary distances and fitting heights for progressive add lenses, Optom Vis Sci 71:401–407, 1994.

However, once the prescription lenses are in the frame, the eye must turn in the direction of the apex of its prescribed prism. The amount of displacement in the spectacle plane will be 0.3 mm for every 1∆ of prescribed prism.

When vertical prism is present, the fitting cross should be raised 0.3 mm for every diopter of base-down prism or lowered 0.3 mm for every diopter of base-up prism.

If the entire amount of vertical prism is prescribed before one eye, the vertical displacement of the fitting cross should be carried out on one lens. But if the vertical prism is split, the displacement of the fitting crosses should also be split in the same proportion.

To be certain of vertical fitting cross positioning with perscription prism, cover the wearer's left eye when measuring the fitting cross for the right eye. Then when measuring fitting cross height for the left eye, cover the wearer's right eye.

Example **20-5**

A prescription reads as follows:

R: +2.75 –1.00 × 180	3∆ base up
L: +2.75 –1.00 × 180	3∆ base down

The frame of choice is adjusted to fit as it should when being worn. Next fitting cross heights are marked on the glazed lenses to correspond to pupil center location. Heights are measured to be as follows:

R: 27 mm
L: 27 mm

What fitting cross heights should be ordered?

Solution

Vertical prism for the right lens is noted. The amount of vertical compensation is calculated as follows:

Vertical prism amount x 0.3 =
        change in fitting cross height in millimeters.

Or in this case

3 × 0.3 = 0.9 mm.

This is rounded off to 1 mm. Because prescribed prism causes the pupil of the right eye to be displaced 1 mm downward, the fitting cross must be moved 1 mm downward as well.

The left lens has an equal but opposite amount of vertical prism. Therefore the prism in the left lens necessitates moving the left fitting cross 1 mm upward. The end result is that the two fitting cross heights are modified and should be ordered as

R: 26 mm
L: 28 mm

Horizontal Rx Prism Changes PD Measurements

When horizontal prism is prescribed, failure to horizontally compensate the MRP placement will cause the eyes to track along the inside or outside edge of the progressive corridor. This greatly reduces the usefulness of the intermediate zone and narrows the field of view for near work.

Example **20-6**

Suppose a prescription reads as follows:

R: –2.25 –0.50 × 180	5∆ base in
L: –2.25 –0.50 × 180	5∆ base in

Using a pupillometer, the monocular PDs are measured as follows:

R: 29.5 mm
L: 30.0 mm

What monocular PDs should be ordered to compensate for the prescribed horizontal prism?

Solution

Noting horizontal prism, the amount of pupil displacement is calculated as follows:

5 × 0.3 = 1.5 mm.

Base-in prism will cause the eye to move outward by an amount equal to 0.3 mm for every diopter of horizontal prism. In this case 5∆ of base-in prism will cause each pupil to be displaced outward by 1.5 mm. The resulting monocular PDs are modified to

R: 31.0 mm
L: 31.5 mm

When Might the Amount of Horizontal Prism Be Modified?

When prism is prescribed in conventional, nonprogressive, multifocal lenses, the PD is not modified to allow for a change in pupil location. This is quite acceptable because the widths of nonprogressive multifocals are so wide in comparison with the corridors of progressive addition lenses that there is little need for modification.

When a prescriber tests for prism, the measuring prism on the phoropter is in front of the spherocylinder lens combination. As the measuring prism is increased in power, the eye responds by turning, leaving its location behind the OC of the refractive lenses. When the eye moves away from the OC of the lens combination, a second prismatic effect, caused by lens "decentration," is induced (Figure 20-30). Practically speaking this second prismatic effect is of no consequence since the measuring prism is taking it into account. But what happens if the refractive MRP location is altered during fitting? When the fitting cross is changed to correspond to the prismatically altered eye position, the decentration prism

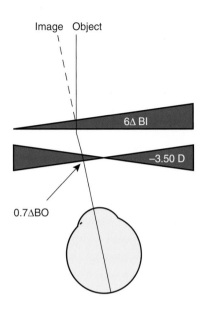

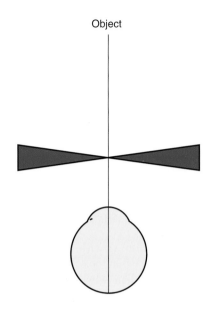

Figure 20-30. A measuring prism in front of the refractive lens will cause the eye to turn outward. As it turns, it leaves its previous location directly behind the optical center of the lens.

(From Brooks CW, Riley HD: Effect of prescribed prism on monocular interpupillary distances and fitting heights for progressive add lenses, Optom Vis Sci 71:403, 1994. Figure 4.)

that was present during refraction disappears. Without decentration prism, the net prismatic effect that was present during refraction has changed. When prescription sphere and cylinder powers are small, this is of minimal consequence. As the refractive power increases, however, the prismatic amount becomes more evident.

Example **20-7**

Suppose a person is wearing or needs a prescription as follows:

> R: –3.50 sphere
> L: –3.50 sphere with 6Δ base-in prism
>   +2.25 add

(Although it may not be advisable to place all prism in front of one eye, we will use this example for simplicity.)

Before refraction the monocular PDs are measured using a pupillometer. There are no refractive lenses in place. The PD measures as follows (Figure 20-31):

> R monocular PD = 31 mm
> L monocular PD = 31 mm

How should the monocular PDs and prescribed prism amounts be modified to allow the eyes to accurately track down the progressive corridor and still maintain the same net prismatic corrective effect?

Solution

Placing 6Δ of base-in prism before the left eye will cause the eye to deviate outward by

$$6 \times 0.3 \text{ mm} = 1.8 \text{ mm},$$

which will be rounded off to 2 mm.

During phoria testing, the eye was looking 2 mm temporally through the –3.50 D refracting lens (see Figure 20-30).

Using Prentice's rule, we see that prism caused by the eye being decentered in relation to the lens is

$$\begin{aligned} \Delta &= cF \\ &= 0.2 \times 3.5 \\ &= 0.7\Delta \end{aligned}$$

Since the lens is minus, prism caused by the eye moving in relationship to the refractive lens is base out. Therefore the net prismatic effect for the eye is

$$(\text{Prescribed } \Delta) + (\text{Decentration } \Delta) = (\text{Total } \Delta).$$

Or in this case

$$6 \text{ base in} + 0.7 \text{ base out} = 5.3 \text{ base in.}$$

To position the progressive zone in front of the eye, the MRP must be moved 2 mm outward. (When the position of the MRP moves, so does the fitting cross location. The fitting cross is directly above the MRP.) When the MRP moves outward, the finished spectacle lens prescription will no longer duplicate the refractive situation. This is because the 0.7Δ of decentration prism caused by the –3.50 D lens no longer exists (Figure 20-32). To maintain the same total prismatic effect, the prescribed prism must be reduced from 6Δ base in to 5.3Δ base in.

The PDs are ordered as follows:

> R monocular PD = 31 mm
> L monocular PD = 33 mm

It is helpful to note that when the MRP is moved in the direction of eye deviation, there will always be a reduction of prescribed prism for minus lenses and an increase in the amount of prescribed prism for plus lenses. In other words:

- For minus lens: *reduce* the Rx prism by an amount equal to the calculated decentration prism.

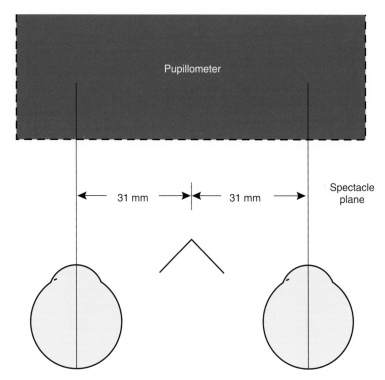

Figure 20-31. A pupillometer normally measures the interpupillary distance with no lens correction in place and with the eyes in a straight-ahead position.

(From Brooks CW, Riley HD: Effect of prescribed prism on monocular interpupillary distances and fitting heights for progressive add lenses, Optom Vis Sci 71:403, 1994. Figure 5.)

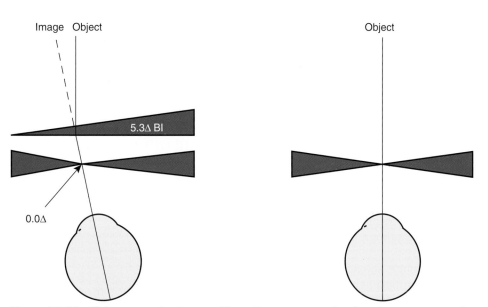

Figure 20-32. If the monocular interpupillary distance were to be altered to compensate for prismatically induced eye movement and correct progressive corridor placement, the net effect would be to change the amount of prism in the prescription. The decentration prism resulting from eye movement caused by the measuring prism will no longer be present.

(From Brooks CW, Riley HD: Effect of prescribed prism on monocular interpupillary distances and fitting heights for progressive add lenses, Optom Vis Sci 71:403, 1994. Figure 6.)

- For plus lenses: *increase* the Rx prism by an amount equal to the calculated decentration prism.

When filling an existing prescription, it should be noted that a modification to the Rx prism amount that is done to maintain the prescribed optical effect is no different than changing sphere and cylinder power in response to a change in lens vertex distance (see Chapter 14). Changing the amount of "Rx prism" to compensate for decentration prism does not change the prescription.

Compensating Fitting Cross Height or Monocular PDs for Prescribed Prism

A. How to Compensate Fitting Cross Height for Prescribed Vertical Prism
   1. Measure the fitting cross heights.
   2. Multiply the amount(s) of prescribed vertical prism by 0.3.
   3. If the prism is base down, raise the fitting cross height by the calculated amount. If the prism is base up, lower the fitting cross height by the calculated amount.
B. How to Compensate Monocular PDs for Prescribed Horizontal Prism
   1. Measure monocular PDs using a pupillometer.
   2. Multiply the amount(s) of prescribed horizontal prism by 0.3.
   3. Modify the monocular PD(s) by the calculated amount, increasing the PD for base in prism and decreasing the PD for base out prism.

BOX 20-5

Compensation Used if Modifying the Monocular Interpupillary Distances Produces Clinically Significant Changes in Rx Prism

It is suggested that compensation be considered **clinically significant** if moving the MRP will cause a change in prismatic effect of 0.50Δ or more. A change of at least 0.50Δ will occur if the prescribed prism totals ≥6.00Δ and refractive power in the meridian of movement is ±2.50 D or greater.
1. When horizontal prism is present, find the power of the lens in the horizontal meridian. When vertical prism is present, find the power of the lens in the vertical meridian.
2. Multiply the power in the meridian of eye movement by the change in monocular PD or change in fitting cross height. That is,

$$\Delta = cF$$

where Δ = change in prescribed prism power, c = change in PRP (prism reference point) location in cm, and F = power in the meridian of PRP movement.
3. For minus lenses, subtract this amount from the prescribed prism. For plus lenses, add this amount to the prescribed prism.

SUMMARY

Prescribed vertical prism in progressive add lenses requires that the fitting cross be moved up or down by an amount equal to 0.3 times the prism amount. The direction of movement is opposite from the base direction of the prism.

Prescribed horizontal prism in progressive add lenses requires that the monocular PDs be increased or decreased by an amount equal to 0.3 times the prism amount. The direction of eye and MRP movement is opposite to the base direction of the prescribed prism. Steps to take when modifying fitting cross height are found in Box 20-4, *A*. Steps to take when modifying monocular PD amounts are summarized in Box 20-4, *B*.

Changing the prism amounts should only be done if there would be clinically significant changes to the prescribed prism. This does not happen unless the prescribed prism is greater than or equal to 6.00Δ and the refractive power in the prism meridian is greater than plus or minus 2.50 D. If this is the case, then prescribed prism may be altered according to the summary found in Box 20-5.

REFERENCES

1. Smith JB: Progressive addition lenses in the treatment of accommodative esotropia, Am J Ophthal 99:1, 1985.
2. Kowalski PM, Wang Y, Owens RE et al: Adaptability of myopic children to progressive addition lenses with a modified fitting protocol in the correction of myopia evaluation trial (COMET), Optom Vis Sci 82(4):328–337, 2005.
3. Red dot procedure for marking progressive lenses, Southbridge, Mass, undated, American Optical Corp.
4. Musick J: A better way to fit progressive lenses, Rev Optom 128:66, 1991.
5. Maitenez B: Four steps that led to Varilux, Am J Optom Arch Am Acad Optom 43:441, 1966.
6. Sheedy JE: Correlation analysis of the optics of progressive addition lenses, Optom Vis Sci 81(5):356,358, 2004.
7. Sheedy JE: The optics of occupational progressive lenses, Optom 76(8):432, 2005.
8. Meister D: Understanding prism-thinning, lens talk, vol 26, no. 35, October, 1998.
9. Sheedy JE, Parsons SD: Vertical yoked prism—patient acceptance and postural adjustment, Ophthal Physiol Optics 7:255, 1987.
10. Young J: Progressive problems, 20/20, March 2000.

Proficiency Test

(Answers can be found in the back of the book.)

1. Which factor is normally *not* considered essential in fitting the progressive add lens?
   a. a good pantoscopic angle
   b. short vertex distance
   c. a sufficient vertical frame dimension
   d. good monocular lens centration
   e. specifying the nasal rotation of the progressive channel

2. The fitting cross for a general purpose progressive addition lens would be fitted higher than specified by the lens manufacturer in which of the following cases?
   a. for short individuals
   b. for tall individuals
   c. if the progressive lens is used to inhibit accommodative esotropia in children
   d. where prism imbalance may exist away from the OC
   e. where one eye is higher than the other

3. When children are fit with progressive addition lenses, yet still have the ability to accommodate just as other children do, the fitting cross is usually fit:
   a. at the lower lid.
   b. in the center of the pupil.
   c. 2 mm below pupil center.
   d. 2 mm above pupil center.
   e. 4 mm above pupil center.

4. True or false? Children fitted with progressive addition lenses should not wear those lenses for sports or play.

5. True or false? Progressive lens fitting crosses should be set lower for the first-time wearer to aid in adapting to the lenses.

6. True or false? Prism is verified at a different location on the progressive add lens from where the distance Rx is verified.

7. True or false? The fitting cross is at the major reference point.

8. A synonym for *major reference point* is:
   a. fitting cross.
   b. distance reference point.
   c. prism reference point.
   d. near reference point.
   e. None of these is a synonym for the major reference point.

9. True or false? If a progressive lens design changes as add power changes, the lens is called a multidesign lens.

10. True or false? Adaptation to progressive addition lenses involves changes in the respective eye and head movements used in fixation.

11. Although all of the factors listed below are important in the fitting of progressive addition lenses, which factor has the most influence on wearer satisfaction?
    a. fitting accuracy
    b. brand and style of progressive lens chosen
    c. accuracy of verification
    d. type of lens material selected

12. True or false? In practice the power of the near addition is seldom measured when verifying progressive lenses.

13. Which of the following is *not* a suggested method for viewing the hidden markings on a progressive addition lens?
    a. Hold the lens so that its surface may be viewed in a mirror by reflected light.
    b. Backlight the lens and hold it in front of a black background.
    c. Hold the lens up so that it may be viewed with a fluorescent light source behind it.
    d. Use an instrument especially designed for the purpose that both illuminates and magnifies the lens surface.
    e. All of the above are recommended methods for viewing the hidden surface markings on a progressive addition lens.

14. A frame has been selected for a progressive addition lens wearer. Some of the parameters of the frame and frame fitting are listed below. Which are problematic?
    a. The laboratory order form specifies a binocular distance PD = 65 mm.
    b. The frame is an aviator shape.
    c. After being adjusted, the pantoscopic tilt of the frame is 12 degrees.
    d. None of the above are problematic.

15. True or false? When a wearer does come back with a complaint, the most straightforward way to check for possible problems is to first put the progressive markings back on the lenses and see if they are correct in relation to where they should be when the prescription is worn.

16. Unwanted peripheral cylinder power in a progressive add lens:
    a. decreases with increase in add power.
    b. increases as the add power increases.
    c. is equal to the cyl in the distance Rx.
    d. is independent of add power.

17. True or false? Compared with a soft design, a hard design usually provides a wider area of high visual acuity in the distance portion of the lens.

18. Progressive power can change from distance to near zones in either a rapid or slow fashion. If it changes in a rapid fashion, then which of the following does NOT occur?
    a. The lens has a short progressive corridor.
    b. The intermediate zone width will generally be smaller.
    c. The near zone is generally smaller.
    d. There is more unwanted peripheral cylinder.
    e. Two of the above will not occur.

19. True or false? Distance and intermediate and near zone widths influence each other. When one zone is made larger or wider, the other two zones will become narrower and smaller.

20. True or false? Contour plots record the surface elevation for the front surface of a progressive addition lens.

21. Which of the following are not demonstrated by contour plots?
    a. relative progressive zone width
    b. the presence of a hard or soft optical design
    c. the anticipated amount of unwanted astigmatism in the upper half of the lens
    d. the expected increase or decrease in chromatic aberration throughout the lens
    e. where certain blur zones may fall

22. Would a progressive add lens with spherical upper front surfaces more likely be hard or soft in design?
    a. hard
    b. soft

23. Which lens design is more likely to have higher amounts of peripheral astigmatism?
    a. a lens with a hard design
    b. a lens with a soft design

24. Is a progressive addition lens specifically designed for frames with a narrow B dimension more likely to resemble a hard or a soft design?
    a. a hard design
    b. a soft design
    c. There is no way to tell.

25. Is a presbyopic emmetrope who is used to crystal clear distance vision more likely to complain about a progressive addition lens with a hard design or one with a soft design?
    a. one with a hard design
    b. one with a soft design
    c. There is absolutely no way to make this kind of prediction.

26. Which lens type listed below does NOT require a free-form type of lens generating to make the lens?
    a. position-of-wear progressives
    b. lenses with the add power split between front and back lens surfaces
    c. lenses that are personalized with the width of the progressive zone based on wearer eye movement preferences
    d. progressives made with atoric curves
    e. progressives made as semifinished lenses and completed in the laboratory
    f. All of the above require a free-form type of lens generating to make the lens.

27. Position-of-wear lenses are able to correct or compensate for all but which of the following?
    a. a difference in the vertex distance between the refraction and the wearer's glasses
    b. a pantoscopic tilt of the lenses that was not present during refraction
    c. a changing base curve requirement based on lens power
    d. varying amounts of induced oblique astigmatism in the two power meridians of a spherocylinder lens using an atoric surface
    e. Position-of-wear lenses can correct for all of the above.

28. True or false? Near variable focus lenses are used for small office environments, and all have 50% of the add power in the upper portion of the lens.

29. Near variable focus lenses have a power degression. Degression is:
    a. the difference between prescribed distance and near power, but going from near to far.
    b. the range in power of a variable focus lens from the total near power of the lens to the power found at the top of the lens.
    c. the range in power from the near portion to the midlevel of the lens.
    d. the range in power from the near portion to the fitting cross.

30. A near variable focus lens design will be used for presbyopes with all different amounts of add power. How many power ranges do near variable focus lenses have for each particular brand?
    a. 1
    b. 2
    c. 3
    d. as many as there are add powers
    e. All of the above responses may be correct.

31. Suppose a variable focus lens made by a certain manufacturer comes with a recommended power range of 1.25 D for wearers who have a +2.25 add. This particular wearer has a distance correction of −0.50 +0.75 × 090 for both right and left lenses and a +2.25 add. What power would be verified in the upper portion of the lens?

32. A near variable focus lens has a +1.25 −0.50 × 010 power in the upper portion of the lens. It has a power of +2.75 −0.50 × 010 in the lower portion of the lens. What is the degression (power range) of the lens?
    a. +0.75 D
    b. +1.25 D
    c. +1.50 D
    d. +1.75 D
    e. +2.75 D

33. True or false? Near variable focus lenses are all fit exactly like standard progressive addition lenses, measuring monocular PDs, and placing the fitting cross in the center of the pupil.

34. True or false? No occupational progressive lenses meant for small offices and computers come with distance powers in the top of the lens-only intermediate powers.

35. Using the rule of thumb* for prism thinning of progressive addition lenses, how much prism thinning would be expected for the following two prescriptions?
    a. R and L distance powers: +3.00 -0.75 × 090
       add power: +2.25
    b. R and L distance powers: -3.00 sphere
       add power: +1.00

36. For the progressive addition lens pair listed below, how much yoked base-down prism would be appropriate for thinning the lenses using the rule of thumb?

$$+3.00 \; -0.75 \times 130$$
$$+3.00 \; -0.75 \times 040$$
$$\text{add} \; +1.50$$

    a. 0.75Δ
    b. 1.00Δ
    c. 1.25Δ
    d. 1.50Δ
    e. none

37. For the progressive addition lens pair listed below, how much yoked base-down prism would be appropriate for thinning the lenses using the rule of thumb?

$$-3.50 \; -0.50 \times 180$$
$$-3.50 \; -0.50 \times 180$$
$$\text{add} \; +2.00$$

    a. 1.00Δ
    b. 1.50Δ
    c. 1.75Δ
    d. 2.00Δ
    e. none

38. A prescription reads as follows:

$$+2.00 \; \text{D sph} \; 3\Delta \; \text{BD}$$
$$+5.00 \; \text{D sph} \; 3\Delta \; \text{BU}$$
$$\text{add} = +2.25$$

Fitting cross heights measure:

$$\text{R: 20 mm}$$
$$\text{L: 20 mm}$$

What fitting cross heights would need to be ordered to compensate for the prescribed vertical prism?

---

*Remember, the rule of thumb is not what one would necessarily expect to receive from an optical laboratory with a computer program that custom calculated the amount based not only on distance and near power, but also on the size and shape of the frame

39. A prescription reads as follows:

$$-1.25 -0.50 \times 180 \text{ sph } 5\Delta \text{ BI}$$
$$-1.25 -0.50 \times 180 \text{ sph } 3\Delta \text{ BI}$$
$$\text{add} = +2.25$$

Monocular PDs:

R: 30 mm
L: 30.5 mm

What monocular PDs would need to be ordered to compensate for the horizontal prescribed prism? Would the prism amount need to be changed? If so, how much?

40. A prescription reads as follows:

$$-5.00 \text{ D sph } 3\Delta \text{ BI}$$
$$-5.00 \text{ D sph } 3\Delta \text{ BI}$$
$$\text{add} = +2.00$$

Monocular PDs:

R: 31 mm
L: 31 mm

The PDs and fitting cross heights were measured without lenses in place, and there was no manifested tropia (i.e., the eyes did not appear to be turned outward).
A. Based on the Rx prism, would you modify any of the PDs when ordering the progressive addition lenses? If so, how?
B. If you modify any of these dimensions, should you also modify the prism amount? If so, how?

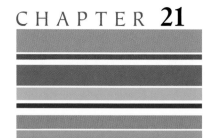

CHAPTER **21**

Anisometropia

W hen left and right lenses in a prescription are significantly different from one another, problems can occur that are primarily a result of the spectacle lenses causing the two images of the same object to differ from one another. This chapter examines those problems and then presents possibilities for their solution.

INTRODUCTION

Anisometropia is when there is a difference in refractive power between the left and right eyes. Anisometropia can work to an individual's favor in presbyopia. When one eye is emmetropic and needs no correction and the other is somewhat myopic, such a person can avoid the need for reading glasses. One eye is used to see for distance vision, the other for near. In fact such a situation is often created in contact lens wear and is called mono-vision. One contact lens contains a weak near correction instead of a distance correction so that a presbyopic individual can avoid having to wear glasses for reading.

On the whole, however, a significant amount of aniso-metropia ends up creating problems. With young children, an unnoticed difference in refractive error between the two eyes can result in the blurred eye failing to develop good visual acuity—a condition termed amblyopia. An amblyopic eye will be unable to obtain 20/20 vision, even when the refractive error is fully corrected. So it is important to correct for anisometropia as soon as it is detected.

When anisometropia is corrected with spectacle lenses, problems are not always over. The spectacle lenses themselves can create difficulties. Spectacle lenses worn at a distance from the eye will magnify or minify everything viewed through the lens. Different lens powers magnify different amounts. When one lens has different power than the other lens, the image of an object seen through the right lens is not the same size as the image of that same object seen through the left lens. The brain tries to fuse these two images into one single object.

Spectacle lenses have prismatic effects that increase with increasing lens power. Viewing an object below the optical center of a low-powered lens creates only a little image displacement. But viewing that same object at that same distance below the optical center of the other more

highly powered lens may cause a more significant displacement of the image. Since the two images appear to be at different locations, the two eyes have to turn downward by differing amounts to keep from seeing double.

This chapter talks primarily about those problems that arise as a result of anisometropia and what can be done to overcome them with spectacle lenses.

ANISEIKONIA

Aniseikonia is a relative difference in the size and/or the shape of the images seen by the right and the left eyes (Figure 21-1). This image size difference can be a result of the eyes themselves or can be produced by the optics of the correcting lenses.

Types of Aniseikonia
Physiologic Aniseikonia
Aniseikonia occurs in a limited but useful amount even for individuals with eyes that are identical to one another. Suppose a person turns their eyes to the left to look at an object. The right eye will be slightly farther away from the object than the left eye. The image of the object in the right eye will be slightly smaller than the image see by the left eye. These size differences give clues that help in localizing the object in space. This type of aniseikonia is expected and is referred to as *physiologic (or natural) aniseikonia*. Any other aniseikonia present to a clinically significant degree is an anomaly and is called *anomalous aniseikonia* or just plain *aniseikonia*. Anomalous aniseikonia can be caused by either the anatomic structure of the eye, or by the optics of either the eye or the correcting spectacle lens.

Symmetrical Aniseikonia
One eye may see an image that is symmetrically larger than the other eye (i.e., it is equally larger in every meridian). This is called *symmetrical aniseikonia* (Figure 21-2). Another type of aniseikonia is still symmetrical, but has a meridional size difference in a meridian of one eye compared with that of the other eye. This is called *meridional aniseikonia*. Meridional aniseikonia can be in either horizontal or vertical meridians or may be found in an oblique meridian (Figure 21-3).

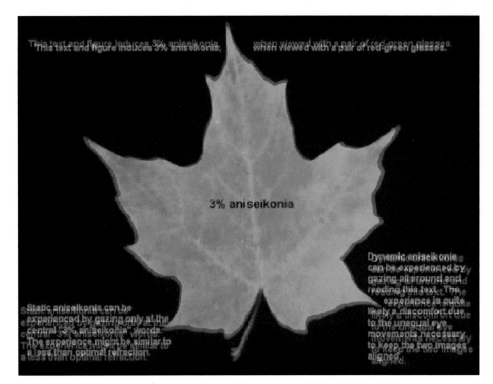

Figure 21-1. This figure will only be realistic if viewed through red-green anaglyph glasses. With red-green glasses on, the eyes will try to fuse both images as one, simulating what happens to a person with aniseikonia.

(From de Wit GC, Remole A: Clinical management of aniseikonia, Optom Today 43(24):39-40, 2003.)

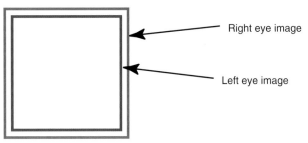

Figure 21-2. Symmetrical aniseikonia occurs when the image of one eye is equally larger in every meridian than the image seen by the other eye.

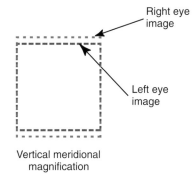

Vertical meridional magnification

Asymmetrical aniseikonia is when there is a progressive increase or decrease across the visual field. The image for one eye will get progressively larger across the visual field (Figure 21-4). This does not occur naturally, but occurs when a flat prism is placed before the eye. Distortion is caused by plus and minus spectacle lenses. This is due to the variable base-towards-the-center effect of plus lenses and base-towards-the-edge prismatic effect of minus lenses. Such variable magnification creates a form asymmetrical aniseikonia. This was shown in Chapter 18, Figure 18-11 as pincushion and barrel distortion.

Anatomic Versus Optical Aniseikonia

When aniseikonia is caused by the anatomic structure, it is referred to as *anatomic aniseikonia*. Anatomic aniseikonia can be caused by an unequal distribution of the retinal elements (rods and cones) of one eye compared with the other.

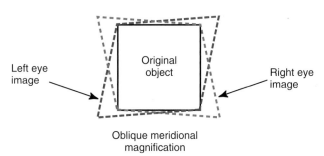

Oblique meridional magnification

Figure 21-3. Meridional aniseikonia is still symmetrical, but has a meridional size difference in a meridian of one eye compared with that of the other eye. Meridional aniseikonia can be in either horizontal or vertical meridians. In the top illustration, the aniseikonia is vertical. Meridional aniseikonia may also be found in an oblique meridian, as shown in the bottom illustration.

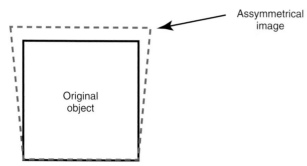

Figure 21-4. Asymmetrical aniseikonia is when there is a progressive increase or decrease across the visual field. The image for one eye will get progressively larger across the visual field, as shown in this figure.

Aniseikonia may also be caused by the optics of the eye or the optics of a correcting lens. When aniseikonia is a result of the optics of the eye, it is called *inherent optical aniseikonia*. When it results from an outside source, as from correcting ophthalmic lenses, it is called *induced aniseikonia*.

Spectacle Magnification: How a Spectacle Lens Changes the Image Size

In this section, we will look only at how a spectacle lens changes the magnification of an image for a single eye. We are not yet comparing differences in magnification between two eyes. The magnification change brought about by a single spectacle lens is called *spectacle magnification*.

Spectacle magnification compares the size of the image seen by a person when wearing glasses with the size of the image seen when that same individual is not wearing glasses. In other words,

$$SM = \frac{\text{retinal image size in corrected eye}}{\text{retinal image in same eye uncorrected}}$$

This is expressed as a ratio, such as 1.04 or 0.96. As percents these would be 4% magnification for a ratio of 1.04 and 4% minification for a ratio of 0.96.

There are two factors within a spectacle lens that contribute to magnification (or minification) of an image. One has to do with the power of the lens, and the other concerns how the lens is shaped. The shape factor has no net power to it, yet can cause a change in magnification. This is like a telescope. A telescope changes the magnification of an object, but since the rays leaving the telescope are parallel, it could be said to have no net power. So think of a spectacle lens as two components:
1. An afocal (telescope-like) component
2. A power component

These components contribute to magnification independently. The afocal components of thickness, index and front curve account for the shape factor; the power

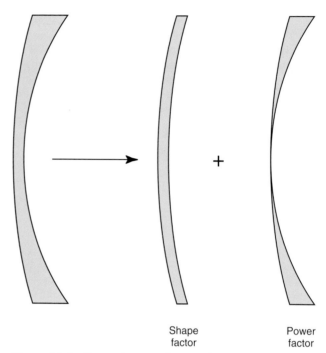

Shape factor   Power factor

Figure 21-5. Spectacle magnification depends upon both the shape of a lens and the lens power. This figure attempts to conceptually separate these two factors to help visualize those two aspects of spectacle magnification.

components of wearing distance and back vertex lens power make up the power factor (Figure 21-5). Their contribution to magnification can be given in the form of an equation for spectacle magnification, which is:

Spectacle Magnification = (Shape factor)(Power factor)

Or

$$SM = \left(\frac{1}{1 - \frac{t}{n}F_1}\right)\left(\frac{1}{1 - hF_v'}\right)$$

Where:
  t = the thickness of the lens in meters, n the index of refraction,
  F_1 = the front surface refractive power of the lens,
  F_v' = is the back vertex power of the lens, and
  h = the distance in meters from the back vertex of the lens to the entrance pupil of the eye. (The entrance pupil is normally assumed to be 3 mm from the front surface of the cornea.)

Here is an example of how spectacle magnification is calculated.*

---

*If the lenses are toric, having a cylinder component, each meridian must be computed separately.

Example **21-1**

What is the spectacle magnification for a +5.00 D CR-39 lens ground on a +10.00 D base curve to a center thickness of 4.6 mm and fit for a 14-mm vertex distance? (Assume that the +10.00 D base curve is the refractive power of the lens surface and neither the nominal nor true base curve.)

Solution

Since the spectacle magnification formula is:

$$SM = \left(\frac{1}{1 - \frac{t}{n}F_1}\right)\left(\frac{1}{1 - hF_v'}\right)$$

Remember that for h, the distance from the back vertex of the lens to the entrance pupil of the eye, we need to add the vertex distance (14 mm) to the distance from the front of the cornea to the entrance pupil of the eye (3 mm) to get the number needed. This is 17 mm, but must be expressed in meters and equals 0.017 m. So we would substitute the following:

$$SM = \left(\frac{1}{1 - \frac{0.0046}{1.498}10.00}\right)\left(\frac{1}{1 - (0.017 \times 5.00)}\right)$$
$$= 1.12752$$

A spectacle magnification of 1.1275 is the same as a 12.75% magnification.

Theoretically, What Was the Best Correction Thought to Be for Preventing Aniseikonia?

To answer this question, we need to know about two types of ametropia.

Axial and Refractive Ametropia

"*Ametropia* is the refractive condition in which, with accommodation relaxed, parallel rays do not focus on the retina.[1]" Ametropia includes myopia, hyperopia, and astigmatism. Ametropia may occur because the axial length of the eye is either too short or too long. This type of ametropia is called *axial ametropia*. On the other extreme, the eyeball may be of normal length, but still ametropic. Then the error is caused by the curves of the refractive components in the eye. In this case the ametropia is called *refractive ametropia*. According to "classical theory" of aniseikonia, the type of ametropia determines how the aniseikonia is corrected.

Producing a "Normal" Image Size (Relative Spectacle Magnification)

Normal image size is customarily taken as the image size for a standard emmetropic eye with a +60.00 refractive power. Suppose another eye, which is ametropic, but corrected with spectacles, produces an image that is larger than the standard. The amount of magnification produced by this eye, relative to the standard eye, is called *relative spectacle magnification*. Expressed as an equation, relative spectacle magnification is:

$$RSM = \frac{\text{image size for a corrected ametropic eye}}{\text{image size for a standard emmetropic eye}}$$

The difference between spectacle magnification (SM) and relative spectacle magnification (RSM) is this:
- Spectacle magnification (SM) compares the image size of *one* eye in both uncorrected and corrected states.
- RSM compares an ametropic but corrected eye with a standard emmetropic eye (that does not need a correction).

It would be desirable to choose the type of refractive correction for myopes, hyperopes, and astigmatics that would produce a normal image size.

Knapp's Law and Axial Ametropia

If the ametropia is axial, optical theory predicted that the image size would be different from that of the normal because the axial length of the eyeball is different from the normal. According to *Knapp's law*, "When a correcting lens is so placed before the eye that its second principal plane coincides with the anterior focal point of an axially ametropic eye, the size of the retinal image will be the same as though the eye were emmetropic.[1]" (It should be noted that for Knapp's law to be fulfilled, the ametropia must be purely axial, and there must be no anatomic aniseikonia present.)

Stated another way, if a person's eye is too long or too short, the image size will be larger or smaller than it would be normally. And Knapp's law says that using spectacle lenses* on such an eye will bring the retinal image size back to normal.

Having explained Knapp's law, it is imperative that we note the following: In spite of what optical theory says, aniseikonia is still present when axial ametropia is corrected with ordinary spectacle lenses that are placed at the theoretically correct position.[2] This appeared to be a result of "differential retinal growth or stretching.[3]" The incongruity between Knapp's law and clinical practice should be kept in mind when reading the rest of the material on aniseikonia. It has important clinical implications when deciding upon appropriate methods of aniseikonia correction.

Image Size for the Axially Ametropic Myope. The uncorrected image size for someone whose myopia is caused by a long eyeball will be larger than the image size for a normal eye. Previously it would have been said

---

*The spectacle lenses referenced in Knapp's law are assumed to be thin, flat lenses. In practice, spectacle lenses are curved, may be thick, and do not necessarily conform to this assumption.

that, according to Knapp's law, spectacle lenses reduce image size and bring it back to normal, eliminating the aniseikonia. Contact lenses, however, are much closer to the principal planes of the eye and do not minify like a minus-powered spectacle lens placed some distance in front of the eye.

When myopic anisometropia is present, optical theory says that we want to return both image sizes back to that of the emmetrope so there will be no magnification differences. Knapp's law would say that in the presence of myopic axial ametropia, spectacle lenses return both images back to normal size. In theory this would make spectacle lenses the correction of choice. However, from a clinical perspective, axial anisometropias were reduced when corrected with contact lenses.[4] Winn, et al also state that contrary to Knapp's law, spectacles "produce significantly greater degrees of aniseikonia than contact lenses.[5]" This suggests that even though the retinal image sizes may be made equal by using spectacle lenses for axially ametropic myopes, making retinal image sizes equal does not mean cortical image sizes will also equate.

Image Size for the Axially Ametropic Hyperope. The same discrepancies between theory and practice exist for the axially ametropic hyperope. The uncorrected image size for someone whose hyperopia is caused by a short eyeball will be smaller than the image size for a normal eye. Theory says that spectacle lenses magnify the image and bring that image size back to normal, whereas contact lenses leave the image size small. According to Knapp's law, the method of choice would be spectacle lenses over contact lenses. But in practice this does not prove to be the case. Contact lenses still prove to be more advantageous. (It should be noted that refractive surgery places the refractive correction at the same location as a contact lens—the corneal plane. Therefore refractive surgery would also be able to reduced aniseikonia in the same manner as would contact lenses.)

Refractive Ametropia and Image Size
If the ametropia is refractive, the uncorrected image sizes will be the same size as the image size for a normal emmetrope. Therefore in correcting an anisometrope with refractive ametropia, we want the image sizes to remain the same. We do not want the refractive correction to magnify or minify the image. Contact lenses are able to correct the error, yet leave the image sizes almost unchanged. Therefore for myopes or hyperopes with refractive ametropia, the method of choice for preventing aniseikonia, both in theory and practice, is contact lenses.

A common indicator for the presence of refractive ametropia is keratometer readings that are significantly different between the two eyes, revealing different front-surface corneal powers for the two eyes. Another indicator of refractive ametropia would be anisometropia in the presence of a developing cataract in one eye.

Anisometropes With Astigmatism. Astigmatism is a form of refractive anisometropia. If spectacle lenses are used for high astigmatism, each meridian will cause a different amount of magnification. Even for high astigmatics who are isometropic,* contact lenses have the advantage of reducing meridional magnification differences. Therefore the method of choice for anisometropes with astigmatism would be contact lenses.

Detecting Clinically Significant Aniseikonia

Although there are both obvious and not so obvious signs and symptoms that may indicate clinically significant aniseikonia, it is sometimes difficult to recognize. Aniseikonia symptoms are often the same symptoms as experienced with uncorrected refractive errors or oculomotor imbalances. The difference is that with aniseikonia, symptoms either are not helped by the correction, or appear after the other problems are corrected.

In addition to those just mentioned, here are some indications of clinically significant aniseikonia:
1. High anisometropia or high astigmatism
2. The presence of certain factors that physically alter the eye, such as pseudophakia, scleral buckling, corneal transplantation, refractive surgery, and optic atrophy[6]
3. Complaints about spatial distortion, such as slanting floors, tilted walls, or ground too close or too far away
4. Better optical comfort when only one eye is used

It is helpful to notice if the symptoms occurred after a prescription change or after the dispensing of new glasses. Assuming the refraction is correct and the lenses verify as they should, when anisometropia is present, aniseikonia is likely. There are several ways to approach the problem.

CORRECTING ANISEIKONIA WITH SPECTACLE LENSES

If an exact amount of aniseikonia is found, modifications to the spectacle lenses that change relative spectacle magnification will be of benefit whether the anisometropia is axial or refractive.[6] This is because there are specific modifications that can be made to spectacle lenses that will change their magnification. Even though contact lenses are usually indicated in the presence of aniseikonia, the patient may not want contact lenses. Changing base curves, lens thicknesses, and vertex distance can still be used with spectacles to correct the aniseikonia.

There are several ways to approach the problem of aniseikonia:

---

*Isometropia is the state of having equal refractive errors of both kind and amount in the two eyes.

1. If you are concerned that aniseikonia might be a problem, but have no clear evidence, use a "First Pass Method."
2. If you are fairly certain aniseikonia is present, want to address it yourself, but have no way of measuring it; then make "directionally correct magnification changes" to each lens individually.
3. Estimate percent magnification differences based on the refractive prescription and change lens parameters accordingly.
4. Measure the percent magnification differences between the two eyes and change the lens parameters accordingly.

Using a "First Pass Method" to Prevent Possible Problems

When there is a concern that aniseikonia might be a problem, there are some things that can be done with frame and lens choices that will reduce magnification differences between lenses that would otherwise occur. This can be done before anything else and will not hurt anything, even if aniseikonia is not a problem at all.

1. Use a frame with a short vertex distance and, if nosepads are present, further reduce the vertex distance.
2. Use a frame with a small eye size. This secondarily reduces vertex distance.
3. Use an aspheric lens design. This usually flattens the base curves.
4. Use a high-index lens material. This will thin plus lens center thickness.

Making "Directionally Correct" Magnification Changes

It is possible to really go after an aniseikonia problem you are fairly certain is present, but have no way of exactly measuring. This is done by making changes to each lens individually in the appropriate direction so as to either reduce or increase magnification. Sometimes it is possible to reduce magnification differences just enough to alleviate the problem, without having an "exact fix." When using this approach, here are two important notes:

1. Remember that the greater the difference in right and left lens power, the greater will the changes need to be to meet the problem. Changes will be to vertex distances, base curves, and lens thicknesses.
2. In your concern about the aniseikonia, do not forget that with presbyopes it may be necessary to correct for vertical imbalance at the same time.

What is done with each lens will depend upon the power of the right and left lenses compared with one another.

- If both lenses are plus, but one more plus than the other, follow the instructions found in Box 21-1.
- If both lenses are minus, but one more minus than the other, follow the instructions in Box 21-2.

BOX 21-1

If Both Lenses Are Plus (Anisohyperopia)

- Choose a frame with a minimum vertex distance.
- Keep the eye size small.

For the Higher Plus Lens	For the Lower Plus Lens
• Flatten the base curve. • Thin the lens. • Decrease the vertex distance.	• Steepen the base curve. • Increase center thickness. If possible try not to go thicker than a match of the thickness of the higher plus lens. • If the edge is thick enough, move the bevel away from the front and toward the back of the lens. (Do not exceed the limits of cosmetic acceptability.) This moves the lens forward in the frame, increasing magnification.

- If one lens is plus and the other minus, follow the instructions in Box 21-3.

Estimating Percent Magnification Differences

It is possible to estimate what the percent differences in magnification are from the prescription itself.* Estimates of how much magnification changes per diopter of power vary. Linksz and Bannon[7] say we can expect 1.5% per diopter of anisometropia when anisometropia is refractive in origin. However, since the ametropia probably has at least some axial component, 1% per diopter is more realistic. One percent per diopter is now considered the rule of thumb.

To correct for estimated aniseikonia, we can figure that if there is a problem, it will probably be between 1% and 2%. How to make exact magnification changes by specifically changing lens parameters will be discussed later in the chapter.

Measuring Percent Magnification Differences

The ideal way to correct for aniseikonia is to measure it directly. Historically the classical method was to use a space eikonometer. A **"space eikonometer"** is used to quantitatively measure image size differences. Space eikonometers are no longer made.

---

*NOTE: Screening devices that are used for estimating percent magnification are not likely to be accurate enough to be effective. Large image size differences result in loss of binocularity and produce no symptoms. Small differences are not accurately measured with screening devices and are the ones that cause the most problems.

An alternative method has been to use appropriate Keystone View stereoscopic cards, preferably in conjunction with the Keystone orthoscope (a stereoscope with "minimum-distortion" lenses). Another more accurate means of testing is the Awaya New Aniseikonia Test (Handaya Co Ltd, Tokyo, Japan).

Once aniseikonia testing is complete it is still necessary to determine which parameters of each lens should be changed by what specific amount. There are tables and nomographs in existence that give expected changes in magnification produced by changes in base curve, lens thickness, vertex distance, and index of refraction.[7]

It is also possible to construct a program using an Excel spreadsheet or the equivalent. Then the formula for spectacle magnification with its shape and power factors can be used directly.[†] Whenever looking at the magnifications for any given pair of lenses, there will typically be a large difference between left and right spectacle lens magnifications. This difference does not have to be reduced to zero. Instead the *difference* between the two spectacle lens magnifications should be reduced by an amount equal to the aniseikonia found between left and right eyes. (Even then, symptoms may disappear with smaller reductions in aniseikonia.)

Fortunately, there is another method that incorporates both testing and lens design into a computer-based software program.

The Aniseikonia Inspector

The Aniseikonia Inspector is a software program that presents a screen as shown in Figure 21-6. The subject wears red-green glasses, and the screen image is adjusted until both halves of the image are of equal size. The Inspector measures for magnification differences in the horizontal, vertical, and diagonal directions.

Once a percentage magnification difference or differences are found and prescription information entered, the program contains a form listing relevant lens parameters, including base curve, thickness, vertex distance, and index of refraction. By changing the parameters that are a part of the spectacle magnification formula, resulting lens magnification percents are seen. Right and left lenses are shown in cross section and also change as lens parameters are altered. The form and/or refractive index of the lens may be modified until suitable left and right lens magnifications result.

Even if it is possible to measure the full percentage differences between left and right eye, it may not be necessary to fully correct those differences. This is especially heartening when attainment of a full magnification difference correction would result in extremely

---

BOX 21-2

If Both Lenses Are Minus (Anisomyopia)

- Choose a frame with a minimum vertex distance.
- Keep the eye size small.
- It is not advisable to change base curves for minus lenses unless there is certainty of what the end result will produce. (If the lens is more minus than −2.00 in power, steepening the base curve alone may not do the expected. Steepening the base curve increases magnification, but also increases the lens bend. This results in increased vertex distance.* Greater vertex distance for minus lenses means increased minification and may produce the opposite of intended results.)

For the Higher Minus Lens	For the Lower Minus Lens
• Decrease the vertex distance for this lens by moving the bevel as far forward as possible. • If a large change in magnification is required, it may be necessary to steepen the base curve considerably. If this is done, then the lens must also be thickened and the bevel moved to the front surface to decrease the vertex distance. Unless this is done, steepening the base curve may not yield the desired results.[†]	• Increase the vertex distance by moving the bevel away from the front of the lens. (Moving it totally to the back is going to look bad.) • Do not thin the lens.

*Each 1 D change in base curve changes vertex distance by approximately 0.6 mm.

[†] Brown WL. The Importance of Base Curve in the Design of Minus Iseikonic Lenses.

BOX 21-3

If One Lens Is Plus and the Other Is Minus (Antimetropia)

- Choose a frame with a minimum vertex distance.
- Keep the eye size small.

For the Plus Lens	For the Minus Lens
• Flatten the base curve. • Thin the lens. • Decrease the vertex distance.	• Decrease the vertex distance by moving the bevel to the front of the lens. • Do not thin the lens.

When one lens is plus in power, some suggest the use of a high-index lens for the higher plus lens. A regular index lens is used for the lower plus. This will reduce thickness, base curve, and secondarily, vertex distance for the higher plus lens.

[†]When constructing a spreadsheet, one must remember that the front curve is the refractive power of the lens and not the 1.53-indexed base curve. A 1.53-index-referenced number may be used if a conversion formula is built into the spreadsheet.

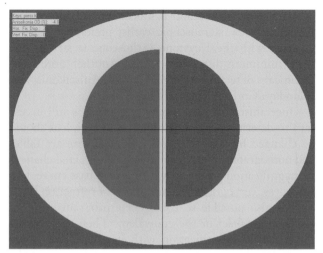

Figure 21-6. This screen simulation from the Aniseikonia Inspector program shows how the right eye would see an image that was smaller than the left.

(From the Optical Diagnostics website: http://www. opticaldiagnostics.com/products/ai/screenshots.html.)

unusual lenses with very thick centers or an inappropriately steep base curve on one of the lenses.

When using this program or when simply making changes in lens shapes to affect magnification in other aniseikonia situations, here are some points to consider. (Refer also to Boxes 21-1 to 21-3.)

1. Just reducing the vertex distance for both lenses will help.
2. Changing the base curve of even one lens may also help. (Reducing the highest base curve to equal the lower base curve can make a big change in magnification difference.)
3. Use an aspheric design. For plus lenses, both base curves will be flatter. This allows a decrease in thickness of the thicker lens. The thinner lens may then be made equal to the thicker lens.
4. Increasing the index of the lens will thin the lens.
5. If the least plus lens is thick enough, it may be possible to move the lens forward in the frame by moving the bevel back on the lens. This increases vertex distance.
6. It is possible to get a bit more of a change in magnification difference in plus lenses by leaving the weaker lens as a nonaspheric lens with a steeper base and using an aspheric design for the stronger lens.
7. Use an antireflection coating on both lenses to reduce lens visibility and any otherwise noticeable differences between the two lenses.

How Helpful Is Correcting for Aniseikonia?

It would be logical to consider just how helpful it is to go to the trouble of making lens changes to correct for aniseikonia when in practice these changes are not always

done. In a study done at Emory Eye Center, Achiron et al[6] compared corrections for 34 anisometropes. They found that modifying lens design to equalize relative spectacle magnification both reduced aniseikonia and improved subjective comfort and performance. At the conclusion of the study, 93% of the study subjects preferred the spectacles that had been modified to correct for aniseikonia over traditional spectacles.

Their results also found that, contrary to Knapp's law, axial anisometropes benefited just as much from modifications to relative spectacle magnification as refractive anisometropes did.

WHAT IS A BITORIC LENS?

It is possible to have a difference in magnification between two major meridians in right and left eyes. Magnification can be changed in each meridian independently.

Normally a cylinder lens has a front surface that is spherical and a back surface that is toric. The toric surface has a different radius of curvature in each of the two major meridians, thereby correcting for the astigmatism. However, it is possible to put a toric surface on the front of the lens *and* on the back of the lens, even if that lens is a sphere. This would happen if one chooses differing front lens curves for the purpose of creating more magnification in one meridian than the other. If this is done, then back surface curves are selected so as to counteract the cylinder power created by the toric front surface. This lens with toric surfaces on both the front and the back is called a *bitoric* lens (Figure 21-7).

PRISMATIC EFFECT OF LENS PAIRS

When depicting the optics of a pair of spectacles, the wearer is normally shown looking directly through the optical center (OC) of both lenses. This situation, of course, occurs only part of the time because the wearer's direction of gaze changes behind the lenses.

When looking to the right or left, upward or downward, because the object viewed is seen through a noncentral lens area, there is a prismatic effect induced by each lens. This prismatic effect is predictable and may be calculated.

If both right and left lenses are equal in all respects, then the prism powers induced by the two lenses for any position of gaze are also equal.

Example **21-2**

A man wearing −3.00 D lenses for both eyes (O.U.) turns his eyes to look at a distant object on his right. In so doing, he looks through a point on his lenses 1 cm to the right of the OCs (Figure 21-8). What is the resultant prismatic effect for each eye?

Figure 21-7. Normally a lens has a sphere curve on both surfaces. This is represented by the first set of power crosses below. The first surface has a power of +9.00 D and the second surface −5.00 D. Ignoring lens thickness, the resulting lens power will be +4.00 D sphere.

Here is a fairly simple example of a bitoric lens. Suppose a lens is supposed to have the same power of +4.00 D. The lens can be made with a cylinder on the front, as shown below. As long as the second surface counteracts the power of the cylinder in the front surface, the lens still has a power of +4.00 D. This lens would produce differing magnifications in each meridian.

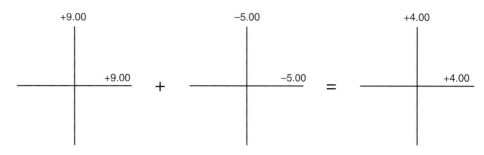

Normal Lens

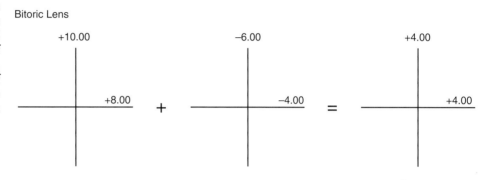

Bitoric Lens

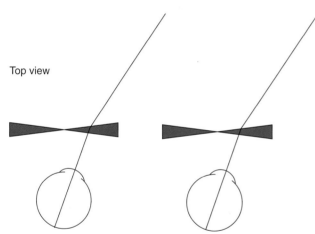

Top view

Figure 21-8. Light from an object at infinity when viewed through the periphery of prescription spectacle lenses is deviated by the prismatic effect of the lenses. When both lenses are of the same power, that deviation is symmetrical. Both rays emerging from the lenses, though deviated, are still parallel. Therefore the eyes neither converge nor diverge relative to one another.

Solution

Using Prentice's rule, it may be seen that:

$$\Delta = cF$$

and in this case

$$\Delta = (1)(3.00) = 3.00$$

Therefore there is 3.00Δ of prism induced by the right lens and 3.00Δ of prism induced by the left. Base direction is base out for the right eye and base in for the left. As seen from Figure 21-8, these effects are both base to the right. As a result, the eyes remain parallel and are forced neither to turn inward (converge) nor outward (diverge) in their orientation to one another.

Anisophoria

Remember that the condition of the eyes whereby a person requires lenses that differ in power—one lens being stronger or weaker than the other—is known as *anisometropia*. When such a person looks at an object through corresponding points on the lenses other than the OCs, the prismatic effects that are induced will be unequal for each eye. This situation is referred to as *anisophoria*.

Example **21-3**

Suppose a prescription of the following power is worn:

> O.D. −7.00 D sphere
> O.S. −3.00 D sphere

What prismatic effects are induced by the lenses for the points 1 cm to the right of the OCs when viewing a distant object located to the right (Figure 21-9)?

Solution

For the right eye, the prismatic effect is found (using Prentice's rule) as:

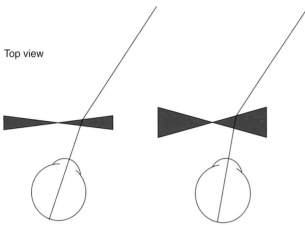

Top view

Figure 21-9. When parallel light from a peripherally viewed object at infinity strikes a pair of spectacle lenses whose powers are unequal, the prismatic effects created at these noncentral lens positions are unequal, causing more deviation for light entering through one lens than through the other. This in turn causes either a convergence or divergence of the eyes, depending on lens powers.

$$\Delta = cF$$
$$\Delta = (1)(7.00) = 7.00\Delta$$

For the left eye, the effect results in 3.00Δ of prism.

In Example 21-2, where both lenses were of identical power, there was no imbalance between the eyes. Both eyes continued to point in the same direction. In Example 21-3, however, the right eye is forced to turn 4.00Δ more than the left. Because the base-out effect overpowers the base-in effect, the net effect for the two eyes is 4.00Δ base out. The eye turns towards the apex of the prism, and the two eyes are forced to converge relative to one another.

Fortunately the eyes are not required to hold this position over long periods of time and quickly adapt to the variations of fixation.

VERTICAL IMBALANCE

When differential prismatic effects are present at varying positions of gaze, resulting from a difference in power between right and left lenses, it is apparent that vertical prismatic effects may also be manifested. The most troublesome situation may occur when reading or close work is attempted over an extended period of time. When the wearer drops the eyes below the OCs of the lens and vertical prismatic effect of unequal values results for the two eyes, the differential prismatic effect induced is referred to as *vertical imbalance*.

To understand vertical imbalance, consider the same person whose prescription was:

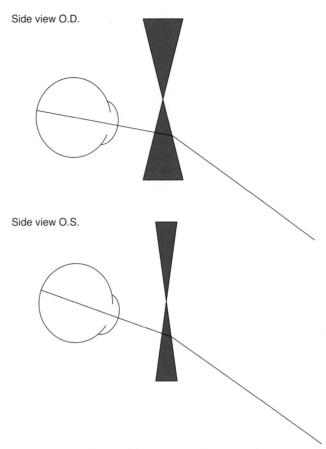

Side view O.D.

Side view O.S.

Figure 21-10. Unequal lens powers also cause the same type of prismatic effect for objects viewed through tops and bottoms of spectacle lenses as is caused when looking through the sides. Unfortunately, the problem created is harder for the eyes to overcome, since turning one eye farther up or down than the other is not a natural paired eye movement.

O.D. −7.00 D sphere
O.S. −3.00 D sphere

If that person now looks 1 cm below the OCs, the prismatic effects induced will be O.D. 7.00Δ base down, and O.S. 3.00Δ base down (Figure 21-10). The net result is 4.00Δ of base-down prism before the right eye.

Who Is Responsible for Correcting Vertical Imbalance?

Vertical imbalance often goes unnoticed throughout the eye examination and dispensing processes. This may happen for a variety of reasons. One major reason, however, is that unless segment and major reference point (MRP) heights are known, the amount of imbalance cannot be determined. These measurements are not known until after frame selection has occurred. Ideally the prescriber should notice the need and call for a correction on the prescription. This does not always happen, however. Therefore unless dispenser and examiner are working in close proximity, the responsibility will rest with the dispenser. The dispenser must first recognize when a vertical imbalance correction is needed.

When Is a Correction for Vertical Imbalance Needed?

The need for a vertical imbalance correction should be questioned when an anisometropic wearer progresses from single vision lenses into multifocals.

For the single vision lens wearer, if the unequal vertical prism proves troublesome with the eyes dropped for reading, simply dropping the head will solve the problem. In this manner, both lines of sight pass through the OCs, where there is a net prismatic effect of zero, alleviating the problem. For the new multifocal wearer, this option is eliminated by the positioning of the segment. To read through the bifocal portion, the wearer *must* lower the eyes and use a noncentral portion of the lens.

Tolerance to vertical imbalance in the reading area varies from person to person. Generally, any time there is a vertical meridian difference greater than 1.50 D in power between right and left lenses, vertical imbalance problems are a possibility; and when power differences are greater than 2-3 D vertical imbalance correction merits consideration. Some individuals with anisometropia are sensitive to the imbalance, whereas others with a higher amount are not bothered. Observing the individual while he or she is reading through the old anisometropic single vision prescription may give a clue as to possible difficulties.

To determine if a vertical imbalance correction may be needed, hand the person a reading card and ask him or her to read something. Notice what the person does when handed the card. If the individual drops the eyes to read, he or she is accustomed to reading with vertical imbalance, and no special compensation may be necessary. If the person drops the head to read, however, reading is being done through the distance OCs to prevent prism imbalance in the lower part of the glasses. These individuals may experience difficulty with a multifocal lens if the imbalance is left uncompensated. In some instances, only partial compensation for the imbalance may be required.

Vertical imbalance corrections are especially critical when the imbalance is of recent onset. This occurs when a person has had either cataract surgery or refractive surgery on one eye only. Both situations create anisometropia, causing a vertical imbalance at near for which a multifocal wearer is unable to compensate. In these cases because adaptation has not occurred over time, the full amount of imbalance correction is indicated.

CORRECTING FOR VERTICAL IMBALANCE

There are several methods of correcting for vertical imbalance, some of which are capable of compensating for more prismatic imbalance than others. The first four on the list attempt to avoid the problem of vertical imbalance. The last four attempt to correct for the problem.

1. Contact lenses
2. Two pairs of glasses
3. Dropping the MRP height
4. Raising the seg height
5. Fresnel press-on prism
6. Slab off (bicentric grind)
7. Dissimilar segs
8. Compensated "R" segs

It should be noted that those who benefit from the correction of vertical imbalance will also benefit from a good choice of lens parameters for offsetting aniseikonia (image size differences). Lens choices for aniseikonia are explained earlier in this chapter.

Contact Lenses

From a purely optical standpoint, one of the best options available for correcting vertical imbalance is the contact lens. The OC of the contact lens moves with the eye. When an individual wears contact lenses, the spectacle lens-induced prismatic difference disappears and the vertical imbalance problem with it.

Two Pairs of Glasses

When anisometropes wear single vision lenses, vertical imbalance seldom surfaces as a problem. This is because single vision lens wearers have the option of dropping the head and looking through the lens OCs instead of just dropping the eyes and looking below the OCs. This means that if an anisometrope decides against multifocal lenses, he or she is not forced to look into the lower portion of the lens where the near segment is located. Thus one option for overcoming vertical imbalance is to have *two pairs of single vision glasses*, one for distance and one for near. When using two pairs of glasses, the reading glasses should be ordered with the OCs lower than normal. This way the wearer looks through the lens OCs. A separate pair of single vision glasses for near does not *correct* for vertical imbalance; it *avoids* vertical imbalance. When ordering two pairs of glasses for this purpose, it is advisable to position the OCs for the near prescription 5 mm below the vertical center of the frames.

Instead of using a regular frame for the near Rx and lowering the OCs, a pair of half-eye frames may be used. In this way, the OCs are lower, even at their normal locations. They do not have to be lowered farther.

Dropping the Major Reference Point Height

Reducing the amount of vertical imbalance at near by dropping the OC or MRP of a multifocal lens pair is used in practice, but is not as optically sound as other options. By dropping the OC, the distance from the OC to the reading level is reduced and so is the prismatic effect at near. Lowering the OC, however, will transfer imbalance from the near portion to the distance portion because gain at near is offset by an increase in imbalance in the upper portion of the lens. Dropping the MRP in multifocals might be successful in borderline cases of imbalance, but is not the best option available.

Raising the Seg Height

By raising the seg height *without* simultaneously raising the height of the distance OC (i.e., the MRP), the wearer will not have to look as far down into the lens at near. If the eyes are not as far from the distance OCs for reading, the vertical imbalance will not be as great.

If the surfacing laboratory moves the distance OC up as the seg goes up, however, then no benefit is derived. If the technique of raising the seg is to be used, it is best to specify not just the seg height but also the MRP height.

Fresnel Press-on Prism

A *Fresnel press-on lens* is made from "thin, transparent, flexible, plastic material which adheres to the surface of an ophthalmic lens when pressed in place.[1]" Thus it is possible to cut a Fresnel press-on prism to fit the lower half of one lens to counteract a vertical imbalance. Placed on the back surface of the ophthalmic lens, the Fresnel prism simulates a slab-off lens. Fresnel lenses for such an application are usually not considered to be a permanent solution, but rather are used on a trial basis to see if the wearer's visual difficulties can be alleviated. (For more on Fresnel lenses, see Chapter 17.)

Slab Off (Bicentric Grinding)

The most common option for correcting vertical imbalance produces a vertical prismatic effect in the lower half of one lens only, beginning at the level of the bifocal segment line. This type of correction is called a *slab off* or *bicentric grind*. It is identified by the presence of a horizontal line across one lens at the level of the segment top.

Slab off is almost always used unless the amount of correction required is less than 1.50Δ. At less than 1.50Δ, it is difficult to control the appearance and placement of the slab line. Fortunately, problems with vertical imbalance do not occur as frequently once vertical imbalance drops below 1.50Δ. Slab off can be made in fairly large amounts. Before using greater than 6Δ of slab off on a given lens, however, it may be advisable to consider using regular (base up) slab off on one eye and reverse slab off (base down) on the other. (Reverse slab off begins at 1.50Δ and progresses in increments of $\frac{1}{2}\Delta$ up to 6Δ.)

Slab off can be custom ground on any lens, whether it is made from glass or plastic.

Slab Off for Fused Glass Multifocals

When bicentric grinding (slabbing off) is done on a fused glass multifocal lens, base-up prism is created in the reading area. Slab-off grinding is done on one lens only. The lens chosen is that which has more minus (or less plus) power in its 90-degree meridian. The process by which this is accomplished is shown and described in Figure 21-11.

One of the greatest advantages of the slab-off method is that a large amount of prism compensation may be made in comparison with other available methods. The completed lens grind produces a relatively inconspicuous line. This line overlaps the flat-top seg line already present on the lens and is partially obscured by it (Figure 21-12). Although any shaped seg, or even no seg at all, may be used in conjunction with bicentric grinding, the flat-top seg gives the best results cosmetically.

For the fused glass lens, the bicentric grind results in base-up prism. Therefore slab off will, by necessity, always be performed on *the most minus or least plus powered lens.*

Slab Off in Plastic Lenses

It is possible to use slab off on any plastic lens, including a progressive addition lens. With plastic the process somewhat resembles that of the glass lens, but is carried out as shown in Figure 21-13.

Slab Off for Progressive Addition Lenses. When slab-off prism is used on a progressive addition lens, the slab line will be on the back surface of the lens. The level of the slab-off line is normally positioned slightly above the near verification circle. The full amount of slab-off correction is usually calculated based on the distance from the prism reference point (*not* the fitting cross) to the center of the near verification circle.

Sheedy reports that slab-off prism on a progressive lens meets with just as much success as slab off on segmented multifocals. As with any slab-off correction, the critical aspect is selection of the candidate and as expected "presbyopia in the presence of anisometropia of greater than 2-3 D in the vertical meridian should trigger slab off consideration. However, we don't consider slab off if the patient is already a successful multifocal wearer with no near-vision complaints. We also tend to avoid slab off in the first-time multifocal wearer, because many anisometropic patients are able to successfully manage the vertical prism. We prefer to use slab off only when it becomes necessary. These patients also often benefit from aniseikonic lens designs—at least equal center thickness and base curves.[9]"

Precast Slab-Off Lenses (the Reverse Slab Lens)[10]

A high degree of skill is required to grind plastic slab-off lenses. The increased need for plastic slab-off lenses and the level of skill required offered an incentive for the development of a suitable precast slab off that could be surfaced in the normal manner. The first precast CR-39 slab-off lens, developed by Aire-o-Lite in 1973,[11] was for a 25-mm round seg. This was followed in 1983 by the Younger Optics Slab-Off lens series.

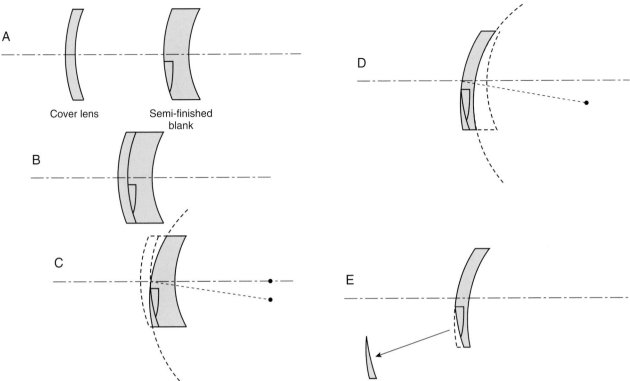

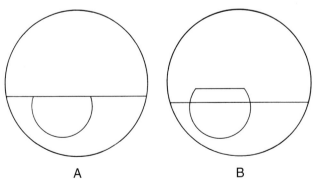

Figure 21-11. Slab-off prism manufacture. **A,** A cover lens is manufactured to have the same inside curve as the base curve of the required semifinished lens blank. **B,** This cover lens is cemented to the semifinished blank. (In actual practice, only one half of a cover lens is required, covering from the center of the lens on down. For instructional purposes, however, the complete cover lens is shown.) **C,** Base-down prism is ground on the front surface of the lens. Glass is surfaced off until only the lower half of the cover lens from the seg line down remains. The dioptric value of the prism is equal to the prescribed amount needed for compensation. **D,** The distance power is surfaced on and the prismatic effect removed during generating (surface grinding). Now the entire lens is once again without prism. **E,** Last, the remaining portion of the cover lens is removed. This wedge-shaped portion is a base-down prism whose value equals that surfaced, as was shown in **C.** The net effect is the addition of base-up prism to the lens from the seg downward.

Figure 21-12. Slab-off prism produces a thin line easily concealed by a flat-top seg. The wider the seg is, the more inconspicuous the line will be. **A,** A bifocal lens is shown. **B,** Shows the correct position for slab-off prism on a flat-top trifocal. The procedure for a trifocal bicentric grind is done from the back in a manner similar to that shown in Figure 21-13 for the plastic lens.

The precast slab-off lens is made using a flat-top 28 lens. The lens blank is large and has the segment in the center so that it may be used for either a right or a left lens (Figure 21-14).

Slab-off prism starts at 1.50Δ and goes up to 6.00Δ in increments of ½Δ. In contrast to conventionally ground slab-off lenses, the precast lenses are a reverse slab. This means that instead of having base-up prism in the area below the slab line, the precast lenses have base-down prism. The slab-off prism is cast molded on the front of the lens so that the semifinished blank can be surfaced on the rear surface in the normal manner (Figure 21-15). In a number of cases, the end result will be a thinner lens.*

---

*For equal plus powers, regular slab-off lenses will be thicker than reverse-slab lenses. Since regular slab off will be placed on the least plus lens, however, added thickness could help equalize left and right lens thicknesses and resulting magnification. For minus powers, the center thickness of both regular and reverse-slab lenses will be equal, but the lower edge of the reverse-slab lens will be thicker than the lower edge of the regular slab-off lens.

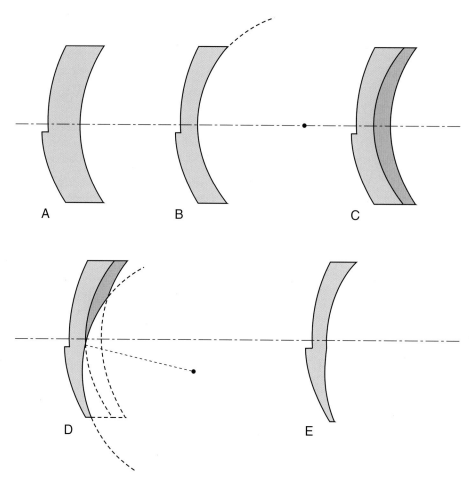

Figure 21-13. The process of bicentric grinding on a plastic lens must be carried out entirely on the rear surface because the front surface contains the one-piece construction bifocal segment area. The process begins with a semifinished lens **(A)**. The semifinished lens is surfaced to the required prescription and is left thick enough for a second prism grind later **(B)**. A liquid resin material is poured into the concave rear surface and allowed to dry. This resin **(C)** serves the same purpose as the cover lens served for the glass lens technique. The lens is then resurfaced at an angle **(D)**. Surfacing a lens at an angle serves to grind on prism. The surfacing tools used are the same as were used in **(B)** so that correct power is maintained. The near portion now contains the proper amount of prism base up and the correct power. Last, the lens is chilled to cause the remaining resin to break away. The upper portion has not been changed since originally surfaced. **E,** The completed lens. It will be noted that with bicentrically ground plastic lenses, the slab line is on the rear surface instead of the front.

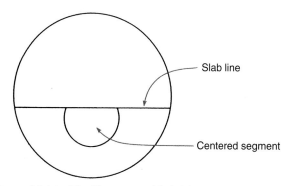

Figure 21-14. The Younger molded slab-off lens has the slab-off prism on the front. Prism is base down instead of the customary base up. The segment is centered so that the blank will work for either a right or a left lens.

With back-surface slab grinds, some segmented multifocal lens wearers experience the sensation of seeing two lines. They see the seg line on the front and the slab line on the back. With precast lenses, the slab line is on the front *with* the seg line. This eliminates the possibility of the wearer seeing two lines. Because reverse-slab lenses use base-down instead of base-up prism, the prism direction and the eye it is worn on is reversed. *The reverse slab is placed on the most plus or least minus, instead of the most minus or least plus.*

There appears to be no difficulty switching wearers from conventional slab off to precast slab off.[12] If a person has more than one pair of glasses, including sunglasses, however, then a possibility exists that all the pairs of

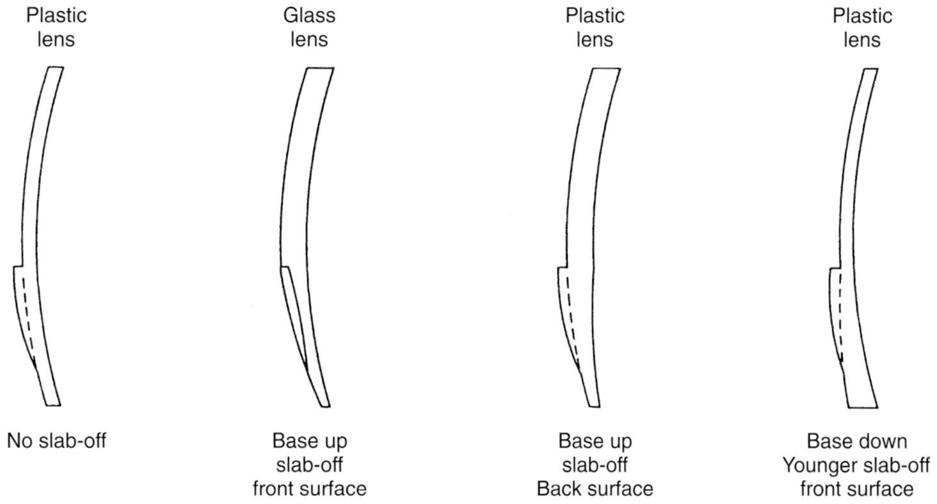

Figure 21-15. Slab-off lenses of plano distance power are compared with one another and with a non–slab-off plastic lens. These cross-sectional drawings show the location of the slab-off grind and how that grind affects lens thickness for a plano lens.

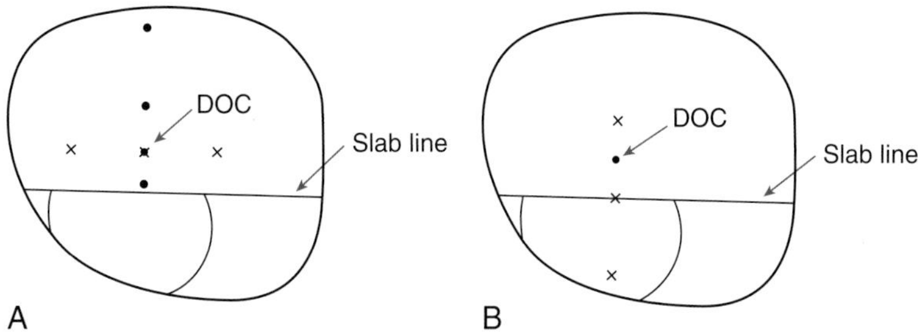

Figure 21-16. A, To verify the amount of slab-off prism present, the three contact points of a lens measure may first be oriented either at the position of the Xs or at the dots. **B,** The second position is shown. For crown glass lenses the difference between these two readings indicates the amount of slab-off prism present. This technique may be used on the back surface for low-index plastic, traditional back-side slab-off if no cylinder is present. It may be used with a cylinder if the lens clock is only held in the 90-degree meridian for both measures.

glasses may have to be switched; otherwise, the wearer could have trouble because of the difference in object displacement between the prescriptions.

Slab-Off Verification

The amount of slab-off prism present may be verified by comparing the seg areas of the slab-off lens with its partner lens through a lensmeter. For a fused glass multifocal lens, a simpler method makes use of the lens clock. The lens clock is first used to find the front curve of the bicentrically ground lens by orienting the contact point horizontally across the lens center in the distance portion paralleling the slab-off line. After noting the base curve, the lens clock is then oriented with contact points perpendicular to the slab-off line. The central contact point of the lens clock is placed directly on the line. For crown glass lenses the difference between these two readings indicates the amount of slab-off prism present (Figure 21-16).

Dissimilar Segs

One possible method of compensating for vertical imbalance in the reading area makes use of prismatic effect induced by the segment of a bifocal lens.

If the bifocal wearer looks through his or her bifocal segment, unless he or she is looking through the segment's OC, the segment (being itself a miniature lens) will produce a prismatic effect. This prismatic effect is separate from that produced by the distance lens.

When both right and left bifocal segs are set at the same heights, having the same power addition, the vertical prismatic effect produced will be the same for both right and left eyes.

Example **21-4**

A wearer looks through points 4 mm below the upper edge of his 22-mm round, symmetrically placed bifocals. If the bifocals have an add power of +2.00 D, how much vertical prism will be induced by the bifocal segment of the lens for each eye?

Solution

Because the two segments are equal in add power and symmetrically placed, both lens segments will produce the same prismatic effect. That prismatic effect may be found by first determining the distance from the segment OC to the point through which the eye looks.

If the lens segment is 22 mm round, the seg OC is 11 mm from the top of the seg. A point 4 mm below the seg top is then 11 − 4 or 7 mm above the segment center.

Having found the location in the seg through which the eye is looking, Prentice's rule may be applied to find the prism produced by the seg at this point. Since

$$c = 7 \text{ mm or } 0.7 \text{ cm}$$

and

$$F = \text{the power of the add, or } +2.00 \text{ D}$$

then

$$\Delta = cF$$
$$= (0.7)(2.00)$$
$$= 1.40\Delta$$

Because the seg power is plus and the point in question is above the center, the base direction will be downward.

The answer is then 1.40Δ base down for each eye.

Example **21-5**

Now assume that the bifocal segments in question are constructed with the segment optical center on the seg line, as was shown in Figure 19-12, *C*. If the add remains +2.00 D and the wearer again looks through a point 4 mm below the top of the seg line, what prismatic effect is induced by the segment?

Solution

Because the seg center is exactly on the upper line, the point in question is 4 mm below the OC. Prentice's rule may again be applied.

$$c = 4 \text{ mm}$$
$$= 0.4 \text{ cm}$$

and

$$F = +2.00 \text{ D}$$

Now

$$\Delta = cF$$
$$= (0.4)(2.00)$$
$$= 0.80\Delta$$

The center of the plus segment is above the area being looked through so the base direction is up. The answer for this style segment is 0.80Δ base up.

Using Seg-Induced Prism to Advantage

Prism induced by the optics of a segment may be used to advantage to counteract vertical imbalance created by distance lenses whose powers are unequal.

Example **21-6**

A distance prescription of:

O.D. –7.00 D sphere
O.S. –4.50 D sphere
Add +2.00 D

is worn with the seg lines 5 mm below the distance OCs (seg drop = 5 mm). If the wearer reads through the lenses at a position 10 mm below the distance OCs, then 7.00Δ of base-down prism is induced by the distance portion of the right lens and 4.50Δ base down by the left. The net result is a vertical imbalance of 2.50Δ base down before the right

eye (or base up before the left). How may this vertical imbalance be corrected by the use of a different segment style for each lens?

Solution

As noted earlier, bifocal segments are small lenses ground onto or fused into the distance portion of a spectacle lens. This smaller "lens" also induces a prismatic effect. The amount of prism induced depends on the power of the seg (the add power) and the distance the reading level is from the seg center.

In this example, the wearer is looking through a point 10 mm below the distance OC. Because the seg line is 5 mm below the distance OC, the wearer will be looking through the seg at 10 – 5, or 5 mm, below the seg line. Because the style seg to be used has not yet been specified, it is impossible to know where the seg OC will be. Hence determination of the amount of prism induced from the seg is not possible. If both segs are of the same style, however, the amount of prism induced by them for the two eyes would be equal, leaving the net imbalance for the lens pair at 2.50Δ base down for the right eye. If two different style segs are chosen, however, the net imbalance could be changed or even eliminated.

To counterbalance base-down prism before the right eye, a pair of segs should be chosen in which the right seg center will be higher than the left seg center. Such a combination will cause more base-down prismatic effect for the left eye than the right.

For simplicity a flat-top seg style whose OC falls 5 mm below the seg top will be chosen for the right eye. When the wearer looks through this position, no prism will be induced by the bifocal segment. To eliminate vertical imbalance, a left seg style must be chosen such that 2.50Δ of prism base down will be induced by the segment at a point 5 mm below the seg top.

Since the power of the segment is known and the desired prism is known (Δ = 2.50), Prentice's rule may be used in transformed fashion to find *c* (the distance from the seg OC to the point in question).

Since

$$\Delta = cF_s$$

then

$$c = \frac{\Delta}{F_s} = \frac{2.50}{2.00} = 1.25 \text{ cms}$$

The seg center must be 1.25 cm (or 12.5 mm) below the point through which the wearer is looking. This in turn means that the seg center should be 17.5 mm below the seg top. A bifocal lens that most closely fulfills these requirements is the A (traditionally referred to as an Ultex A). The A is a semicircular bifocal having a diameter of 38 mm with the seg center 19 mm below the top line (Figure 21-17).

In actuality the vertical segment optical center separation is directly calculated from the vertical imbalance and the power of the near addition. Here the amount of vertical imbalance is 2.50Δ and the add power is +2.00 D. Using Prentice's rule we have

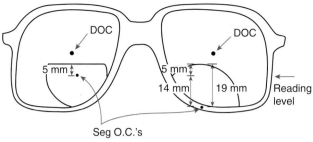

Figure 21-17. Correcting vertical imbalance with dissimilar segments uses prism induced by the segment itself. Prism produced by the segment for a given reading level (depth) varies with the position of the seg OC. Seg OC location is dependent upon bifocal shape so that using segs of two different carefully chosen shapes may serve to correct a vertical imbalance at near.

$$\Delta = cF$$

We know Δ is 2.50 and F is +2.00, so

$$c = \frac{\Delta}{F} = \frac{2.50}{2} = 1.25 \text{ cms or } 12.5 \text{ mm}$$

So the segments must have a vertical difference in their segment optical centers of 12.5 mm. The segment with the highest segment optical center always is placed on the most minus or least plus lens.

Although it is optically possible to use an unusual combination of dissimilar segs to correct high amounts of vertical imbalance, the cosmetic results will not be good. In addition, there are also areas in the field of view of the lens where the wearer is looking through the distance portion of one lens and the seg portion of the other. Using dissimilar segs for other than small amounts of vertical imbalance would normally be considered only when there are financial limitations since dissimilar segs are less expensive than slab off.

Dissimilar Segs for Correcting Low Vertical Imbalances

An excellent combination of segments for correction of small amounts of vertical imbalance is obtained using two differently styled, wide flat tops. Some large flat tops are made with the seg OC 4.5 mm below the line. Others are made with the seg OC right on the line. If a large flat-top 35 made with its seg OC 4.5 mm below the seg line is used for one eye and a flat-top 45 made with its seg OC on the seg line is used for the other, the segs look very much alike, but create a differential vertical prismatic effect (Figure 21-18). This difference of 4.5 mm multiplied by the power of the add gives the amount of vertical imbalance this combination will correct.

For example, if the add is +2.50, the amount of imbalance this combination will correct is

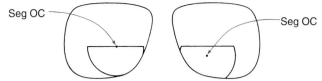

Figure 21-18. Two different styles of large flat-top lenses work well together for correcting small amounts of vertical imbalance. The lower the seg height, the less obvious the differences will be.

$$\text{Prism imbalance corrected} = (0.45)(2.50)$$
$$= 1.125\Delta \text{ of imbalance}$$

It is especially helpful to remember that the subjective symptom of discomfort caused by vertical imbalance may be relieved, even if the full amount of imbalance is not corrected. A pair of large-seg flat tops may be the answer. Remember that if the imbalance is below 1.50Δ, slab off is not a viable option, making this price-worthy dissimilar seg combination a cosmetically acceptable valid alternative. (An important summary explaining the steps in finding correct dissimilar segs is shown in Box 21-4.)

Compensated "R" Segs

A method used for correcting vertical imbalance at near in amounts below 1.5Δ is *compensated "R" segs*. The compensated "R" seg is 22 mm wide and 14 mm deep, being flat at both top and bottom. When resurfaced to create prism in the seg, the lenses are able to compensate for vertical imbalance. This resurfacing process moves the seg OC up in one lens and down in the other (Figure 21-19). The upper limit for the amount of prism produced depends upon the power of the add.

BOX 21-4

Steps in Finding Correct Dissimilar Segs

1. Calculate vertical imbalance at the reading level.
2. Calculate the required distance between seg centers needed to counteract reading level imbalance.

$$\Delta = cF_s \text{ or } c = \frac{\Delta}{F_s}$$

   c = distance between seg centers in centimeters
   F_s = add power (not near Rx)
   Δ = necessary prism

3. Note which lens requires the higher seg OC. (The lens with the most minus or least plus power in its vertical meridian should contain the segment with the higher segment OC.)
4. Choose two seg styles so that, with seg tops at equal heights, the seg OCs will be separated by the required amount. (The required amount is the value c found in Step 2.)

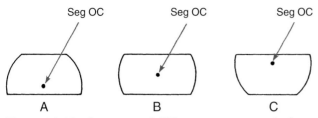

Figure 21-19. Compensated "R" segments are made from ribbon-style segment lenses. The OCs can be lowered or raised (**A**) and (**C**). Optically compensated R segments behave just like dissimilar segments.

Compensated "R" lenses are seldom used and are available only in glass.

DETERMINING THE CORRECT AMOUNT OF COMPENSATION FOR VERTICAL IMBALANCE

The steps needed for determining the needed amount of vertical imbalance are as follows:
1. Select an appropriate frame and measure for bifocal height.
2. Determine the vertical location within the segment where reading will take place. That level is called the *reading level*. (The terms *reading level* and *reading depth* are used synonymously.)
3. Determine the prism amount that is to be used to correct the imbalance.

Bifocal height is determined as was explained in Chapter 5. Reading level may be determined subjectively, objectively, or by calculation.

Determining the Reading Level

Determining the Reading Level Objectively

Reading level may be objectively measured using the correctly sized sample frame. Place tape at the level of the proposed bifocal, occluding the distance portion so that the wearer looks *under* the tape. Then place reading material so as to simulate normal working or reading conditions. Position yourself below the wearer's eye level, almost in line with the reading material. Measure from the bottom edge of the tape to the estimated line of sight (which extends from the center of the pupil to the reading material). Add this value to the seg drop (MRP height minus seg height) to arrive at the reading level.

Determining the Reading Level Subjectively

To determine reading level subjectively, tape the sample frame as described above. This time have the wearer fixate a point at the near working distance. Lower a card from above past the level of the tape until it just barely occludes the fixation point. Note the distance the edge of the card overlaps the tape into the near portion and add this value to the seg drop.

Determining the Reading Level by Calculation

To determine the reading level by calculation, make a judgment as to how far below the seg line most near work will occur. That is to say, estimate how far below the seg line the reading level will be. This estimation allows a certain amount of flexibility. The closer to the line that the reading level is estimated to be, the more likely the imbalance will be "undercorrected." Thus the person doing the calculation can choose to undercorrect the imbalance a certain amount by choosing a higher reading level. In most instances, reading level will be 3 to 5 mm below the seg line. Reading depth will be the seg drop plus the estimated distance that the reading level is below the seg line.

Example **21-7**

The MRPs for a pair of flat-top bifocal lenses are both 23 mm high. The lenses are measured for placement at a seg height of 18 mm. What will the reading depth be?

Solution

An estimate of the reading level position is made for 3 mm below the seg line. This allows the distance between MRP and reading level to be calculated. First, the position of the seg line is determined.

$$\begin{array}{r} 23\text{ mm (position of MRP)} \\ -18\text{ mm (seg height)} \\ \hline = 5\text{ mm (seg drop below MRP)} \end{array}$$

To find the reading depth, 3 mm is added to this value so that the eyes are far enough into the seg area to allow for reading.

$$\begin{array}{r} 5\text{ mm (seg drop below MRP)} \\ +3\text{ mm} \\ \hline = 8\text{ mm (reading depth)} \end{array}$$

METHODS FOR DETERMINING THE PRISM CORRECTION NEEDED

How the Prescriber Determines the Needed Amount of Imbalance Correction

Correcting for a vertical imbalance at near may not necessitate using the full amount of calculated compensation. (How the amount of vertical imbalance is calculated is covered later in this chapter in the section titled Correcting the Full Imbalance by Calculations.) Some individuals with a longstanding vertical imbalance become acclimated to it and through continuous use are able to overcome some of the prismatic effect by vertically diverging the eyes somewhat when reading or performing near tasks. Thus many spectacle lens wearers are able to compensate partially for an imbalance themselves. For example, a person may show a need for 2.00Δ of slab-off prism when actual calculations indicate a need for 3.00Δ. It is possible to test and see how much imbalance is required. This is most easily done if the person is wearing glasses that contain a current, valid distance prescription.

With the individual wearing the correct distance prescription, place tape over the upper portions of the lenses at the actual or theoretical segment line location. This forces the wearer to look below the tape and through the lower area of the lenses at the level where he or she will be reading. A fixation disparity testing unit is held in the reading position and Polaroid filters placed over the glasses. Hold a hand-held vertical prism bar with prisms of increasing power over one of the wearer's eyes. (If a prism bar is not available, loose trial prism lenses may be used.) Incrementally increase the prism amount by moving the prism bar until the fixation disparity target shows proper alignment. This is the correct amount of slab-off prism needed.

If a fixation disparity testing unit is not available, it is possible to position a pen light at the reading level and place a red Maddox rod over one eye. Incrementally increase the prism over one eye with the prism bar until the red line intersects with the white light. This method may yield a larger amount of vertical prism than the fixation disparity method. When imbalance is determined using methods such as these, the prism amount becomes a part of the prescription.

Sometimes a prescription simply indicates the need for slab off, but does not state the amount, leaving it to the dispenser or laboratory to calculate. In many instances, even when the need for slab off exists, it is not part of the prescription. This does not preclude the dispenser from incorporating slab off in the wearer's spectacles, however, since vertical imbalance is a spectacle lens-induced problem.

How to Use a Lensmeter to Determine the Amount of Imbalance

If the wearer's distance prescription has not changed, the amount of imbalance may be determined as follows:
1. Spot the MRPs of the lenses.
2. Having predetermined the reading position, locate the reading centers. This is done by measuring down from the MRPs to the reading level and in by the amount seg inset.
3. Spot the newly located reading centers. (These will correspond to the wearer's near interpupillary distance [near PD] at the reading level).
4. Center one reading center before the lensmeter aperture and read the amount of vertical prism present. Without moving the lensmeter table up or down, slide the glasses over so the second reading center is in front of the lensmeter aperture and measure the vertical prismatic amount at this point.
5. The vertical prism difference between these two vertical prism readings is the full amount of vertical prism imbalance experienced by the wearer.

If the distance prescription has changed, the old glasses cannot be used to measure vertical imbalance.

How an Optical Laboratory Determines the Amount of Imbalance

The optical laboratory determines the amount of slab-off prism by calculation. The chief advantage a laboratory may have is the possible availability of computer software containing the appropriate formula. The laboratory will compute the *full* amount of imbalance. If the dispenser does not specify a reading level, the laboratory will choose one.

CORRECTING THE FULL IMBALANCE BY CALCULATIONS

If the full correction for vertical imbalance is indicated, this may be calculated. There are several methods of calculation that may be used as will be described in the following sections. The methods do not always result in exactly the same answers. As with any decentration problem, difficulty in calculation increases with the complexity of the prescription—the easiest being spheres and the most difficult, spherocylinder combinations. Here are the steps normally used to find the amount of vertical imbalance.
1. Find the reading depth. The reading depth (or reading level) is the seg drop plus the distance from the segment top to the level at which the wearer is expected to read (usually 3 to 5 mm).
2. Find the power of each lens in the 90-degree meridian.
3. Find the prismatic effect at the reading depth of each lens.
4. Find the prismatic difference (vertical imbalance) between the right and left lenses.
5. When using slab-off, determine which lens will receive the imbalance correction.

Using Prentice's Rule to Calculate Vertical Imbalance for Spheres

The traditional methods for calculating vertical imbalance use Prentice's rule. Here this traditional method will be explained, starting with an example of a prescription for spherical lenses.

Example **21-8**

Suppose vertical imbalance at near is to be corrected for the following prescription:

O.D. +3.00 D Sphere
O.S. +0.50 D Sphere
Add +2.00 D
Frame B dimension = 46 mm
Seg Height = 19 mm
Reading level is 4 mm below the seg line.

What is the vertical imbalance at the reading level?

Solution

Begin by finding the reading level. In calculating imbalance, it is helpful to visualize the situation described. Because the B dimension is 46 mm,

$$\text{seg drop} = B / 2 - \text{seg height}$$
$$= 46 / 2 - 19$$
$$= 23 - 19$$
$$= 4$$

Because the reading level is 4 mm below the seg line, it will be 8 mm below the distance OCs. (This is shown in Figure 21-20.)

Use Prentice's rule to determine the vertical prismatic effect at the reading level. In the example problem, the reading level is 8 mm below the OC so the vertical prismatic effect for the right eye is:

$$\Delta_v = cF$$
$$= 0.8 \times (3.00)$$
$$= 2.40\Delta$$

The base direction is up since the lens is plus. (Since we are only concerned with vertical prismatic imbalance, the horizontal prismatic effect is not needed and does not need to be calculated.)

The vertical prismatic effect at the left reading center is calculated in the same manner as for the right:

$$\Delta_v = cF$$
$$= 0.8 \times (0.50)$$
$$= 0.40\Delta \text{ Base Up}$$

Therefore the vertical imbalance is the difference between the left and right vertical components at the reading level.

$$
\begin{array}{r}
2.40\Delta \text{ base up O.D.} \\
- \ 0.40\Delta \text{ base up O.S.} \\
\hline
= 2.00\Delta \text{ base up O.D.}
\end{array}
$$

The full correction for vertical imbalance must counteract 2.00Δ base up before the right eye at near. This may be done by:

1. Either placing 2.00Δ of base-up prism before the left eye at near, or
2. Placing 2.00Δ base-down prism before the right eye at near.

The choice depends on the method of compensation used. If the imbalance were corrected using conventional slab-off prism, the slab-off correction would be placed before the most minus or least plus lens. In this case the least plus is the left lens.

Using Prentice's Rule to Calculate Vertical Imbalance for Spherocylinders

Spherocylinders at 90 Degrees or 180 Degrees

Calculation of vertical imbalance at near for spherocylinders is fairly straightforward when the cylinder axes are at 90 or 180 degrees.

Example **21-9**

Calculate the imbalance for the following prescription:

$$\text{O.D. } +4.00 - 0.50 \times 180$$
$$\text{O.S. } +2.00 - 1.25 \times 180$$
$$\text{Add } +2.00 \text{ D}$$
$$\text{Seg drop} = 4 \text{ mm}$$
Reading level is 5 mm below the segment line.

Solution

1. First we find the distance from the optical center of the lens to the reading level. This is the seg drop plus the distance from the segment line to the reading level. In this case it would be

$$\text{Reading depth} = 4 \text{ mm} + 5 \text{ mm}$$
$$= 9 \text{ mm}$$

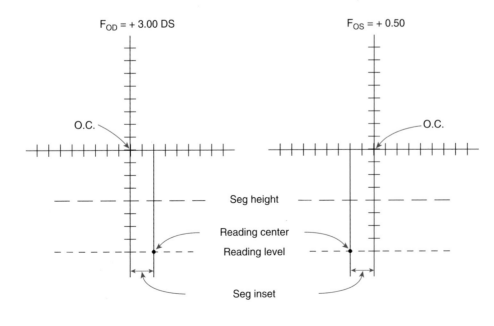

$F_{OD} = + 3.00 \text{ DS}$ $F_{OS} = + 0.50$

O.C.   O.C.

Seg height

Reading center
Reading level

Seg inset

Figure 21-20. Reading center location is specified from two dimensions. The lateral position is dictated by the near interpupillary distance, which determines seg inset, and the vertical position is ascertained by reading level.

2. Next find the power of each lens in the 90-degree meridian. This can be done by placing the prescription on power crosses as shown in Figure 21-21. For the right lens the power in the 90-degree meridian is +3.50 D. For the left lens the power in the 90-degree meridian is +0.75 D.
3. Now we use Prentice's rule to find the vertical prismatic effect at the reading level. For the right lens this is

$$\Delta = cF$$
$$= 0.9 \times 3.50$$
$$= 3.15\Delta$$

Since the lens is a plus lens and we are looking below the optical center, the base direction is base up. The prismatic effect is 3.15Δ base up.
   For the left lens

$$\Delta = cF$$
$$= 0.9 \times 0.75$$
$$= 0.675\Delta$$

The prismatic effect is 0.675Δ base up.
4. Since both lenses have a base up prismatic effect, the prismatic difference is found by subtracting the two numbers.

3.15Δ base up – 0.675Δ base up = 2.475Δ base up

The imbalance is rounded to 2.50Δ base up and is written as 2.50Δ base up O.D. (It could also be expressed as 2.50Δ base down O.S.) Do not confuse the imbalance with the correction!

The slab-off correction used will be base up, so it will be placed on the eye with the most minus or least plus power in the 90-degree meridian. For this prescription the slab-off goes on the left lens.

Example **21-10**

Calculate the imbalance for the following prescription:

O.D. –4.00 –1.00 × 180
O.S. +1.00 –0.50 × 180
Add +1.50 D
Frame B dimension = 34 mm
Seg height = 14 mm
Reading level is determined to be 4 mm below the top of the bifocal line.

Solution

First find the reading level. This is done by finding the seg drop and adding it to the distance from the segment line down to the reading level. Segment drop is

Drop = B/2 – segment height
= 34/2 – 14
= 17 – 14
= 3 mm

The segment drop of 3 mm is added to the 4 mm distance to the reading level, which totals 7 mm.
   Next we find the power of each lens in the 90 degree meridian. For the right lens the power in the 90 degree meridian is -5.00 D. For the left lens this will be +0.50 D.
   For the right lens the vertical prismatic effect for a distance 7 mm (0.7 cm) below the distance optical center is found by using Prentice's rule.

$$\Delta = cF$$
$$= 0.7 \times 5$$
$$= 3.5 \ \Delta \text{ base down}$$

The direction is base down because the lens is minus and we are looking below the optical center.
   For the left lens the prismatic effect will be

Figure 21-21. To calculate vertical prismatic effect for spherocylinder lenses with axes at 90 or 180 it helps to place the lens powers on a power cross. The power in the 90 degree meridian then becomes easy to see.

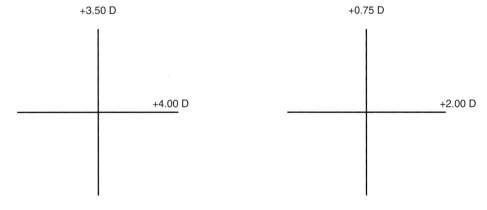

+3.50 D

+4.00 D

+0.75 D

+2.00 D

$$\Delta = cF$$
$$= 0.7 \times 0.5$$
$$= 0.35 \, \Delta \text{ base up}$$

The prism direction is base up because we are looking through the lower half of the lens and the lens is plus in power. To find the amount of imbalance we will need to add the two prism amounts. This is because one base direction is base down and the other base up. The total amount of *imbalance* can be expressed as either

3.85 Δ base down, right eye, or
3.85 Δ base up, left eye

The amount of *correction* must be an equal and opposite amount. Either 3.85 Δ of base up is placed on the right eye, or 3.85 Δ base down on the left eye. Regular slab off prism is base up. So the slab off correction would be placed on the right eye. (Traditional slab off prism is always placed on the most minus or least plus eye. The right eye is the most minus eye.)

Planocylinders and Spherocylinders, Axes Oblique (Exact Calculations for the Traditional Method)
Calculating imbalance for planocylinders whose axes are oblique requires considerably more calculations to achieve the best result. One way of doing this is to use the same calculations as outlined in Chapter 16 in the section on Decentration of Cylinders Oriented Obliquely and Horizontal and Vertical Decentration of Oblique Cylinders.

Calculating the prismatic effect of the distance lens at the reading center for spherocylinders is done by first calculating the prismatic effects caused by the sphere component, then calculating the prismatic effects caused by the cylinder component. The prismatic effects found in the two separate operations are then added together. The calculations required to use this method are feasible, but difficult, and are seldom used in clinical practice.

Using the Cosine-Squared Method and Prentice's Rule to Find Vertical Imbalance
The cosine-squared method is a shortcut method for finding vertical imbalance when a prescription has oblique cylinder. Results obtained using this method are not as exact, but the method is much faster and considerably easier. This method allows one to find a total lens power for the 90-degree meridian quickly. To use this method, follow these steps:
1. Find the "power*" of the oblique cylinder in the 90-degree meridian of the right lens using the formula:

$$F_{90cyl} = F_{cyl} \cos^2 \theta$$

---

*Actually, there is only power in the meridian 90 degrees away from the cylinder axis (i.e., in the power meridian of the cylinder). This formula will accurately give curvature for a nonaxis meridian. As stated before, this traditionally used method gives close, but not exact, approximations.

where

F_{90cyl} = power of the cylinder in the 90 degree meridian

F_{cyl} = power of the cylinder

θ = axis of the cylinder

2. Add the power of the cylinder in the 90-degree meridian for the right lens to the power of the sphere for the right lens ($F_{90cyl} + F_{sph}$).
3. Repeat steps 1 and 2 for the left lens.
4. Either (A) multiply each power by the reading depth distance and then find the prismatic difference between the two (a longer method), or (B) find the power difference between the right and left lenses and then multiply this difference by the reading depth distance (a shorter method).

Example **21-11**

Calculate the vertical imbalance for the following prescription using the cosine-squared method:

O.D. +3.00 +2.50 × 030
O.S. +0.50 +1.00 × 135
Add +2.00
The flat top bifocal segment has a seg drop of 3 mm.
The reading level is 5 mm below the segment top.

Solution
1. To find the power of the cylinder in the 90-degree meridian, use:

$$F_{90cyl} = F_{cyl} \cos^2 \theta$$
$$= (+2.50)\cos^2 30$$
$$= (+2.50)(0.75)$$
$$= +1.875 \, D$$

2. Adding the power of the cylinder in the 90-degree meridian (+1.875 D) to the sphere power (+3.00) gives:

$$+3.00 + 1.875 = +4.875 \, D$$

3. Repeating for the left lens results in:

$$F_{90cyl} = F_{cyl} \cos^2 \theta$$
$$= +1.00 \cos^2 135$$
$$= (+1.00)(0.50)$$
$$= +0.50 \, D$$

for the cylinder power in the 90-degree meridian.

Total lens power in the 90 degree meridian $= (F_{90cyl} + F_{sph})$
$$= (+0.50) + (+0.50)$$
$$= +1.00 \, D$$

4. For this step, proceed in one of two ways. The first way, though somewhat longer, is that used in earlier examples.
   A. Multiply each 90-degree lens power by the reading depth distance in centimeters. We know the lens power in the 90-degree meridian, but not the reading depth. The reading depth is 5 mm below the segment line and the segment line has a drop of 3 mm. This places the reading

level 8 mm (0.8 cm) below the distance optical center. Now we can find vertical prismatic effect.

For the right lens this is:

$$(4.875)\ (0.8) = 3.9\Delta \text{ base up}$$

For the left lens this is:

$$(1.00)\ (0.8) = 0.8\Delta \text{ base up}$$

The total vertical imbalance at the near point is the difference between these two vertical prismatic effects.

$$
\begin{array}{r}
3.90\Delta \text{ base up O.D.}\\
\underline{-0.80\Delta \text{ base up O.S.}}\\
=3.10\Delta \text{ base up O.D.}
\end{array}
$$

To shorten the process, we use the second option:

B. Find the difference between right and left lens powers. In the 90-degree meridians these differences are:

$$(+4.875) - (+1.00) = +3.875 \text{ D}$$

Next multiply the power difference by the reading depth in centimeters:

$$(3.875)\ (0.8) = 3.10\Delta \text{ base up O.D.}$$

Both of these ways of finding the imbalance result in the same amount of vertical imbalance.

(For a summary of how to calculate vertical imbalance using the cosine-squared method, see Box 21-5.)

Remole's Method

In a series of articles[13,14,15,16,17], Arnulf Remole exposes some deficiencies in the traditional methods for calculating vertical imbalance. Remole points out a basic problem with using Prentice's rule. This problem stems back to Prentice's original supposition. Prentice presented his rule in "the context of a single, hypothetically thin lens.[18]" His rule works correctly when used in context. However, prismatic effect at a given point on a lens is also influenced by lens thickness and base curve.

The second problem has to do with the amount each eye turns downward. To find vertical imbalance in the traditional manner we must determine a reading level. To calculate imbalance, we assume that both eyes turn downward equally, looking through a reading level that is the same distance below the optic axis for both right and left eyes. Yet we know that unequal vertical prism is induced by unequal left and right lens powers. This causes the two eyes to turn downward by different amounts. This will place them at slightly different distances from their starting points and not at the same reading level.

Remole presents an alternate method for finding prismatic effect that takes lens thickness, base curve, and

unequal vertical turning of left and right eyes into consideration. It shows how aniseikonia and vertical imbalance are related and how correcting for aniseikonia has a direct influence on the amount of vertical imbalance correction that may be required.

Prismatic Effect and Magnification Are Related

Magnification is the result of a changing prismatic effect across a lens. The equation for spectacle magnification is employed when calculating magnification with aniseikonia. This equation takes both base curve and lens thickness into account. Changing either base curve or lens thickness causes a change in magnification. Remole uses spectacle magnification to more accurately find prismatic effect at a given point on a lens.

Normally the entrance pupil of the eye is used when calculating spectacle magnification for aniseikonia purposes. Here is the conventional formula as previously described when discussing aniseikonia.

$$
SM = \left(\dfrac{1}{1-\dfrac{t}{n}F_1}\right)\left(\dfrac{1}{1-dF'_v}\right)
$$
$$
= (S)(P_{stat})
$$

BOX 21-5

Calculating Vertical Imbalance Using the Cosine-Squared Method

1. Find the reading depth.

   Reading depth = seg drop + 5 mm (usually)

2. Find the "power" of the oblique cylinder in the 90-degree meridian of the right lens using the formula:

   $$F_{90cyl} = F_{cyl}\cos^2\theta$$

   where
   F_{90cyl} = power of the cyl in the 90-degree meridian
   F_{cyl} = power of the cylinder
   θ = axis of the cylinder

3. Add the power of the cylinder in the 90-degree meridian for the right lens to the power of the sphere for the right lens.

   $$(F_{90cyl} + F_{sph})$$

4. Repeat Steps 2 and 3 for the left lens.
5. Find the power differences between right and left lenses and then multiply this difference by the reading-depth distance.

Where

SM = static spectacle magnification
t = center thickness
F_1 = front surface lens power
n = refractive index
d = distance from the back surface of the lens to the entrance pupil of the eye (usually vertex distance plus 3 mm)
F_v' = back vertex lens power
S = shape factor
P_{stat} = static power factor

Remole uses P_{stat} to point out that this is the power factor for an eye that is not moving. However, when calculating spectacle magnification when the eye is moving, Remole maintains that the more logical point of reference is the center of rotation of the eye. "Because the entrance pupils of the eye move as the eye rotates, they can't be used as reference points. Instead the center of rotation must be used.[13]" This changes the formula for the eye when it is no longer in the straight-ahead position. The formula then becomes a "dynamic spectacle magnification formula" so that it reads:

$$G = \left(\frac{1}{1 - \dfrac{t}{n}F_1} \right) \left(\frac{1}{1 - sF_v'} \right)$$
$$= (S)(P_{dyn})$$

Where

G = dynamic spectacle magnification
t = center thickness
F_1 = front surface lens power
n = refractive index
s = distance from the back surface of the lens to the center of rotation of the eye
F_v' = back vertex lens power
S = shape factor
P_{dyn} = dynamic power factor

So "in dynamic spectacle magnification, primary image sizes are determined with reference to the centers of rotation rather than the entrance pupils.[13]"

Example **21-12**

For a pair of lenses made from Trivex lens material, use Remole's method to find the prismatic effects for right and left lenses for a reading level 10 mm below the distance optical centers. Then determine the vertical imbalance between the two eyes. The distance from the back of the lens to the center of rotation of the eye is 27 mm. Here are the lens parameters.

Right lens:

> Power = +2.00 D sphere
> Index of refraction = 1.53
> True base curve = +6.30*
> Center thickness = 3.2 mm

Left lens:

> Power = +4.00 D sphere
> Index of refraction = 1.53
> True base curve = +8.34
> Center thickness = 4.4 mm

Solution

In solving a problem like this, remember that the reading level of 10 mm is the level at the back vertex plane of the lens where the object ray strikes the lens. This 10-mm measurement is represented by m, the object eccentricity (Figure 21-22). Unless the lens has a power of zero, this point is not the point through which the image ray appears to be coming. The prismatic effect of the lens causes the eye to turn from this point. The distance from the center of the lens to the image point is called the image eccentricity, represented by m'.

To find the prismatic effect using object and image eccentricities, we first need to find the dynamic spectacle magnification.

Dynamic spectacle magnification is:

$$G = \left(\frac{1}{1 - \dfrac{t}{n}F_1} \right) \left(\frac{1}{1 - sF_v'} \right)$$

For the right lens, dynamic spectacle magnification is:

$$G_{OD} = \left(\frac{1}{1 - \dfrac{0.0032}{1.53}(+6.30)} \right) \left(\frac{1}{1 - (0.027)(+2.00)} \right)$$
$$= (1.01335)(1.05708)$$
$$= 1.0712$$

The object angle (a) is the angle between the optical axis and a line from the object point to the center of rotation of the eye (see Figure 21-22). This angle may be calculated since m is known and so is s. Remember,

m is the object projection on the back vertex plane of the lens. (In this case m equals the reading level.)

s is the distance from the back vertex plane of the lens to the center of rotation of the eye.

Therefore from the geometry of the figure we know that:

$$\tan a = \frac{m}{s}$$

---

*Since Trivex has an index of 1.53, the true base curve is also the refractive power of the front lens surface. If the index of refraction was any other index than 1.53, it would be necessary to convert the true base curve to refractive power before entering it in the equation as F_1.

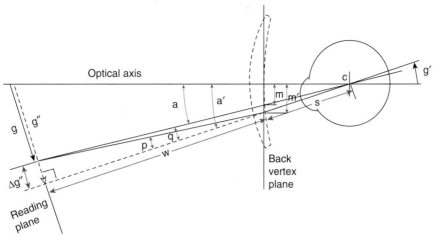

Figure 21-22. In this drawing, the eye is looking through an off-axis point and experiencing prismatic effect. The object in the reading plane is denoted by g and the image of that object by g′. The difference in object and image size resulting from dynamic spectacle magnification is denoted by Δg″.

The angle made by the object projection as it goes through the center of rotation of the eye (denoted by c) is abbreviated as a. The projection of the image of that object has the abbreviation a′. The letter q is the difference between the object and image angles, a and a′.

The letters m and m′ are the object and image projections of a and a′ on the back vertex plane of the lens. m is called the object eccentricity; m′ is called the image eccentricity. The working distance is w; s is the stop distance.

The letter p is the angle formed by the chief ray from the object point and the projection of the chief ray entering the eye. The diagram is not to scale.

(From Remole A: New equations for determining ocular deviations produced by spectacle corrections, Opt Vis Sci 77(10):56, 2000.)

And we can find a by taking the inverse tan of $\dfrac{m}{s}$.
In other words,

$$a = \tan^{-1}\frac{m}{s}$$

In our example this angle is:

$$
\begin{aligned}
a &= \tan^{-1}\frac{m}{s} \\
&= \tan^{-1}\frac{10}{27} \\
&= \tan^{-1} 0.37037 \\
&= 20.32314°
\end{aligned}
$$

This means that if the lens had a power of zero, the eye would turn 20.3 degrees to view the object.

To find the prismatic effect caused by the lens we need to find out how much the lens displaces the image of that object. Therefore we need to find the image angle a′. To find this angle, we need to know m′. And to find m′, we need to know how much the image of the object was magnified. This is found by multiplying the magnification factor, G, by the object eccentricity, m. So

$$m' = Gm$$

For the right lens this is:

$$
\begin{aligned}
m' &= (1.0712)(10) \\
&= 10.712 \text{ mm}
\end{aligned}
$$

Knowing m′, we can find a′, the image angle. Using the same method as we did for the object angle, we have:

$$
\begin{aligned}
a' &= \tan^{-1}\frac{m'}{s} \\
&= \tan^{-1}\frac{10.712}{27} \\
&= \tan^{-1} 0.39674 \\
&= 21.64021°
\end{aligned}
$$

The difference between these two angles is the prismatic effect caused by the lens. In degrees this is:

$$q = a' - a$$

where q is the angle the eye deviates (angle of ocular deviation) from where it would be looking without a lens in place. This is prismatic effect in degrees. For the right lens this is:

$$
\begin{aligned}
q &= 21.64021° - 20.32314° \\
&= 1.31707°
\end{aligned}
$$

To convert this to prism diopters, we use the definition of a prism diopter. So

$$q_{PD} = 100 \tan q$$
$$= 100 \tan 1.31707$$
$$= 100(0.02299)$$
$$= 2.30\Delta$$

So the prismatic effect for the right eye at the 10-mm reading level is 2.30 prism diopters, base up.

For the left eye the procedure is repeated.

Dynamic spectacle magnification is:

$$G = \left(\cfrac{1}{1 - \cfrac{t}{n} F_1} \right) \left(\cfrac{1}{1 - sF'_v} \right)$$

$$G_{OS} = \left(\cfrac{1}{1 - \cfrac{0.0044}{1.53}(+8.34)} \right) \left(\cfrac{1}{1 - (0.027)(+4.00)} \right)$$
$$= (1.02457)(1.12108)$$
$$= 1.14862$$

The object angle (a) for the left eye is the same as for the right. But the image eccentricity (m) will change as will the image angle (a').

$$m' = Gm$$

For the left lens, image eccentricity is:

$$m' = (1.14862)(10)$$
$$= 11.4862 \text{ mm}$$

And the image angle for the left lens is:

$$a' = \tan^{-1} \frac{m'}{s}$$
$$= \tan^{-1} \frac{11.4862}{27}$$
$$= \tan^{-1} 0.38635$$
$$= 23.04562°$$

For the left eye, the prismatic effect in degrees is:

$$q = 23.04562° - 20.32314°$$
$$= 2.72248°$$

In prism diopters this is equal to:

$$q_{PD} = 100 \tan q$$
$$= 100 \tan 2.72248$$
$$= 100(0.04755)$$
$$= 4.76\Delta$$

So the prismatic effect for the left eye at the 10-mm reading level is 4.76 prism diopters, base up.

The vertical imbalance between left and right eyes is:

4.76Δ base up − 2.30Δ base up = 2.46Δ base up left eye

Shortening the Procedure. It is possible to shorten the procedure some by finding the image angles (a') for both right and left eyes. But instead of converting these angles to prism diopters, subtract the two angles first. Then convert to prism diopters. Here is how it would work for the above example. We find this *relative prismatic effect* (relative q) as the difference between right and left image angles in degrees.

$$\text{relative } q = (\text{eye with greater } a') - (\text{eye with lesser } a')$$
$$= (23.04562°) - (21.64021°)$$
$$= 1.40541°$$

This relative difference in degrees is then converted into prism diopters.

$$q_{PD} = 100 \tan (\text{relative } q)$$
$$= 100 \tan 1.40541$$
$$= 100(0.02453)$$
$$= 2.45\Delta$$

Since the greater plus power is on the left eye, the imbalance is 2.45Δ base up left eye. This agrees with what was found earlier.

Note that this amount of vertical imbalance is greater than would be found using Prentice's rule. Prentice's rule would have given 2Δ base up left eye as the imbalance.

For a summary of how to find vertical imbalance using Remole's method, see Box 21-6.

Remole has also presented a method for determining prismatic effect for any point on a lens in the presence of oblique cylinder using magnification ellipses. He states that "For determining differential prismatic effects in cylindrical lenses, the methods based on the dynamic spectacle magnification and magnification ellipses are far easier than the multiple vector methods. . . . They can be applied to all types of spectacle lenses as well as to iseikonic corrections.[14]" (For more on this topic see Remole A: A new method for determining prismatic effects in cylindrical spectacle corrections, Optom Vis Sci 77:4, 2000.)

Comparing Results: Remole's Method Versus Prentice's Rule

Results obtained using Remole's method will not yield the same results as found using Prentice's rule. Because Remole's method takes both lens thickness and base curve into consideration, it would be expected to give more accurate results. So how do the two compare?

Fortunately, "The conventional application of Prentice's rule can be applied to most low and moderate anisometropic minus lens corrections without producing clinically significant errors.[13]" However, "The differential prismatic effects found with minus lenses by using the exact formula are smaller than the estimate made by Prentice's rule, whereas with plus lenses, the prismatic

Finding Vertical Imbalance Using Remole's Method

1. Find the dynamic spectacle magnification (G) for both right and left lenses.
2. Determine the proposed reading level for the wearer, if not already known.
3. Find the object angle (a) for the reading level in degrees.
   a. Object angle can be found knowing that:

$$\tan a = \frac{m}{s}$$

   m is the object projection on the back vertex plane of the lens. (In this case, m equals the reading level.)
   s is the distance from the back vertex plane of the lens to the center of rotation of the eye.
   b. Therefore to find a, we use:

$$a = \tan^{-1}\frac{m}{s}$$

4. Use the dynamic spectacle magnification (G) and the object eccentricity (a) to find the image eccentricity (a') in degrees for each eye.
   a. For each eye, image eccentricity (a') along the back vertex sphere is equal to object eccentricity (a) times the dynamic spectacle magnification (G), or a' = aG.
5. Find the difference between the image angles for right and left lenses.

relative q = (eye with greater a') − (eye with lesser a')

6. Convert this degree measure into prism diopters.

$$q_{PD} = 100\tan (\text{relative } q)$$

This is the amount of vertical imbalance for the two eyes.

effects are larger.[13]" In fact, "The conventional application of Prentice's rule to anisometropic plus lens corrections will often result in large errors.[13]"

Simply put, ". . . the textbook application of Prentice's rule will underestimate the differential prismatic effect for plus lens corrections and overestimate the effect for minus lens corrections.[13]"

Reducing Aniseikonia Will Also Reduce Vertical Imbalance

When aniseikonia is present, one lens has a different power than the other. This means that in the periphery of the higher-powered lens, there is more prismatic effect. By changing parameters, such as base curve and lens thickness, magnification changes and, as we have seen in the previous section, so does prismatic effect.

This means that, hypothetically, if we are able to make right and left lenses have the same magnification,* we will also eliminate vertical imbalance. "Furthermore, the absence of prismatic effect will apply to the entire binocular field, which presents an enormous advantage over a slab-off lens.[13]"

However, as Remole himself points out, this will not usually be the case because the clinically measured amount of aniseikonia is usually less than the calculated amount. Thus the calculated amount of aniseikonia will not be fully corrected. But it does mean that any amount of correction for aniseikonia will lessen the need for as much vertical imbalance correction.

In summary:
1. Reducing aniseikonia will reduce the amount of vertical imbalance correction needed.
2. Reducing aniseikonia may reduce the vertical imbalance a sufficient amount so that the remaining imbalance is not clinically significant enough to require correction.

DESIGNING A LENS TO CHANGE THE APPEARANCE OF A BLIND EYE

Normally, lens power is used only to correct refractive error and prism power to alleviate problems with binocular vision. Yet there is another use for power, prism, and even tint that has nothing to do with refractive error. It can also be used to improve the cosmetic appearance of a blind or prosthetic (artificial) eye.

A skilled ocularist will be able to match the color and appearance of the artificial eye's iris and sclera to that of the seeing eye. But because of a condition of the eye socket, an artificial eye may look abnormal, even when eye colors are well matched. If further cosmetic surgery will not help, cosmetics may be improved with spectacle lenses. Lenses used for cosmetic purposes are not part of the prescription. They may be determined by the dispenser at the time of frame selection.

Changing the Apparent Size of the Eye

Lenses have the optical effect of magnifying if they are plus or minifying if they are minus. When a plus lens magnifies, it not only causes the world to look larger to the wearer, but the wearer's eyes will also look bigger to everybody else. Normally, dispensers try to reduce this effect by using aspherics to flatten and thin the lens. Yet sometimes it may be advantageous to make a nonseeing eye look bigger *intentionally*.

---

*This magnification needs to be the dynamic spectacle magnification as calculated with reference to the eyes' centers of rotation, not the static spectacle magnification; the dynamic spectacle magnification is a greater magnification than the normally calculated (static) spectacle magnification.

Using Spheres

If a person has lost an eye and had it replaced with a prosthetic eye, the artificial eye may match the color of the seeing eye perfectly. The artificial eye may have a sunken appearance, however, making it look smaller. To correct this effect, hold up plus trial lenses in front of the prosthetic eye until it looks closer in size to the seeing eye. When a good match is achieved, use the experimentally found power. Likewise, if the nonseeing eye looks too big, minus power can be used to make it appear smaller.

Using Cylinders

Planocylinders may be used to change only the horizontal or only the vertical size of the eye. For instance, sometimes even when the horizontal dimension of the eye looks normal, the vertical depth of the palpebral fissure* of the nonseeing eye may be smaller than that of the seeing eye. To make the fissure look larger vertically, a plus cylinder, axis 180 may be used. To find the correct power, hold plus cylinders up in front of the eye until the desired cosmetic effect is achieved.

Tilting the Cylinder to Change Lid Slant

In some instances, the eyelids of the prosthetic eye may appear slanted. When a cylinder lens is rotated around its axis, it will cause a horizontal line to tilt. A plus cylinder will cause a straight line to tilt against the direction of rotation, whereas a minus cylinder will cause a line to tilt with the direction of rotation. When deciding whether to use plus or minus cylinder, the deciding factor is magnification.

To determine the optimal axis placement, hold the cylinder lens in front of the eye (preferably using a trial frame) and turn the axis until the slanted lids match the straight lids.[20]

Summary

1. The apparent overall size of the eye may be changed using plus or minus sphere lenses.
2. By using planocylinder lenses, the size of the eye may be increased or decreased in one meridian (the power meridian of the cylinder). The magnification in the meridian 90 degrees away (the axis meridian) will remain unaffected.
3. Rotating a planocylinder lens away from the horizontal or vertical meridian causes tilt. If eyelids look unnaturally tilted, place a cylinder lens in front of the nonseeing eye and rotate the cylinder axis until the eyelids look more like the normal eye.

*The palpebral fissure is the area between the upper and lower eyelids.

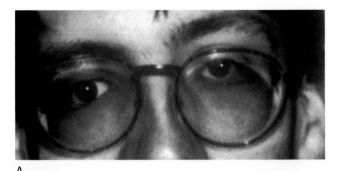

A

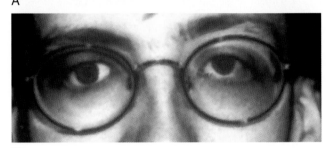

B

Figure 21-23. A, The artificial eye is this person's right eye. It appears low in comparison with the left eye. **B,** An attempt has been made to cosmetically alter the appearance of the eye. This has been done by placing 10Δ of base-down prism in the right lens. To help prevent a thick lower edge on the right lens, a frame should be chosen with a narrow vertical dimension. To help camouflage lens thickness, the lenses have been given an antireflection coating.

(Courtesy of Laurie Pierce, Tampa, Fla.)

Using a Lens to Camouflage Scars or Deformities

Sometimes a nonseeing eye is scarred or disfigured, but not to the point where a patch would be worn. In this case a lens should be selected that will decrease the visibility of the eye. Tinting may be applied to the lens as either a solid or a gradient tint. An antireflection coating should not be used. Keep in mind that tinting both lenses will decrease the wearer's vision at night. Cosmetic considerations should not rule over safety considerations.

Changing the Apparent Location of an Eye

Trauma causing the loss of an eye can also cause the displacement of the socket. This makes the prosthetic eye appear higher or lower than the seeing eye. If the blind or prosthetic eye is lower or higher or appears to turn inward or outward compared with the seeing eye, its apparent location may be altered by using prism.

The base direction of the prism used will always be placed in the direction that the eye is physically displaced. In other words, if the eye appears too high, use base-up prism. If the eye turns in, use base in. If this is done, then to an observer, the wearer's eye will appear to be displaced toward the apex of the prism. Such prism is called *inverse prism* because it is opposite to what would normally be prescribed for a seeing eye.

Example **21-13**

Suppose a right prosthetic eye is physically displaced downward as in Figure 21-23, *A*. How could the eye be made to look more normal?

Solution

Increasingly larger amounts of base-down prism are held in front of the prosthetic eye until, with 10Δ of base-down prism, the eye appears more evenly placed relative to the seeing eye. To prevent having the right lens appear thick at the bottom, use a frame with a small vertical size (small B dimension. To make the prism less obvious, an antireflection coating should be used.

It is possible to split the prism unevenly between the left and right eyes. If the prism is split, the *maximum* amount of vertical prism should not exceed 4Δ in front of the seeing eye. Exceeding 4Δ may cause postural changes and errors in the perceived location of objects. In this case one might use 7Δ base down before the right eye and 3Δ base up before the left eye.

Table 21-1 summarizes the use of lenses for cosmetic effects.

TABLE 21-1
Using Lenses to Achieve a Desired Cosmetic Effect

Problem	Desired Cosmetic Effect	Lens Solution
Eye looks small.	Make the eye look bigger. 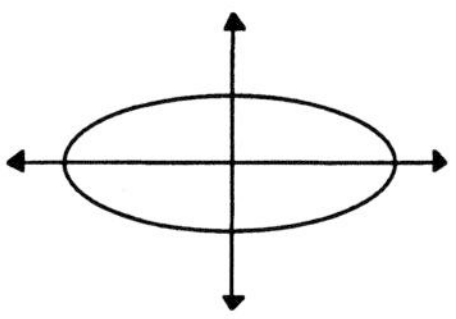	Use a plus sphere lens.
Eye looks large.	Make the eye look smaller. 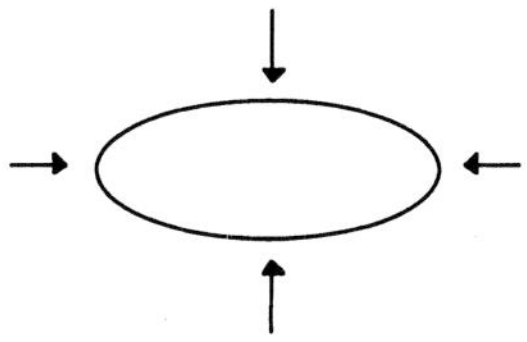	Use a minus sphere lens.
Eye not open as wide as the seeing eye. (Fissure looks too small vertically.)	Widen the fissure vertically. 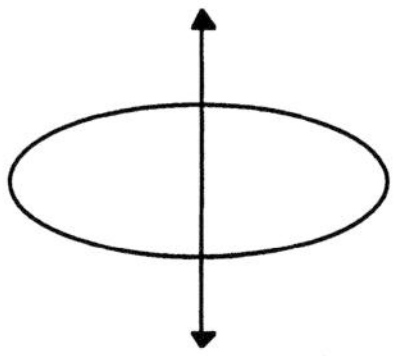	Use a plus cylinder, axis 180.
Eye open wider than the seeing eye. (Fissure looks too large vertically.)	Close the eye somewhat. 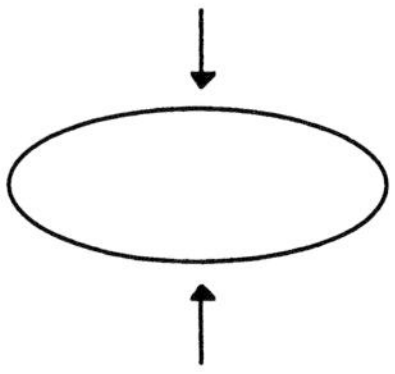	Use a minus cylinder, axis 180.
Eye looks too small horizontally.	Widen the horizontal appearance of the eye. 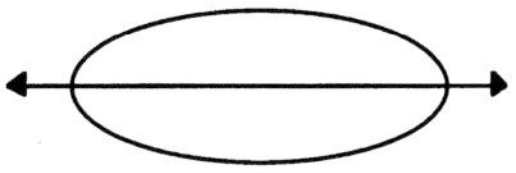	Use a plus cylinder, axis 90.

Continued

TABLE **21-1**
Using Lenses to Achieve a Desired Cosmetic Effect—cont'd

Problem	Desired Cosmetic Effect	Lens Solution
Eye looks too wide horizontally.	Narrow the horizontal appearance of the eye.	Use a minus cylinder, axis 90.
Eye looks too low.	Raise the apparent height of the eye.	Use base-down prism.
Eye looks too high.	Lower the apparent height of the eye.	Use base-up prism.
Eyelid is slanted.	Cause the rotated appearance of the lid to change in tilt and match the horizontal look of the seeing eye.	Rotate plus cylinder axis against the direction of desired tilt or rotate minus cylinder axis with the direction of desired tilt.
Eye has unsightly appearance or scarring of the lids or orbital area.	Reduce visibility of the eye.	Use tinted lenses—solid tint for overall masking, gradient tint to mask the upper areas. If tints are not used, avoid antireflection coatings.

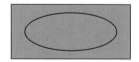

Plus Cylinder Axis

Minus Cylinder Axis

REFERENCES

1. Hofstetter HW, Griffin JR, Berman MS et al: The dictionary of visual science, ed 5, Boston, 2000, Butterworth-Heinemann.
2. Rabin J, Bradley A, Freeman RD: On the relation between aniseikonia and axial anisometropia, Am J Optom & Physiol Optics 60:553-558, 1983.
3. Bradley A, Rabin J, Freeman RD: Nonoptical determinants of aniseikonia, Investig Ophthalmol Vis Sci 24(4):507, 1983.
4. Winn B, Ackerly RG, Brown CA et al: Reduced aniseikonia in axial anisometropia with contact lens correction, J Ophthalmic Physiol Opt 8:341-344, 1988.
5. Winn B, Ackerly RG, Brown CA et al: The superiority of contact lenses in the correction of all anisometropia, Transactions BCLA conference:95, 1986.
6. Achron LR, Witkin NS, Ervin AM et al: The effect of relative spectacle magnification on aniseikonia, JAOA 69(9):591-599, 1998.
7. Linksz A, Bannon RE: Aniseikonia and refractive problems, Int Ophthalmol Clin, 5(2):515-534, 1965.
8. Stephens GL, Polasky M: New options for aniseikonia correction: the use of high index materials, Optom Vis Sci 68(11):899-906, 1991.
9. Sheedy JE: Answer to reader query: slab-off in progressive addition lenses? Opt Dispensing News 223, 2005.

10. Brooks CW: Understanding Lens Surfacing, Boston, 1992, Butterworth-Heinemann, p 290.

11. Drew R: CR-39 slab-off lenses: now ready cast, Optic Manage 13:23, 1984.

12. Rosen K: Premolded slab-offs bring results, Optic Manage 13:32, 1984.

13. Remole A: Determining exact prismatic deviations in spectacle corrections, Opt Vis Sci 76(11):783-795, 1999.

14. Remole A: A new method for determining prismatic effects in cylindrical spectacle corrections, Opt Vis Sci 77(4):211-220, 2000.

15. Remole A: New equations for determining ocular deviations produced by spectacle corrections, Opt Vis Sci 77(10):555-563, 2000.

16. Remole A: Compensating for vertical anisometropic imbalance by the positioning of segment centers, Opt Vis Sci 78(7):539-555, 2001.

17. Remole A: The theory of object and image eccentricities: a new dimension in ophthalmic optics, Opt Vis Sci 80(10):708-719, 2003.

18. Remole A: Correspondence: new equations for spectacle induced ocular deviations: responses to some typical questions, Opt Vis Sci 78(7):481, 2001.

19. Remole A: A new method for determining prismatic effects in cylindrical spectacle corrections, Opt Vis Sci 77(4):220, 2000.

20. Flynn MF, Hosek DK: Cosmetic ophthalmic lenses: prescribing them for patients with ocular prostheses, Opt Today 3:49, 1995.

Proficiency Test

(Answers can be found in the back of the book.)

1. A form of aniseikonia occurs in a limited but useful amount in those whose eyes are identical to one another—both eyes may not have refractive error, or both may have identical refractive error. This form of aniseikonia is used to help in determining the location of an object in space and is called:
   a. symmetrical aniseikonia
   b. anatomic aniseikonia
   c. optical aniseikonia
   d. axial aniseikonia
   e. physiologic aniseikonia

2. A person is wearing the following prescription:
   R: +3.00
   L: +0.50
   a. The right lens is made from CR-39 plastic of index 1.498, is 4.3 mm thick, and has a front surface refractive power of +8.50 D. Both lenses are worn at a vertex distance of 13 mm. What is the spectacle magnification for the right lens?
   b. The left lens is 2.0 mm thick, is also made from CR-39 plastic, has a front surface refractive power of +6.00 D, and is also worn at a 13-mm vertex distance. What is the spectacle magnification for the lens?
   c. What is the difference in spectacle magnification resulting from the right and left spectacle lenses?

3. True or false? The amount of magnification produced by an ametropic eye compared with the image size produced by a "standard emmetropic eye" is called relative spectacle magnification.

4. If an eye has axial ametropia and is too long or too short, the image size will be larger or smaller than it would normally be. According to Knapp's law, using spectacle lenses on such an eye will bring the retinal image size back to normal. Which of these statements about Knapp's law is correct?
   a. Knapp's law is not just theory. It can be depended upon clinically.
   b. Knapp's law does not always hold true in clinical practice.

5. True or false? Aniseikonia symptoms are often the same as those experienced with either uncorrected refractive error, or oculomotor imbalances. The difference is that with aniseikonia, symptoms either are not helped by the correction, or appear after refractive and oculomotor problems are corrected.

6. Which of the following lens and frame options will **NOT** help to reduce the possibility of aniseikonia becoming a problem?
   a. Use a frame with a short vertex distance.
   b. Use a frame with a small eye size.
   c. Use lenses with steepened base curves.
   d. Use an aspheric lens design.
   e. Use a high-index lens material.

7. A wearer has anisometropia, and both right and left lenses are plus in power. One lens is higher plus than the other. To reduce aniseikonia, all of the following responses are appropriate **EXCEPT ONE**. Which possibility is *not* appropriate?
   a. Thin the higher plus lens.
   b. Steepen the base curve of the higher plus lens.
   c. Choose a frame with a minimum vertex distance.
   d. Increase the center thickness for the lower plus lens.

8. One lens is plus and the other minus. We want to minimize aniseikonia. All of the following are *wrong* things to do **EXCEPT ONE**. Which one is the **correct** thing to do?
   a. Steepen the base curve of the plus lens.
   b. Increase the vertex distance for the minus lens by moving the bevel to the back part of the lens edge.
   c. Thin both lenses.
   d. Choose a frame with a smaller vertex distance.
   e. Use a frame with a larger eye size.

9. One possibility for determining the percent magnification difference between right and left lenses is to estimate what this difference might be based on the spectacle lens prescription. This is done using a rule of thumb that multiplies a certain percent by the difference between the spectacle lens prescription for left and right eyes. At the time of this writing, the preferred closest rule of thumb is:
   a. 0.5% magnification difference for each diopter of anisometropia.
   b. 1.0% magnification difference for each diopter of anisometropia.
   c. 2.5% magnification difference for each diopter of anisometropia.
   d. 3.5% magnification difference for each diopter of anisometropia.

10. Here are some statements about the value of modifying spectacle lenses to lessen aniseikonia. Which of these statements is most accurate?
    a. Compensating for aniseikonia by modifying the spectacle lenses is of no value.
    b. Compensating for aniseikonia by modifying the spectacle lenses is only of minimal value since it is seldom done in practice.
    c. Compensating for aniseikonia by modifying the spectacle lenses has about a 50-50 chance of making a subjectively noticeable difference from the wearer's perspective when compared with no compensation for aniseikonia.
    d. Compensating for aniseikonia by modifying the spectacle lenses makes a subjectively noticeable difference for a significant majority of wearers when compared with no compensation for aniseikonia.

11. What is a bitoric spectacle lens?
    a. A bitoric spectacle lens is one that has two lens curves on one surface of the lens.
    b. A bitoric spectacle lens is one with aspheric surfaces on both the front and back of the lens.
    c. A bitoric spectacle lens is one with two curves on the front and two curves on the back of the lens.
    d. A bitoric spectacle lens is one with an aspheric front surface and an atoric back surface.

12. Vertical imbalance situations are most troublesome to the wearer when they are:
    a. long standing.
    b. of recent origin.

13. Contact lenses are used to overcome vertical imbalance because:
    a. Spectacle lenses create vertical imbalance at near, but contact lenses do not.
    b. Contact lenses have vertical imbalance, but that imbalance is smaller and therefore not troublesome.
    c. Contact lenses can be made with prism ballasting on one lens to correct for vertical imbalance.
    d. Contact lenses are not used to overcome vertical imbalance problems.

14. Tolerance to vertical imbalance in the reading area varies from person to person. Generally, any time there is a difference of between _____ and _____ of refractive power between right and left lenses, possible vertical imbalance problems merit consideration.
    a. 0.50 D and 1.00 D
    b. 1.00 D and 2.00 D
    c. 2.00 D and 3.00 D
    d. 3.00 D and 4.00 D

15. Listed below are several options for vertical imbalance. Choose the correct response for how the option overcomes (or does not overcome) the problem of vertical imbalance.
    a. ___contact lenses
    b. ___two pairs of glasses
    c. ___dropping the MRP height
    d. ___raising the seg height
    e. ___Fresnel press-on prism
    f. ___slab off (bicentric grind)
    g. ___dissimilar segs
    h. ___compensated "R" segs
    1. This option provides an equal but opposite amount of prism to counteract the imbalance.
    2. The imbalance is still present, but this option allows the wearer to look through areas of the lens where imbalance is either not problematic, or not as problematic.

3. Imbalance is no longer present with this option.

4. This option presents a compromise situation where vertical imbalance is reduced at near, but increased in the distance.

5. This option is of no help in correcting or avoiding imbalance and should not be used.

16. True or false? The best correction for vertical imbalance at near caused by the spectacle lens correction of anisometropia is always the full calculated amount of prismatic effect induced at the reading center.

17. When a slab-off correction is used on a bifocal lens, the slab-off line:
    a. is always on the same lens surface as the bifocal line.
    b. is always on the opposite side of the lens surface as the bifocal line.
    c. may be on either the same, or the opposite side as the bifocal line, depending on segment style.

18. True or false? A slab-off correction can be used with a progressive addition lens.

19. Slab off for a fused glass multifocal lens pair is always ground on the:
    a. most plus or least minus lens.
    b. stronger of the two lenses.
    c. most minus or least plus lens.
    d. thicker lens.
    e. dominant eye.

20. A reverse slab lens:
    a. has the slab-off prism correction on the same lens as it would be for a fused glass bifocal lens, but the prism is base down in effect.
    b. has base up created in the distance portion only.
    c. is the only possible choice for a 25-mm round seg plastic lens.
    d. has prism on the most plus or least minus lens.
    e. none of the above is a correct response

21. A prescription reads as follows:
    O.D. −3.50 −1.00 × 090
    O.S. −5.50 −1.50 × 090
    add +2.00 D
    Using the traditional method for calculating vertical imbalance, how much vertical imbalance is present for a reading level 10 mm below the distance OCs?
    a. 1.10Δ base down O.D.
    b. 2.00Δ base down O.S.
    c. 2.00Δ base down O.D.
    d. 2.50Δ base down O.S. and 0.50Δ base up O.D.
    e. none of the above

22. A prescription reads as follows:
    O.D. +5.00 −2.00 × 180
    O.S. +3.00 −2.00 × 090
    Would there be vertical imbalance manifested at a reading level 10 mm below the OCs?
    a. yes
    b. no

23. Using traditional methods for calculating vertical imbalance, *how much* slab-off prism would have to be ground on *which lens* to correct vertical imbalance completely at a point 10 mm below the distance OC for the following prescription?
    O.D. +2.75 D sphere
    O.S. −2.75 D sphere
    a. 2.75Δ base down O.D.
    b. 0.00
    c. 5.50Δ base up O.D.
    d. 5.50Δ base up O.S.
    e. none of the above

24. What amount of vertical imbalance at the reading level is created by the following lens correction (the reading level is 10 mm below the distance OC)? (Use traditional methods of calculation to find your answer.)
    O.D. +3.00 +1.00 × 180
    O.S. +1.00 +0.75 × 180
    a. 2.00Δ
    b. 5.75Δ
    c. 2.25Δ
    d. Not enough information is given.
    e. Enough information is given, but none of the above is correct.

25. Here is a prescription for an individual who will be wearing a slab-off correction:
    R: +4.50 sphere
    L: +1.00 sphere
    Add = +2.00
    On which eye would the slab-off prism be placed for each of the following lenses?
    a. fused-glass flat-top 28 bifocal
       1. right
       2. left
       3. cannot be made
    b. CR-39 plastic Executive bifocal
       1. right
       2. left
       3. cannot be made
    c. Younger precast slab-off flat-top 28 bifocal
       1. right
       2. left
       3. cannot be made

26. a. What is the vertical imbalance to the nearest quarter diopter for the following prescription, assuming that the reading level will be 4 mm down into the bifocal? (Again, use traditional methods for calculating imbalance.)

R: –6.00 – 1.00 × 180
L: –0.50 – 0.50 × 180
Add = +2.25
Seg height = 18 mm
A = 50 mm
B = 40 mm
Distance between lenses = 18 mm
PD = 64 mm

b. The slab off is to be used with an Executive bifocal. The slab off should be placed on which lens?
1. right
2. left

27. A prescription reads as follows:

R: –5.50 – 2.50 × 030
L: –2.50 – 1.50 × 160
Add: +2.00
Frame B dimension = 48 mm
Seg height = 20 mm

If the assumption is that the reading level is 5 mm below the seg line, what amount of vertical imbalance is present in the lens pair? (Use the cosine-squared method for calculating the imbalance and give the answer to the nearest quarter diopter.)
a. 3.25Δ
b. 3.50Δ
c. 4.00Δ
d. 4.50Δ

28. A prescription reads as follows:

R: +4.25 – 0.50 × 105
L: +0.50 – 1.25 × 065
Add: +2.25
Frame B dimension = 44 mm
Seg height = 19 mm

If the assumption is that the reading level is 5 mm below the seg line, what amount of vertical imbalance is present in the lens pair? (Use the cosine-squared method for calculating the imbalance and give the answer to the nearest quarter diopter.)
a. 3.25Δ
b. 3.50Δ
c. 4.00Δ
d. 4.50Δ

29. A wearer has a prescription for a pair of glasses with powers of:

R: –1.00 – 0.25 × 175
L: –7.50 – 2.50 × 025

The slab-off line is to be placed on a pair of progressive add lenses at a level of 7 mm below the PRP. The reading level is assumed to be 4 mm below the slab line. Using the cosine-squared method, how much vertical imbalance would be present at the reading level?

30. Vertical imbalance must be corrected for a reading level 10 mm below the distance OC for the following prescription:

R: O.D. +4.50 D sphere
L: O.S. +2.75 + 0.50 × 180
Add: +2.50 D
seg drop = 5 mm

What combination of dissimilar segs could be used?
a. 1 and 2   1. 22-mm round
b. 2 and 3   2. 38-mm round
c. 3 and 4   3. flat-top 22 or 25 or 28 or 35 (all with seg centers 5 mm below the seg line)
d. 1 and 3
e. 2 and 4   4. flat-top 45 or Executive (seg center on the line)

31. In the previous question, which seg style is used on the left eye?
a. 22 round
b. 38 round
c. flat-top 22 or 25 or 28 or 35
d. flat-top 45 or Executive

32. Find the theoretical dissimilar segment pair which will correct 2.80Δ of vertical imbalance for a prescription with a +2.00 D add power.
a. 1 and 2   1. 22-mm round seg
b. 2 and 3   2. 38-mm round seg
c. 3 and 4   3. flat-top 22 or 25 or 28 or 35 (all with seg centers 5 mm below the seg line)
d. 1 and 3
e. 2 and 4   4. flat-top 45 or Executive

33. A person wears a prescription of:

O.D. +1.00 − 0.75 × 180
O.S. −3.00 − 0.50 × 180
add +2.00 D

and reads at a level 8 mm below the distance OC.

a. How far apart would the segment optical centers of two dissimilar segs have to be separated from each other to correct fully for vertical imbalance calculated using traditional methods?
1. 13 mm
2. 15 mm
3. 19 mm
4. 20 mm
5. none of the above

b. Even though this would work optically, would it normally be considered an acceptable cosmetic solution to the problem?

34. True or false? Reducing the amount of aniseikonia can also reduce the amount of vertical imbalance correction needed for a prescription with anisometropia.

35. True or false? Two spectacle lenses have the same power, but their base curves and center thicknesses are different. For a point 10 mm below their distance centers these two lenses may not have the same prismatic effect.

36. For a high plus, anisometropic correction, how will vertical imbalance calculated using Remole's method compare with the amount of vertical imbalance calculated using Prentice's rule?

a. The calculation using Prentice's rule will yield the higher amount of imbalance.

b. The calculation using Remole's method will yield the higher amount of imbalance.

c. Both methods will yield the same amount of imbalance.

37. A blind, prosthetic left eye is physically lower than the right, seeing eye. Otherwise, the two eyes match perfectly. What could be done to give a better overall appearance?

a. Use a plus lens in front of the left eye.

b. Use a minus lens in front of the left eye.

c. Use base-up prism in front of the left eye.

d. Use base-down prism in front of the left eye.

38. A right, prosthetic eye has a palpebral aperture that is larger than the left, seeing eye. The horizontal dimension of the aperture is definitely not larger than the seeing eye. What would be your first trial lens option for the prosthetic eye?

a. a plano, plus cylinder lens, axis 180

b. a plano, plus cylinder lens, axis 90

c. a plano, minus cylinder lens, axis 180

d. a plano, minus cylinder lens, axis 90

e. a plus sphere lens

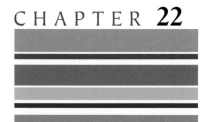

C H A P T E R **22**

Absorptive Lenses

O ne of the most misunderstood areas in ophthalmic dispensing is absorptive or "tinted" lenses. Myths and folk tales about the harmful or therapeutic effects of certain hues persist. This may create confusion, even for the dispenser, who may develop a personal philosophy about absorptive lenses through a combination of learned facts and educated guesses or who may simply yield to the changing tides of fashion and let the wearer have whatever most pleases him or her.

Yet it is the responsibility of the person engaged in eye care to know as much as possible about the subject of absorptive lenses. This chapter provides a thorough introduction.

CLASSIFICATION

Absorptive lenses are classified by *two variables*. The first is *the tint of the lens* itself, and the second is *the lens transmission*. Tints of the same basic color are labeled by a variety of names, depending on the manufacturer or in the case of plastic lenses, the name of the dye used to tint the lens. Differences of shade are sometimes discernible when two manufacturer's products are held side by side. For this reason, a record of the lens source should be entered on the wearer's record so that a replacement lens will match the original.

The relative absorption of a lens is most often denoted as either percent transmission or percent absorption. (Twenty percent transmission is the same as 80% absorption.)

Absorption used to be denoted by a letter, such as A, B, C, or D, or by a number, such as 1, 2, or 3. The higher the number or the further down the alphabet, the darker the tint will be.

Because this system was developed for tinted glass lenses that change transmission with increasing thickness, specific transmission will vary for different powered lenses having the same number or letter designation. Because this system still has limited usage, the dispenser must be aware of these potential differences.

Problems of Uniform Transmission Inherent in Pretinted Glass Lenses

It should be noted that the specified transmission for a pretinted glass lens applies to a 2-mm thick plano lens.

Any departure from this thickness will give rise to changes in transmission. The individual who was previously wearing a C tint in a +2.00 D glass lens may therefore find the same tint irritatingly dark when the prescription is changed to +3.50 D.

Glass lenses that vary in thickness from one area to another will also show proportional changes in transmission. The high minus lens will have a lighter central portion, darkening rapidly towards the periphery (Figure 22-1, *A*); the plus lens shows a darkened central zone with the tint lightening to the normally expected shade at the periphery (Figure 22-1, *B*). Perhaps the most unusual is a high, near plano minus cylinder lens. In this case a lighter band runs across the lens corresponding to the location of the minus cylinder axis (Figure 22-1, *C*). Fortunately, few absorptive lenses require glass lens material, making the problem an infrequent occurrence.

THE EFFECT OF VISIBLE AND NONVISIBLE LIGHT ON THE EYE

Light is electromagnetic radiation found in the wavelength range that includes infrared (IR), visible, and ultraviolet (UV) radiation. Not all of these wavelengths cause an activation of photoreceptors that produce vision (Figure 22-2). Light is interpreted as color according to the length of the light wave that strikes the retina.

The visible spectrum is considered to be between 380 and 760 nm.[1] (However, light with a wavelength as short as 309 nm may be seen if it is of sufficient intensity. Light having sufficient intensity and a wavelength as short as 298 nm could be seen if it were not absorbed by the crystalline lens before reaching the retina.)[2]

Much of the "light" in the UV and IR regions of the spectrum that strikes the eye never reaches the retina. Instead it is absorbed by the cornea, aqueous humor, crystalline lens, or vitreous humor of the eye. If too much of this "light" is absorbed by the individual eye structure in sufficient quantity or over an excessively lengthy period, it can be potentially harmful.

The Effects of Ultraviolet Radiation

"Light," or more properly, electromagnetic radiation with a wavelength shorter than 400 nm, is known as UV

526

radiation. UV radiation can be further subdivided into four regions.[3]
1. UVA 315 to 380 nm
2. UVB 290 to 315 nm
3. UVC 200 to 290 nm
4. UV Vacuum 100 to 200 nm

UVA radiation has the longest wavelength band and, relatively speaking, is the least harmful of the three radiation bands. It causes the skin to tan. UVB has shorter wavelengths and a higher energy than UVA. If present in sufficient quantity, long enough duration, or both, UVB causes sunburn, photokeratitis, cataracts, and retinal lesions. UVC is still higher in energy, but is effectively filtered out by the earth's ozone layer. UV Vacuum is present outside the earth's atmosphere, but is filtered by the atmosphere. The shorter the wavelength, the more biologically harmful the radiation will be.

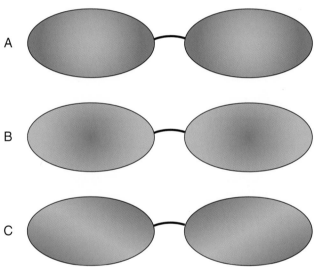

Figure 22-1. Glass lenses with the tint right in the material will vary in transmission as the thickness of the lens varies. **A,** A high minus prescription will be lightest in the middle and darken toward the edges. **B,** A high plus prescription will be darkest in the middle and lighten toward the edges. **C,** A plano, high minus cylinder will be lightest along the cylinder axis. Here the minus cylinder axis for the wearer's right eye is about 140; for the left eye it is about 40. This only occurs with high cylinders when the tint is within the glass itself.

There are a number of negative effects attributed to excessive exposure to ultraviolet radiation. The question becomes what constitutes "excessive exposure?" The answer is not simple. Single, high level amounts of UV can be damaging—but so can long-term, low-level amounts of UV exposure.

UV radiation is a normal component of sunlight, but the amount reaching the earth has been increasing with the thinning of the atmospheric ozone layer. The ozone layer normally filters out a large portion of shorter wavelength UV radiation.

UV radiation from sunlight is more intense between the hours of 10 AM and 2 PM with 60% of total UV radiation taking place during these hours.[1] The total annual amount of UV radiation is greater in geographic regions closer to the equator, and the amount of UV radiation increases in intensity at high altitudes.

Sand and snow increase the amount of UV radiation an individual receives because sand reflects 20% to 30% of UV light. Fresh snow reflects 85% to 95% of the light that strikes it as compared with only 3% for grass.[4] This makes UV protection for skiers absolutely essential.

Other sources of UV radiation include UV-type lamps and welding.

Ocular Damage Caused by Ultraviolet Radiation
An example of ocular damage caused by a single dose of high-level UV radiation is a *welder's burn*. In a welder's burn, the cornea and conjunctiva absorb UV light between 210 and 320 nm.[1] The excessive exposure to these UV wavelengths results in inflammation of the cornea and conjunctiva known as *photokeratitis*. The same photokeratitis may result from exposure during snow-related activities and is referred to as "*snow blindness*." It takes approximately 6 hours after a burn has occurred before the onset of pain. Fortunately, although the symptoms of grittiness, intense light sensitivity, excessive tearing, redness, and difficulty in opening the eyes are severe, in most cases the cornea heals, and symptoms are gone in 6 to 24 hours.

An example of ocular damage caused by long-term, cumulative, low doses of UV radiation is *the formation of cataracts*. People who live where UV radiation is high (at high altitudes or in desert or tropical areas) develop cataracts earlier in life. As an example, those who live in an

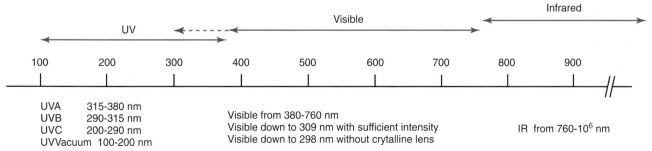

Figure 22-2. The light spectrum: ultraviolet, visible, and infrared.

area where the average amount of sunlight exposure is 12 hours have four times the amount of cataract formation compared with those who live in areas with a daily average of 7 hours.[5]

Welder's burn and cataracts are not the only eye-related problems induced by UV radiation. Another serious problem is retinal damage, particularly for the *aphake* (person without a crystalline lens) since the lens no longer absorbs light between 300 and 390 nm, but allows it to fall on the retina. This light is not only refracted somewhat differently, failing to produce as good an image, but now is absorbed by the retina, causing it to fluoresce.[6] This causes somewhat of a veiling glare effect. The glare effect is not the main problem since the sensitive, unprotected macular area of the retina can develop swelling from the UV and short blue spectrum (400 to 500 nm)[7] rays. In time this is followed by degeneration of the sensitive macular area. This degeneration is known as *age-related maculopathy* (ARM) or *macular degeneration*.

Though UV and short-wavelength retinal damage is normally associated with age, it should be noted that because children have more transparent crystalline lenses, their lenses allow some UV light to be transmitted to the retina.[8]

Protecting the retina from UV light is imperative. For aphakes it is an absolute necessity. Today cataract surgery is followed by the implantation of an intraocular lens to replace the cataract-clouded crystalline lens. Individuals who have an intraocular lens implant are called *pseudophakes*. Although presently used intraocular lens implants are UV absorbing, UV protection is still advisable.

A *pterygium* is a growth of tissue that begins on the white of the eye and extends onto the cornea. With continued growth it can travel to the center of the cornea, blocking clear vision. There is a correlation between the incidence of pterygia and UV exposure. A similar condition known as a *pinguecula* may also be UV related. A pinguecula manifests itself as a yellowish thickening of the conjunctiva, usually on the nasal side of the cornea.

Drugs That Heighten Ultraviolet Damage

Certain drugs increase the amount of damage that can be done by UV radiation. These include, but are not limited to, sulfonamides, tetracyclines, certain diuretics, tranquilizers, and oral contraceptives. This means that in addition to those effects of UV radiation that have already been discussed, individuals taking these drugs are more prone to sunburn and skin cancer. Individuals known to be taking these medications should be advised to use UV protective eyewear and use sunscreen for skin protection when appropriate.

Who Should Have Ultraviolet Protection?

UV damage to the eye is known to be cumulative over time. Reduction in ozone layer levels means that

---

BOX 22-1

Individuals With a Greater Need for Ultraviolet (UV) Protection

THOSE WITH THE FOLLOWING CONDITIONS:
- Beginning cataracts
- Macular degeneration
- Pterygia
- Pinguecula
- Aphakia
- Pseudophakia

THOSE WHO ARE TAKING MEDICATIONS, INCLUDING:
- Sulfonamides
- Tetracyclines
- Diuretics
- Tranquilizers
- Drugs for hypoglycemia
- Oral contraceptives

(This list is only a sampling of drugs that may increase UV damage. It is by no means all inclusive.)

THOSE IN THE SUN UNDER THE FOLLOWING CONDITIONS:
- Outdoors between 10 AM-2 PM in summer
- Outdoors long hours (especially children at play)
- Snow skiing
- Sun bathing
- In high-altitude conditions
- Near the equator

PERSONS WHO ARE AROUND UV SOURCES, INCLUDING:
- Welders
- Those working near UV lamps, such as dentists and dental technicians
- Those in industries that use UV radiation

---

exposure to UV radiation is higher than in years past. Because UV radiation affects everyone over time, the best way to reduce UV-related eye disease is to wear UV-absorbing spectacles and sunglasses early in life. Environmental and job-related factors place certain individuals at an even greater risk. For example, skiers in high mountainous areas are at particularly high risk because there is less atmospheric filtering of UV radiation at higher altitudes, and snow reflects about 85% of the UV light that strikes it. The eyebrows and even hats do not provide the protection that they normally would because of reflected light.

Factors regarding protection from UV light are summarized in Box 22-1. Regardless of special factors that heighten the danger of UV light, studies conclude that "All sex and racial groups would benefit from simple methods to avoid ocular sun exposure.[9]"

Eyewear That Blocks Ultraviolet Radiation

There are a number of lens options available to protect against UV radiation. Some require special ordering, but many lenses come with UV filtering as a basic part of the lens.

1. *Lenses with the UV filter directly in the lens material*—The first lenses that were developed specifically to block UV light had a yellowish cast. As manufacturing methods and chemistry improved, the yellow disappeared.

2. *Lenses with the UV filter in the coating*—Now many lenses come with a protective coating that have a secondary UV-blocking effect. These include all polycarbonates and many high-index plastic lenses.

3. *Lenses with a dyed-in UV filter*—Plastic lenses can be made UV inhibiting by immersion in a hot UV dye in the same manner as is used to tint a lens.

4. *Polarizing lenses*—Good quality polarizing lenses block UV radiation, though the polarization process has nothing to do with blocking UV light.

5. *Photochromic lenses also have UV-blocking properties.* In their darkened state, photochromic lenses are considered sufficiently protective against UV light.

6. *Lenses that go beyond UV protection*—There are lenses designed to go beyond simple UV protection. They also block out short wavelength (primarily blue) visible light. These are generally referred to as "glare control lenses" and are described later in this chapter.

Checking for Ultraviolet Absorption

Lens transmissions are often checked using a photometer. Though photometers are helpful (Figure 22-3, *A*), at the time of this writing, they should not be totally relied upon for absolute UV measurements. As Torgersen[3] points out, photometers typically:

- Are not able to accurately determine absolute UV transmittance.
- Disproportionately weight the waveband of 360 to 400 nm.
- Do not cut off at the UVA limit of 380 nm, but measure on up through 400 nm.
- Are affected by the power of the lens.

It is therefore advisable for the practitioner to be very familiar with the absorptive properties of individual lens materials.

It should be remembered that the dyes used to make a regular plastic lens into a UV-blocking lens are only good for a finite number of applications before they must be replaced. Even when ordered, it is feasible that UV protection may be inadvertently overlooked in the laboratory. Photometers are still helpful to determine if dyes have been applied. Transmission may also be measured using a Humphrey automated lensmeter (Figure 22-3, *B*). If no UV meter is available, there is a crude test that can be performed to see if the lens is blocking UV light:

Place the lens in question on top of an unedged photochromic lens, such as a Transitions lens. (A plastic photochromic lens is more UV dependent than a glass photochromic lens.) Expose the two lenses to sunlight.

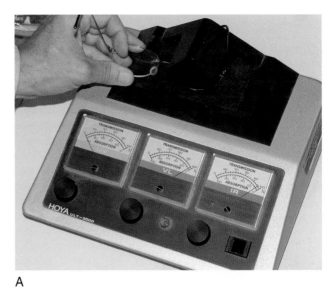

A

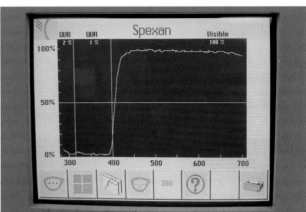

B

Figure 22-3. A, Lenses ordered with ultraviolet (UV) absorption should be checked using a UV meter. This light transmission meter measures UV, visible (VL), and infrared (IR) light. The lenses being measured are blocking all UV light and are transmitting most of the visible and infrared radiation. **B,** It is possible to check the transmission of a lens using a Humphrey Model LA360 Lens Analyzer. This autolensmeter allows both an on-screen display and a printout.

If the photochromic lens darkens under the lens that is supposed to be filtering UV light, the lens being tested is not filtering UV light adequately.

Selecting a Frame

Here is what to look for when selecting a frame for sunglasses or for serious protection against UV radiation. The frame should have a large lens area. It should be fit close to the face with minimum vertex distance. Wraparound frame styles are better still. Note: When wraparound styles are used for prescription eyewear, the prescription may need to be compensated for lens tilt (see Chapter 18). To get maximal protection, a cap or hat with a large visor or brim will help considerably. (For a summary of UV protection options, see Box 22-2.)

Options for Protecting the Eyes From Solar Ultraviolet (UV) Radiation

HEADGEAR WEAR
- Sun visor
- Cap
- Wide-brimmed hat

PRESCRIPTION LENSES
- Lenses specifically made to be UV blocking
- Polycarbonate lenses
- High-index lenses with a UV-absorbing coating
- UV-dyed plastic lenses
- Photochromic lenses
- Glare control-type lenses
- All quality polarizing lenses

EYEGLASS FRAMES THAT HAVE THE FOLLOWING:
- A short vertex distance
- Face form

SUNGLASSES WEAR
- UV-absorbing sunglasses
- Lenses that cover a large area
- Wraparound sunglasses

Ultraviolet Index

The UV Index is a measure of UV radiation. The U.S. Weather Service and the Environmental Protection Agency, along with the World Health Organization, use a UV index on a scale of 1 to 11+ with intensities from low to very high. The index is categorized as follows:

UVI	Exposure Level
0 1 2	low
3 4 5	moderate
6 7	high
8 9 10	very high
11 and greater	extreme

Any UV index will vary from day to day and place to place. The intent of a UV index is to make the general public aware of UV radiation levels and encourage eye and skin protection.

The Effects of Infrared Radiation

At the present time, there is little conclusive evidence in the literature that would indicate any undesirable effects resulting from the IR component in sunlight in ordinary viewing.

Previously, it was thought that the solar retinitis caused by the intense exposure of looking directly at the sun for a long period of time was a result of the heat-producing IR component alone. Scientists at the Medical College of Virginia, however, found the eye to be 800 times more susceptible to damage from the blue end of the spectrum than from the near IR. It appears that solar retinitis is due to a combination of photochemical damage from short wavelength (UV and blue) radiation and thermal damage from long wavelength IR.[1]

IR radiation, when combined with UV radiation and blue light, can adversely affect the crystalline lens. Over a prolonged period of time, this will cause opacification. This lens opacification is commonly referred to as "glass blower's" or "furnace men's" cataract.

Common sources of IR are direct sunlight; molten substances, such as glass and metal; arc lamps; and IR lamps.

In looking at the transmission curve of a given lens, remember that simply because there is a drop in the transmission of IR in the region nearest the visible spectrum, there may not be this same absorption in the longer wavelength IR region. Many lenses that absorb strongly in the near IR transmit a great deal in the longer wavelengths. Therefore if a lens is to be chosen for IR absorption characteristics, a transmission curve showing the full range of the IR spectrum is needed.

The heat produced by IR radiation will cause the eye to be more easily damaged when exposed to UV radiation.[1] Therefore though not scientifically verified, it would seem that a sun lens that practically eliminates UV radiation while also blocking IR to the same degree that it blocks visible light would be desirable. Examples of commercially available lenses that block IR are NoIR and IREX lenses.

REQUIRED AMOUNTS OF ABSORPTION

Practitioners are continually asked how dark a tinted lens should be for best protection or how light a fashion tint must be to not adversely affect the wearer's vision. The answer is considerably more complex than might be expected since much depends on the activities for which the lens is to be used.

If the only object is the comfort of the wearer, then the decision is often subjective and is fairly accurately determined through the wearer's past experience. Other factors, however, must be considered as well. As far as actual improvement of vision, Miller[6] found that for high levels of illumination, sufficiently dark sunglasses will improve visual discrimination for certain types of targets, but not for others. In other words, for high illumination, a person's ability to see clearly may be helped by dark lenses, and his or her visual comfort most certainly will improve.

How Much Tint Is Enough?

Normal transmission for sun lenses is generally between 15% and 30%. A sun lens that transmits more than 30% may not help the average wearer enough in full sunlight.[10] Sun lenses that transmit less than 15% may present problems because of reflected glare from the back surface. These problems can be eliminated by using a back-surface antireflection (AR) coating.

According to ANSI Z80.3-2001 sunglass standards, general purpose sun lenses used for driving should not be darker than 8%, although for special purposes, such as skiing, mountain climbing, or use on the beach, transmission may go as low as 3%.[11]

At the lower end of the transmission spectrum, it was found that acuity increased with a 10% neutral density filter.* But for persons more than 40 years of age, vision worsened if the filter was any darker than 10%.[12]

It should be noted that people who are exposed to sunlight for long periods of time on a continual basis will require sun lenses that transmit 15% or less. Hecht, et al[10] found that a single exposure to ordinary bright sunlight for 2 or 3 hours caused dark adaptation to start 10 or more minutes later than usual and then slowed the process itself so that normal night vision was not reached until several hours later than usual.

For example, if a person (such as a lifeguard) is exposed to bright sunlight every day for long periods of time, his or her dark adaptation does not return to what it used to be even after a full night's darkness. If this continues for 10 days of unprotected high exposure to sunlight, it will impair dark adaptation to such an extent that 3 or more days of nonexposure are required for dark adaptation to return to its previous level. This loss of dark adaptation can be prevented by wearing sunglasses that allow only a transmission of between 10% and 15%. For the person exposed to bright sunlight, wearing commercially available cosmetically tinted lenses that transmit 35% to 50% of the light will not prevent impairment of dark adaptation.[12] In fact "it is strongly recommended that sunglasses transmitting 10% or less of visible light be used by all persons who, while working in bright sunlight during the day, will be expected to perform critical night duties soon afterward.[10]" In short anyone who has a job that requires seeing well at night must wear sunglasses if they are exposed to bright sunlight for 2 or more hours a day.

The Hazards of Too Much Tint

As just discussed, there are certain situations where a large amount of *absorption* is quite desirable. By the same token, there are also circumstances in which a maximum of light *transmission* is desirable. When considering darker fashion tints, wearers should be warned of the reduction in visual acuity in dimly lit conditions.

Tinted Lenses and Night Driving

A commonly occurring situation that demonstrates the hazards of too much tint for existing conditions is night driving. At night with eyes adapted to a light intensity of 0.1 mL through a clear glass windshield, the visual acuity of an individual who normally sees 20/20 will be reduced to 20/32. This is not because of looking through

---

> ## BOX 22-3
>
> **Effect of Lens and Windshield Tint on Visual Acuity**
>
> Day vision = 20/20
> Night vision = 20/32
> Night + 82% transmitting pink tint = 20/40
> Night + tinted windshield = 20/46
> Night + tinted windshield + 82% transmitting pink tint = 20/60

Data from Miles PW: Visual effects of pink glasses, green windshields, and glare under night driving conditions, Arch Ophthalmol 52:15-23, 1954.

---

the windshield, but rather is simply a result of reduced illumination. Any tinted material between the observer's eye and the object being viewed will further reduce acuity. Even an 82% transmitting pink tinted lens worn at night reduces acuity to 20/40. A green-tinted windshield by itself reduces acuity to 20/46. The combination of tinted windshield and tinted lens, however, reduces acuity to 20/60 (Box 22-3).[13] The level of tint desirable is therefore a function of the circumstances under which it is to be worn.

It should be obvious that a lens tinted only slightly more than the lightest available shade quickly becomes a potential hazard under circumstances, such as night driving, that may otherwise be considered normal. This was reinforced by a German study[14] that found windshield tinting to reduce night driving hazard detection distances by 10%. Allen[15] also found that a person wearing lenses having a 70% transmission at night ended up being much closer to an object on a highway before being able to see that object than when they were not wearing tinted lenses.

Another factor in the determination of the amount of tint permissible is age. As age increases, performance differences observed while wearing certain optical filters decreases. In other words, a person's ability to work effectively under a situation of reduced illumination decreases as he or she ages.

In spite of evidence to the contrary, some wearers insist that a light tint at night is helpful in reducing the glare of oncoming headlights. This is likely due to the ability of a tint to reduce some internal lens reflections. An antireflection coating is better at reducing internal lens reflections. Rather than using tinted lenses, an AR coating will reduce oncoming headlight annoyance and will increase the wearer's contrast sensitivity by increasing available light.

COLOR CHARACTERISTICS

During the past several years, there has been a phenomenal increase in available frame styles. Previously, certain types of frame styles went in and out of fashion. Now,

---

*A neutral density filter is gray and absorbs light evenly across the visible spectrum.

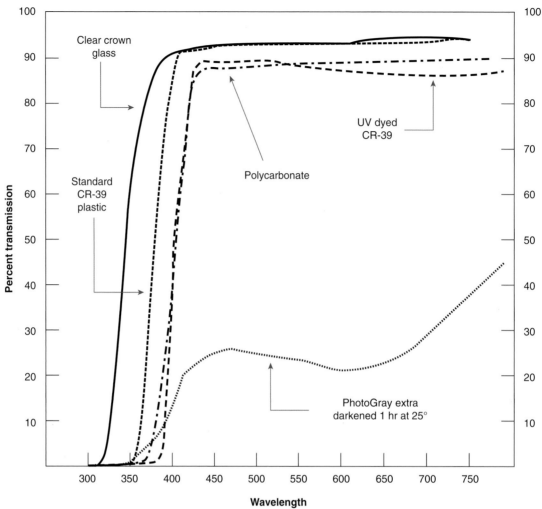

Figure 22-4. Transmission of ultraviolet radiation for standard ophthalmic lens materials. The polycarbonate lens material listed has an antiscratch coating standard for polycarbonate prescription lenses. Polycarbonate lens' UV blocking properties are a result of the coating on the material and not the material itself. (Transmission curves from: Spectral transmission of common ophthalmic lens materials, St Cloud, Minn, 1984, Vision-Ease, pp 1, 16; from Photochromic ophthalmic lenses, technical information, Publication #OPO-232, Corning, NY, 1990, Corning Inc, p 5; and from Pitts DG and Kleinstein RN: Environmental vision, Boston, 1993 Butterworth-Heinemann.)

however, a full range of designs is being used. More recently this effect has also been seen regarding lens tints since there are many different shades and hues of lenses available. Because of this multiplicity of available colors, analysis of each one's merit becomes increasingly difficult. This section presents characteristics of the major lens colors in an attempt to address this problem.

Clear Crown Glass and CR-39 Plastic

Crown glass and CR-39 plastic both transmit approximately 92% of visible light. The 8% not transmitted is lost through reflection. All UV light below 290 nm is absorbed by crown glass (Figures 22-4 and 22-5). Unfortunately, from a practical standpoint, it is the UV from 290 on up to the visible light that can be more disturbing.[6] Most UV light below 290 in the UVC and UV

Vacuum ranges, though the most damaging to the eye, will have already been absorbed by the atmosphere.

Crown glass transmits IR in the same proportion as it does visible rays.

CR-39 plastic used in normal spectacle lens wear contains a UV inhibitor that does not block all UV light, but does block UV light below 350 nm.

Pink

Pink is a tint that has been widely used in the past and continues to be used, but in a limited amount. The lightest shades are referred to synonymously as pink, rose, or sometimes, flesh.* Pink tints have a uniform transmis-

---

*Brand names used when glass lens tints were popular include Soft-lite (B & L) and Cruxite (AO).

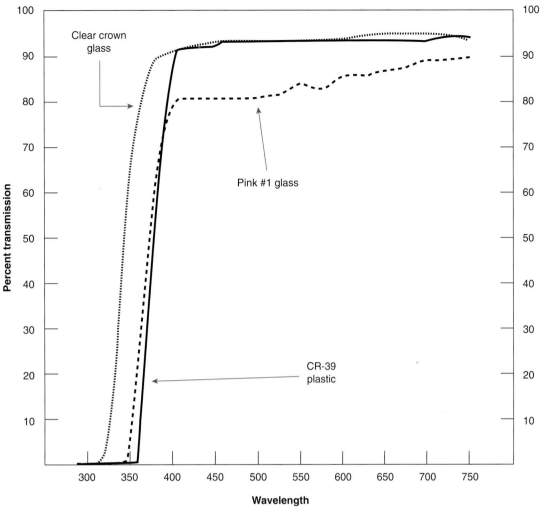

Figure 22-5. Transmission curves for clear crown glass, clear CR-39 plastic, and a #1 crown glass pink tint. Note how closely the transmission curve for the pink matches the curves for the clear. Because the pink has a relatively flat, horizontal curve across the visible spectrum, there should be no disturbance to relative color perception. (From: Spectral transmission of common ophthalmic lens materials, St Cloud, Minn, 1984, Vision-Ease.)

sion across the visible spectrum (see Figure 22-5) and therefore do not cause any color distortion for the wearer.

Pink tints are occasionally used for unfavorable indoor lighting situations, such as bright fluorescent lighting or glare in the work area. The best solution to those problems is a change in lighting, rather than an indoor tint. Glare problems may be due to internal reflections within the lenses. This occurs most often in low minus corrections (see the section in this chapter on antireflection coatings). Light tints do reduce some of the reflections encountered, but not nearly as effectively as an antireflection coating. Many wearing light tints would be better helped with a simple antireflection coating.

It is not advisable to use an indoor tint much darker than 80% because of interference with perception and reaction time when worn at night or under very dim illumination.

Yellow

Yellow-tinted lenses (Figure 22-6) are especially subject to myth and speculation. Can people see better with yellow lenses? After reviewing the literature, Bradley states, "... probably not. Dozens of studies all report the same basic result: visual performance through yellow filters is approximately the same as vision through a spectrally neutral filter with the same absorption and this is generally slightly worse than with no filter at all. A select few studies have shown that vision through yellow filters is slightly better than vision through transmission-matched spectrally neutral filters, but these studies fail to show that vision through a yellow filter is superior to vision without any filter.[16]"

Yet in certain circumstances, if the background color surrounding a specific object, such as the blue sky, can be altered by a filter, then it is possible to increase contrast and make the object being viewed easier to

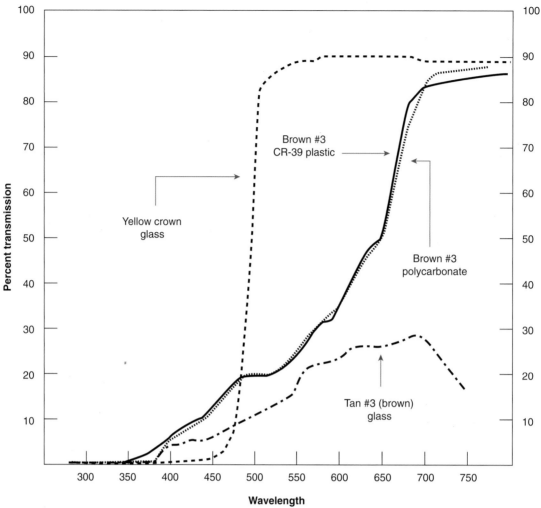

Figure 22-6. Transmission curves for yellow and brown tints. Yellow has a characteristic sudden drop in transmission between 500 and 450 nm. Brown also shows a drop, but that drop is spread over a larger part of the visible spectrum. Note how dyed plastic and polycarbonate lenses transmit the long end of the spectrum, including the infrared. It is possible to use lens dyes that absorb in the infrared region of the spectrum, if desired. (Yellow crown glass and tan #3 [brown] glass transmission curves are redrawn from: Spectral transmission of common ophthalmic lens materials, St Cloud, Minn, 1984, Vision-Ease, pp 9, 10. Brown #3 CR-39 and polycarbonate transmission curves from Pitts DG and Kleinstein RN: Environmental vision, Boston, 1993, Butterworth-Heinemann.)

perceive.[17] "It has been argued that yellow lenses have the advantage that they selectively darken the bright blue sky without reducing the luminance of green, yellow, and red targets on the ground.[16]" For example, yellow lenses are traditionally used in competitive shooting. Many sportsmen believe their shooting ability is improved by a yellow tint. Even so, one of the earliest studies of 136 marksmen done in overcast daylight conditions found that only one individual showed a marked improvement. The author concluded that "the benefit of yellow lenses depends entirely upon the individual; some may be helped while others may be hindered.[18]" More sophisticated variations of shooting lenses, such as Corning's Serengeti Vector lenses, continue to be used for competition shooting.

Yellow lenses have been advocated for driving in haze or fog. Even though any lens, including a yellow lens, that absorbs light in the blue end of the spectrum can be helpful in reducing glare from light scattered by the atmosphere, this does not extend to fog situations. In contrast to atmospheric gases, fog is not as selective in the wavelength of light it scatters.[18]

Yellow lenses have on occasion been suggested for use in night driving. This is not advisable and should not be encouraged. *Any* tint that cuts down on already dim illumination further reduces visual acuity, offsetting any reduction in headlight glare. The best solution for headlight glare at night is an AR-coated prescription that is up to date. Uncorrected refractive error will cause glare at night. This up-to-date lens prescription should be AR

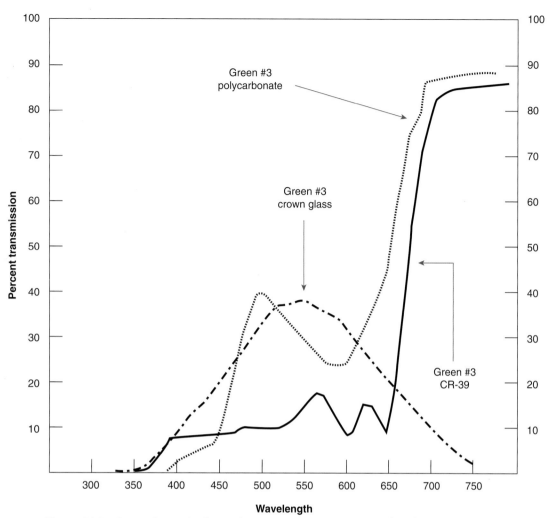

Figure 22-7. Green absorptive lenses have a transmission curve with a characteristic "hill" in the middle of the visible spectrum. Green glass lenses are good ultraviolet and infrared absorbers. Plastic and polycarbonate lenses, however, transmit light in the long visible end and infrared region of the spectrum. This is characteristic for dyed plastic materials in any color unless a specific infrared absorber has been added to the dye. (Transmission curves from Spectral transmission of common ophthalmic lens materials, St Cloud, Minn, 1984, Vision-Ease, and from Pitts DG and Kleinstein RN: Environmental vision, Boston, 1993, Butterworth-Heinemann.)

coated to further reduce glare caused by reflections within the spectacle lens itself.

Two brand names that have been traditionally associated with yellow lenses are Hazemaster (AO) and Kalichrome H (B & L).

Brown

Brown or gray-brown lenses are most often used for sun lenses in Germany and other middle-European countries.[19] Brown lenses have some of the same characteristics as yellow lenses in that there is a higher absorption of shorter visible wavelengths (see Figure 22-6). By reducing the transmission of the blue end of the spectrum, brown lenses, like their yellow counterparts, are also commonly thought to improve contrast on bright,

hazy, or smoggy days. If this is the intent, a specialized lens may be more appropriate.

Green

Green sun lenses have a transmission curve that closely approximates the color sensitivity curve for the human eye. They were first made popular through use in the military, but have now been fairly well replaced by the neutral gray lens. The green-tinted glass lens obtains its color and characteristic transmission curve from ferrous (iron) oxide. There is good absorption for the green glass lens in both the IR and UV regions (Figure 22-7). When a lens is vacuum coated to a green tint, the IR absorption is acceptable, but not quite as good as the tinted glass lens.

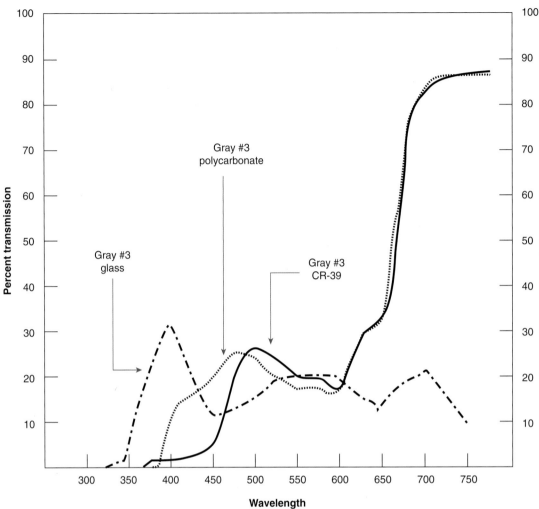

Figure 22-8. In the visible region from approximately 400 to 700 nm, the gray lens gives a fairly even transmission curve, making color perception closer to what would be perceived without absorptive lenses. (Transmission curves from: Spectral transmission of common ophthalmic lens materials, St Cloud, Minn, 1984, Vision-Ease, and from Pitts DG and Kleinstein RN: Environmental vision, Boston, 1993, Butterworth-Heinemann.)

A plastic lens dyed green to approximately the same shade as its glass counterpart exhibits poor absorption in the IR region. This characteristic is not atypical for dyed plastic lenses of other shades as well. Most dyed plastic lenses do not absorb well in the long wavelength, visible, and infrared regions of the spectrum.

Gray

Gray is a tint most popular for sun protection—and with good reason. Perhaps the best aspect of gray is its evenness of transmission through the whole visible spectrum (Figure 22-8). This characteristic allows colors to be seen in their natural state relative to one another. For this reason, neutral gray is quite satisfactory for use by those with color vision deficiencies. Gray lenses will not help a color-defective individual in his or her perception of colors, but neither will it cause further misjudgment of colors as often happens to a color-defective individual when wearing lenses having a transmission that varies

across the visible spectrum. Persons with normal color vision are able to adapt to most color changes caused by colored lenses, but color defectives do not have this adaptive ability. To the color defective, this may increase color-judgment errors or cause some objects to appear with unusual or unnatural colors when other than neutral gray lenses are worn.

Colored Filter Lenses for Color Defectives*

A color-defective individual lacks one of the three different types of retinal cones. So a person lacking in the cones that are sensitive to longer wavelength (red) light cannot differentiate red from green. Likewise a person lacking cones sensitive to the green area of the visible

---

*Much of the information in this section is taken from Bradley A: Special review: colored filters and vision care, Part I, Indian J Optom 6(1):13-17, 2003.

spectrum will have a similar red-green color discrimination problem.

Using a filter that selectively absorbs certain colors but not others will change the intensity of those colors, making it possible for a color defective to use light intensity cues to tell one color from another that may not have been previously distinguishable. These intensity differences are helpful when intensities can be compared with and without the specialized filter.

Factors Favoring the Use of Colored Filter Lenses for Color Defectives

As just stated, colored filters will allow a color-defective individual to use intensity cues to discriminate between two otherwise indistinguishable colors. A red filter will make a green object look dimmer than a red object. Selective filters for this purpose have been attempted with colored contact lenses, such as the red X-chrome lens worn on one eye or the ChromaGen contact lens available in different colors, depending upon defect type.* Filter contact lenses are placed on one eye only so that when closing first one eye, then the other, intensity variations are comparable. Some spectacle lens color filters are placed in only one sector of a spectacle lens so that a comparison of how the object appears can be made by moving the head. The object can be viewed first without, then with the filter.

Certain filters cause other colors to appear more vivid to a color defective because of the manner in which perceived colors shift in appearance when viewed through the filter.

Negative Effects of Using Colored Filter Lenses for Color Defectives

Colored filters worn over both eyes for the purpose of helping certain colors to be better distinguished by color defectives can cause problems. This is because colors that were distinguishable before may now be confused when viewed through the filter.

Even a colored filter, such as the X-Chrom contact lens, worn over one eye is not without a down side. One problem is that objects may appear to glisten.[†] A second problem is that when there is a difference in intensity between the two eyes, moving objects may appear to be wrongly located as to how far away they appear.[‡] Sheedy points out that "The red contact lens may drastically improve performance on pseudoisochromic plates (used to test color vision), but the improvement is spurious and does not properly represent the small improvement in real world performance.[20]"

SUNGLASSES

According to Pitts and Kleinstein,[1] the ideal pair of sunglasses should do the following:
1. Reduce the intensity of sunlight for optimum visual comfort and visual performance.
2. Eliminate parts of the optical spectrum that are not required for vision and are hazardous to the eyes.
3. Provide enough protection while being worn during the day so that the wearer's dark adaptation and night vision are preserved at night.
4. Maintain normal color vision and allow the wearer to distinguish traffic signals quickly and correctly.
5. Resist impact and scratching and only require a minimum of care.

Sunglasses must meet the same impact-resistance requirements as any other spectacle lenses, whether they are for prescription or nonprescription use. The test for impact resistance is the ability to withstand the impact of a $\frac{5}{8}$-inch steel ball dropped from 50 inches.

There are four categories of sunglass lenses listed in the ANSI Z80.3-2001 sunglass and fashion eyewear standard. These are listed in Table 22-1.

The standard does not give specific examples of applications for the categories, but following are some basic descriptions:
- *A cosmetic lens*—Generally speaking this lens is more for fashion than function.
- *A general purpose lens*—This is the category used for sunglasses normally used by most individuals.
- *A very dark special purpose lens*—This lens is appropriate for situations of very intense light, such as for mountain climbing.
- *A strongly colored special purpose lens*—This type of lens might filter certain spectral colors more heavily than others.

Food and Drug Administration (FDA) guidelines for nonprescription sunglass lenses include requirements concerning color. These are based upon the American National Standards requirements for sunglass and fashion eyewear.* Color requirements are put in place because of traffic signal recognition needs. Since sunglasses are sold over-the-counter to anyone, they must be made safe for anyone. (European and Australian standards allow some of these tints to be sold that would not be permitted in the United States, but require warning labels, such as "Not suitable for driving" and "Not suitable for persons with defective color vision.[21]") Color defective individuals[†] can have their perception of color significantly altered by certain tints in a lens. Color

---

*ChromaGen filters also come in the form of spectacle lenses.
[†]This is called binocular luster.
[‡]This is called the Pulfrich phenomenon.

---

*FDA optical transmission requirements are based on ANSI Z80.3 Ophthalmic-Nonprescription Sunglasses and Fashion Eyewear Requirements.
[†]A red-green color-defective individual (a protanomalous or deuteranomalous person) may have some varying ability to discriminate red from green. A red-green "color blind" individual (a protanope or deuteranope) cannot tell red from green.

TABLE **22-1**
Nonprescription Sunglass and Fashion Eyewear

| | | Mean UV Transmittance | | | |
| | | UVB (290-315 nm) | | UVA (315-380 nm) | |
Primary Function and Shade	Light Transmittance	Normal Use	High and Prolonged Exposure Use	Normal Use	High and Prolonged Exposure Use
A cosmetic lens or shield (light)	Transmission of greater than 40%	0.125 Tv max	1% max	Tv max	0.5 Tv max
A general purpose lens or shield (medium to dark)	Transmission of between 8% and 40%	0.125 Tv max	1% max	Tv max	0.5 Tv max
A special purpose lens or shield (very dark)	Transmission between 3% and 8%	1% max	1% max	0.5 Tv max	0.5 Tv max
A special purpose lens or shield (strongly colored)	3% minimum transmission	1% max	1% max	0.5 Tv max	0.5 Tv max

"Mean UV Transmittance" refers to the average transmittance for all wavelengths in the stated range (either UVA or UVB).
"Tv" refers to visible transmittance. So the allowable UVB transmittance for a general purpose lens intended for normal use would be 0.125 of the maximum visible transmittance of the lens. So if a lens transmits 40% of the light, the maximum UVB transmittance would be 0.125 × 40 or 5%. However, if the lens has a visible transmittance of 10%, the maximum allowable UVB transmittance would be 0.125 × 10 or 1.25%.
Data from: ANSI Z80.3-2001: American national standard for ophthalmics—nonprescription sunglasses and fashion eyewear—requirements, Merrifield, Va., 2002, Optical Laboratories Association p 18.

normal individuals would not have their ability to discriminate traffic signal colors affected by the same tints that would confuse a color-defective individual. The FDA's document, *Guidance Document for Nonprescription Sunglasses* states[22]:

"Traffic Signal Recognition provisions contained in ANSI Z80.3 were developed with the color defective person in mind. Approximately 8% of the male population and less than 3% of the female population have some type of color deficiency. Therefore, some of the requirements of this section of the standard may be overly stringent for color normal individuals."

This may be one reason why over-the-counter sunglass standards do not apply to prescription sunglass lenses. However, this places a larger burden of responsibility upon the prescriber and dispenser for dispensing prescription sunglass lenses.

For example, Bradley[23] shows that both yellow and brown lenses fail to meet the ANSI Z80.3 (and FDA) standards for nonprescription sunglass lenses. Yet these tints are readily available in prescription eyewear, and brown is a commonly used prescription sunglass lens tint. So whereas such a tint may not make traffic signal colors unrecognizable for a color-normal individual, a color defective would not be able to discriminate a red from green traffic light signal adequately.

What does this mean? This means that the dispenser should not knowingly dispense sunglass or fashion lenses

to a color-defective individual that would not conform to FDA standards for nonprescription sunglass and fashion eyewear.

DYEING PLASTIC LENSES

Plastic lenses offer great versatility in tinting since they may be dyed to almost any color and may also be made as light or dark as desired. The clear plastic lens is simply dipped in a dye solution of the desired color. The longer the lens is left in the dye, the darker the tint. As the dye is absorbed over the surface area of the lens, good-quality, well-cured plastic lenses result in a tint of a uniform density independent of lens power and variation in lens thickness. The tint is not lighter in the thinner portions nor darker in the thicker, as when tinted glass is used. However, a plastic lens that has not been properly cured when cast molded during manufacture may produce a certain amount of splotchy unevenness of color when they are dyed.

Gradient Lenses

Gradient lenses have a dark upper portion that gradually lightens toward the lower lens sections. Gradients are nicely produced in plastic (Figure 22-9). A gradient tint is accomplished by immersing the whole lens upside down in the dye. The lens is repeatedly immersed and removed from the solution, each time to a slightly different level on the lens. The bottom of the lens is in the

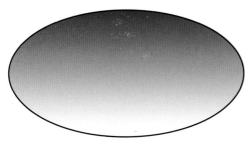

Figure 22-9. A gradient lens varies in transmission over the surface of the lens.

tinting solution only occasionally, whereas the upper section remains longer, absorbing more of the color. A poor-quality gradient lens results when the lens is not dipped evenly and continuously. Poor-quality gradients show a fairly sharp demarcation line between upper and lower sections, whereas the better-quality lenses demonstrate no specific cutoff. Both lenses of a given pair must also lighten evenly from top to bottom to prevent differences in transmission between the two eyes at any one level on the lenses.

Changing and Matching Colors

Plastic lenses that have been tinted may be bleached out again and retinted if a tint has proven unsatisfactory as long as they have not been subsequently antireflection coated. Clear lenses may be tinted at any time. For example, when a person decides to change to a new frame, even though the prescription remains unchanged, the old pair may be tinted for fashion or sun wear.

When only one tinted lens is to be replaced, it is not always easy to match the previous tint of the other lens. One method used to create a match between two lenses is to bleach out the old lens and redye it with the new one. Even then an exact match can be difficult because the lens materials from the two lenses may not take dyes in the same manner.

Dyeing Polycarbonate and High-Index Lenses

Polycarbonate lenses must be antiscratch coated to be usable for ophthalmic purposes. With polycarbonate lenses, dyeing of the lens occurs within the antiscratch coating. Antiscratch coatings are not uniformly permeable to dyes. Dyeing some of the harder coatings dark enough to reach a sunglass tint may not be possible. A few polycarbonate suppliers have a selection of pretinted polycarbonate lenses. These lenses have the tint within the polycarbonate material itself. The lens can then be further darkened by additional tinting.

High-index plastic lenses dye more slowly than CR-39 lenses and may require special processing. Especially dark tints may not be easy to achieve, depending on the type of material used. It should also be noted that the resulting color of the tint may not be the same for high-index plastics as for a CR-39 sample lens. (Some high-index plastics cannot be dyed at all.)

LENS COATINGS

The practice of coating ophthalmic lenses varies widely from country to country. It is not at all uncommon for dispensers who edge their own lenses to maintain a stock of coated-lens blanks. In the United States, keeping a stock of plastic, AR-coated lenses is becoming more commonplace. In countries where hardening of glass lenses is not required, dispensers commonly stock AR-coated glass lenses.

Coatings represent an area that can greatly increase wearer satisfaction. Those who educate themselves in the area and can apply that information will find the benefits rewarding. Here are a few interesting possibilities.

Scratch-Resistant Coatings (SRCs)

Because of the tendency of plastic lenses to scratch more easily than glass lenses, manufacturers have developed processes of coating the plastic lens to develop more surface hardness and thus more resistance to scratching. SRC lenses are not specifically designed to reduce lens reflections. SRC plastic lenses, however, do exhibit some reduction of lens reflections. This means that they will have a higher light transmission compared with a non-SRC lens. An uncoated CR-39 plastic lens transmits about 92% of the incident light. By antiscratch coating the lens, transmission may increase to just short of 96%.

Scratch-resistant coatings are also called antiscratch coatings or hard coatings.

How Scratch-Resistant Coatings Are Applied

Antiscratch coatings may be applied during manufacture or in the optical laboratory. The quality of available coatings varies. If the lens is to be antireflection coated, the quality of the hard coating is essential to the success of the antireflection coating.[24] Here are the two main ways that hard coatings are applied:

1. Thermally Cured Hard Coatings.* With this hard coating process, lenses are dipped in a "varnish" and removed from the varnish at a consistent rate to control thickness of the coating. The lenses are then thermally cured or "baked" over an extended period of time.[25] This method is commonly used by lens manufacturers.

2. UV-Cured Hard Coatings. Scratch-resistant coatings can be applied using a system that spins the coating on the lens. It then uses UV light to cure the coating.

---

*There is a similar, but certainly not equal, method that has been used at the retail level. It is not very satisfactory. In this process, the lens is mounted on a tool that spins the lens. A liquid material is dripped onto the lens, and the lens is either allowed to dry by itself, or is transferred to a small oven for curing. In some cases the finished product introduces problems with the stability of the coating that can outweigh the slight increase in scratch resistance that the process affords. Because most plastic lenses now come with a manufacturer-applied hard coating, this process is falling into disuse.

The coating unit is normally enclosed in a positive pressure area to ensure a dust-free environment. The type of liquid coating material used will vary, depending upon lens material and whether or not the lens is to be tinted later. (There is a trade-off between coating hardness and tintability.) UV curing is done in seconds. This makes it considerably faster than the hours-long thermal curing process. At the time of this writing, UV curing is the method of choice for surfacing laboratories. A coating unit is essential for surfacing laboratories that process polycarbonate lenses.

Front Side Only or Both Sides?

Antiscratch coatings may be applied to only the front side of a lens or to both sides. SRC lenses that come factory finished (i.e., stock lenses) will usually be coated on both front and back surfaces. If a lens is semifinished and must be surfaced on the back side to obtain the needed power, however, it will be antiscratch-coated only on the front unless the laboratory applies a back-surface coating.

Since the front surface is most susceptible to scratching, one-side-only antiscratch coatings may be justifiable. If the wearer (and dispenser) is expecting front and back antiscratch protection on regular plastic lenses, however, it may be necessary to ask for it.

Care of Scratch-Resistant-Coated Lenses

Lenses with antiscratch coatings should not be exposed to excessive heat; approximately 200° F is a safe upper temperature limit. (Obviously the better quality coatings will do better under stressed conditions.) Therefore a certain amount of care should be taken when heating the frame for the insertion of lenses. It is not advisable to immerse coated plastic lenses in a hot salt bath. An air blower is the safer alternative to help prevent possible surface crazing. (In fact there are so many situations where a hot salt or hot beads frame warmer can damage lenses that dispensers should use hot air for frame warming exclusively.)

Damage to the coating of a lens may not appear immediately. At the time, the effect of mistreatment by exposure to intense heat in the dispensary may not make the lens appear any different. With use and exposure to sunlight, heat, and agents in the environment, however, the weakening initiated in the dispensary may cause the coating to fail at a later date. Most coating failure is reported by the wearer as an inability to clean the lens sufficiently. The wearer will report a film on the lens that no amount of cleaning will remove. On examination the surface of the lens is lightly crazed and may have an oily or lightly frosted appearance. As would be expected, cheaply applied coatings are most subject to failure.

Cleaning Lenses With Scratch-Resistant Coatings

Cleaning instructions for SRC lenses are basically the same as for regular CR-39 lenses. Namely, rinse the front and back surfaces with water to remove small particles. Dry the lenses with a soft, clean cloth or a tissue, such as Kleenex. Do not wipe the lenses when they are dry. If lenses are to be cleaned dry, the best solution is to use the same type of cleaning cloth as is used for antireflection-coated lenses.

Note: There is disagreement over whether or not to use tissues on plastic lenses. If the lens surface is dirty and dry, using a dry tissue may cause circular microscratches on a lens surface. If the lens surface has been washed or rinsed clean, drying the lens with a tissue will cause no harm.

Antifogging and antistatic agents are compatible with scratch-resistant coatings. As always it is best to keep the spectacles in a soft, lined case when not being worn.

Identifying Scratch-Resistant-Coated Lenses

It may be possible to identify an SRC lens by seeing if water beads on the surface as it does on a waxed car. Another test is to mark the surface with a water-soluble marking pen. An antiscratch coating can cause the mark to look streaky or blotchy.[26] These tests may detect most, but not all, antiscratch coatings successfully. It is almost unnecessary to check for the presence of a scratch-resistant coating since it may generally be presumed that most plastic lenses now come with such a coating.

Color Coatings

An absorptive coating may be added to a lens through the use of a metallic oxide applied to the lens in a vacuum. There are several advantages to these coatings.

Color coatings may be removed and the lens recoated to a new color or different transmission. This helps if the coating wears or if the existing color or darkness no longer meets the wearer's changing needs.

A characteristic of the color-coated lens that should not be overlooked is the smoothness of its transmission curve. Transmission curves for color-coated lenses are generally more even across the visible spectrum than either internally tinted glass or dyed plastic. In addition, coatings continue to absorb the longer wavelengths in the near-IR region of the spectrum in roughly the same proportion as they do in the visible spectrum.

In the past, it has been said that color-coated lenses should not be wiped when dry, but rather washed or cleaned with a damp cloth and dried with a soft cloth. Fortunately, color coatings are becoming more durable because the same advancing technology used for antireflection coatings are now beginning to be used for color coatings.

Color Coating of Glass Lenses

Color coatings are definitely advantageous for glass lenses since the coating is uniform in density, regardless of the lens prescription. Color-coated lenses have a predictable transmission, whereas lenses where the color is added to the molten glass exhibit a darker tint as the glass thickens. As a result, a C tint could be considerably darker in a higher plus lens than in a plano sample. Color-coated glass lenses do not have this problem.

Because coated lenses are made from clear lenses, coated lenses are available in a wide range of colors and transmissions. This is especially advantageous for glass multifocals since multifocals that have the color directly within the glass are only available in limited tints and transmissions.

Color Coating of Plastic Lenses

Because plastic lenses are normally dyed to achieve their tint, color coatings are not usually associated with plastic lenses. However, CR-39 plastic, high-index plastic, and polycarbonate lenses can also be color coated. Since dying high-index and polycarbonate lenses may have occasional limitations, color coatings offer a versatile alternative.

Antireflection Coatings

An AR coating is a thin, clear layer or layers applied to the surface of a lens. Its purpose is to: (1) reduce unwanted reflections from the lens surface and (2) increase the amount of light that actually passes through the lens to the eye.

Lens Reflections Vary According to Index of Refraction

When light strikes the front or back surface of a lens, a certain percentage of the light is reflected back from the surface. This light is seen by an observer and could be described as a "window effect," such as light seen reflecting from the surface of a window (Figure 22-10). The amount of light that is reflected is predictable and depends upon the index of refraction of the lens. (See the Absorptive Lens Calculations section at the end of this chapter for more on this subject.) The higher the index of refraction, the more light is reflected. For this reason, those who wear high-index lenses will like their lenses much better with an antireflection coating that removes these annoying reflections. As can be seen in Table 22-2, a low-index CR-39 plastic lens reflects 7.8% of incoming light, but a high-index plastic lens can reflect 14.1% or almost twice as much. This can have an effect not only on how the lenses look, but how they perform at night with only 85.9% of incoming light being transmitted.

Five Troublesome Lens Reflections

There are basically five reflections that present potentially disturbing reflected images to the wearer's eye (Figure 22-11). These reflections are caused by light coming from an image that does not go directly into the eye, but is first reflected from one or more surfaces of the spectacle lens.

Under certain circumstances, a light or object from behind can be seen by the spectacle lens wearer. This situation is shown in Figure 22-11, *A* and *B*. In Figure 22-11, *A*, light is reflected from the back surface of the lens and enters the eye, whereas in Figure 22-11, *B*, light is reflected from the front surface of the lens. For normal spectacle-lens wearers, this is most noticeable at night when illumination is low, and there is a bright source of light from behind. For those wearing sunglasses, reflections from behind may even be visible during the day. This is because the image illustrated in Figure 22-11, *A* will not be attenuated by the dark sunglass lens as are objects viewed through the front of the lens.

The reflected images illustrated in Figure 22-11, *C* through *E* will appear as "ghosts" of objects viewed through the front of the lens. They are much less intense than the object itself, but under certain conditions, are readily noticeable. Ghost images can be most easily seen at night by looking at a source of light, such as a street

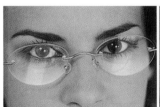 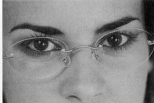

A   B

Figure 22-10. AR coating removes the "window effect" by extinguishing reflections from the lenses, as seen here in photos comparing how rimless lenses look with **(A)** and without **(B)** an AR coating. (From Zeiss ET: Coatings-product facts, publication MI 9054-1198, Carl Zeiss.)

TABLE **22-2**
How Surface Reflections Vary According to Lens Refractive Index

Lens Material	Refractive Index	% Reflection from Front Surface	% Reflection from Back Surface	Total % Reflected from Both Surfaces	Total % of Light Transmitted
CR-39 plastic	1.498	3.98%	3.82%	7.8%	92.2%
Crown glass	1.523	4.30%	4.11%	8.4%	91.6%
Polycarbonate	1.586	5.13%	4.87%	10.0%	90.0%
A high-index plastic lens	1.66	6.16%	5.78%	12.0%	88.0%
A higher-index plastic lens	1.74	7.29%	6.76%	14.1%	85.9%

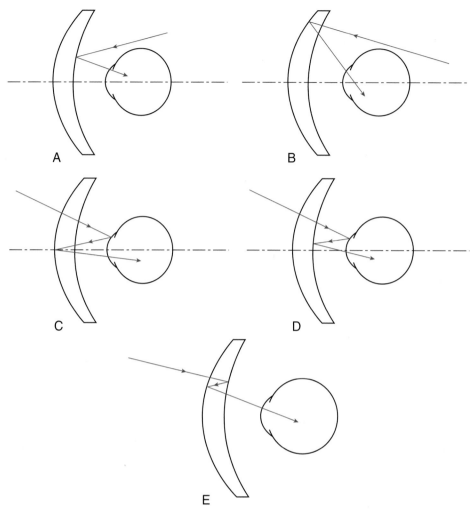

Figure 22-11. Five reflections of spectacle lenses that may prove troublesome to the wearer. It is possible to lessen the effect of reflections **(B)**, **(C)**, and **(E)** with a tinted lens. However, all reflections are virtually eliminated using an antireflection lens coating. A coated lens is the method of choice for reducing lens reflections rather than the use of a light lens tint. (From Rayton WB: The reflected images in spectacle lenses, J Optical Soc Amer 1:148, 1917.)

light. By turning the head while still looking at the street light, it is often possible to see one or more "ghosts" of the light trailing off to one side. These ghost images are caused by the reflections illustrated in Figure 22-11, *C* through *E*.

In addition to reflections seen by the wearer, there are reflections of light sources and other objects seen on the lens surface by an observer. Regardless of source, all reflections are reduced considerably by AR coatings.

Often a person will request a tint for indoor glare conditions when he or she would be best helped by an AR coating. Although a tint may help somewhat, an AR coating is superior. It will be noted that in Figure 22-11 all but one of the troublesome reflections travel through the lens at least once. The reflected images are therefore reduced by a light tint within the lens. But they are not reduced as much as they would be if an AR coating was used.

Uncoated crown glass transmits 92% of the incident light. If even a single-layer AR coating is used, transmission jumps to approximately 98%.[27] If a multilayer antireflection coating is used, transmission is increased to more than 99%.[28] (It should be noted that these figures are for light entering the lens from the straight-ahead position. Light striking the lens at an angle will be reflected slightly more.)

The Theory of Antireflection Coatings
According to optical theory, for a single-layer AR coating to reduce reflections, an AR coating must meet two conditions: the *path condition* and the *amplitude condition*.

The Path Condition. Very simply stated, the path condition determines what the optical thickness of a single-layer coating film must be. To achieve the desired effect, the film must be either one fourth of a wavelength thick or odd multiples of one fourth of a wavelength (i.e., one fourth, three fourths, five fourths, and so forth). As light strikes the single layer–coated lens surface, some of the light will reflect from the coating surface and some from the lens surface (Figure 22-12). This causes the two reflected waves of light to be out of phase with each other, causing destructive interference and preventing reflection (Figure 22-13).

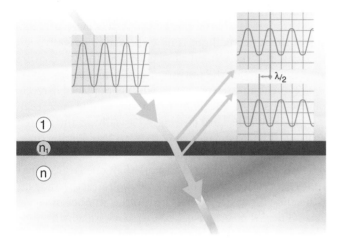

Figure 22-12. When light strikes a surface with a single-layer AR coating having the correct thickness, the reflected light from the two surfaces will be one half wavelength out of phase. (From: Coatings, ophthalmic lens files, Paris, 1997, Essilor International.)

The Amplitude Condition. The amplitude condition requires that the amplitude of the light waves in the lens material and in the film be equal. This is required so that the destructive interference of the two reflected waves will be complete, as shown in Figure 22-13, where the two sine waves combine to form the zeroed-out straight line. The distance from the top to the bottom of the wave must be the same. This can be achieved by controlling the index of refraction of the film. The relationship between the index of refraction of the lens material and the film coating must be:

$$n_{film} = \sqrt{n_{lens}}$$

The index of the film must be equal to the square root of the index of the material being coated. This relationship is derived from reflection factors (ρ) between air and film

$$\rho_1 = \left[\frac{n_F - 1}{n_F + 1} \right]^2$$

and between film and lens.

$$\rho_2 = \left[\frac{n_L - n_F}{n_L + n_F} \right]^2$$

The reflection factors must be equal for the amplitude condition to be fulfilled. In other words,

Constructive Interference

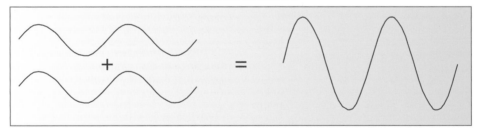

Destructive Interference

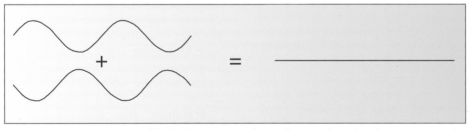

Figure 22-13. Two waves of light that are exactly in phase with each other, as seen at the top left, will constructively interfere with each other. The resulting amplitude of the combined light is enhanced as seen at the top right. Two waves of light which are out of phase, as seen on the lower left, will destructively interfere with each other and when added together are extinguished, as shown by the line on the right.

$$\left[\frac{n_F - 1}{n_F + 1}\right]^2 = \left[\frac{n_L - n_F}{n_L + n_F}\right]^2$$

which reduces to

$$n_F = \sqrt{n_L}$$

Example **22-1**

What would the ideal refractive index be for a single-layer antireflection coating applied to a high-index lens if the lens has an index of refraction of 1.6?

Solution

Since the lens has an index of refraction of 1.6, the ideal index of the single-layer AR coating would be the square root of 1.6.

$$n_F = \sqrt{n_L}$$
$$= \sqrt{1.6}$$
$$= 1.265$$

Therefore the ideal single-layer antireflection coating would have an index of refraction of 1.265.

Why Single-Layer Antireflection Coatings Are Not 100% Effective. If both the amplitude and path conditions are exactly fulfilled for every wavelength, there would be minimal reflections from the lens with close to 100% of light passing through to the eye. This is not the case, however, because of limitations in available coating materials that are both hard enough and of the proper refractive index.

Another reason why single-layer AR coatings are not 100% effective is because the correct coating thickness for yellow light, which falls in the center of the visible spectrum, is not the correct thickness for blue and red light, which fall at either ends of the visible spectrum. This is the reason why, for certain angles of viewing, single-layer AR-coated lenses have a purplish cast. Since yellow light is found at the approximate midpoint of the visible spectrum and is also the color to which the eye is most sensitive, it has been chosen as the optimum wavelength for which the conditions should be fulfilled. For that reason red and blue, which have longer and shorter wavelengths than yellow, do not fulfill these conditions as well.* They are reflected more than the yellow. Red and blue reflections combine to give a bluish-purple cast to a single-layer AR-coated lens.

Initially, AR coatings were only available as single-layer coatings. This posed certain limitations on the effectiveness of the coating. Now that multilayer coatings are the norm, AR-coated lenses are more attractive,

more efficient, more scratch resistant, and considerably easier to clean.

Multilayer-Coated Lenses

From an optical point of view, using more than one layer helps to solve the problem of a single-layer coating that is ideal only for yellow light. Stated in oversimplified terms, if another layer of a different specifically determined refractive index is added, more of the remaining light that would otherwise be reflected is allowed to pass through; if a third layer is added, even more light would pass through. If a lens is coated properly, a large percentage of the reflected light is now allowed to pass through the lens. But the optical aspects of a multilayer coating are only a part of the purpose for multiple layers.

A typical multilayer-coated lens is not placed directly on the lens. The lens is first coated with a primer, then hard coated. This hard coating is basically an antiscratch coating. The next layer is chosen to provide maximal adhesion between the hard coating and the AR coating. The AR coating is applied as more than one layer; sometimes alternating layers of high and low refractive index.[29] Efficiency is not directly related to the number of layers used. The AR coating is then sealed in with a hydrophobic (water-repelling) top coat (Figure 22-14). Many newer coatings are so efficient in repelling smudges that the surface is slippery enough to require the depositing of a temporary "overlayer*" so that the lens will not slip during the edging process.[30]

The Relationship Between Antireflection and Scratch-Resistant Coatings. AR coatings will adhere to a lens *better* if the lens has a high-quality antiscratch coating. Antiscratch coatings are now considered essential for good adherence of the coating and reduction in damage to the coating.

Here is an analogy that describes how an antiscratch coating supports the AR coating: "AR coatings are hard and brittle. By comparison, plastic lenses are soft and spongy. Think of a single paper tissue (representing the AR coating) lying on a soft feather pillow (representing the lens). If you poke your finger at the tissue it easily rips. If you place a single tissue on a hard desk and try poking it with your finger, the tissue remains intact and undamaged. The analogy holds with AR coated lenses. The organic hard coat (over the lens and under the AR coating) supports the thin brittle AR coating much as the hard desk supports the paper tissue.[31]" This explains why AR coatings were successful on glass lenses before they were on plastic lenses. Glass is a very hard substrate and an excellent support for the thin, brittle AR coating layers.

Matching the Antireflection Coating to the Substrate. The best way to be sure that an AR Coating will perform well is to engineer it for the material upon

---

*In addition to wavelength differences for incoming light, lens material will have different indices of refraction for each wavelength. (See the Chromatic Aberration section of the chapter titled Special Lens Designs.)

*This overlayer, called the Pad Control System, is used with the Crizal Alizé AR coating.

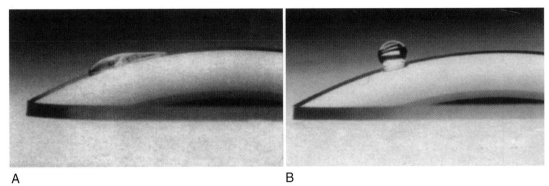

Figure 22-14. The lens on the left does not have a water-repelling top coat, and the water droplet spreads out on the lens. The lens on the right does. The hydrophobic coating causes water to bead up and slide off more easily, keeping the lens cleaner. (From Bruneni J: AR and other thin film coatings, Eyecare Business p 50, 2000.)

which it will be placed. A number of manufacturers are doing just that. The basic lens material is chosen, such as ordinary CR-39. Then a primer and hard coating selected that will work well with both the lens and the AR coating. The lens is sold with the coating already on it.

However, for other than single vision lenses, this may not be able to be controlled as well. There are a large number of variables. This is especially true in the U.S. market where there are a diversity of wholesale optical laboratories supplying different brands of lenses made from a variety of lens materials. A semifinished lens may come with one type of antiscratch coating already on the front surface. The optical laboratory applies another type of antiscratch coating to the back of the lens after surfacing. Now the coating laboratory must apply an AR coating to both surfaces, have it stick to both surfaces and perform well. Best results are possible if these variables are known. The AR Council recommends that if the lenses are being edged "in house" and sent out for coating, that the coating laboratory be informed of the type of lens material, the lens brand, and the type of hard coating being used.[32]

To overcome the diversity of lens materials and hard coatings, manufacturers have addressed the problem by developing a special scratch coating that "can be applied to any nonglass lens, whether the lens is already scratch coated or not.[33]" This provides a known, uniform base upon which an AR coating can be applied so that inequities from chemical and physical differences in factory-applied and lab-applied coatings can be eliminated. Another approach is to totally strip the existing lens of the existing scratch coating and begin again on the base lens material. Others do not apply their coating to any lens that they have not manufactured themselves.

Impact Resistance and Antireflection Coating. When a plastic lens is coated, the impact resistance normally decreases. (For more on this topic, see Chapter 23.) However, by engineering the coating specially for the material, some high-index plastic lenses are able to be made with 1.0-mm center thicknesses and still pass the FDA drop ball test because the lenses have a special "cushioned" scratch coating that absorbs shock.[33]

Reflex Colors

Multilayer AR coatings do not have the old purplish cast so characteristic of single-layer lens coatings. Instead most have a blue, green, or blue-green appearance. The reflex color itself is not an indication of the quality of the coating. However, if the lens has a reflex color that changes from one section of the lens to another, that is an indication of an unevenly applied coating. Reflected color "can be tuned by adjusting the layer thickness in the multilayer AR stack.[34]"

It is possible to cause a coating to have any one of a range of different reflex colors and still be an efficient coating. It is also possible to produce a coating with practically no color, resulting in a faint gray reflex,[35] which is not very pleasing visually and does not "announce" that the lens is an AR lens. In short the manufacturer's goal is to produce a lens with a faint reflex having an aesthetically pleasing color.

Antireflection Coating of Pretinted Lenses

Pretinted lenses, be they glass or plastic, may also be AR coated. This is quite advantageous in several situations. It should be remembered that once a dyed lens has been AR coated, it cannot be either bleached to a lighter color, or redyed to a darker color unless the AR coating is stripped from the lens.

Antireflection Coatings Make Lightly Tinted Lenses More Acceptable at Night. If a person desires a light tint in his or her lenses yet it is believed that night vision might be hindered, AR coating the lens can return the lens to its previous nontinted transmission. For example, a light tint may reduce lens transmission for a CR-39 lens from the normal uncoated 92% transmission to 88%. By eliminating front and back surface reflections, AR coating the lens will bring the transmission up to about 95% transmission—better than the transmission in the uncoated state. For night driving, any reduction in illumination will result in a loss of acuity.

If a Specific Tint Transmission Is Required. If a dyed plastic lens is to be AR coated, it must first be dyed 10% to 15% darker than the transmission desired, then bleached back to the intended tint. This ensures that lens color is buried deeper in the lens. Because of the intense cleaning process used in AR coating, some of the tint near the surface of the lens will be removed. Tinting the lens darker and then removing some of the tint near the surface with neutralizer ahead of time prevents the 5% to 7% lightening that will otherwise occur during the cleaning process.

Unfortunately, at present writing, the application of an AR coating may occasionally change the existing color of tints. The color may lighten, shift in hue, or become unmatched in the application process. These effects are unpredictable as to exactly how and when they will occur.[36]

Antireflection Coating of Sunglasses. AR coating of sun lenses reduces mirrorlike reflections from the back surface. Sun lenses may be AR coated to advantage. For example, the wearer may find reflections from the back surface of the sun lens disturbing. This is a genuine complaint because of the brightness of purely reflected light coming from behind, contrasted to the darkened image of the object being viewed through the sun lens. (See Figure 22-11, *A*, showing this reflection.) An AR coating allows the majority of light coming from behind the wearer to pass on through the lens without being reflected back into the eye.

Opinion on whether to AR coat the front of the lens is mixed. Some say that an AR coating on the front surface of the lens is not recommended because, when combined with the color of the sun lens, the AR coating leaves an objectionable residual color.[37] However, when residual color can be controlled, then the recommendation is to coat both surfaces because "light is also reflected at a lower intensity at the back side of the front surface . . . [and] . . . will give sunglass customers peak performance and the greatest comfort.[38]"

Antireflection Coating of Photochromics. A photochromic lens may be AR coated. AR coating of photochromics will increase both the maximum *and* the minimum transmission by a certain amount. The lens will transmit more light in both the lightened and the darkened state. *Color* coatings, however, should be applied only to the *rear surface* of a photochromic lens since the added tint cuts out many of the rays that activate the lens-darkening mechanism. The lens will not darken properly when color coated on the front.

A Side Comment on Tinted Contact Lenses

It has long been observed by contact lens fitters that the tint in a contact lens does not seem to have the same effect on light reduction for the wearer as does a tinted spectacle lens. The reason for this lies with the reduction of surface reflections when the contact lens is worn.[39]

If a clear contact lens is measured for light transmission in air, it will transmit about 91.2% of the incident light. This is because about 7.8% of the light is reflected from the front and back surfaces, and 1% is absorbed by the contact itself. But if the same contact lens is placed on the eye, the back surface only reflects 0.2% because of the tears, and the front surface only reflects 1.5% more than the front of the eye would without the contact lens. This combined with the 1% absorption of the lens material means that a clear contact lens transmits 97.3% of the incident light. In essence it is as if the contact lens had been AR coated. Therefore a lightly tinted contact lens will transmit more light than a non–AR-coated, clear spectacle lens.

Pros and Cons of Antireflection Coatings

The *pros* of an AR-coated lens are both subjective ones noticed by the wearer and objective ones seen by an observer.

Pros. Subjective advantages noticed by the wearer include better light transmission, decreased glare, and improved night vision. There is also a loss of the starlike flare from self-illuminated objects such as headlights, tail lights, and street lamps (Figure 22-15), resulting in better visual performance at night.[40] For progressive addition lens wearers, the distracting "tails" that appear on illuminated digital dashboard accessories are also reduced.

Objective advantages include the loss of surface lens reflections (the *window effect*). Without lens reflections, the wearer's eyes become more visible (see Figure 22-10). Because edge reflections are reduced and the lens appears less visible, AR coatings make thick lenses appear thinner.

What used to be the biggest "con" for AR-coated lenses can now be a "pro." That has to do with cleaning of the lenses. Because the single or multilayer AR coating only works if it is the first thing that light strikes when entering the lens, any dirt, water, or skin oils will reduce the effectiveness of the coating. What this means is that a very small smudge on an AR-coated lens will be much more visible to the wearer. This is because the smudge will not only be visible in and of itself, but because the AR coating will not work there, reducing light transmission through the smudge by approximately 4%. Recognizing this AR developers have worked hard to make their lenses much more cleanable. They have accomplished this with the addition of a hydrophobic top coat that repels water and oils (see Figure 22-14). In fact these top coatings are so good at repelling liquids that they are not able to be marked with a normal marking pen. Instead they must be marked with either a china marker or a Staedtler permanent overhead transparency marker. "Permanent" marks are later removed using alcohol. Because of these hydrophobic properties, the newer types of AR coatings make the lenses much easier to clean than uncoated lenses.

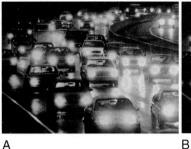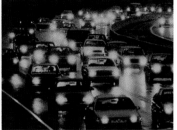

A   B

Figure 22-15. Night driving is where many experience a notable difference between uncoated **(A)** and AR-coated **(B)** lenses. (From Zeiss ET: Coatings-product facts, publication MI 9054-1198, Carl Zeiss.)

A large "pro" for AR coatings are that, given the choice of a good coating or no coating, studies are showing that people are choosing the AR-coated lenses by a wide margin.[40,41]

Cons. Smudges are more visible than with uncoated lenses. AR coatings exaggerate the contrast between clean and dirty areas.

Caring for an Antireflection-Coated Lens

AR coatings are much tougher than they used to be. They are not, however, as tough as the surface of a normal spectacle lens. Certain precautions need to be taken to keep them in good condition. They include the following:
1. Avoid using ultrasonic cleaners.
2. Avoid salt or bead frame warmers.
3. Avoid excessive heat. (This includes the interior of hot automobiles.)
4. Avoid caustic chemicals and sprays, such as acetone, ammonia, chlorine, hair spray, and other aerosols.
5. Avoid marking lenses with heavy inks.

Cleaning the Antireflection-Coated Lens

There are ways to correctly clean lenses and there are cleaning procedures that should be avoided. Lenses should be cleaned at least once a day.

Correct Ways to Clean Antireflection-Coated Lenses. Here is a simple sequence for cleaning AR-coated lenses without using a cleaner specifically made for AR-coated lenses[42]:
1. Rinse the lenses with lukewarm water.
2. Clean using a mild dishwashing liquid or hand soap. Soap should not contain a hand cream. That will cause the lenses to smear. Rub soap on both sides of the lens for about 5 seconds. (It is helpful to wash both lenses and frames at the same time.)
3. Rinse the soap off with tap water.
4. Dry with a soft, clean cloth, such as a cotton towel.

Naturally a cleaner designed specifically for cleaning AR-coated lenses will give excellent results. From time to time it is still worthwhile to use a soap or detergent on both frames and lenses, with lots of running water, to keep the frames clean, too.

There are soft cloths specifically made for use with AR-coated lenses that allow the lens to be cleaned dry. These work very well for throughout the day and are especially handy when there is no soap and water available. These cleaning cloths should be washed periodically with laundry soap and water, but do not use fabric softener.[43]

Things to Avoid When Cleaning Antireflection-Coated Lenses. There are certain treatments and cleaners that should not be used on the AR-coated lens. Antistatic and antifog agents put a layer of coating on the lens. Some regular lens cleaners also leave a coating on the surface. Any layer on top of the coating reduces its effectiveness. The safest policy is to use a cleaner specifically designed for AR-coated lenses.

The newer the type of AR coating, the more it may be treated like an ordinary lens.

As with any lens, AR-coated lenses should not be exposed to household spray cleaners, chemicals, ammonia, chlorine, and hair spray.[43]

Antifog Coating

Antifog coatings are used for individuals who are constantly going into and out of changing temperature environments or who are exposed to other environmental conditions that would fog lenses. Wearers who may appreciate antifog coatings include cooks, ice skaters, and skiers. Antifog coatings can be made as permanent coatings applied directly to the lens during manufacture. To produce the antifogging properties, the lens is coated with a resin film that absorbs moisture. "When the absorption reaches the saturation point, the interfacial activator [within the resin] changes water droplets into a thin outer layer of water.[44]" It is much more common to find permanently applied antifog coatings in sport eyewear, such as swimming goggles. Prescription lenses with an antifog coating are not always available. When available they are limited to single vision lenses.

Fortunately, there are sprays and drops that can be applied to ordinary spectacle lenses to reduce fogging, such as Zero-Fog lens treatment by OMS Opto Chemicals. Although Zero-Fog claims to be compatible with AR coatings, not all antifog sprays or drops are.

Mirror Coating

A mirror coating can be applied by a vacuum process to the front surface of the lens, causing the lens to have the same properties as a two-way mirror. When applied as a full-mirror coating, the observer is unable to see the wearer's eyes and sees his or her own image reflected from the lens. The wearer is able to look through the lens normally. There is, of course, a reduction in the transmission of the lens simply because of the high percentage of light reflected.

Mirror coatings alone do not reduce the amount of light coming through the lens to the level of regular sunglasses. Mirror coatings may be used in combination with a tinted lens to provide more protection from intense sunlight than the mirror coating alone can provide.

Metallized and Dielectric Mirror Coatings[45]

Mirror coating can be applied as a metallized or a dielectric coating.

Metallized coatings apply a thin layer of metal on the front of the lens. They both absorb and reflect light. Each metal used has its own coloration that is transferred to the lens. Some metals allow more color variation by controlling the thickness of the coating. Metallized coating can be applied as:

1. Full-mirror coatings that hide the wearer's eyes.
2. Gradient mirrors that are highly reflective at the top and decrease in reflectance toward the bottom.
3. Double gradient mirrors that have maximum reflectance at top and bottom, with less along the midline. These are often used for snow and water sports.
4. Flash coatings that may have only a hint of reflectance.

Dielectric coatings reflect certain wavelengths selectively. They transmit more light through to the wearer than metallized coatings. Dielectric coating can reflect just one color or be applied in a way that causes the lens to change color when seen from different angles.

Edge Coating

Lenses may be edge coated to reduce the concentric rings visible to the observer. The idea of edge coating is to apply a color to the bevel area of a lens that matches the frame, camouflaging the edge. Many times edge coatings look "funny." This is because they are usually applied with a small brush, then hardened in an oven. If the job is not done well, if an inappropriate frame is chosen, or if the color match is poor, the net effect can be worse than no coating at all.

There are many suitable alternatives to edge coatings. These include the following:

- Polishing the edge of the lens
- Rolling the edge of the lens
- AR coating the lens
- Using a lens of higher refractive index to reduce edge thickness
- Using any combination of the above

THE PHOTOCHROMICS

A major breakthrough in the area of absorptive lenses took place in 1964[46] with the invention of Corning's PhotoGray photochromic lens. A photochromic lens changes in its transmission when exposed to light.

Glass Photochromic Lenses

For glass lenses, the darkening process occurs as a result of silver halide crystals within the glass that are activated by UV and short visible radiation of wavelengths between 300 and 400 nm.

The photochromic process is similar to that which takes place when light strikes photographic film emulsions, also containing silver halide crystals. With the crystals "trapped" in the glass, however, the darkening process is reversible. The glass photochromic lens will not wear out with repeated darkening and lightening cycles, although over time the lenses do not lighten indoors like they do when new. "Within a year indoor light transmission percentage is in the low 70s.[47]"

In the United States the most generally used *glass* photochromic lens is the PhotoGray Extra lens. This lens has a range from 85% to 22% transmission, allowing it to double as a sunglass lens for most purposes. (It should be kept in mind, however, that under fluorescent lighting, a photochromic lens will not always lighten to its lightest transmission. Neither do lenses darken as well when driving.) See Figure 22-16 for examples of glass photochromic faded and darkened transmission curves.

Plastic Photochromic Lenses

Photochromic lenses are now preponderantly plastic. Plastic photochromics are available in a variety of brands and colors. Instead of using an inorganic material, such as the silver halide crystals used for glass lenses, plastic photochromics use organic dyes.

How Plastic Photochromics Are Made

Plastic photochromics can be made in a variety of ways. These include, (but are not limited to)[48]:

- Imbibition
- In Mass
- Multimatrix
- Dip Coating
- Front Surface Coating
- Transbonding

At the time of this writing, the first two methods are the most commonly used.

Imbibition Surface Technology. The primary example of the lens type made using imbibition surface technology is the Transitions photochromic lens. Transitions lenses are made by starting with a clear plastic lens. It can be plastic material very much like CR-39 or other organic lenses. Each lens manufacturer is responsible for making their own lens using compatible lens materials. These lenses are then sent to a facility where their surfaces are infused (imbibed) with photochromic material using a proprietary manufacturing process.

The evenly distributed photochromic material results in an even color density over the entire lens as it darkens.

In-Mass Technology. In-mass technology mixes the photochromic dyes into the liquid lens material before the lens has been formed. This has been the standard technology for the manufacture of glass lenses. The

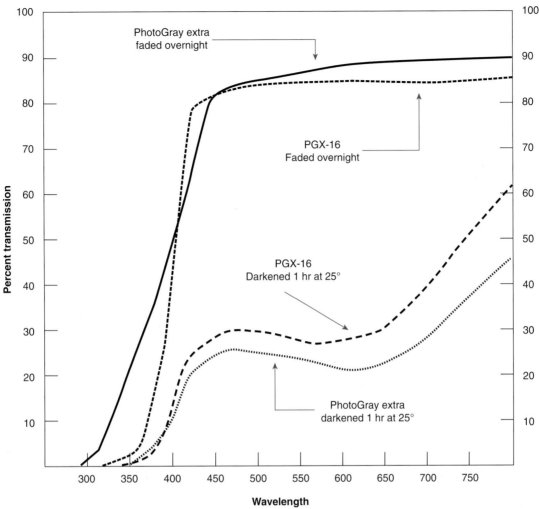

Figure 22-16. PhotoGray Extra, like crown glass, has an index of refraction of 1.523. The PGX-16 is the equivalent of PhotoGray Extra in a 1.6 index glass material. As can be seen, their transmission curves are very similar, with the PGX-16 having a somewhat smaller faded or darkened range compared with the standard PhotoGray Extra material. (From: 1.6 index photochromic lenses, preliminary technical information, Publication #OPO-245, Corning, NY, 1991, Corning Inc. and Photochromic ophthalmic lenses, technical information, Publication #OPO-232, Corning, NY, 1990, Corning Inc.)

disadvantage in glass is that the photochromic material reacts throughout the lens. This causes the thicker edges of a minus lens to darken more than the thinner center does. But with plastic material, primarily only the photochromic material positioned near the surface of the lens reacts. A high-minus glass photochromic lens may give a very slight "bull's-eye" effect. A high-minus plastic photochromic lens does not produce the same effect. In fact proponents of in-mass technology point out that as the organic dyes wear out near the surface and do not darken as fully, the dye slightly deeper in the lens is then activated by the now entering UV rays. The deeper dyes take over the darkening function, thus extending the photochromic life of the lens. Corning SunSensors and Rodenstock ColorMatic lenses are examples of a lens made with this type of manufacturing technology.

Dip Coating, Front-Surface Coating, and Transbonding. Although imbibition and in-mass tech-

nologies are preponderant, photochromic plastic lenses can be made in other manners. A lens may be *dip coated* and then cured with a heat process. Another method is to *coat the front surface of the lens*. A third process called *transbonding* is used with polycarbonate and high-index lenses. This process uses surface treatments in combination with a series of ophthalmic grade layers.[48]

Multimatrix.[49] Kodak Insta-Shades photochromic lenses use a process they refer to as *Multimatrix*. This process begins with a clear lens that has a 1-mm layer bonded to it. The bonded layer contains the photochromic dye.

Advantages and Disadvantages of Photochromic Lenses

Over time plastic photochromics wear out and glass photochromics fail to fully lighten in their faded state. The amount of time that it takes to wear the lens out depends on the cumulative number of hours that the lens is exposed to UV radiation. In other words, the more the lens is worn outdoors, especially during high sunlight conditions, the faster it will wear out. This causes problems when only one lens needs to be replaced. It is not advisable to replace one lens even if the other lens is less than 1 year old because the two lenses will age differently.

Although photochromics are becoming more able to perform like a sun lens in their darkened state, they still are not able to replace sunglass lenses. The primary example of why they do not function as efficiently as a sun lens is the way they are unable to darken well behind the windshield of a car. Although a full-range photochromic lens responds to both UV and visible light, because a person driving a car is shaded from direct sunlight and shielded from much UV radiation by the windshield, the lens will not fully darken in normal driving conditions. Glass windshields have a plastic laminate between front and back glass layers that helps retain fragments of glass during an accident. The plastic layer has UV absorbers to keep the plastic from being degraded by UV light. Those wanting photochromic lenses of any type should be informed that the lens will not darken as deeply when driving. The upside to all of this is that since photochromic lenses use UV light in their activation process they are good UV absorbers and furnish UV protection to the eyes.

Factors Influencing Photochromic Performance

There are several variables that influence photochromic transmission and darkening speed. Some affect only glass photochromics and others both glass and plastic:
1. Light intensity (both glass and plastic)
2. Temperature (both glass and plastic)
3. Previous exposures (exposure memory) (glass)
4. Lens thickness (glass)

It may be noted that the glass lens hardening process can also affect glass photochromic lens performance. The method of choice for hardening of photochromic glass lenses is chemical tempering.*

Light Intensity

Although exposure to UV and visible light is the condition that influences photochromic lens transmission most, several other factors contribute to lightening and darkening. A photochromic lens is made to return to its lighter state by exposure to red light or IR radiation. This is referred to as *optical bleaching*.

Temperature

Heat will also bleach the lens. This is referred to as *thermal bleaching*. As a consequence, photochromic lenses do not darken as much on hot days as they do on cold days.

Taking advantage of this characteristic makes it possible to make photochromic lenses fade faster indoors by running warm tap water over them for 30 seconds. This is likely only necessary in certain rare circumstances (e.g., when the wearer is having photographs taken).

Exposure Memory

Glass photochromics achieve their full changing range and speed only after a "breaking-in" period. This is a consequence of the cumulative effect that takes place; the lenses have *exposure memory*, meaning they respond to light in proportion to accumulated total recent exposures. Put away unused for long periods of time, a glass photochromic lens will lose its exposure memory and have to be broken in again to obtain rapid, complete cycling. For this reason, a well-used glass photochromic lens will darken at a faster rate than an identical, new lens. When only one lens is being replaced in a pair of glasses, this can present a rather curious effect.

Glass photochromic lenses rarely return to their maximum transmission during ordinary wear.[50] Therefore another problem with replacing only one lens is that the older lens will be darker in its lightened state than the new lens.[†]

Lens Thickness

Transmission of glass photochromics is also influenced by *lens thickness*. A PhotoGray Extra lens will darken down to 22% transmission if 2 mm thick, but can get as dark as 11% if 4 mm thick.[51] Even though the transmission varies with thickness, the noticeable variation from edge to center found in high-plus or high-minus tinted glass sun lenses is not present.

---

*Because of federal requirements, glass photochromic lenses must be hardened by some method. There are two primary methods for hardening a glass lens. Fortunately, heat hardening of lenses has practically fallen into disuse. Heat hardening a photochromic lens causes it to lighten slower and reduces its transmission in the indoor lightened state. It also reduces transmission of the lens in the darkened state at higher outside temperatures. The amount of this reduction depends on the color and type of lens, but can be significant enough to be visibly noticeable. This causes the heat-tempered lens to be darker for night activities than the chemical-tempered lens. Chemical tempering is the method of choice for photochromics.

[†]To cause both old and new glass photochromic lenses to have the same shade and behave in a more nearly identical manner, an old glass photochromic lens may be returned closer to its original state in one of two ways.
1. When the new lens is hardened, the old lens may be rehardened as well. The temperature change cycle helps equalize their differences. This proves to be the most effective method and is the one recommended by the manufacturer.
2. If retempering the old lens with the new is not feasible, the old lens may be boiled in water for 2 hours. This boiling process thermally bleaches the lens, returning it closer to the condition of the newer one. The same bleaching effect may also be produced by placing the lens in an oven set for 212° F (again the boiling point of water) for an equal time. A heat lamp may also be used.

Most plastic photochromics are not influenced by thickness.

Photochromic lenses now come in a wide variety of materials including polycarbonate, trivex, and high index. They are also available with polarization.

Photochromic Ultraviolet Absorbing Properties

Photochromic lenses are good absorbers of UV radiation. In their darkened state, glass photochromic lenses generally absorb 100% of UVB radiation and 98% of UVA radiation. The darkened state is the normal situation where UV protection would be needed.

Plastic photochromics have effective UV absorption properties as well.

Coating a Photochromic Lens

In the past, AR coatings used to interfere with the performance of plastic photochromic lenses. With changes in both coatings and lenses, this is not the problem it used to be. AR coatings will not reduce the range of the photochromic cycles. As with any lens, it will increase the transmission in both the lightened and darkened states. In the lightened state, this may be significant. In the darkened state, because of the light absorbed going through the lens, the difference will only amount to a little more than a 1% decrease in darkening—hardly noticeable to the wearer.

Colors for Photochromic Lenses

Photochromic lenses can be made in a variety of colors. Most photochromic lenses begin with one color and change to a darker shade of that same color. It is also possible to make a photochromic lens that starts with one color in the lightened state and darkens to a different color. These lenses have been available in the past and may reappear in the future.

POLARIZING LENSES

Glare from reflecting surfaces is one problem that is only partially alleviated by regular absorptive lenses. Glare is commonly caused by reflections from water, snow, highways, and metallic surfaces. A normal absorptive lens reduces the intensity of light evenly, which also reduces reflected glare. Yet a normal absorptive lens leaves the glare at the same level relative to the surroundings as it was before. Light reflected from a smooth, nondiffusing surface is peculiar in that for the most part it has been *polarized* through the reflection process.

How Polarizing Lenses Work

Ocean waves vibrate up and down as they travel, as is evidenced by the up-and-down motion of a floating cork. A light wave is not so restricted and is free to vibrate up and down, sideways, or obliquely. In other words, in their nonpolarized state, light waves vibrate perpendicular to the direction in which the light is traveling, but

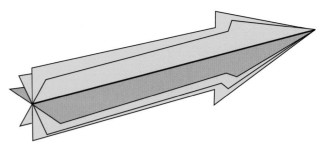

Figure 22-17. Light waves are not restricted to one direction of vibration. Light from a single source can vibrate in the vertical plane, in the horizontal plane, and in any plane in between simultaneously.

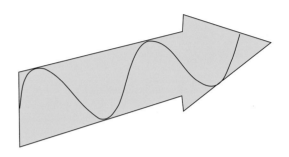

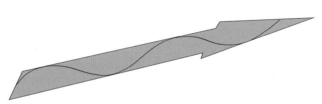

Figure 22-18. Polarized light vibrates in only one plane. The light at the top is vibrating vertically; the light at the bottom, horizontally. Polarized reflected light from water, sand, or snow is horizontally vibrating light.

with no particular degree orientation (Figure 22-17). The process of polarization, however, causes the vibration direction to be restricted. Instead of vibrating in just any direction, polarized light will be vibrating only in one plane (Figure 22-18).

When light strikes a horizontal *reflecting* surface, it becomes partially polarized with the major direction of vibration being in the horizontal plane (Figure 22-19).

If light strikes the surface of a *refracting* material, such as water or glass, most of the light will be refracted as it strikes the surface of the water and go on into the water. The rest of the light will be reflected. There is an angle of incidence of the light striking a surface where not just some, but all of the reflected light will be polarized. This angle is called Brewster's angle (Figures 22-19 and 22-20). See Box 22-4 for more on Brewster's angle.

To reduce the intensity of reflective glare more than that of surrounding objects, a filter that absorbs the horizontally vibrating components of light would be useful. Such a filter is available for ophthalmic use and

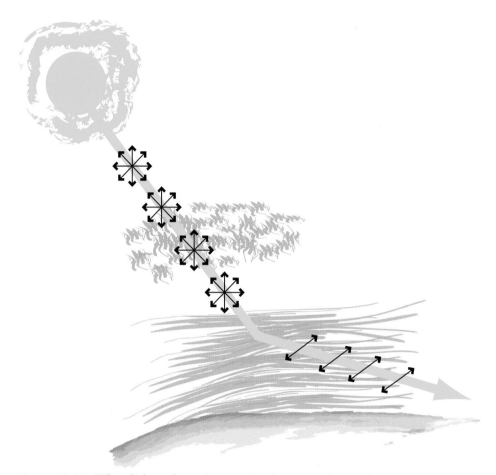

Figure 22-19. When light strikes a horizontal reflecting surface, such as water or sand, it becomes partially polarized with the major direction of vibration being in the horizontal plane.

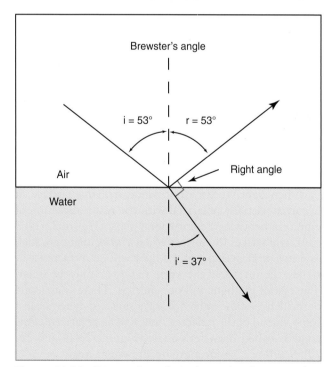

Figure 22-20. Brewster's angle is the angle where complete polarization of reflected light occurs. At Brewster's angle, the reflected and refracted rays are 90 degrees away from one another.

is made from a sheet of polyvinyl acetate (PVA). The PVA is first stretched to five times its normal length in one direction. Then it is dipped in iodine. The iodine is absorbed into the chains of molecules in the PVA. These darkened lines create the polarizing filter. This filter may be "sandwiched" between two layers of cellulose acetate butyrate (CAB) (Figure 22-21).[52] This is how thin, plano polarizing lenses are made. For prescription lenses, the polarizing sheet is mounted between hard resin or polycarbonate material. Alternately, it can be mounted on one layer of CAB material and molded directly into a plastic lens during the lens casting process.

Polarized ophthalmic lenses are oriented so as to extinguish the horizontally vibrating component of light, hence reducing the intensity of light reflected from horizontal surfaces. Although reflected glare is not eliminated, it is much reduced in comparison with other objects in the visual field.

Because the polarizing element in the lens must be oriented to extinguish horizontally vibrating light, the lens blank may not be rotated (Figure 22-22). This necessitates custom grinding the rear surface of the lens so that both the direction of polarization and the cylinder axis are correct. In other words, all nonplano lenses must be individually surfaced, including single vision lenses.

BOX 22-4

Brewster's Angle

When light strikes a refracting surface, most light is refracted into the media, and some is reflected. The reflected light is partially polarized until it reaches a certain angle when it is completely (linearly) polarized. This angle is where the reflected light and the refracted light are at right angles to one another. This angle is called the *angle of polarization* or *Brewster's angle*.

The angle of polarization happens when the reflected light is at right angles to the refracted light (see Figure 22-20). The angle of polarization is measured as the angle of incidence (*i*) of light striking the surface when the right angle's condition for reflection and refraction is met. Figuring out what this angle of incidence will be is done using Snell's law. Snell's law says that the index of the first media (*n*) times the sine of the angle of incidence (*i*) is equal to the index of the second media (*n'*) times the sine of the angle of refraction (*i'*). This is written as:

$$n \sin i = n' \sin i'$$

We know that for Brewster's angle the reflected light and the refracted light are at right angles to one another, which means that:

$$r + i' + 90 = 180$$

where *r* is the angle of reflection and *i'* is the angle of refraction.

This equation reduces down to:

$$i' = 90 - r$$

We also know that for reflected light the angle of incidence and the angle of reflection are always the same. In other words:

$$i = r$$

This means that we can substitute *i* for *r* so that:

$$i' = 90 - r$$

becomes

$$i' = 90 - i$$

Going back to Snell's law and substituting 90 − *i* for *i'*, results in:

$$n \sin i = n' \sin(90 - i)$$

From trigonometry, we know that:

$$\sin(90 - i) = \cos i$$

so that Snell's law can now be written as:

$$n \sin i = n' \cos i$$

then changed algebraically to:

$$\frac{\sin i}{\cos i} = \frac{n'}{n}$$

Using mathematical principles, we know that if:

$$\sin = \frac{\text{opposite}}{\text{hypotenuse}}$$

and

$$\cos = \frac{\text{adjacent}}{\text{hypotenuse}}$$

then

$$\frac{\sin}{\cos} = \frac{\dfrac{\text{opposite}}{\text{hypotenuse}}}{\dfrac{\text{adjacent}}{\text{hypotenuse}}}$$
$$= \frac{\text{opposite}}{\text{adjacent}}$$
$$= \tan$$

So now:

$$\tan i = \frac{n'}{n}$$

If the first media is air, then n = 1 and the equation becomes:

$$\tan i = \frac{n'}{1}$$

$$\tan i = n'$$

In this equation *i* is Brewster's angle.

Usually we already know the refractive index of the media and want to know Brewster's angle (*i*). We can find *i* by using the inverse tan.

$$i = \tan^{-1} n'$$

EXAMPLE
What is the angle at which any reflected light will be completely polarized when light strikes water?

SOLUTION
Using the formula for Brewster's angle allows us to find the angle of complete polarization. Knowing that water has a refractive index of 1.33, we can find the angle of incidence that corresponds to Brewster's angle and produces complete polarization of all reflected light.

$$i = \tan^{-1} n'$$
$$= \tan^{-1} 1.33$$
$$= 53 \text{ degrees}$$

For water Brewster's angle is 53 degrees. This is shown in the figure. Note that the angle of reflection and angle of refraction are at 90 degrees to one another. This always occurs for Brewster's angle.

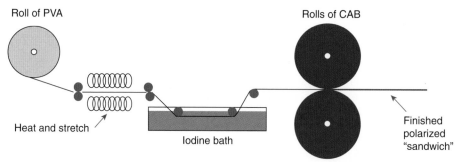

Roll of PVA

Rolls of CAB

Heat and stretch

Iodine bath

Finished polarized "sandwich"

Figure 22-21. A polarized filter is made beginning with a sheet of PVA. This sheet is stretched to five times its normal length in one direction. Then it is dipped in iodine, and the iodine is absorbed into the chains of molecules in the PVA. These darkened lines create the polarizing filter. This filter is then "sandwiched" between two layers of CAB. (From Young J: Polar process, 20/20 p 88, 2002.)

Figure 22-22. This finished, uncut polarizing lens has two notches cut out on the side so that it is clear how the lens should be oriented to maintain the intended polarizing properties.

If an ideal polarizing filter is oriented properly and all incoming light is horizontally polarized, then all of the light would be extinguished. However, if the filter is tilted, then some light will get through. When the filter is 90 degrees away from where it should be, all of the horizontally polarized light will come through the filter. The amount of light that comes through depends upon the orientation of the polarizing filter. This amount is predictable and may be found using Malus' law. (For more on Malus' law, see Box 22-5.) If the polarizing lens is not oriented along the 180-degree meridian, not all horizontally polarized light will be absorbed. And if a person is wearing a polarizing filter and tilts his head to one side, the filter will not absorb as much of the horizontally polarized light. The more the head is tilted, the less horizontally polarized light is absorbed.

When Should Polarizing Lenses Be Used?

Polarizing lenses offer advantages in a number of different situations and can be recommended for the following reasons:

1. *To decrease driving fatigue and increase driving safety*—Because much of the light reflected from large pavement areas is polarized, those who do a lot of daytime driving will benefit from polarizing lenses. There is also polarized light that reflects off the inside of the windshield from the dashboard or from objects on the dashboard. This is an intensely distracting glare that will be almost totally eliminated with polarizing sunglasses.
2. *For fishing and for boating on the water*—Reflected light from the surface of water makes it hard to see below the surface. Wearing polarizing lenses not only removes the discomfort of reflected glare, but makes it easier to see below the surface.
3. *For more visual comfort at the beach*—Sand and water are both sources of polarized glare. Polarizing lenses are especially helpful here.
4. *So that colors are not bleached out*—Reflected polarized light produces a veiling glare. This veiling glare causes colors to appear less vivid. When glare disappears, colors return.
5. *So that bright, snowy days are not as blinding*—Snow is highly reflective. It is also polarizing. Those who are out working or driving in the snow will benefit from using polarizing lenses. (Note: Polarizing lenses may not be as advantageous for skiers as one might think. Skiers' heads tilt far to the left and right when skiers turn and lean. This makes the polarizing filter less effective when the frame front is no longer oriented parallel to the ground and causes changes in brightness.)
6. *To block UV radiation*—Virtually all prescription polarizing lenses, both glass and plastic, are made to block UV radiation. This is not a function of the polarizing filter, but rather foresight on the part of the manufacturers. UV filtering is a big advantage, since the same surfaces that normally reflect light in a polarized manner also reflect a high percentage of UV light.
7. *Polarizing lenses are good sunglasses*—Polarizing lenses should be considered for ordinary sun lens wear.

BOX 22-5

Malus' Law

A polarizing filter has an absorption axis and a transmission axis. If an ideal polarizing filter is oriented with its absorption axis along the 180, it will extinguish all horizontally polarized light. This means that the transmission axis of this same filter will be at 90 and will allow all vertically polarized light to pass through. When the filter is tilted somewhere between these two positions, only a certain percentage of horizontally polarized light comes through the filter.

Malus' law is a predictor of how much polarized light will be transmitted by an obliquely oriented polarizing filter. It is expressed by the equation:

$$I_x = I_0 \cos^2 \theta$$

I_x is the intensity of the light transmitted through the filter, I_0 is the original intensity of the entering light, and θ is the angle of tilt with *reference to the transmission axis*. The equation for the traditional form of Malus' law is based on the transmission axis, not the absorption axis. For polarizing ophthalmic lenses the absorption axis is oriented at 180. The transmission axis is at 90.

EXAMPLE

A polarizing filter used in a lens has its absorption axis oriented along the 180-degree meridian. We will assume that it is an ideal filter and will absorb all horizontally polarized light. The polarizing lens is being worn by a person who tilts his head 30 degrees. What percent of horizontally polarized light will now be allowed to pass through the tilted filter?

SOLUTION

Assuming that we have 100% of incoming horizontally polarized light striking the filter, then the intensity of the irradiating (incoming) horizontally polarized light (I_0) is 1. Remember that Malus' law is based on the transmission axis. When the wearer tilts his head 30 degrees the transmission axis of the lens is 60 degrees away from the horizontally polarized light. Therefore using Malus' law:

$$\begin{aligned} I_x &= I_0 \cos^2 \theta \\ &= 1 \cos^2 60 \\ &= 0.25 \end{aligned}$$

Therefore the intensity of the horizontally polarized light passing through the filter is 25%. So tilting the head while wearing polarizing lenses will allow 25% of polarized reflected light to pass through, making the tilted lens a less effective glare filter.

There are many cases of polarizing glare that occur routinely during outdoor activities. A surprising number of individuals would benefit.

Polarizing lenses are made in most lens styles—not just single vision lenses, but bifocals, trifocals, and progressive addition lenses as well. They are available in glass, photochromic glass, plastic, photochromic plastic, polycarbonate, and high-index plastic. Colors and tints are available, including mirrored and iridescent. Polarizing lenses may also be AR coated.

Precautions With Polarizing Lenses

There are some instances where polarizing lenses create unique situations. Here are a few:

1. Since windshields are tempered, the tempering process induces intentional stress into the material. This stress may be visible through polarizing lenses in much the same way the stress is visible through the crossed polarizing filters of a polariscope (colmascope) used to check for impact resistance of glass lenses (see Chapter 23).

2. Some skiers believe polarizing lenses make snow conditions harder to judge. In addition, as the skier tilts from side to side, the polarizing lens tilts. The percentage of horizontally polarized light reflected from the surface of the snow and absorbed by the polarized lenses will vary, depending upon the angle of tilt. This will cause an ongoing change in the intensity of the reflected light.

3. Golfers also sometimes find polarizing lenses make judging the condition of the course more difficult since the smooth grass surface causes a certain amount of polarization of reflected light.

4. The instrument panels in some cars use LCDs (liquid crystal displays) to display information. An LCD display is polarized. If the LCD is horizontally polarized, polarizing sunglasses will extinguish the display. To see how this works when wearing polarizing lenses, turn the display of an LCD display watch 90 degrees. The time display will disappear. Or when pumping gas while viewing the display on the gas pump, tilt your head sideways and see the numbers fade out.

5. Pilots experience a number of adverse situations when wearing polarizing lenses, some of which can be dangerous.
   a. Polycarbonate windshields in many aircraft have stress patterns. These patterns become visible and may be distracting when wearing polarizing lenses.
   b. Some airplane cockpits, like some car instrument panels, may have polarized numbers or images that can disappear when viewed through polarizing lenses.
   c. Much of the light from an oncoming aircraft that makes it visible is reflected light from the metallic surfaces of the plane. Much of this reflected light is horizontally polarized. When this reflected light is eliminated by horizontally polarizing sunglasses, the oncoming aircraft may not been seen as soon as it would otherwise have been.

Two Methods for Demonstrating Polarizing Lenses

It is helpful to explain how polarizing lenses work to a prospective buyer. But it is much better to show them with a first-hand demonstration. Here are two methods that show how polarizing lenses affect light. (There are also commercially available demonstration units.)

It is possible to take two plano polarizing lenses and, by holding one before the other with their polarizing axes crossed at 90 degrees, eliminate all incoming visible light rays. What one polarizing lens does not extinguish the other will. To demonstrate how polarizing lenses work with this method, hold one lens still, then rotate the other lens back and forth 90 degrees. Watch objects viewed through the lenses dim out completely, then brighten up as the lens is rotated back.

(*Caution*: When crossed sheets of polarizing material or lenses are not quite 90 degrees apart, only a small portion of the light is admitted. Herein lies a potentially dangerous problem. Some wearers may be inclined to use your demonstration system with one polarizing lens and one sheet polarizer, or two pairs of polarizing glasses, for viewing an eclipse of the sun. Unfortunately, Clark[53] reports that plastic sheet polarizers are inefficient polarizers of IR radiation—as are most spectacle lenses. Therefore an inordinate amount of heat-producing IR reaches the retina and, especially when combined with UV or short wavelength blue light could be damaging. Direct viewing of an eclipse, even with highly absorptive lenses, is *never* advisable.)

A second method for demonstrating how polarizing lenses work uses a pair of glasses with polarizing lenses and a glossy magazine.[54] Place the magazine on a flat surface with a light source in the background. With the glossy magazine between you and the light source, the magazine will show a reflecting glare. Move around until the glare is maximal. Now turn the glasses 90 degrees so that the lenses are vertically aligned, instead of horizontally as when worn. View the magazine through one of the lenses. Now slowly rotate the glasses until they are horizontal again. As the glasses are rotated, the glare on the magazine will decrease.

GLARE CONTROL LENSES

Polarizing lenses correct reflective glare. There are other types of glare that polarizing lenses alone cannot eliminate, however. Glare problems are corrected by addressing the type of glare experienced. For our purposes, we will divide glare into two types: (1) discomfort glare and (2) disability glare. These two types of glare are similar in cause, but different in their effect upon vision. *Discomfort glare* is a "glare which produces discomfort, but does not necessarily interfere with visual performance or ability.[55]" *Disability glare* "reduces visual performances and visibility [and] may be accompanied by discomfort.[55]"

Discomfort Glare

Discomfort glare may occur when the eyes try to cope with high and low light intensities in a relatively small viewing area. The eyes have difficulty adjusting to both lighting situations simultaneously. Discomfort glare is best corrected by a change in environmental factors. Individuals working at a computer screen placed in front of a bright window experience discomfort glare from the surrounding area. The problem is corrected by repositioning the computer or shading the window. Discomfort glare is also experienced when viewing a television in a dark room. When an individual must look back and forth between vastly different illuminations, discomfort is experienced. Put another way, stray light that reduces visual comfort but does not interfere with resolution is called discomfort glare.[56]

Disability Glare

Disability glare occurs when stray light interferes with contrast, making it difficult to resolve an image. Stray light washes out the image on the retina in the same manner that strong overhead lighting degrades the image of a slide on a projector screen.

If the stray light causing glare were made up of just polarized light, it could be eliminated using a polarizing filter. If the stray light causing problems were to originate from a light source of only one color, a selectively absorptive lens capable of filtering out only that one color would be able to screen out the offending light, restoring the quality of the image.

Factors That Cause Disability Glare

There are many situations that cause disability glare. For example, dazzlingly bright oncoming headlights can obscure a dark road, making it nearly impossible to see someone in dark clothing walking along the side of the road. In addition, there are factors that can cause or increase disability glare. One such factor is the presence of a cataract. If the crystalline lens begins to cloud and fog up like a dirty windshield, disability glare can increase. Oncoming headlights at night are bad enough when viewing the scene through normal eyes. When those same intense headlights are passing through a cloudy, light-scattering cataract, the effect is considerably magnified.

Another cause of increased glare may be related to the absorption of UV light by the crystalline lens. As the crystalline lens of the eye absorbs UV and short wavelength visible light between the range of 310 and 410 nm, it fluoresces, giving off light with a wavelength near 530 nm.[57] Contact lens practitioners will see the pupil giving off a greenish-yellow cast when viewing the eye with a UV lamp. This is really fluorescence of the crystalline lens as seen through the pupil.

Additional Protection from Glare Using Side Shields

The person who is especially sensitive to glare, such as someone with corneal scarring, may benefit from the use of side shields. These shields may be tinted and attached to prescription spectacles.

A wraparound frame is like a frame with built-in side shields. Wraparound frames are available in regular sunglasses or in specialty filters, such as NoIRs or Solar Shields. Many of these specialty filters are made to be worn by themselves or over conventional eyeglasses.

Using Absorptive Filters That Block Short Wavelengths

The effects of UV radiation on the retina are known and have been discussed in an earlier section of the chapter. In addition to UV light, there are some damaging effects of blue light reported.[58,59] However, the amount of light needed to cause such retinal damage is not found in the natural environment.[60] There is enough short wavelength light generated by ophthalmic instruments to cause ocular damage with sufficient exposure.[61] However, there are normally filters used in these instruments to prevent such damage.

In an attempt to slow the development of certain degenerative diseases, such as macular degeneration and retinitis pigmentosa, practitioners sometimes use lenses that block both UV and blue light.

Another rationale for using a lens that blocks short wavelength light is to try to increase contrast. When a blue object is viewed through a lens that filters blue, the object does not disappear but looks darker. A darker object against the same background will have a higher border contrast. For this reason, lenses that filter out short wavelength light are said to increase contrast.

Lenses Made to Block Short Wavelengths and Control Glare

Several lenses made their appearance in the 1980s that have been used in an attempt to control glare. Some of these lenses have been used heavily by low-vision practitioners and by those who see a large proportion of older wearers.

Glare Control CPF Lenses

Corning developed a series of photochromic lenses referred to as Glare Control CPF lenses. This line of lenses has since been acquired by and is sold through Winchester Optical.* They are specialty photochromic lenses made using a unique manufacturing process.

CPF lenses begin with photochromic material that is surfaced for the prescription and edged for the frame. Afterwards the lens is "fired" by heating the lens in a hydrogen atmosphere. This reduces the silver halide crystals near the surface of the photochromic lens to elemental silver. Left in this condition, wavelengths critical for causing the photochromic change would be blocked, and the lens will not darken. Therefore the front surface of the lens must be reground to remove the altered layer. The altered back layer that gives the lens its unique spectral-absorbing properties remains in place.

There are several series of these lenses, each with a coded name, such as the CPF 527. The letters "CPF" stand for "Corning protective filter." The number indicates the wavelength below which light is absorbed. (For the CPF 527 lens, all UV and visible light up to 527 nm is absorbed by the lens.)

CPF lenses are described and compared in Table 22-3. Some of their transmission curves in lightened and darkened states are shown in Figure 22-23.

None of these Glare Control lenses are to be worn for night driving.

Glare Control Dyes

There are some glare control "colors" available in lens dyes. This is a less expensive option, whereby clear plastic lenses may be tinted to the desired absorptive characteristics. To work as anticipated, the tint should not just match an expected lens color. The absorptive properties of the dyed lens should also fulfill the desired transmission requirements.

Nonprescription Options for Controlling Glare

Well-known nonprescription filters available for controlling glare are available from NoIR Medical Technologies.† These are wraparound glasses that come in sizes allowing them to be used alone or on top of prescription eyewear. There are many options available. NoIRs vary in the amount of light absorbed, the selectivity of that absorption across the spectrum, and the resulting physical color of the lens. However, according to one study[62] that reviewed 318 patients from three low-vision centers, when NoIRs were used, 89% of low-vision patients chose either the #101 or #102 NoIR filters.

Disadvantages of Glare Control-Type Lenses

There are certain disadvantages associated with lenses that block the short-wavelength visible spectrum. One of the greatest disadvantages of these lenses is their effect on color vision. The amount and type of color confusion will vary, depending upon the lens. The more of the visible spectrum that is absorbed by the lens, the greater will be the effect on color vision.

For the color-normal individual, there may be no color confusion induced for lenses that absorb moderately in the blue end of the spectrum. There may be mild confusion for lenses, such as the BluBlocker,[63] that absorb more of the visible spectrum.

---

*Winchester Optical, Winchester, MA 01890.

†NoIR Medical Technologies, P.O. Box 159, South Lyon, MI 48178.

TABLE 22-3
Comparison of Lenses in the CPF Glare Control Series

Lens Name	Color, Light Transmission, Description	Activities and Eye Disorders for Which the Lens Is Often Chosen
CPF 450X lightened | darkened	Transmission range: 68%-20%	The X series of lenses are made for general use and minimal color distortion while still blocking UV and minimizing short wavelength exposure.
CPF 511X lightened | darkened	Transmission range: 53%-15%	
CPF 527X lightened | darkened	Transmission range: 33%-15%	
GlareCutter lightened | darkened	Transmission range: 18%-6%	
CPF 450 lightened | darkened Available in progressives	Lighter color Moderate blue filtering Turns from a lemon yellow inside (67%) to a brown outside (19%)	Reading Television Helping with glare from fluorescent lighting
CPF 511 lightened | darkened	Turns from a yellow-amber inside (44%), to a brown outside (14%)	Developing cataracts Aphakes and pseudophakes Macular degeneration Corneal dystrophy Optic atrophy Sometimes glaucoma or diabetic retinopathy
CPF 527 lightened | darkened	Turns from an orange-amber inside (32%), to a brown outside (11%)	Same as for CPF 511
CPF 550 lightened | darkened	Turns from an orange-red inside (21%), to a brown outside (5%) Overall light transmission low both indoors and out	Intense sensitivity to light Poor dark adaptation Retinitis pigmentosa
CPF 550-XD lightened | darkened	Mahogany brown color: extremely dark 9% inside 4% outside (XD stands for extra dark.) Note: Lenses are too dark to meet FDA standards for daytime driving.	Extraordinary photophobia Aniridia Achromatopsia

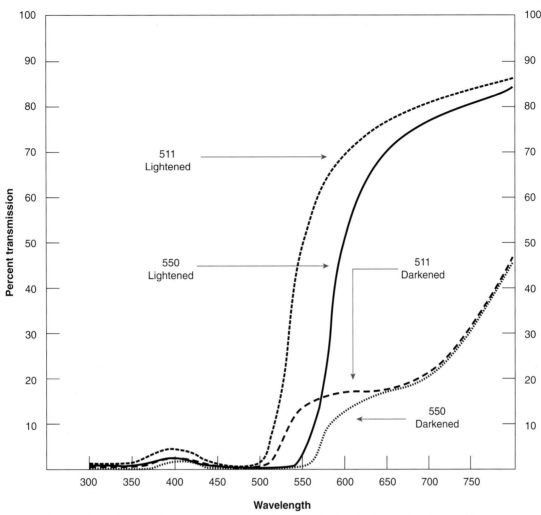

Figure 22-23. Transmission curves for two of the standard series CPF Glare Control lenses. Note that CPF lenses block all wavelengths below the identifying number for the lens (i.e., for the 550 lens, no light with a wavelength shorter than 550 nm is transmitted through the lens). Spectral transmission curves for the CPF 527 lens (not shown in the figure) fall between the transmission curves for the 511 and 550 lenses. (From: Corning Glare Control lens manual, OPM 190, Corning, NY, 1991, Corning Inc.)

Color discrimination will be more noticeably affected for individuals who already have a color deficiency. Scores on standardized color testing decreased notably for color defectives. In some cases, this can affect the color defective's ability to identify traffic signals quickly.

The expectation with glare control lenses is that visual performance will improve. However, improvements in visual performance by individuals who would be considered candidates for these type of lenses is not a given. In fact there may be no statistically significant difference in visual acuity or contrast sensitivity with the glare control-type lens compared with a neutral density filter of the same transmission.[64,65] Reported improvement in vision is more of a subjective assessment on the part of the wearer. Therefore decisions on which lenses to use are usually made by the individual subjectively comparing two or more appropriate lens types.

Clinically, glare control lenses continue to enjoy popularity, especially in practices specializing in low vision. Although not everyone with glare problems or degenerative eye disorders may find the lenses beneficial, those who do wear them report a subjective improvement in vision and satisfaction.

SPECIALTY ABSORPTIVE LENSES

Glass Blower's Lenses

Glass blowers prefer an absorptive lens that filters out the yellow band of the spectrum so that they may more clearly see what is happening to the color of the heated glass without it being marked by the yellow flame. This function is fulfilled with a glass *didymium filter* lens. Didymium lenses are dichroic, meaning the lens will appear rose colored in natural and incandescent lighting, but aqua under fluorescent lighting. Didymium lenses used in glass blowing *are not welding glasses,* even though there are some welding glasses that contain didymium.

X-Ray Lenses

Lenses used for x-ray protection are made from a 1.80 index, heavy glass material. This particular glass is softer than regular glass and is prone to scratching. (Note: Just because a lens may have an index of refraction of 1.8 does not mean that it protects against x-rays.) X-ray protective lenses are not capable of being chemically hardened. They cannot be heat tempered using normal ophthalmic air hardening equipment. X-ray protective lenses can be heat tempered at a lower temperature. But since most air hardening equipment does not have adjustable temperature capabilities,[66] the wearer must sign a waiver acknowledging that these lenses are not impact resistant.

ABSORPTIVE LENS CALCULATIONS

How Index of Refraction Affects the Transmission of a Spectacle Lens (the Fresnel Equation)

The amount of light that is reflected when light goes from one media to another is determined using the Fresnel equation. The Fresnel equation is:

$$I_R = \left[\frac{n'-n}{n'+n}\right]^2 \times I$$

where n' is the index of refraction of the second media, n is the index of refraction of the first media, I is the amount of incident light, and I_R is the amount of incident light that is reflected.

Example **22-2**

What percentage of light can we expect an absolutely clear CR-39 plastic lens to transmit if it has an index of refraction of 1.498?

Solution

Using the Fresnel equation, we substitute the index of air, which is 1, for n, and the index of CR-39 plastic for n'. The amount of incident light is 100% or 1. Therefore the amount of incident light that is reflected equals:

$$I_{R(Front)} = \left[\frac{n'-n}{n'+n}\right]^2 \times I$$
$$= \left[\frac{1.498-1}{1.498+1}\right]^2 \times 1$$
$$= \left[\frac{0.498}{2.498}\right]^2 \times 1$$
$$= [0.1994]^2 \times 1$$
$$= 0.0398$$

Reflected light expressed as a percentage is

$$R_F = 100(I_R).$$

Therefore reflected light from the front surface of the lens will be:

$$R_F = 100(0.0398) = 3.98\%$$

To determine how much light is reflected from the second surface, we run through the equation again. This time the value of the incident light is not 100% or 1. Instead it is:

$$I = 1 - 0.0398 = 0.9602$$

Therefore

$$I_{R(Back)} = \left[\frac{n'-n}{n'+n}\right]^2 \times 0.9602$$
$$= \left[\frac{1-1.498}{1+1.498}\right]^2 \times 0.9602$$
$$= \left[\frac{-0.498}{2.498}\right]^2 \times 0.9602$$
$$= [-0.1994]^2 \times 0.9602$$
$$= 0.0398 \times 0.9602$$
$$= 0.0382$$

Expressed as a percent, the light reflected from the back surface is:

$$R_B = 100(0.0382) = 3.82\%$$

Because of reflection from the front surface, only 96.02% of the light ever reaches the second surface of the lens. At the second surface, 3.82% of the light is reflected. This means that total light transmitted through the lens will be 96.02% − 3.82% = 92.2%.

Why High-Index Lenses Work Best With an Antireflection Coating

High-index lenses work much more to the wearer's satisfaction if they are AR coated. The reason can be seen when figuring the percentage of light transmitted by a high-index lens.

Example **22-3**

How much light is transmitted by an absolutely clear, uncoated plastic lens having an index of refraction of 1.66?

Solution

Using the Fresnel equation, the index of air remains as 1, and 1.66 is used for n'. Therefore

$$I_{R(Front)} = \left[\frac{n'-n}{n'+n}\right]^2 \times I$$
$$= \left[\frac{1.66-1}{1.66+1}\right]^2 \times 1$$
$$= \left[\frac{0.66}{2.66}\right]^2 \times 1$$
$$= [0.248]^2 \times 1$$
$$= 0.0616$$

and

$$R_F = 100(0.0616) = 6.16\%$$

This means we have already lost more than 6% of the light to reflection from the first surface. Next we find the amount of light that is incident on the second surface.

$$I = 1 - 0.0616 = 0.9384$$

Therefore

$$
\begin{aligned}
I_{R(Back)} &= \left[\frac{n'-n}{n'+n}\right]^2 \times 0.9384 \\
&= \left[\frac{1-1.66}{1+1.66}\right]^2 \times 0.9384 \\
&= \left[\frac{-0.66}{2.66}\right]^2 \times 0.9384 \\
&= [0.248]^2 \times 0.9384 \\
&= 0.0616 \times 0.9384 \\
&= 0.0578
\end{aligned}
$$

This means that the percent of light reflected from the back surface is:

$$R_B = 100(0.0578) = 5.78\%$$

If 93.84% of the light strikes the second surface and 5.78% is reflected from that surface, then the total light transmitted through the lens will be 93.84% − 5.78% = 88.06%.

The uncoated higher-index plastic lens in the example transmits only 88% of the incident light in its clear state. This is the same transmission as a lightly tinted crown glass or CR-39 plastic lens. Fortunately an AR coating will bring the lens back up to nearly 100% transmission. When these greater-than-normal lens reflections are eliminated with AR coating, the high-index lens becomes much more cosmetically appealing. AR-coated high-index lenses also perform better at night than uncoated high-index lenses. This is because more light is transmitted, and less glare from oncoming lights is encountered.

Why Coating Fused Glass Multifocals Help to Reduce Segment Visibility

Fused glass multifocal segments are made from a glass material having a higher refractive index than the distance portion of the lens. This means that the segment will reflect more light than the distance portion, increasing its visibility. By applying an AR coating, both parts of the lens transmit close to 100%. The difference in percent transmission between the distance lens and the segment is less, making the lens segment less noticeable.

Why a Tinted Glass Lens Becomes Darker When Its Plus Power Increases (Lambert's Law of Absorption)

When a lens material contains its tint in the melt or resin, the amount of light transmitted will change with a change in thickness. The amount of change is predictable using Lambert's law of absorption. Lambert's law of absorption states[67] that:

1. As light passes through a homogeneous substance of a given thickness, the same percentage of light is absorbed regardless of the intensity of the incident light.
2. The intensity of transmitted light varies as an exponential function of the length of the light path in the absorbing medium.

The first part of the law means that if a given thickness of absorptive material absorbs 50% of dim light, it will absorb 50% of bright light as well. The same percentage of light will be absorbed, regardless of how dim or bright the light is.

The second part of the law says that as the thickness of the absorbing medium doubles, the effect is equal to squaring the transmission factor for the original thickness. If the thickness triples, the effect is cubed, and so on.

Example **22-4**

Suppose a 1-mm thick lens has a transmission factor (q) of 0.9. This means that, ignoring reflections, if light strikes the lens, 90% of the light comes out the other side. If reflections are ignored, what would the transmission of a lens made of the same material be if it had a 2 mm thickness?

Solution

If the intensity of light entering the first millimeter of lens material is 100% or 1, the intensity of light leaving the first millimeter is:

$$
\begin{aligned}
I_1 &= I_0(q) \\
&= 1(0.9) \\
&= 0.9
\end{aligned}
$$

Next light enters the second millimeter with an intensity of 0.9. After passing through the second millimeter, the intensity of light leaving the second surface is:

$$
\begin{aligned}
I_2 &= I_1(q) \\
&= 0.9(0.9) \\
&= 0.81
\end{aligned}
$$

In other words, the second millimeter absorbs 90% of the light leaving the first millimeter, which was also 90%. Ninety percent of 90% is 81%. (This is the same as 0.9 squared.) Therefore 81% of the original oncoming light will make it through this 2-mm thick lens.

Expressing Lambert's Law As an Equation

To make Lambert's law into an equation, we see that if:

$$I_1 = I_0(q)$$

and

$$I_2 = I_1(q)$$

then

$$I_2 = I_0(q)(q) = I_0(q)^2$$

I_0 is the original amount of incident light, I_1 is the amount of incident light remaining after leaving the first layer, I_2 is the amount remaining after leaving the second layer, and q is the transmission factor for the thickness of the layer. Continuing the logic, we see that if we have x layers, then the amount of incident light remaining after the xth layer will be:

$$I_x = I_0(q)^x$$

and the percentage of light transmitted will be:

$$T_x = 100[I_0(q)^x]$$

How to Take Reflections into Consideration When Using Lambert's Law

If reflections are considered, then the amount of incident light that enters the first surface after reflection is:

$$I_0 = I - I_R$$

I in the original intensity of entering light, I_R is the intensity of the reflected light, and I_0 is the intensity of light entering the first layer (after reflection).

Total lens transmission will be:

$$T = T_x - R_B$$

Where T_x is the total percent transmission leaving the last layer (or back of the lens), R_B is the light reflected from the back surface, and T is the total percentage of light transmitted from the lens with both reflection and absorption considered.

Example **22-5**

A tinted crown glass lens has a transmission factor of $q = 0.9$ for each millimeter of lens thickness. If the lens has an index of refraction of 1.523 and is 3.0 mm thick, what is the transmission of the lens?

Solution

The intensity of the light reflected from the front surface of the lens is:

$$I_{R(Front)} = \left[\frac{n' - n}{n' + n}\right]^2 \times I$$
$$= \left[\frac{1.523 - 1}{1.523 + 1}\right]^2 \times 1$$
$$= 0.043$$

The intensity of light entering the lens ("first layer") is:

$$I_0 = 1 - 0.043$$
$$= 0.957$$

The intensity of light at the back surface of the lens (leaving the last layer) before back surface reflection occurs is:

$$I_x = I_0(q)^x$$

or

$$I_3 = (0.957)(0.9)^3$$
$$= 0.698$$

The percent transmission leaving the last layer before reflection is:

$$T_x = 100(I_x)$$
$$= 100(0.698)$$
$$= 69.8\%$$

The intensity of light reflected at the last layer is:

$$I_{R(Back)} = (0.698)\left[\frac{1 - 1.523}{1 + 1.523}\right]^2$$
$$= (0.698)(-0.207)^2$$
$$= (0.698)0.043$$
$$= 0.03$$

Therefore the total percent transmission for light leaving the lens is:

$$T = T_x - R_B$$
$$= 69.8\% - 3.0\%$$
$$= 66.8\%$$

Ultimate Transmission

The ultimate transmission (T_u) is found by multiplying the transmissions of each element through which light passes to determine ultimately what transmission results.

$$T_u = (T_1) \times (T_2) \times (T_3) \ldots \text{etc}$$

(such as 3 lenses lined up one behind another.)

Example **22-6**

An individual is driving a car with a lightly tinted windshield having a transmission of 85%. He is wearing sunglass clip-ons with a 20% transmission over a pair of lightly tinted spectacle lenses with an 87% transmission. What percentage of incoming light gets through to the eye?

Solution

To find ultimate transmission, multiply all of the transmissions together. In this case

$$T_u = 0.85 \times 0.20 \times 0.87$$
$$= 0.15$$

Therefore the ultimate transmission of light through this "system" is 0.15 or 15%.

Opacity

Opacity is the reciprocal of transmission. (When calculating opacity, transmission is *not* expressed as a percentage.)

$$O = \frac{1}{T}$$

Example **22-7**

What is the opacity of a lens having 67% transmission?

Solution

Since transmission is not expressed as a percentage, then:

$$O = \frac{1}{0.67} = 1.49$$

The opacity of the lens is 1.49.

Example **22-8**

Suppose an individual is wearing absorptive spectacle lenses having a transmission of 80%. She gets into a car with a tinted windshield. The windshield has a transmission of 80%. In this situation, what percentage of the light is transmitted to the eye? What would our answer be if expressed as opacity?

Solution

We are seeking the ultimate transmission of the combination of elements. In this case it is:

$$\begin{aligned} T_u &= (T_1) \times (T_2) \\ &= (.8) \times (.8) \\ &= 0.64 \text{ or } 64\% \end{aligned}$$

The opacity of this combination would be:

$$\begin{aligned} O &= \frac{1}{T} \\ &= \frac{1}{0.64} \\ O &= 1.56 \end{aligned}$$

Optical Density

Using transmissions makes figuring odd thicknesses difficult. Densities, however, are additive. Densities are the log of the opacity and are expressed as:

$$\text{optical density} = \log_{10}(\text{opacity})$$

which is the same thing as:

$$D = \log O$$

and can also be expressed as:

$$D = \log \frac{1}{T}$$

Since

$$\begin{aligned} \log \frac{1}{T} &= \log 1 - \log T \\ &= 0.0 - \log T \end{aligned}$$

Therefore

$$D = -\log T$$

Example **22-9**

If a lens has a transmission of 0.90 for each millimeter of thickness, what is its optical density per 1/10 mm and what is the transmission for 1/10 mm?

Solution

First, we find the optical density for 1 mm.

$$\begin{aligned} D &= -\log T \\ &= -\log 0.90 \\ &= 0.0457575 \end{aligned}$$

Now we can find the optical density for 1/10 mm. Density (*D*) for 1/10 mm is:

$$\frac{0.0457575}{10} = 0.00457575$$

The optical density for 1/10 mm is 0.00458.

Now to find the transmission for $1/10^{th}$ mm we convert from optical density back to transmission. We know that

$$D = -\log T$$

and that the density of $1/10^{th}$ mm is 0.00458.
Therefore

$$-\log T = 0.00458$$

So

$$\log T = -0.00458$$

Taking the antilog of −0.00458 we find

$$T = 0.99$$

So 1/10 mm has a transmission of 99%.

Laser Protective Eyewear Specified in Optical Density
When transmission of a lens is a very small number, optical density of the lens will be large. As an example, when the transmission of a lens is 1% (or .01), the density of that lens is 2.0. For this reason, many times occupational safety tints or laser safety tints are specified in terms of optical density instead of percent transmission.

As an example, in Figure 22-24 laser protective eyewear used around Argon lasers is shown to have

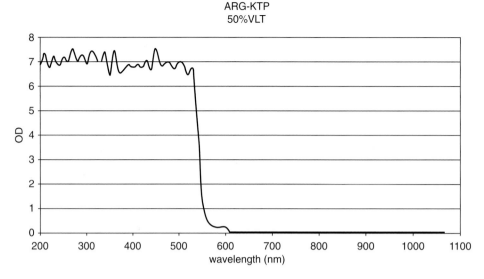

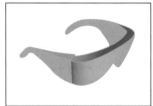

Figure 22-24. Laser protective eyewear uses optical density instead of transmission to specify the absorbency of the filter. The higher the density, the more the radiation is absorbed. (From http://www.noirlaser.com/filters/arg.html, NoIR Laser Co, LLC, 6155 Pontiac Trail, South Lyon, MI, 48178, 8/16/2005.)

a high optical density for wavelengths from 200 to 532 nm. This high optical density protects the wearer in the wavelength zone for Argon lasers. However, the optical density drops back to almost zero above 600 nm. Light above 600 nm can be seen easily. In a graph that uses optical density such as the one shown in Figure 22-24, the high areas of the graph indicate the wavelength areas of most protection.

REFERENCES

1. Pitts DG, Kleinstein RN: Environmental vision, Boston, 1993, Butterworth-Heinemann.
2. Goodeve DF: Vision on the ultraviolet, Nature 134:416-417, 1934. (As cited by Pitts DG, Kleinstein RN: Environmental vision, Boston, 1993, Butterworth-Heinemann.)
3. Torgersen D: UV radiation and the eye, lab talk, 1998. (Also Pitts DG, Kleinstein RN: Environmental vision, Boston, 1993, Butterworth-Heinemann.)
4. Pitts DG: Ultraviolet protection—when and why? Prob Optom 2:97, 1990.
5. Brilliant LB, Grasset NC, Pokhrel RP et al: Associations among cataract prevalence, sunlight hours, and altitude in the Himalayas, Am J Epidemiol 118:239, 1983.
6. Miller D: Effect of sunglasses on the visual mechanism, Surv Ophthal 19:38, 1974.
7. Young RW: The family of sun-related eye diseases, Optom Vis Sci 71(2):125-144, 1994.
8. Reme CJ, Reinboth J, Clausen M et al: Light damage revisited: converging evidence, diverging views? Graefes Arch Clin Exp Ophthalmol 234(1):2-11, 1996 as cited by Bradley A: Special review: colored filters and vision care, part II, Indiana J Optom 7(1):2, 2004.
9. West Sheila K et al: Sunlight exposure and risk of lens opacities in a population-based study: the Salisbury eye evaluation project, JAMA 280:714-718, 1998.
10. Hecht S, Hendley C, Ross S et al: The effect of exposure to sunlight on night vision, Am J Ophthal 31:1573, 1948.
11. ANSI Z80.3-2001: American national standard for ophthalmics-nonprescription sunglasses and fashion eyewear-requirements, Merrifield, Va, 2002, Opt Lab Assoc.
12. Peckham RH, Harley RD: Reduction in visual acuity due to excessive sunlight, Arch Ophthalmol 44:625, 1950.
13. Miles PW: Visual effects of pink glasses, green windshields, and glare under night driving conditions, Arch Ophthal 52:15, 1954.
14. Waetjen R, Schiefer U, Gaigl A et al: Influence of windshield tint and tilt on recognition distance under mesopic conditions, German J Ophthalmol 1:424-428, 1992.
15. Allen MJ: Highway tests of photochromic lenses, J Am Optom Assoc 50:1023-1027, 1979.
16. Bradley A: Special review: colored filters and vision care, part II, Indiana J Optom 7(1):2-4, 2004.
17. Wolffsohn JS, Cochrane AL, Khoo H et al: Contrast is enhanced by yellow lenses because of selective reduction of short-wavelength light, Optom Vis Sci 77(2):73-81, 2000.

18. Luckiesh M, Moss E: The science of seeing, New York, 1937, D Van Nostrand Co.

19. Reiner J: Farbige brillenglaser unter besonderer berucksichtigung der modefarben, Augenoptiker 30:41, 1975.

20. Sheedy J: Dispensing tip: tinted lenses for color blindness, Opt Dispensing News, 248:2005.

21. Dain S: Sunglasses and sunglass standards, Clin Exp Optom 86(2):87, 2003.

22. Guidance document for prescription sunglasses, U.S. Department of Health and Human Services, Food and Drug Administration, Center for Devices and Radiological Health, Division of Ophthalmic Devices, Office of Device Evaluation, Rockville, Md, October 9, 1998.

23. Bradley A: Special review: colored filters and vision care, part I, Indiana J Optom 6(1):13-17, 2003.

24. LaLuzerne J (with Quinn D): Hard coating chemistry can make or break your AR coating, LabTalk pp 16-20, 2003.

25. Coatings, ophthalmic lens files, Paris, 1997, Essilor International.

26. Lee BK: Tints and coatings—physical considerations, Problems Optom 2(1):176, 1990.

27. Dowaliby M: Practical aspects of ophthalmic optics, Chicago, 1972, The Professional Press Inc.

28. Hoya multicoat lenses, Torrance, Calif, Hoya Lens of America Inc.

29. McQuaid RD: Reflections of antireflection films, JAOA 68(3):196, 1997.

30. Pénaud B: Crizal Alizé, a unique combination of performances for anti-reflective lenses that are less sensitive to smudge and easier to clean, Points de Vue (50):55-57, 2004.

31. Ellefsen E: Advances in anti-reflection coating technology, LabTalk p 8, 2001.

32. http://www.arcouncil.org, 2004, AR Council, 2417 West 105th Street, Bloomington, MN 55431.

33. Bruneni JL: AR and other thin film coatings, Eyecare Business p 52, 2002.

34. Transitions, publication U2S123, St Petersburg, Fla, Transitions Opt.

35. Drew R: Ophthalmic dispensing, the present-day realities, Newton, Mass, 1990, Butterworth-Heinemann.

36. Bell-o-gram, Bell Optical Laboratory, Oct/Nov 1992, p 1.

37. Bruneni JL: Ask the labs, Eyecare Business 10(3):47, 1995.

38. Culbreth G: To AR, or not to AR sunwear . . . that is the question, LabTalk p 26, 2002.

39. Barron C, Waiss B: An evaluation of visual acuity with Corning CPF 527 lens, J Am Optom Assoc 58:50, 1987, as cited by Pitts DG, Kleinstein RN: Environmental vision. Boston, 1993, Butterworth-Heinemann.

40. Ross J, Bradley A: Visual performance and patient preference: a comparison of anti-reflection coated and uncoated spectacle lenses, JAOA 68(6):361-366, 1997.

41. Bachman WG, Weaver JL: Comparison between antireflection-coated and uncoated spectacle lenses for presbyopic highway patrol troopers, JAOA 70(2):103-109, 1999.

42. Sheedy JE: How to present AR coating to your patients, Staff CE Workbook, Optom Today pp 7-13, 1998.

43. An eyecare professional's guide to AR, 2002, AR Council.

44. Bruneni JL: Ask the labs, Eyecare Business 10(4):41, 1995.

45. Karp A: Mirror image lenses and technology, 20/20 Magazine p 54, 2005.

46. Young JM: Photochromics: past & present, Optical World p 16, 1993.

47. Bruneni JL: The new photochromics, Eyecare Business p 52, 2003.

48. Evaluating plastic photochromics, lenses and technology, 2002, Jobson Publications.

49. Morgenstern S: Keeping up with photochromic technology, Vis Care Prod News p 62, 2005.

50. Garner LF: A guide to the selection of ophthalmic tinted lenses, Aust J Optom 57:346-350, 1974.

51. Photochromic ophthalmic lenses, Corning, NY, Corning Glass Works, Publication OPO-232 3/90.

52. Young J: Polar process, 20/20 p 88, 2002.

53. Clark BA: Polarizing sunglasses and possible eye hazards of transmitted radiation, Amer J Optom Arch Amer Acad Optom 46:499-509, 1969.

54. Bittan C: The story of polarizing lenses, Opt Manage 5(12):19-23, 1976.

55. Hofstetter HW, Griffin JR, Berman M, Everson R, Dictionary of visual science and related clinical terms, ed 5, St Louis, 2000, Butterworth-Heinemann.

56. Rosenberg R: Light, glare, and contrast in low vision care, In Faye E, editor: Clinical low vision, Boston, 1984, Little, Brown and Co.

57. Klang G: Measurements and studies of the fluorescence of the human lens in vivo, Acta Ophthalmol Suppl 31:1-152, 1948. (As cited by Miller: Surv Ophthal 19:38-44, 1974.)

58. Harwerth RS, Sperling H: Prolonged color blindness induced by spectral lights in rhesus monkeys, Sci 174:180-184, 1975. (As cited by Dain S: Sunglasses and sunglass standards, Clin Exp Optom 86(2):77-90, 2003.)

59. Ham WT, Mueller HA, Sliney DH: Retinal sensitivity to damage from short wavelength light, Nature 260:153-155, 1976. (As cited by Dain S: Sunglasses and sunglass standards, Clin Exp Optom 86(2):77-90, 2003.)

60. Sliney DH, Wolbarsht M: Safety with lasers and other optical sources, New York, 1980, Plenum. (As cited by Dain S: Sunglasses and sunglass standards, Clin Exp Optom 86(2):77-90, 2003.)

61. Schoolmeesters B, Rosselle I, Leys A et al: Light-induced maculopathy, Bull Soc Belge Ophtalmol 259:115-122, 1995. (As cited by Dain S: Sunglasses and sunglass standards, Clin Exp Optom 86(2):77-90, 2003.)

62. Maino JH, McMahon TT: NoIRs and low vision, J Am Optom Assoc 57(7):7, 1986.

63. Thomas RS, Kuyk TK: D-15 performance with short wavelength absorbing filter in normals, Am J Optom Physiol Opt 65:679-702, 1988.

64. Barron C, Waiss B: An evaluation of visual acuity with Corning CPF 527 lens, J Am Optom Assoc 58:50-54, 1987. (As cited by Pitts DG, Kleinstein RN: Environmental vision, Newton, Mass, 1993, Butterworth-Heinemann.)

65. Lynch DM, Brilliant R: An evaluation of the Corning CPF 550 lens, Optom Monogr 75:36-42, 1984. (As cited by Pitts DG, Kleinstein RN: Environmental vision, Newton, Mass, 1993, Butterworth-Heinemann.)

66. X-Cel Optical Co: Filter glass available from X-Cel Optical. http://www.x-celoptical.com/Occupational%20Eyewear%20Protection.htm, accessed 2/3/2006.

67. Hofstetter HW, Griffin JR, Berman M, Everson R: Dictionary of visual science and related clinical terms, ed 5, St Louis, 2000, Butterworth-Heinemann.

Proficiency Test

(Answers may be found in the back of the book.)

1. True or false? The longer the wavelength of the UV rays, the greater the likelihood of biologic damage.

2. True or false? Single, high-level amounts of UV radiation can be damaging, but the eye is able to recover from long-term, low-level amounts of UV exposure without being affected.

3. True or false? A person's ability to work effectively under a situation of reduced illumination increases with age.

4. True or false? Coatings for plastic lenses are purely for scratch resistance and have no AR properties.

5. True or false? When a tint and an AR coating are both desired, plastic lenses should be dyed before they are AR coated.

6. True or false? Although in certain instances acuity may increase when a 10% neutral-density filter is worn in bright sunlight, persons older than age 40 years experience poorer vision if the filter is darker than 10%.

7. True or false? Normal transmission for average sunglasses runs between 15% and 30%.

8. True or false? Exposure to sunlight over an extended period of time will reduce the time needed for the eye to dark adapt.

9. True or false? Yellow tints help nighttime driving because they eliminate blue haze.

10. True or false? With AR coatings, it is possible to have any one of a range of reflex colors or no color at all and still produce an efficient coating.

11. True or false? The quality of the AR coating is not indicated by the evenness of the reflex color of the coating.

12. True or false? An AR coating will make a lightly tinted lens perform better at night than it otherwise would perform with the tint but no AR coating.

13. True or false? The process of adding an AR coating to a tinted plastic lens sometimes changes the color of the tint.

14. True or false? AR coating the back surface of a pair of sunglasses is not advisable because it lets more light through the lens.

15. True or false? An AR-coated lens is best cleaned in office by using an ultrasonic cleaner.

16. True or false? An AR-coated lens is helped by use of an antifog or antistatic agent.

17. True or false? Mirror coating provides good protection from sunlight if combined with a tint, but allows more UV and IR than a nonmirror-coated lens of equal transmission.

18. For which type of entering light is an AR coating most effective?
    a. for light that is entering the lens from straight ahead
    b. for light that is entering the lens from an angle
    c. AR coating is equally effective for incoming light, regardless of whether it is entering from straight ahead or obliquely.

19. True or false? An antiscratch coating is usually affected by exposure to antifog and antistatic agents.

20. True or false? UV or color dyeing a plastic photochromic lens makes the photochromic aspects of the lens work better.

21. True or false? Lenses that absorb the short end of the visible spectrum may help reduce some types of glare.

22. True or false? In denoting the amount of light absorbed by the lens, if numbers, such as 1, 2, 3, are used, the higher the number, the more light is allowed to pass through the lens.

23. True or false? There is no such thing as a "glare control dye."

24. True or false? Glare control-type lenses will not cause a decrease in scores on standardized color testing for color defectives.

25. All of these lenses are vacuum coated to the equivalent of a "gray #3" tint. Which lens will be the darkest?
    a. +7.00 D
    b. plano
    c. -7.00 D
    d. It depends on whether edge or center is being considered.
    e. All will be equally dark.

26. For a neutral gray glass sun lens of plus power with the tint in the glass, as plus power increases,
  a. the transmission increases.
  b. the absorption decreases.
  c. the transmission decreases.
  d. the transmission stays the same.
  e. Both a and b are correct.

27. Which UV radiation has the longest wavelength?
  a. UVA
  b. UVB
  c. UVC

28. Which of the following may not be caused by or increased in severity by excessive exposure to UV radiation?
  a. photokeratitis
  b. cataracts
  c. diabetic retinopathy
  d. age-related maculopathy
  e. All of the above may be caused by or increased in severity by excessive exposure to UV radiation.

29. Rank the following lenses in order, beginning with the lens that absorbs the most short wavelength visible and UV radiation and concluding with the lens that absorbs the least short wavelength visible and UV radiation.

  1. coated polycarbonate lenses   a. 2,4,1,3
  2. crown glass lenses   b. 3,1,2,4
  3. CPF 550 lenses   c. 1,4,2,3
  4. uncoated CR-39 plastic lenses   d. 3,1,4,2
     e. 3,4,1,2

30. Glass blower's cataract is believed to be caused by:
  a. UV radiation.
  b. short-wavelength visible light.
  c. IR radiation.
  d. both UV radiation and short-wavelength visible light combined.

Match the color to the most appropriate characteristic for that color.

31. Light Pink _____
32. Yellow _____
  a. blue absorbing
  b. advisable for night driving
  c. selective absorption of red
  d. good UV and IR absorption
  e. even absorption across the visible spectrum

Match the color to the most appropriate characteristic for that color.

33. Gray _____
34. Green _____
  a. recommended for bright, hazy days
  b. good for color defectives
  c. highly absorbing of yellow light
  d. highest transmissions of visible light found in the middle of the visible spectrum
  e. selectively cuts out blue light, leaving the rest of the visible spectrum

From the list below pick the most applicable lens to match the following characteristics:

35. poor IR absorption _____
36. tint varies with thickness _____
  a. dyed plastic lens
  b. heat-treated lens
  c. tinted glass lens
  d. vacuum-coated lens
  e. No lens listed matches.

37. A color-deficient individual will readapt to the induced color changes for which of the following lenses?
  a. brown
  b. CPF-550
  c. yellow
  d. a and c above
  e. none of the above

38. As a secondary effect, antiscratch coatings will:
  a. reduce lens reflections somewhat.
  b. increase lens reflections somewhat.
  c. neither increase nor decrease lens reflections.

39. What is the most effective method to use when attempting to match a new glass photochromic replacement lens with an older glass photochromic lens?
  a. Reharden the old lens with the new.
  b. Boil the old lens 2 hours.
  c. Expose both lenses to a UV lamp for 1 hour.

40. A person has new lenses and has been wearing them for a month. She now decides she would like to have them AR coated. The lenses are lightly scratched. If the lenses are then AR coated:
  a. the scratches will be more evident.
  b. the scratches will not show up as much.
  c. the AR coating will not affect the appearance of the scratches.

41. A pair of glasses with SRC lenses is best adjusted using:
a. a forced-air frame warmer.
b. a salt bath.
c. Either unit will work equally well and not be a problem for the lenses.

42. Disregarding impact resistance and taking only transmission characteristics into consideration, which method is best for hardening a photochromic lens?
a. heat tempering
b. chemical tempering
c. There is no difference in the finished product.

43. What color lens is "Kalichrome H"?
a. gray
b. green
c. pink
d. blue
e. yellow

44. A glass absorptive lens with the tint in the glass has a lighter horizontal area running the full width of the lens. What might the prescription be?
a. -4.00 sphere
b. +4.00 sphere
c. Plano -4.00 × 180
d. Plano +4.00 × 180
e. +4.00 -4.00 × 135

45. The tint may be removed and reapplied for which types of lenses?
a. vacuum-coated lenses
b. internal-tinted lenses
c. plastic lenses
d. a and c above
e. none of the above

46. Which of the following lenses should *not* be AR coated?
a. lightly tinted glass lenses
b. sun lenses
c. glass photochromic lenses
d. All of the above may be AR coated.
e. None of the above should be AR coated.

47. First-generation, single-layer AR-coated lenses had a bluish-purple cast when they were held at certain angles. This occurs because to most nearly fulfill path and amplitude conditions and still achieve a maximal antireflective effect over a large area of the visible spectrum a specific wavelength had to be chosen. That wavelength corresponded to which color?
a. yellow
b. blue
c. red
d. bluish purple
e. All wavelengths equally fulfill path and amplitude conditions.

48. The problem of annoying internal lens reflections occurs most often in:
a. high plus-powered clear lenses.
b. low minus-powered clear lenses.
c. SRC clear lenses.
d. AR-coated clear lenses.
e. sun lenses.

49. Pick out the correct combination of causes contributing to the rapid darkening of a photochromic lens.
a. 1, 3, 4   1. IR
b. 2, 3, 5   2. UV
c. 1, 4   3. previous exposures
d. 2, 5   4. cold
e. 2, 3, 4   5. heat

50. A polarizing ophthalmic lens should be oriented so as to eliminate:
a. vertically vibrating waves.
b. horizontally vibrating waves.
c. obliquely vibrating waves.
d. all vibrating waves.
e. Orientation is unimportant.

51. A prescription-ground polarizing lens is characterized by:
a. silver iodide crystals.
b. a coating process.
c. a mixing into the molten glass.
d. a frosting process.
e. a stretched sheet of polyvinyl alcohol.

52. What glare source(s) will not be helped by "glare control" lenses?
a. glare from smooth surfaces
b. glare caused by fluorescence of the crystalline lens
c. glare caused by a developing cataract
d. glare from both high and low intensities occurring in a small area

53. If a lens has an index of refraction of 1.66, what is the ideal index of refraction for a single-layer AR coating?

54. Two lenses are placed back-to-back. One has a transmission of 50%; the other has a transmission of 40%. What percent transmission do they have together?

55. If a perfectly clear, uncoated lens has an index of refraction of 1.73, what percent of the incoming light would be transmitted out the back of the lens?

CHAPTER 23

Lens Materials, Safety, and Sports Eyewear

Lens material and eye safety in the workplace and for sports or recreational activities are all interrelated. In this chapter the characteristics of lens materials are considered. This leads logically to a discussion of appropriate frames and lens materials in eye protection.

LENS MATERIALS

The variety of materials that can be used for lenses has increased substantially during the past few years and promises to continue to expand. With choices abounding, the practitioner needs to know the unique characteristics of each lens material so that a proper match between the needs of the wearer and the best possible material occurs. Ophthalmic lenses are made from glass and plastic. Glass lenses are often referred to as *mineral* lenses, whereas if a lens is made from plastic, it is said to be from *organic* material.

Crown Glass

The material traditionally used for spectacle lens wear for several hundred years has been glass. Glass works well for ophthalmic materials because it resists scratching and is not easily affected by environmental factors. The main disadvantages of glass are weight and impact resistance. To pass United States requirements for impact resistance, glass must be hardened.

The most commonly used clear glass lens material is made from a type of *crown glass* having an index of refraction of 1.523. This material is low in chromatic aberration.

High-Index Glass

There are higher index glass lens materials available that will reduce lens thickness for higher powered prescriptions. Index 1.60 lenses are readily available in spherical and aspheric designs and in segmented and progressive multifocals. *Corning Clear 16* is able to be surfaced to a 1.5-mm center thickness and, after hardening, is impact resistant enough to pass Food and Drug Administration (FDA) standards.

There are fused flat-top bifocals available in indexes up to 1.70, and single vision lenses in still higher indexes. Even though there is a 1.90 index glass available, it is generally not used in the United States because it cannot be hardened and thus will not meet impact resistance standards.

Unfortunately, high-index glass lenses are composed of materials with a higher specific gravity, making them heavier. In countries where there are not impact resistance requirements, this is not a problem since they can be ground very thin anyway. But with the thicknesses needed to achieve a sufficient impact resistance, a prescription must be fairly strong in order for high-index glass lenses to be both thinner and lighter than crown glass. What the dioptric value should be for a high-index glass lens to exhibit the expected advantages of both thickness *and* weight will depend upon the specific gravity of the material used. When glass was the main material used, the rule of thumb was that high index became lighter than crown glass for lenses more than −7.00 D.

High-index glass lens materials generally have Abbé values close to that of polycarbonate. Chromatic aberration is measured in terms of an Abbé value. The lower the Abbé value, the higher the chromatic aberration. Chromatic aberration can result in color fringes being visible at high-contrast borders. An example of a high-contrast border would be the black and white keys of a piano. Fortunately, when lenses are fit properly, most problems with chromatic aberration can be minimized so that they do not pose a problem.

Plastic Lenses

CR-39

For years the most commonly used plastic lens material was CR-39. CR-39 was developed by PPG Industries. "CR" stands for Columbia Resin, and the number 39 denotes the type of Columbia Resin used. CR-39 lens material processes well in the laboratory. For years CR-39 was used without antiscratch coating. Now, however, most CR-39 lenses come with an antiscratch coating, making the material much more scratch resistant. CR-39 lenses that must be surfaced are less likely to have an antiscratch coating on the back side unless one is ordered. (Segmented multifocals and progressive addition lenses are examples of lenses that must be surfaced.)

Plastic lenses are roughly half the weight of crown glass lenses. For low velocity, large mass objects, such as a softball, chemically tempered lenses perform somewhat better than CR-39 lenses in their impact resistance ratings. For smaller, high velocity, sharply pointed objects, CR-39 lenses perform better than chemically tempered glass. (It should be noted that glass is weakened more by scratching than is CR-39 plastic.) Keep in mind, however, that for impact resistance there are a number of other plastic lens materials that outperform both chemically tempered glass and CR-39 plastic. Impact resistance will vary according to the type of plastic used.

CR-39 plastic lenses do not fog up as easily as glass lenses. Whereas welding or grinding spatter will pit or

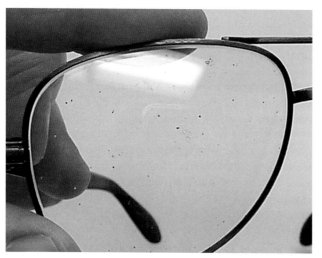

Figure 23-1. Welding or grinding spatter will pit or permanently stick to glass lenses, as shown here. It does not adhere to plastic lens material.

permanently stick to glass lenses, it does not adhere to plastic lens material (Figure 23-1).

High-Index Plastics

CR-39 plastic lenses have an index of refraction of approximately 1.498. This is the lowest refractive index material used for spectacle lenses. For minus lenses of equal powers and center thicknesses, the higher the index of refraction of a lens material, the thinner the lens edge can be made. Therefore high-index plastic lens materials will have both a weight and a thickness advantage over CR-39. They are an attractive alternative.

High-index plastic comes in a variety of materials. When considering the virtues of a high-index lens, the materials should not only be compared on the basis of index of refraction alone, but also on the basis of weight, impact resistance, finished lens thickness, Abbé value (chromatic aberration), and ease of production. Table 23-1 gives a comparison of some of these characteristics for a few representative materials.

Table 23-2 gives a summary of the impact-resistance characteristics for many of the currently available lens materials.

Polycarbonate

Polycarbonate lens material is soft and requires an anti-scratch coating. However, the very softness of the material contributes to its high-impact resistance. Instead of breaking on impact, the softer polycarbonate material is more likely to absorb a blow and just dent. When safety is the primary concern, polycarbonate has traditionally been the number one choice. (Safety is the primary concern for children, monocular individuals, people

---

TABLE **23-1**
A Representative Comparison of Lens Materials

Lens Material	Refractive Index (n)*	Density†	Thickness† (Minus Lens Center Thickness)	Abbé Value§
CR-39 plastic	1.498	1.32	2.0	58
Crown glass	1.523	2.54	2.0-2.2	59
Trivex	1.532	1.11	1.0-1.3	43-45
Spectralite	1.537	1.21	1.5	47
Polycarbonate	1.586	1.22	1.0-1.5	29
Polyurethane	1.595	1.34	1.5	36
Corning Clears 16 (glass)	1.60	2.63	1.5	42
High-Index plastic	1.66	1.35	1.0-1.7‖	32
	1.71	1.4		36
Thin & Lite 1.74 High-Index plastic	1.74	1.46	1.1	33
High-Index glass[30]	1.7	2.97	2.0-2.2	31
	1.80	3.37		25
	1.90¶	4.02		30.4

*The higher the refractive index, the thinner the edge of a minus lens.
†The lower the density, the lighter the lens.
‡Lens thickness is based on the thinnest lens that will both maintain U.S. impact resistance requirements and stability (will not warp). Thicknesses are approximate and may vary with lens coatings.
§The higher the Abbé value, the less the chromatic aberration.
‖Depends upon if lenses are single vision stock or surfaced and whether AR coated.
¶Cannot be chemically tempered for impact resistance and will not pass FDA requirements.

TABLE **23-2**
Relative Impact Resistance of Various Ophthalmic Materials

Lens Material	Comments
Untreated crown glass	Because of Food and Drug Administration regulations, untreated crown glass is not used for ophthalmic eyewear in the United States.
Heat-Treated crown glass	Heat-treated glass loses much impact resistance when it is scratched. In fact against the impact of small, high-velocity objects, a badly scratched untreated glass lens is more impact resistant than a badly scratched, heat-treated lens.
Chemically tempered crown glass	Against the impact of large, slow moving objects, such as a softball, chemically tempered lenses are more impact resistant than CR-39 plastic. Against the impact of small, high velocity objects, however, the CR-39 plastic lens is the more impact resistant.
CR-39 plastic	An uncoated CR-39 lens ranks as shown here. If this lens is coated, however, the impact resistance tends to be reduced. Just how much depends on the type of coating that is used.
High-Index plastic	High-index plastics are made from a variety of materials and, although they vary in their impact resistance, have been classed as only being as strong as CR-39.[23] Keep in mind that there are subgroups in this category. Many of the newer high-index plastics perform well enough to be thinned to 1.0 or 1.5 mm thickness. As with CR-39, impact resistance of high-index lenses is decreased with the addition of antireflection coatings.
	Polyurethane lenses appear to perform fairly well in impact resistance.
Polycarbonate, Trivex, and NXT materials	Impact resistance for polycarbonate, Trivex, and NXT lens materials exceeds other commonly used prescription lens materials. Antireflection coating does reduce impact resistance of these lenses by varying degrees, depending upon the type of missile impacting it. Eye care practitioners should be attentive to new information on these lenses before assuming that they are equal in all situations.

with good acuity in one eye only, and those who are purchasing safety or sports eyewear.)

Because polycarbonate lenses are so much safer than conventional lenses, the eyewear purchaser should be informed of the availability of safer lens materials and given the opportunity to choose a lens that affords better protection.

Trivex Lenses

Trivex lens material is a very impact-resistant lens material. It was developed by PPG Industries, the developers of CR-39 material. Trivex processes fairly easily and takes a lens tint easily. The lens material was originally for military use as a plastic material to provide excellent safety characteristics for windows in combat vehicles and good optics.[1] PPG Industries promotional materials attribute the "tri" in Trivex to a triperformance lens material; meaning it offers a triple combination of superior optics, impact resistance, and ultra light weight.

Trivex rivals polycarbonate in impact resistance. It is the lens of choice for drill-mounted lenses because it does not crack or split at the drilled hole. Some laboratories will warrant no other material than Trivex for drill-mounted lenses.

The lens is very light weight, having a density of 1.11. Even though the index of 1.53 is just a bit higher than crown glass, it may be thinned to 1 mm so that thickness and weight are seldom an issue. The Abbé value of 43 to 45 is less than CR-39, but higher than its rival, polycarbonate. It maintains a good resistance to damage from chemicals.

NXT Material[2]

There are other lens materials that continue to be developed that will add much to the ophthalmic lens market in the coming years. An example of one such material with some potential for more ophthalmic use is called NXT. NXT was developed in the early 1990s under a U.S. government contract to develop a new bullet-proof material. The resulting lens is a light-weight material that is extremely strong and also compatible with photochromic pigments and with polarization. It has already been used in sun and sport eyewear, helmet visors for motorcycles, airline cockpit door view ports, ballistic police shields, and vehicle door armor.

NXT has an index of refraction of 1.53, a density of 1.11, an Abbé value of 45, and is highly flexible. It is reported to be compatible with low-powered sphere and cylinder prescription lens powers.

Laminated Lenses

Lenses that are made from two or more layers of material are called *laminated lenses*. Lamination can be used for several purposes. Before dyed plastic lenses, clear glass lenses were sometimes laminated with a thin layer of tinted glass to give an even tint across the lens. Polarizing lenses have a stretched polarizing film sandwiched between two layers of regular lens material to cut out reflected glare. Lamination can also be used to increase impact resistance.

Effect of Lens Coatings on Impact Resistance

When a plastic lens is either scratch resistance coated or antireflection (AR) coated, the impact resistance of the lens decreases. This seems opposite to what would be expected.

Both scratch resistance and antireflection coatings are harder than the plastic lens material to which they adhere. When a lens breaks, the break starts at the weakest point. If a plastic lens is hit by an object, the lens may flex, but may not break. If the coating is harder than the lens, however, as the lens flexes, the harder (more brittle) coating cracks before the uncoated lens. When the coating is strongly bonded to the lens, the energy that is concentrated in the first crack is released. The released energy travels through the lens and may cause it to break.

Corzine et al[3] used a static load form of testing* and compared uncoated CR-39 lenses with (1) scratch resistance-coated lenses, (2) five-layer AR-coated lenses, and (3) lenses that had been prepared for antireflection coating but not coated. The mean fracture loads required to break the lenses in each category were as follows:

Lens Type	Fracture Load
Uncoated CR-39	587
Scratch resistance coated CR-39	505
AR coated CR-39	465
AR prepped but not coated CR-39	609

As can be seen from the results, the weakening of the lens is due to the coating itself, not by the process the lens is subjected to in preparation for coating.

In another study, Chou and Hovis[4] tested coated CR-39 *industrial* lenses for impact resistance using the Canadian Standards Association ballistic test protocol. They concluded that AR coating produced such poor impact resistance that they were "unsuitable for use in spectacles that are intended to provide even minimal impact protection in industrial, sports, or other environments."[4] They also concluded that CR-39 lenses with just scratch resistance coatings do produce adequate protection for these environments.

The weakening of a plastic lens by an AR-coated lens is not limited to CR-39 material. Weakening would be expected to occur in some degree with other lens materials that are softer than the more brittle AR coating.

Effect of Surface Scratches on Impact Resistance

A scratched lens surface reduces impact resistance. The scratch introduces a weak spot on the lens and creates a sort of "fault line." The scratch provides an easy area for stress to build during impact, making breakage more likely. To better imagine how this works, think about how panes of glass are "scored" with a diamond so that they may be broken along the scored line.

Contrary to intuition, scratches on the back surface of a lens will reduce lens impact resistance *more* than front surface scratches. Glass or CR-39 lenses with front surface scratches were reduced in impact resistance by 20%, whereas CR-39 lenses with back surface scratches were reduced in impact resistance by 80%.[5]

GENERAL EYEWEAR CATEGORIES

We can divide eyewear into three broad categories:
- *Dress Eyewear*
  Dress eyewear is eyewear that is designed for everyday use.
- *Safety Eyewear*
  Safety eyewear is designed to meet higher standards of impact resistance since it will be worn in situations that could be potentially hazardous to the eyes.
- *Sports Eyewear*
  Sports eyewear is designed to protect the eyes and/or enhance vision in specific sports situations. What is appropriate will vary dramatically, depending upon the sport.

REQUIREMENTS FOR DRESS EYEWEAR*

There are a number of industry and government agencies that have a direct impact on the business of eyewear. All are important to the dispenser in ensuring that the wearer is receiving a product that is within the expectations of the ophthalmic industry and government regulatory agencies. The following sections list the agencies involved and how they affect the dispensing of eyewear.

Food and Drug Administration

There did not used to be any impact resistance requirements for dress ophthalmic lenses. In most places in the world, there still are not. It is possible to surface glass lenses as thin as 0.3 mm and still have the lenses be wearable. The lenses look wonderfully thin and are still optically excellent. But they afford little protection for the eyes and in many situations end up becoming a hazard to the wearer.

For that very reason, the United States Food and Drug Administration (FDA) began mandating impact resistance for dress ophthalmic lenses in 1971. Since then all eyeglass and sunglass lenses must be impact resistant, except when the optometrist or physician finds that they will not otherwise fulfill the patient's visual requirements. If the lens cannot be rendered impact resistant, this must be recorded in the patient's record, and the patient must also be notified in writing.

---

*Static load testing is where an increasing amount of pressure is applied to the lens until the lens finally breaks.

*Much of the material from this section and the following section on Safety Eyewear is from Brooks CW: Essentials for ophthalmic lens finishing, St.Louis, 2003, Butterworth-Heinemann.

When May Nonimpact-Resistant Lenses Be Dispensed?

Some dispensers may assume that a written agreement having the patient assume responsibility makes it possible to dispense nonimpact resistant lenses. This does not ensure freedom from liability. Here is the way the FDA responds to three frequently asked questions on dispensing nonimpact-resistant lenses.[6]

Q. Under what circumstances may retailers dispense lenses that are not impact resistant?

A. Lenses that are not impact resistant may be dispensed when a physician or optometrist determines that impact-resistant lenses will not fulfill the visual requirements of a particular patient. The physician or optometrist directs this in writing and gives written notification to the patient.

Q. Can a retailer supply a nonimpact-resistant lens if a patient requests it or if the patient/customer agrees to assume all responsibility?

A. No. Nonimpact-resistant lenses may be provided only when the physician or optometrist determines that impact-resistant lenses will not fulfill the visual requirements of the patient.... In such cases the physician or optometrist must give notice in writing to the patient, explaining that the patient is receiving a lens that is not impact resistant.

Q. May a physician or optometrist prescribe nonimpact-resistant lenses for a patient for purely cosmetic reasons?

A. No. If medical problems are related to cosmetic considerations, however, the physician or optometrist may invoke special exemption provision of the regulation based on professional judgment. For example, if the patient's prescription cannot be filled by impact-resistant lenses because the physician or optometrist knows from previous experience that the weight of the heavy lenses may cause headaches, undue pressure on the bridge of the nose or ears, pressure sores, etc., the physician or optometrist may find that the visual requirements of the patient cannot be met by use of impact-resistant lenses.

For lenses to qualify for impact resistance, they must meet certain qualifications.

Must Dress Ophthalmic Lenses Have Minimum Thickness?

Formerly, dress ophthalmic lenses had a minimum thickness requirement of 2.0 mm. Now there is no thickness requirement, regardless of lens material. Impact resistance requirements are performance based, and the lens must be capable of withstanding a predetermined amount of impact. If that requirement can be met with lenses that are thinner than 2.0 mm, the lens is acceptable. Today there are many lenses that can meet current impact resistance requirements and still be below 2.0 mm, including some types of glass lenses.

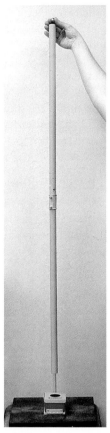

Figure 23-2. A drop-ball tester drops a steel ball on the front surface of a lens from 50 inches.

Impact Resistance Test Requirements

The standard "referee test" for determining impact resistance suitability for dress ophthalmic lenses is the drop ball test. This test is very specific in how it should be administered. However, the FDA states that this does not inhibit the lens manufacturer from using equal or superior test methods to test for impact resistance.

The Drop Ball Test

To be judged acceptable, a lens is first placed front side up on a neoprene gasket. It must be capable of withstanding the impact of a five-eighth-inch steel ball weighing 0.56 oz, dropped from a height of 50 inches (Figure 23-2).

When Should the Drop Ball Test be Performed?

Glass lenses must be tested after the lens has been edged and hardened and before it is placed in the frame. Plastic lenses may be tested in the "uncut-finished" stage before they have been edged.

Drop-Ball Testing of Glass Lenses

With few exceptions, all glass lenses must be hardened *and* individually subjected to the drop ball test. Only lenses that could be damaged by the test are exempt. These lenses must still be hardened, but do not need to be tested. Glass lenses that are exempt from testing are:

1. Raised multifocal lenses (These are lenses that have a ledge area on the lens, such as an Executive lens.)
2. Prism segment multifocals
3. Slab-off lenses
4. Lenticular cataract lenses
5. Iseikonic (size) lenses
6. Depressed-segment one-piece multifocals
7. Biconcave, myodisc, and minus lenticular lenses
8. Custom laminate lenses (such as polarizing lenses)
9. Cement assembly lenses

Individual Versus Batch Testing

Batch testing is the practice of selectively testing a statistically significant number of lenses in a manufactured group. This avoids having to individually test lenses that could sustain damage by the test itself. The practice of batch testing is permitted for:

1. Plastic lenses.
2. Nonprescription lenses, such as mass-produced sunglass lenses.

Glass, plano-powered sunglass lenses that are individually produced in a finishing laboratory must still be individually drop-ball tested.

Who Does Batch Testing?

The lens manufacturer normally does batch testing. When this is done, plastic lenses that are edged in a finishing laboratory do not have to be individually tested or batch tested in the finishing laboratory. Batch testing for semifinished lenses is done for a certain minimum thickness. If these lenses are surfaced to *less* than what was considered minimum thickness, they are no longer within the batch. They would need to be individually tested.

If the lens is altered after having been received from the manufacturer, as when it is sent out for AR coating, then the lens is no longer warranted by the original lens manufacturer. There are a great many types of coatings that could be applied to the lens. Each of these coatings will affect the impact resistance of the lens differently.

Typically the AR coating laboratory will batch test lenses being coated in their laboratory. To do this, they will use lenses of the same material and minimum thickness as those being sent to them for coating. It is the responsibility of the finishing laboratory to be in communication with the company that applies the coating to determine that testing requirements have been fulfilled.

Defining "Manufacturer"

There are a large number of participants involved in the process of making a pair of glasses. One company makes the lenses, another may surface the lenses, a third may edge the lenses, and someone else could coat the lenses. Who then is the manufacturer of the finished eyeglasses? Although in a lawsuit, each participating party is likely to be named, final responsibility lies heavily with the unit that performed the final process on that lens. Here is how the FDA responds to the question.

Q. In terms of the regulation, who is the manufacturer?
A. The manufacturer is the person who puts the lens in the form ready for its intended use or who alters the physical or chemical characteristics of the lens by such acts as grinding, heat treating, beveling, or cutting. For the purpose of this regulation the term "manufacturer" includes a company that imports eyeglasses for resale.[6]

In this chain of manufacturing events, the question of record keeping may arise. Here is how the FDA poses and answers this question.

Q. What are the record keeping requirements on partially finished lenses furnished by one manufacturer for completion by another?
A. Records must be kept to show how lenses were rendered impact resistant, when and how they were tested for impact resistance, and by whom in the processing chain these actions were accomplished.[6]

This means that if the retailer is the manufacturer, then the record keeping requirements of the manufacturer apply. Retailers also have a 3-year requirement of keeping the names and addresses of persons buying prescription eyewear.

The Dispenser's Role in Record Keeping

To ensure that all regulations have been met and that ophthalmic lenses are safe, the FDA requires that records be kept for 3 years after the purchase of eyeglasses. Records that must be kept consist of records of the sale or distribution of prescription eyewear, including the names and addresses of people buying prescription eyewear. (Records do not have to be kept for individuals buying nonprescription eyewear.)

If the dispenser has an in-house laboratory, record keeping requirements for a manufacturer apply. These requirements include:

1. Copies of invoice(s), shipping document(s), and records of sale or distribution.
2. Results of impact-resistance testing (drop-ball test results).
3. A description of the test method and of the test apparatus used.

Federal Trade Commission

The Federal Trade Commission (FTC) was established to prevent unfair business practices, such as deceptive advertising and monopolies. In the 1980s the FTC began to look at the ophthalmic industry. After two series of investigative studies known as Eyeglasses I and Eyeglasses II, prescription release rules were formulated for spectacle and contact lenses. The spectacle lens aspects of these rules will be considered here.

Eyeglasses I

In 1978 the FTC concluded their Eyeglasses I investigative study with a spectacle lens prescription release rule.

This rule requires that patients be given a copy of their spectacle lens prescription so that they may fill that prescription wherever they desire. The prescription is to be given immediately after the eye examination is completed, whether or not the patient asks for the prescription. A new written prescription is also to be given even if the change is too small to require a change in eyeglasses or if there is no change at all since the previous eye examination. The Eyeglasses I prescription release rule listed minimal information to be included in the prescription: sphere power, cylinder power and axis (if any), prism (if any), and the signature of the prescribing optometrist or physician.[7]

Eyeglasses II

In 1989 the FTC did a more complex investigative study that was primarily concerned with restrictions on practice ownership by people who were not optometrists, ophthalmologists, or opticians.

Eyeglasses II rules no longer list minimal information needed for a spectacle lens prescription. Therefore prescribers are at liberty to include whatever they consider important for the patient's visual welfare on the prescription. This could include lens material, specific lens styles, and instructions for wear. For example, suppose a patient has one eye with normal vision and one with very little usable vision. In this instance in which eye protection is important, including polycarbonate lens material on the prescription may reduce the possibility of prescriber liability in the event of eye injury.

An expiration date is usually a part of the prescription. (Although duplication of an existing pair of glasses may be done without restrictions, the dispenser has an ethical obligation to inform such a person of the importance of regular eye examinations. Eye disorders and diseases are not always accompanied by pain and so may not be readily apparent. Contrary to what is often believed, state laws do not set a time limit, such as 2 years, on the length of time an eyeglass prescription may still be filled. "Most states do not have a requirement for an expiration date on spectacle Rx's, although they do not prohibit a doctor from indicating one. Where states do have laws, the concern has been primarily to regulate how short the time limit should be, not how long. In states where this subject is not regulated, it is left to the discretion of the doctor.[8]")

Like Eyeglasses I, Eyeglasses II continues to prohibit disclaimers written on the prescription, such as "Not responsible for accuracy of ophthalmic prescription materials obtained from third-party dispensers."

American National Standards Institute Recommendations for Prescription Ophthalmic Lenses

The main points of the American National Standards Institute (ANSI) Z80.1 recommendations for prescription ophthalmic lenses are summarized in Appendix A.

The ways in which many of these standards are verified are found in Chapter 6.

It must be kept in mind that in the case of prescription lenses, these parameters are recommendations only—not requirements. Practitioners may choose to allow more latitude than the standard requires in some instances, or they may request more accuracy in a given area in other instances. The document itself summarizes it best:

"The standard remains a recommendation. Therefore it is the specific intent of the Z80 Committee that this standard not be used as a regulatory instrument.[9]"

SAFETY EYEWEAR

Safety eyewear has been an extremely important factor in reducing eye injuries. Now that safety eyewear is a must in industry, eye injuries most often occur because of a failure to wear eye protection at the time of the accident or because the wrong kind of eye protection was worn. Today the most likely eye injury situation occurs when workers are wearing safety eyewear without side shields.[10]

ANSI Establishes Safety Eyewear Standards

The standards used for safety lenses and frames are agreed to and put forth by the ANSI. The ANSI Z80.1 standards for prescription eyewear are not a regulatory instrument. However, the ANSI Z87.1 standard for safety eyewear has become just that. Here is how it happened.

OSHA Regulates Safety Eyewear Standards

The Occupational Safety and Health Administration (OSHA) is the federal agency charged with regulating safety practices in the workplace and in educational settings. OSHA rulings have the same power as law. Visits to a workplace are often unannounced, and violations of OSHA regulations discovered at the time of the inspection can result in both mandates to correct the violation and substantial fines.

Rather than beginning anew with a set of eye and face protection requirements OSHA has chosen to adopt the Z87.1 standards already set forth by ANSI as their standards. Therefore the ANSI Z87.1 standards are a federal requirement.

Because it would be difficult to list every situation in which eye protection must be worn, OSHA has instead chosen to place the burden on education and industry by simply stating that "protective eye and face equipment shall be required where there is a reasonable probability of injury that can be prevented by such equipment.[11]"

Impact Requirements for Safety Eyewear

At the time of the writing, the most recent ANSI Z87.1 requirements for safety eyewear were published in August 2003. The previous 1998 standard had a single set of requirements for all safety eyewear. The 2003 standard has two levels of safety standards. One level is called *basic impact*; the other, *high impact*. The Z87.1 1998 standard is identical to the basic impact level for the 2003 standard.

Basic Impact Requirements for Safety Eyewear

Because there are two levels of safety eyewear, why would anyone want to wear a basic-impact lens when high-impact lenses are available?

In a number of work situations, workers are cleaning their glasses constantly (e.g., places with a lot of dust and places in which liquids or mists are present). In these situations, plastic and polycarbonate lenses may scratch. Glass lenses withstand scratching better and will not have to be replaced constantly. Badly scratched lenses are irritating to wear and, if vision is impaired, may create a safety hazard. So even though glass lenses are not able to pass the high impact requirement, in the absence of a material that has the same scratch resistance, basic-impact glass lenses may be the more appropriate lens.

Basic Impact Thickness Requirements

For a number of years, thickness requirements for prescription safety lenses have been a minimum of 3.0 mm. The exception has been for plus lenses that have a power of +3.00 D or higher in the most plus meridian of the distance portion of the lens. The reason for the exception is because high plus lenses are much thicker in the center. Therefore these lenses may be thinned to a 2.5-mm minimum edge thickness and still remain strong because of their overall thickness. These standards remain as thickness requirements for the 2003 basic-impact category of Z87 safety eyewear.

Basic Impact Testing Requirements

The testing requirements for basic-impact safety lenses are similar to those for dress ophthalmic lenses. Dress lenses are required to withstand the impact of a five-eighth-inch steel ball dropped from 50 inches. Basic-impact safety lenses must withstand the impact of a 1-inch steel ball dropped from 50 inches.

Basic Impact Marking Requirements

Basic-impact safety lenses must be marked with the manufacturer's logo or identifying mark. The markings are applied after edging. In-house laboratories that do their own edging of safety lenses must mark the lenses. Marks on the surface of the lens should be out of the line of sight. They usually appear at the center of the top of the lens or in the upper, outer corner. If the lens is other than a clear lens, it may require an additional marking (Figure 23-3). A summary of these marking requirements are found in Table 23-3. Remember, a lens that is thick enough to be classed as a safety lens and strong enough to pass safety lens impact testing is not acceptable as a safety lens until it is marked with the required manufacturer's identification.

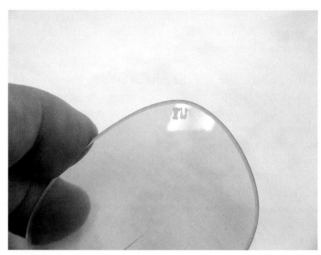

Figure 23-3. The marking identifying a lens as a safety lens.

Warning Labels for Basic-Impact Lenses

Basic-impact safety glasses are not as impact resistant as high-impact safety glasses. The person wearing the lenses needs to know this. Therefore a warning must accompany basic-impact eyewear. That warning is in the form of a notice included with the basic-impact eyewear and is intended for the wearer. The notice must say that the lenses meet the basic impact requirements, but should not be relied upon for protection from high-impact exposure.

High Impact Requirements for Safety Eyewear

Though it may seem opposite to the expected, high impact requirements allow the lenses to be made thinner than basic-impact lenses. However, the tests that high-impact lenses must withstand are more stringent than those for basic-impact lenses.

High Impact Thickness Requirements

The thickness requirement for high-impact safety lenses is a minimum of 2.0 mm. This includes both prescription and nonprescription (plano) safety lenses.

High Impact Testing Requirements

High-impact safety lenses must pass a high velocity impact test. In this test, the lens is mounted on a special holder and must be capable of withstanding the force of a one-fourth-inch steel ball traveling at 150 feet/sec.

High Impact Marking Requirements

High-impact safety lenses are marked in the same manner as basic-impact lenses, except that they are to be additionally marked with a plus (+) symbol, not just the manufacturer's logo (Table 23-4).

Comments on Multilayer Antireflection Coating and Safety Lenses

As previously mentioned, AR coatings generally reduce impact resistance of a lens compared with the impact

TABLE **23-3**
ANSI Z87.1 Lens Marking Requirements

Lens Type	Requirement*	Basic Impact Example	High Impact Example
Clear lenses	Manufacturer's monogram and sometimes +	JO	JO+
Tinted (absorptive) lenses except for special purpose lenses	Manufacturer's monogram, shade number, and sometimes +	JO 2.5	JO+2.5
Photochromic lenses	Manufacturer's monogram, "V" for variable shade, and sometimes +	JO V	JO+V
Special purpose lenses (Special purpose lenses provide eye protection while performing visual tasks that require unusual filtering of light. Examples include didymium-containing lenses, cobalt-containing lenses, uniformly tinted lenses, and lenses prescribed by an eye specialist for particular vision problems.)	Manufacturer's monogram, "S" for special purpose, and sometimes +	JO S	JO+S

*All markings must be legible and permanent and placed so that interference with the vision of the wearer is minimal.

TABLE **23-4**
Safety Lens Requirements

	Basic Impact	High Impact
Thickness	3.0 mm 2.5 mm if power is +3.00 D or greater	2.0 mm
Marking (See also Table 23-3)	Manufacturer's logo	Manufacturer's logo +
Impact testing	1-inch steel ball dropped from 50 inches	1-inch steel ball dropped from 50 inches and ¼-inch steel ball traveling at 150 feet/sec

resistance of that same lens in an uncoated state. The amount of reduction will depend upon the lens material and the type of AR coating used. This is an important factor with safety lenses.

Chou and Hovis[12] tested 2- and 3-mm thick polycarbonate lenses for penetration with an industrial sewing machine needle mounted in a cylindric aluminum carrier. The lenses were tested with and without a multilayer AR coating. (All lenses had scratch-resistant coatings.) They confirmed that polycarbonate lenses are more susceptible to penetration by sharp, high-speed missiles than blunt missiles. They also found that reducing lens center thickness and applying a multilayer AR coating further reduces penetration resistance. Their conclusion was that 2-mm thick polycarbonate lenses and the use of multilayer AR coating on polycarbonate lenses should be discouraged for industrial eye protectors where sharp missile hazards are possible.

In a second article, Chou and Hovis[13] tested the Hoya Phoenix brand of Trivex lenses using a pneumatic gun to propel a 6.35-mm steel ball at the center of 2- and 3-mm thick lenses, with and without multilayer AR coatings. They found that multilayer AR coatings significantly reduce the impact resistance at both dress and industrial

thicknesses. They concluded that when multilayer AR coated, these lenses should not be used in industrial or sports eye protectors, particularly at 2-mm center thickness where there is a high risk of exposure to high-energy impacts.

Safety Frames

In 1989 the ANSI standards for safety frames dropped specific design requirements, including groove design. Instead requirements are performance based. Safety frames must withstand certain specific impact tests that are not required of normal dress frames. Frames are placed on a head model. When impact occurs, the frame cannot break. Nor can the frame or lens come into contact with the eye.

The first test used to test safety frames is the *high velocity impact test*. This test simulates a high velocity, low mass object. In the high velocity impact test, a series of one-fourth-inch steel balls traveling at 150 feet/sec are directed at 20 different parts of the glazed frame* (Figure 23-4). A new frame is used for each impact. Neither the

*A glazed frame is a frame with lenses. In this case the lenses are plano in power.

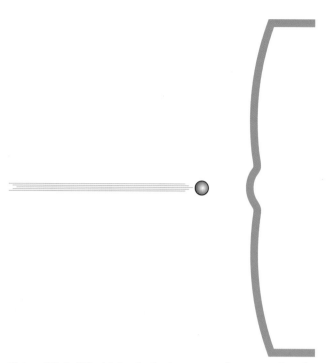

Figure 23-4. The high velocity impact test fires a one-fourth-inch steel ball at 150 feet/sec at a frame or lens.

Figure 23-5. The high mass impact test drops a pointed, 1-inch diameter projectile onto safety eyeglass frames from 51.2 inches to test their suitability for use as Z87 safety frames.

frame nor the lens can break, nor can the lens come out of the frame.

The second test simulates the impact of a large, pointed, slow moving object. In this *high mass impact test*, a pointed, conical-tipped projectile, 1 inch in diameter, weighing 17.6 oz is dropped 51.2 inches through a tube and onto the eyeglasses (Figure 23-5). When the projectile strikes the frame, the lens must not break, nor come out of the frame.

Marking Safety Frames

With safety requirements, a clear distinction between "dress" frames and safety frames must be kept in mind. *Dress* frames are those worn for everyday purposes. No matter how sturdy the construction of a dress frame, it is still not a safety frame unless it passes the required tests and is specifically marked as being a safety frame. Without these markings, the frames are not safety frames. These markings are size, the manufacturer's trademark, and the all-important Z87 or Z87-2 marking on both temples and front, indicating compliance with ANSI Z87 standards.

Safety frames intended for use with 2.0-mm thick high-impact lenses must be tested for 2.0-mm thick lenses. When successfully designed and tested, these frames are marked "Z87-2," instead of just "Z87." The "2" signifies that the frame is suitable for 2-mm lenses (Box 23-1). All frames that are marked Z87-2 must be capable of retaining both basic-impact 3.0 lenses and high-impact 2.0 lenses. Thus all new safety frames can be expected to bear the Z87-2 markings.

BOX 23-1

Safety Frame Marking Requirements

FRONTS
1. A-dimension (eye size)
2. DBL (Distance between lenses)
3. "Z87" to indicate frame compliance with basic-impact standards or Z87-2 to indicate frame compliance with high-impact standards (Z87-2 frames may be used for both basic- and high-impact lenses.)
4. Manufacturer's identifying trademark

TEMPLES
1. Overall length
2. "Z87" to indicate frame compliance with basic-impact standards or Z87-2 to indicate frame compliance with high-impact standards
3. Manufacturer's identifying trademark

Defining Safety Glasses

Safety frames should only be used with safety lenses. Some safety frames are less expensive than regular dress frames. However, *regular lenses must not be put into a safety frame,* even to save the wearer money. A pair of regular

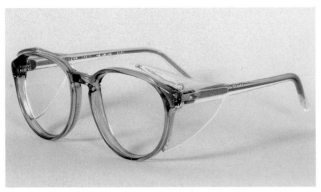

Figure 23-6. Side shields provide protection from flying fragments coming from a different work area and from the immediate area when the wearer turns his or her head.

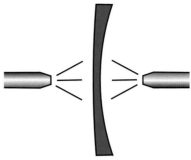

Figure 23-7. When air strikes front and back surfaces of a lens that has been heated just below the softening point, it "freezes" the outside, setting up a controlled internal stress that makes the lens more impact resistant.

"dress" lenses placed in a safety frame may give the wearer the impression that they are wearing safety glasses. A safety frame with dress-thickness lenses is no more safety eyewear than a dress frame with safety lenses. Eyeglasses are not safety glasses until both the frame and lenses are in compliance.

Lenses that are made thicker for added safety should not be placed in a pair of regular frames. If safety is important enough to warrant thick lenses, it is important enough to warrant safety or sports-type frames. "Safety" lenses in regular frames can give the wearer a false sense of security and the mistaken impression that this is a "safe" prescription. *Under no circumstances should a pair of lenses be marked as safety and placed in a nonsafety frame.*

Side Shields

Now that eye protection is required and used in many settings, eye injuries that happen to people wearing safety glasses often occur from the side. There is special attention called to this in the preface to the ANSI Z87.1 2003 safety eyewear standards with the statement, "This standard recognizes the Bureau of Labor Statistics study that revealed the need for angular protection, in addition to frontal protection, in eye and face protectors worn in the occupational setting.[14]"

Side shields may be removable or permanent (Figure 23-6). Most people would rather not wear side shields if given the choice. If side shields are constantly required, then permanent side shields are logical. Removable side shields have the advantage of being able to be taken off when working in a nonhazardous situation. The drawback is that removable side shields often end up not being worn.

Side shields are not universally interchangeable. A removable side shield designed for one particular type of frame cannot be expected to provide the ANSI-standard-approved protection required if used on a different type of frame.

Hardening of Glass Lenses

Glass lenses are not impact resistant enough to pass the FDA-mandated impact test unless they are hardened. There are currently two methods of hardening glass lenses. One uses a heat-treating process and the second a chemical-tempering process. Not all types of glass are capable of being tempered. Glass lenses that are not capable of being hardened may only be used in the United States if no other type of lens material is acceptable for the visual needs of the wearer.

Scratched lenses are more likely to break than unscratched lenses, regardless of the method used to harden a lens. Scratches introduce weak points on the lens. A scratched heat-tempered lens looses more of its impact resistance than a scratched chemically tempered (or *chemtempered*) lens. For maximal safety, scratched lenses should be replaced.

Heat-Treating Process

Heat treating is done by placing the edged glass lens into a small kiln where the temperature is high enough to almost bring the glass to the softening point. The lens is left in the kiln for about 2 or 3 minutes. The exact amount of time depends upon:

1. Lens thickness.
2. Type of glass.
3. Lens tint.

To help determine a still more accurate length of time a lens is left in the kiln, lens weight may also be considered.

The lens is removed from the heat and cooled rapidly by blowing forced air against both front and back surfaces (Figure 23-7).

To understand how this process could cause an increase in impact resistance, remember that as glass heats, it expands and becomes more like a liquid. When the hot lens is struck by cool air against its outer surfaces, the outer surfaces "freeze." The inner part of the lens cools more slowly. As it is cooling, it is trying to contract. But the outer part of the lens is already "frozen" and refuses to shrink further. This creates an inner pull on the lens, inducing stress. Part of the stress is surface compaction or squeezing called *maximum compressive stress*. Another part of the stress is called *maximum tensile stress*. This stress creates strength in the same way that

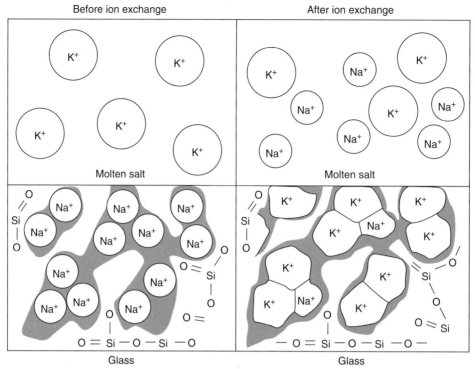

Figure 23-8. In chemtempering, smaller sodium (Na) or lithium (Li) ions from the glass are replaced by larger potassium (K) ions from the molten salt.

the tightened spokes on a bicycle wheel add strength to the rim. These forces result in a compression of the lens surface. The depth from the outside surface of the lens where compressive stress and tensile stress meet is called the *depth of compression.*

The advantage to heat treating is that it is fast. The disadvantage is that the heat-tempered lens is not as impact resistant as a lens that is chemically tempered.

Chemical Tempering

Glass lenses are chemically hardened by immersing them in molten salt. The salt used for clear crown glass and tinted crown glass lenses is potassium nitrate (KNO_3). During the process of chemical tempering, smaller sodium (Na) or lithium (Li) ions from the glass are drawn out of the lens surface and replaced by larger potassium (K) ions from the salt (Figure 23-8). This crowds the surface, setting up a surface tension that "squeezes" the lens. This surface tension increases impact resistance by creating compressive stresses. The actual amount of compressive stress is 28 to 50 kg/mm², compared with 6 to 14 kg/mm² for heat-tempered glass.[15]

The salt used to temper a photochromic lens is different from the salt used for crown glass lenses. Salt used for photochromic lenses is a mixture of 40% sodium nitrate ($NaNO_3$) and 60% potassium nitrate (KNO_3). Both of these salts are hazardous in dry or molten states. Salts are available in both commercial and reagent grades. Reagent grade is more expensive, but being purer, does not require conditioning and prevents salt-related problems.

If the proportion between salts is incorrect or if the salt is contaminated or has been used too long, the lenses will have problems. Lenses may break in the bath, come out hazy, or show hairline cracks. Processing a crown glass lens in a salt bath intended for photochromic lenses will cause the lens to craze, showing a meshwork of hairline surface cracks (Figure 23-9).

Salt needs to be replaced on a regular basis. As salt pH rises above neutral, some salt should be removed and replaced with new salt to lower the pH. When sediment builds up in the bottom of the tank, all of the salt should be replaced.

To chemically temper crown and tinted glass lenses together, the temperature of the salt is 450° C ± 5° C (842° F ± 9° F). To temper photochromic glass lenses, the salt is heated to 400° C ± 5° C (752° F ± 9° F).[16]

If the temperature of the bath is not exact, there will be problems with photochromic lenses being off-color, splotching, or not lightening or darkening properly.

The Chemical Tempering Process. Lenses are cleaned and placed in a lens holder. That holder is held above the bath to allow the lenses to preheat, preventing breakage caused by extreme temperature changes. The lenses are then immersed in the molten salt bath for 16 hours.* (By using a special process it is possible to

---

*It is possible to leave the lenses over the weekend for 64 hours. Impact resistance drops slightly, but the amount of drop is normally insignificant.

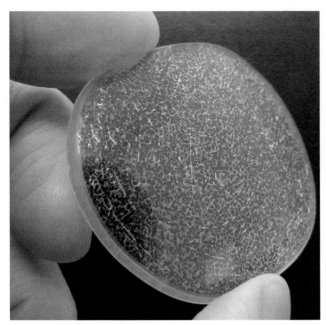

Figure 23-9. A crown glass lens mistakenly placed in a photochromic salt bath will craze.

chemically harden standard photochromic lenses in 2 hours.*) At the end of the cycle, the lenses are again held above the bath. The postbath cool times are the same as the preheat times. Lenses are then removed from the unit, allowed to cool at room temperature, then rinsed in hot water to remove the salt.

Chemically hardened crown glass lenses are more impact resistant than thermally hardened crown glass lenses and maintain their strength better, even when scratched. They will not warp during the chemical tempering process, as do some lenses during the heat-tempering process. Because their internal tensile stress is less than that of a heat-tempered lens, chemtempered lenses may be re-edged or resurfaced without breaking.

If a pair of chemically tempered glass lenses has been removed from a broken frame and reshaped for a new frame, the lenses should be rehardened. (Heat-tempered lenses should never be re-edged on an edger or hand edger unless they have been dehardened† first.)

Compared with heat tempering, chemical tempering of crown glass lenses is clearly the method of choice.

Determining Whether a Glass Lens Has Been Hardened

Determining if a lens has been heat treated is possible by viewing it between two crossed polarizing filters. An instrument with a light source and two crossed polarizing filters made for this purpose is called a *colmascope* or *polariscope*. Viewed through a colmascope, a heat-treated lens will show a Maltese-cross pattern (Figure 23-10). A perfectly shaped Maltese-cross pattern does not mean that the lens is any more impact resistant than a lens showing a misshapen Maltese cross. Rotating the lens while viewing it though the colmascope will cause the Maltese cross to change in appearance anyway. This pattern shows up because surface compression in a heat-treated lens is nonuniform.[17]

Chemically tempered lenses have an even surface compression and therefore show no stress patterns when viewed through crossed polarizing filters. A chemically tempered lens can only be identified by taking the lens out of the frame and immersing it in a glycerin solution while viewing it between crossed polarizing filters. A chemically hardened lens will show a halolike, bright band around the edge of the lens. Because of the time-consuming inconvenience of this process, everyone depends upon the notification enclosed with the finished spectacle lenses as ensurance that the lens has been chemically hardened.

Effect of Re-edging of Glass Lenses on Impact Resistance

Edging a plastic lens does not significantly affect impact resistance. However, edging or re-edging a glass lens that has already been hardened will affect impact resistance. May a hardened glass lens be re-edged and then worn? Here is the FDA's response to the question.

Q. May a glass lens, after it has been chemically or thermally treated for impact resistance, be processed further in any way?

A. Lenses that are treated for impact resistance by induced surface compression may be re-edged or modified for power. However, the beneficial effects of surface compression may be substantially reduced. Such lenses must be retreated and tested before they are dispensed to the patient.[6]

Effect of Drilling and Grooving on Glass Lens Impact Resistance

Drilled glass lenses that are heat treated are not safe to wear. They may pass the drop ball test in their unmounted state, but the compounded stress brought about by the mounting causes the mounted lenses to fail too easily.

Drilled lenses that are chemically tempered will pass the drop ball test and are not as affected by drill mounting as are heat-treated lenses. Nevertheless, glass lenses are seldom used in a drill mounting, even when chemically tempered.

In fact glass lenses are seldom used with grooved lenses either. In 1993 Optical Laboratories Association Technical Director George Chase addressed the glass lens grooving and drilling issue in an OLA Tech Topics paper. He indicated that even though drilled and grooved

---

*The 2-hour photochromic process is used for PhotoGray Extra, PhotoBrown Extra, PhotoGray II, and PhotoSun II.
It may not be used for PhotoGray, PhotoBrown, PhotoSun, PhotoGray Extra 16, or PhotoBrown Extra 16.
†A heat-tempered lens is "dehardened" by heating it as if it were to be heat tempered again. When the lens comes out of the furnace, the cold air is turned off and the lens allowed to cool slowly.

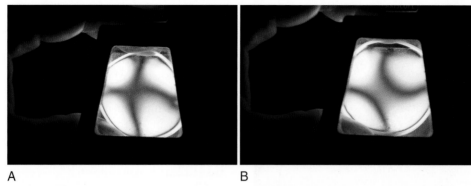

A   B

Figure 23-10. **A** and **B,** A heat-treated lens may be identified by the characteristic Maltese-cross pattern seen when the lens is viewed through the crossed polarizing filter of a colmascope. The symmetry of the Maltese-cross pattern is not the important factor. As a lens is rotated, the pattern seen will vary, as seen in the above two photos of the same lens seen in two different angles of rotation between the polarizing films.

TABLE **23-5**
ASTM Standards Applicable to Ophthalmic Dispensing

Standard Identification Number	Year of Revision	Sports Covered by the Standard
ASTM F513	2000	Standard specification for eye and face protective equipment for hockey players
ASTM F659	1998	Standard specification for skier goggles and face shields
ASTM F803	2003	Standard specification for eye protectors for selected sports
		These sports are listed as racquet sports (such as racquetball, badminton, and tennis), women's lacrosse, field hockey, basketball, baseball, and soccer
ASTM F910	2004	Standard specification for face guards for youth baseball
ASTM F1587	1999, reapproved 2005	Standard specification for head and face protective equipment for ice hockey goaltenders
ASTM F1776	2001	Standard specification for eye protective devices for paintball sports

glass lenses would normally pass the drop ball test, the unprotected, exposed lens edges were likely to chip or microcrack with normal use, reducing impact strength. If drilled or grooved glass lenses are to be made, the OLA encourages optical laboratories to first obtain a waiver from the person ordering the lenses.[18] If the laboratory wants a waiver from the dispenser, it is a clear indication that the dispenser should not be using glass lenses for a drill mount or groove mounted frame.

EYE PROTECTION FOR SPORTS

The appropriate selection of eyewear for sports is increasingly important. Correct eyewear selection may improve performance in the sport and at the same time protect the wearer. At the present time, there are only certain standards specifically designed for sports eye protection.

An increase in litigation following eye injuries has served to raise the consciousness of eye care practitioners who are now more aware of the need for providing appropriate information on eye protection customized to patient needs.

American Society for Testing and Materials

As the name implies, the American Society for Testing and Materials (ASTM) develops standards for testing and for materials. There are several ASTM standards that apply to ophthalmic dispensing. These are shown in Table 23-5.

These standards describe tests that must be used to evaluate the ability of the eyewear to withstand and protect from the impact of common equipment used in the chosen sport. Examples would be balls and rackets.

The standard most often encountered in an eye care practice is the F803 standard. This is called *F803 standard specification for eye protectors for selected sports.* It is especially applicable since it applies to many of the most popular sports, such as baseball, basketball, soccer, and tennis.

ASTM Product Marking

ASTM sports eyewear product marking includes (1) marking on the eyewear, (2) a label or tag, and (3) specific warnings about product use.

Marking on the Eyewear. ASTM standards include required product marking. For example,[19] all ASTM F803-approved eyewear must be marked with:

1. The manufacturer's identity marking.
2. The eye protector model identity.
   Label or Tag. In addition, it should include a label or tag with the following information:
1. Week and year of manufacture
2. The protector size and also guidance concerning the age and gender of the wearer that the protector has been designed for
3. A clear statement on the package as to the sport or sports for which the protector was designed
   Specific Warnings to Accompany ASTM-Approved Eyewear. There should be specific warnings listed. (These warnings are important for dispensers to know because they are generally applicable for safety and sport eyewear). Warnings include, but are not limited to, the following:
1. Lenses should be replaced when scratches become troublesome or if cracks appear at the edges.
2. If the eye protector is severely impacted, short of failure, then the degree of protection provided will be reduced, and the eye protector must be replaced. Failure to do so may result in permanent injuries to the eye.
3. If a lens pops out because of impact during play, the wearer should stop playing and have the protector replaced.
4. If the eye protector is stored at cold temperatures, it should be allowed to return to room temperature before use.
5. Instruction as to the cleaning and antifog agents that may be used should also be included.
   There is not just one type of protector that is intended for F803 protection. F803 protection can be in 4 different types. These are listed in Box 23-2.
   Other Cautions With Sports Eyewear. Frames that are designed to be worn with lenses should not be worn without lenses even if designed for safety or sport. Small, fast moving balls may elongate and penetrate the empty lens opening, even if the opening is smaller than the ball.

When even a large ball, such as a soccer ball, strikes the eye, the blunt trauma can produce a shock wave impact that causes the eyeball to distort then rebound with a large amount of force resulting in severe damage. So even though a large ball would not seem like it would be able to damage an eye surrounded by the bony structure of the skull, it still can. Sports eyewear protection is still important.

If spectacle lenses are worn under protective eyewear, then polycarbonate lenses should be worn in the spectacles.

Custom Eyewear Needs for Individual Sports

Each sport has certain unique visual demands. Some demands may be met by simply providing appropriate sunglasses. Others may require a specialized prescription that includes a uniquely positioned multifocal segment. A number of sports and their hazards and problems are listed in Table 23-6, along with recommended solutions. Yet as with occupational needs, there is not always a single "cookbook answer" for every individual's sports vision needs. Each situation should be discussed and any corrective or protective eyewear designed to meet the needs of that particular individual. However, there are certain common themes that recur in sports eyewear.

Themes in Sports Eyewear

Sports eyewear can be confusing because of the large number of sports and sports situations possible. Here are some general statements about sports eyewear that help in getting an overall picture:

- Virtually all sports demand highly impact-resistant lenses made from such materials as polycarbonate.
- Helmets are required when there is danger of head injury.
- Outdoor sports call for UV protection, and when intense sunlight is a factor, sun lenses are appropriate.
- Most sports using round balls call for ASTM F803-approved protectors. These include baseball, basketball, soccer, and any racquet sports, such as tennis or badminton.
- Underwater sports for those dependent upon their prescription need special in-mask or in-goggle prescription adaptations.
- Billiards and pistol shooting may require prescription changes.
- Golf, flying, and shooting may require relocation of multifocal segments and/or optical centers.
- Bicycling and billiards may require changes in the positioning of the frame front.

PROVIDING BEST CHOICES AND PREVENTING LIABILITY

The Dispenser's Obligation in Helping Choose the Most Appropriate Product

The process of dispensing eyewear is one that involves helping the wearer choose the best product for a particular need. This may include absorptive lenses, high-index and aspheric lenses, specialized multifocal lenses, eyewear for certain sports or hobbies, or protective eyewear. Thus

BOX 23-2	
Four Types of F803 Sport Protectors	
Type I	The front piece is molded as one unit—lens or lenses and front together
Type II	A unit with lens(es) separate from the frame front and then assembled; the lenses are either plano or prescription lenses
Type III	A protector without a lens
Type IV	A full or partial face shield

TABLE 23-6

Problems, Hazards, and Recommended Solutions for Sports Eyewear

Problems and Hazards	Recommended Solutions
BADMINTON	
1. Danger from birdie and racquet.	1. Wear ASTM F803-approved sports protectors with polycarbonate lenses.
2. Brightness of outdoor environment.	2. Use sun lenses when appropriate.
BASEBALL	
1. Hazard of ocular injury from the ball.	1. Batters should wear a batting helmet with attached face shield. Others should wear ASTM F803-approved sports protectors with polycarbonate lenses when playing other positions. Little League players can use a reduced injury factor ball.[24] Youth baseball use ASTM F910 standard specification for face guards when appropriate.
2. Brightness of outdoor environment.	2. Wear sun lenses when appropriate.
BASKETBALL	
1. Eye hazard from other player's fingers, elbows, etc.	1. Wear ASTM F803-approved basketball protectors with polycarbonate lenses.
BICYCLING[25]	
1. Head or eye injury from a fall.	1. Wear a bicycle helmet. Use strong frames with polycarbonate lenses.
2. Dust, sand, or small object blown into the eyes.	2. For nonprescription eyewear, wraparound frames and lenses are helpful. Drop-in frame fronts may be added, if desired.
3. UV radiation.	3. Add UV protection to glasses (will be included with polycarbonate lenses).
4. Inability to see vehicles from behind without looking backward.	4. Use special small mirror mounted on the spectacle frame.
5. Brightness of outdoor environment.	5. Wear sunglasses when appropriate.
6. Bent-over position forces eyeglass wearers to look over the top of their frames.	6. Select frames that can be set high on the face. Use adjustable pads and adjust the glasses high.
BILLIARDS	
1. Viewing the ball on the table must be done through the very tops of the lenses.	1. For conventional frames, choose a frame that is high on the face, has a thin upper rim, and may be adjusted upward. Use a frame specially designed for billiards. Such a frame is thin rimmed, sits high on the face, and has retroscopic tilt.
2. Presbyopia can keep the field of view unclear.	2. Prescribe a small amount of additional plus power. Since most viewing is done 1-2 meters away, the additional plus required may be as small as +0.25 D, but usually not greater than +0.75 D.[26] This can be given in the form of a distance prescription increased in plus by this amount. If bifocals are used in this same lens, the bifocal segment should be low set, and the add power decreased in plus by an equal amount to compensate for the increased plus found in the distance.
BOATING	
1. Glare from the water.	1. Use a polarizing lens, which also blocks UV light.
2. There is intensified UV radiation from both overhead and reflected UV light.	2. Use a sunglass lens that cuts out all UV light below 400 nm. Wear a hat with a brim or a visor.
3. Glasses that drop from the face or are knocked off will sink and be lost.	3. Use a well-fitting frame, possibly one that has cable temples. Consider using an athletic strap when boating. Some have used floats that attach to the temples.
FLYING	
1. Overhead dials and gauges are difficult to read with a normal presbyopic correction.	1. Inform the pilot of the existence of occupational double-segment lenses. However, many presbyopic pilots prefer progressive addition lenses. Progressive addition lenses are a good choice because of the various distances at which near gauges and dials must be viewed.

TABLE **23-6**
Problems, Hazards, and Recommended Solutions for Sports Eyewear—cont'd

Problems and Hazards	Recommended Solutions
2. Bright daylight flying reduces dark adaptation at night.	2. Use sunglasses with frames that are large and have short vertex distances or that wrap around. Select lenses that transmit 10%-15% of the light. Do not use polarizing lenses.
FOOTBALL[24] 1. Eye injury from the ball or other players.	1. Wear an approved helmet with face guard or cage. Additional protection is possible using eye protection, such as Liberty's Helmet Specs worn under the helmet and behind the guard or cage.
GOLF 1. Bifocals and other normal presbyopic corrections may interfere with viewing the ball during swing.	1. Use single vision lenses. Use one, small round bifocal segment only: for right-handed players, on right; for left-handed players, on left. Position segment either in extreme upper temporal corner or extreme lower temporal corner. (It is best to mark the glazed lenses with a colored marking pen where the segment will be positioned. Have the wearer use a golf club and simulate the playing situation ahead of time.)
2. Frame interferes with vision.	2. Use thin-rimmed, rimless, or nylon cord frames. Avoid frames with thick, wide temples.
3. UV exposure.	3. Wear a hat with a brim or visor. Add UV protection to glasses.
4. Brightness of outdoor environment.	4. Wear sun lenses when appropriate, but know that some golfers avoid sunglasses because of interference with viewing the contour of the course. Know that polarizing lenses will decrease the golfer's ability to read the contour of the course. Polarizing lenses for golf may not be appropriate or appreciated.
HANDBALL 1. Danger from ball.	1. Use ASTM F803-approved sports eye protectors with polycarbonate lenses.
HOCKEY: ICE[24] 1. Danger from pucks and sticks.	1. Use helmet with full-face wire or polycarbonate face protector approved by the ASTM F513 standard for Eye and Face Protective Equipment for Hockey Players or by the Canadian Standards Association. Avoid half shields and form-fitting goalie masks.
HOCKEY: STREET, FLOOR, OR FIELD[24] 1. Danger from pucks and sticks.	1. Use helmet with full-face wire or polycarbonate face protector approved by the ASTM F513 standard for Eye and Face Protective Equipment for Hockey Players or by the Canadian Standards Association. Use ASTM F803-approved eye protectors with polycarbonate lenses.
LACROSSE: WOMEN'S 1. Danger from ball and players' sticks.	1. Use ASTM F803-approved eye protectors intended for women's lacrosse with polycarbonate lenses.
2. Brightness of outdoor environment.	2. Wear polycarbonate sun lenses in conjunction with protective eyewear when appropriate.
MOTORCYCLING[25] 1. Head and/or eye injury from a fall.	1. Wear a motorcycle helmet with face shield. If helmets are not used, vented goggles should be. Venting is to prevent fogging.
2. Dust, sand, or small object blown into the eyes.	2. Use strong frames and polycarbonate lenses. Wraparound frames and lenses are helpful.
3. UV radiation.	3. Add UV protection to glasses (will be included with polycarbonate lenses).
4. Brightness of outdoor environment.	4. Wear sun lenses when appropriate.

Continued

TABLE 23-6

Problems, Hazards, and Recommended Solutions for Sports Eyewear—cont'd

Problems and Hazards	Recommended Solutions
MOUNTAIN CLIMBING	
1. Increased exposure to UV radiation because of less atmospheric absorption.	1. Use UV-absorbing goggles that eliminate all wavelengths below 400 nm.
2. Brightness of outdoor environment.	2. For high altitudes where brightness is especially excessive, use sun lenses with approximately 5% transmission and a wraparound design or use sunglasses with side shields (often leather).[26]
PAINTBALL	
1. Danger of paintball injury to eyes.	1. Wear ASTM F1776 eye protective devices for paintball sports.
RACQUETBALL	
1. Danger from ball and opponent's racquet.	1. Use ASTM F803-approved eye protectors intended for racquetball with polycarbonate lenses.
RIDING[24]	
1. When riding in other than open areas: brush or twigs.	1. Use polycarbonate lenses. (Riding helmets should conform to ASTM standards, but do not include eye protection.)
2. UV exposure.	2. If dress eyewear is worn for riding, polycarbonate lenses should be chosen.
3. Brightness of outdoor environment.	3. Wear sun lenses when appropriate.
RUNNING	
1. Sweating and slipping eyeglasses.	1. Use a sweatband. Use comfort cable temples or an eyeglass headband. For low prescription powers try simply not wearing eyeglasses.
2. Fogging.	2. Be certain that the frames do not ride on the cheeks. If eyeglasses are not antireflection coated, use an antifogging agent.
3. UV exposure.	3. Wear a hat with a brim or visor. Add UV protection to glasses or wear sunglasses with UV protection.
SHOOTING: PISTOL[27]	
1. Danger of reverse discharge of powder.	1. Use polycarbonate lenses.
2. Need for large field of view.	2. Use large (even 62-mm A dimension and above) metal aviator frames.
3. Need for improved contrast and/or reduced glare.	3. Traditional shooter preference for overcast days is an amber tint. This is not a recommendation, since there is no proven correlation between shooting performance and an amber tint. For those who so desire, Corning makes a Serengeti lens designed specifically for the competition shooter called Vector. It is available in "sport orange" for all-weather use and "sport vermilion" for heavily overcast and misty days. Both are photochromic, antireflection coated, and are available in plano or prescription. Each shooting situation should be evaluated and judgment made on individual need using the principles outlined in Chapter 22.
4. Pistol shooting has a unique need for focusing on the pistol sights rather than on the target. This can be troublesome for presbyopes.	4. Early presbyopes should use a specifically designed device that is mounted to spectacle frames. It consists of a diaphragm mounted before the dominant eye and an occluder mounted before the nondominant eye. As an alternative, punch a 1- to 2-mm hole through a piece of electrical tape using a 1/32-inch nail. Mount the tape with pinhole directly in the line of sight. Late presbyopes should use an add power prescribed for the distance from the spectacle plane to the pistol sights. For accuracy it is more important for the sight to be in focus than the target. That add may be fit as: a. A single vision "near Rx." b. A bifocal mounted very high on the sighting, eye (in a shooting stance the sight is seen through the bifocal and the upper part of the target is viewed through the distance lens). c. An add lens mounted in the flip-up portion of a double-front frame. The nondominant eye usually has an occluder in the flip-up portion.

TABLE 23-6
Problems, Hazards, and Recommended Solutions for Sports Eyewear—cont'd

Problems and Hazards	Recommended Solutions
SHOOTING: RIFLE[27]	
1. Danger of reverse discharge of powder.	1. Use polycarbonate lenses.
2. Blurring of the front sight of the rifle. (Some presbyopes are bothered by this problem.)	2. Convert to a telescopic sight where no accommodation is required.
3. Need for improved contrast or reduced glare.	3. See Shooting: pistol.
4. The dominant eye does not correspond to the dominant hand, making sighting with the dominant eye impossible.	4. Specially designed gun stocks are available.
SHOOTING: SHOTGUN[27]	
1. Danger of reverse discharge of powder.	1. Use polycarbonate lenses.
2. Stock jolts against frame.	2. Do not fit frame too low. Choose a frame with a flat lower edge.
3. Need for improved contrast or reduced glare.	3. See Shooting: pistol.
4. During aiming the line of sight passes through the upper nasal part of the lens and, for lenses with high distance powers, causes a prismatic effect that may create problems. Some progressive addition lenses may be problematic when viewing through this upper nasal section of the lens.	4. Use contact lenses, or if spectacles are used, mark the location of the line of sight on the spectacle lens and have the laboratory place the optical center of the lens at this location. (To prevent binocular problems, the optical center of the other lens must be moved to the same vertical position and outward temporally to achieve the binocular interpupillary distance.) If progressive addition lenses are to be worn, avoid using the softer design progressive addition lenses that allow asphericity to flow into the upper peripheral areas of the lens.
SKIING	
1. Exposure to UV radiation resulting in "snow blindness" (burning and photophobia from photokeratitis).	1. Use lenses that eliminate all wavelengths below 400 nm.
2. Wind and flying snow.	2. Wear ASTM F659 approved ski goggles. Some are designed to hold prescription lenses. Some have double lenses to reduce fogging.
3. Blurring from bifocal or trifocal segments for presbyopes.	3. Use a single vision lens. To reduce fogging, use lens materials other than glass. Glass is also not appropriate since lenses with higher impact resistance should be used.
4. Brightness of outdoor environment.	4. Protective sun lenses are appropriate. It may be helpful to avoid polarizing lenses. Some skiers believe that it hinders judgment of snow conditions. Also as the body tilts, the polarizing lenses will vary in their absorption of horizontally polarized light.
SNORKELING AND SCUBA DIVING[28]	
1. Eyeglass prescription needed to see clearly.	1a. Use a removable mask insert. The insert is like a "frame front" that attaches to the front surface of the mask.
	1b. Cement lenses to inside of mask as follows: With the mask in place, mark the front of the mask as if taking monocular interpupillary distances as described in Chapter 3. Calculate the correct lens power for the vertex distance from the eye to the face mask surface (see Chapter 14). Order lenses for the corrected distance prescription with plano front base curves. (Minus lenses work well, but plus lenses have problems because, with plano front curves, they would essentially be worn backward.) Cement the lenses to the inside of the mask with clear epoxy or UV curing cement.
2. The inside of the mask fogs.	2. Use an antifogging lens cleaner. (Note: Some antifogging agents may evaporate into the mask chamber and cause eye irritation or even corneal erosion.[29] If agents are used, they should be allowed to dry thoroughly before wearing the mask or goggles.)
3. Presbyopes encounter difficulty seeing near objects clearly.	3. Use a specially designed multilens or bifocal mask. The multilens mask has distance and near prescription in the mask, whereas the bifocal mask has only near lenses in the lower half. Bond a near add lens to the lower left-hand side of the mask.

Continued

TABLE 23-6

Problems, Hazards, and Recommended Solutions for Sports Eyewear—cont'd

Problems and Hazards	Recommended Solutions
SOCCER	
1. Danger from ball or collisions with other players.	1. Use ASTM F803-approved protective eyewear for soccer with polycarbonate lenses.
SQUASH	
1. Danger from ball and opponent's racquet.	1. Use the appropriate ASTM F803-approved eye protectors.
SWIMMING	
1. Water gets in the eyes and water changes the refractive power of normal spectacles, making underwater wear of normal spectacles unproductive.	1. Use swimming goggles. Goggles may be fit with powered lenses. Base curves of lenses in contact with water must be plano to retain the intended power characteristics both above and below the water. Order goggles with interchangeable, premanufactured refractive power (usually minus-powered spherical equivalents). Contact lenses may be worn underneath plano goggles.
2. Swim goggles fog up.	2. Use a goggle with back-surface antifogging properties. (See also under Snorkeling and Scuba Diving above.)
TENNIS	
1. Danger from ball and racquet.	1. Use the appropriate ASTM F803-approved eye protectors with polycarbonate lenses.
2. Brightness of outdoor environment.	2. Wear polycarbonate sun lenses when appropriate.
VOLLEYBALL	
1. Being hit with the ball.	1. Use ASTM F803-approved protective eyewear with polycarbonate lenses.
2. When played outdoors, bright sunlight and reflections from sand or water can be a hindrance and a hazard from UV exposure.	2. Use polycarbonate sun lenses with UV protection in an appropriate F803 protector.
WATER SKIING	
1. Water spray gets in eyes.	1. Use a goggle similar to a swim goggle but with holes in the sides to prevent fogging. Use swimming goggles and drill 3/16- to ¼-inch holes temporally in the sides.
WRESTLING	
1. Eye protection currently not conducive to the sport.	1. Monocular individuals or individuals with good correctable acuity in one eye only should avoid wrestling.[24]

(*Note:* When polycarbonate material is listed, it should be noted that there may be other highly impact resistant material that may also be suitable.)

it becomes the responsibility of the dispenser to provide each individual with sufficient information so that an informed decision may be made. The dispenser has a "duty to inform" about the availability of eyewear alternatives that provide optimal eye safety in the particular wearing conditions applicable for that individual.

When lawsuits involving eyewear occur, the case is usually made on the basis of either product liability or negligence.[20]

Product Liability

Product liability means that the product was not up to accepted standards. What those standards are depends on the type of eyewear.

- For dress eyewear, determine if the drop ball test was administered when appropriate.
- For safety eyewear, the critical factor is determining if Z87 standards were met—particularly thickness standards.
- For sports eyewear, the critical factor is faulty design or failure to meet impact resistance expectations. If ASTM standards are appropriate, was this type of eyewear chosen so that those standards were met?

Negligence

To prove negligence, it must be shown that, "the defendant practitioner did not conform to the standard of care expected of like practitioners acting under the same or similar circumstances. Practitioners are expected to exercise reasonable prudence and demonstrate the minimum degree of learning and skill possessed by members of the profession in good standing.[20"]

In the case of a dispenser this would include:

- Failure to recommend the most appropriate material.
- Failure to inform the wearer about decreased impact resistance of other materials compared with the most suitable material.
- Failure to verify that materials received were in accordance with standards required for materials ordered.

Responsibility for Recommending the Most Appropriate Lens Material

One of the most important decisions an eyeglass wearer will make relates to the safety of the product. According to Classé,[20,21] there are five general classes of persons for whom safety is of great importance. These are the following:

1. Monocular individuals (For sports an individual should be considered as "monocular" if the weaker eye has a corrected visual acuity of less than 20/40.)
2. Athletes
3. Children
4. People with occupations that put them at risk for ocular injury
5. Individuals whose eyes have a reduced capacity to withstand ocular trauma, including aphakes and pseudophakes, high myopes, those who have undergone refractive surgery, and those who have had previous eye injuries

It is the dispenser's responsibility to identify these individuals, make them aware of their need for eye protection, and recommend the most impact-resistant lens material available. In some cases this will involve recommending a certain type of frame as well.

Whether or not the practitioner deems the prospective lens wearer in need of high-impact-resistant lenses, each person should be informed of the availability of the safest lens product. The person can then make a personal decision on the matter.

Suppose a person is not informed of the availability of the safest lens product and subsequently has a severe eye injury. In such a case it is easy for the wearer to say, "If I had been told about this lens, I would have chosen it, and this would never have happened to me."

In instances where a person has an eye examination but requires no refractive correction, the examiner who takes a thorough case history will note the need for protective eyewear. If protective eyewear is needed, that need is not limited to full-time eyeglass wearers. The need for safety or sports eyewear includes the need for plano safety or sports eyewear.

If a prescriber strongly believes that a certain lens material should be used for a given eyewear function,

then that material should be written on the prescription, making it required.

To prevent liability, everyone purchasing eyewear should be informed of the safest lens products.

Responsibility for Recommending Safety or Sports Frames

If eyeglasses are to be worn for contact sports or for activities hazardous to eyes, wearers need to know about options available. If these options are not brought to the wearer's attention, the wearer may assume that his or her "dress wear" frames and lenses will provide all the protection needed.

The following are some situations that may require safety or sports eyewear[22]:

- Working with lawn or garden equipment, such as string trimmers, shredders, or chain saws
- Working with shop equipment, such as power saws, drills, or grinders
- Working with hazardous liquids, such as acids or alkalis or with sprayers
- Engaging in contact sports or sports using balls or racquets

It should be obvious that anytime a safety frame is needed, impact resistance in a lens is also of highest priority.

Any lens or frame safety information explained to the wearer should be noted in the record and dated, as should the wearer's final selection of lens material and frame.

Responsibility to Inspect the Finished Product

When newly fabricated spectacles are returned from the laboratory, it is the dispenser's responsibility to inspect the finished product. If the lens is classified as a safety or sports product, it must comply with all the requirements outlined by ANSI or ASTM standards.

It is to be expected that if an eye injury occurs, all these factors will be checked for the injured by their legal council. If any ANSI or ASTM standards are unmet, it is obvious that either (a) an inspection was never done, or (b) that inspection was done incompetently or inadequately.

REFERENCES

1. Chaffin R: Trivex: a new category of lens material, Opti World 30(243):34, 2001.
2. www.nxt-vision.com, 2005, Intercast.
3. Corzine JC, Greer RB, Bruess RD et al: The effects of coatings on the fracture resistance of ophthalmic lenses, Optom Vis Sci 73:8, 1996.
4. Chou R, Hovis JK: Durability of coated CR-39 industrial lenses, Optom Vis Sci 80(10):703-707, 2003.
5. Torgersen D: Impact resistance questions and answers, OLA Tech Topic p 4, 1998.
6. Snesko WN, Stigi JF: Impact resistant lenses questions and answers, HHS Publication FDA 87-4002, U.S. Department of Health and Human Services, Public Health

Service, Food and Drug Administration, Center for Devices and Radiological Health, Rockville, Md, 1987.

7. Classé JG, Harris MG: "Doctor, I want a copy of my . . ." how to handle requests for Rx's and records in the light of eyeglasses II, Optom Manage 24:19, 1989.

8. Bruneni, JL: Ask the labs, Eyecare Business p 28, 1998.

9. ANSI Z80.1-2005 American national standard for ophthalmic- prescription ophthalmic lenses- recommendations, Optical Laboratories Association, Fairfax, VA, 2006, Fairfax, Va, 2006, Optical Laboratories Association.

10. Eye protection in the workplace, U.S. Department of Labor Program Highlight, Fact Sheet No. OSHA 93-03, GPO: 1993 0-353-374

11. General Industry, OSHA Safety and Health Standard (29 CFR 1910), Washington, DC, 1981, U.S. Department of Labor, Occupational Safety and Health Administration.

12. Chou BR, Hovis JK: The effect of multiple antireflective coatings and center thickness on resistance of polycarbonate spectacle lenses to penetration by pointed missiles, Optom Vis Sci 82(11):964-969, 2005.

13. Chou BR, Hovis JK: Effect of multiple antireflection coatings on impact resistance of Hoya Phoenix spectacle lenses, Clin Exp Optom 89(2): 2006.

14. American national standard practice for occupational and educational personal eye and face protection devices, Z87.1-2003, Des Plaines, Ill, 2003, American National Standards Institute Inc, American Society of Safety Engineers.

15. Krauser RP: Chemtempering today, Corning, NY, 1974, Corning Glass Works.

16. Chemtempering photochromics, publication OPO-5-3/79MA, Corning, NY, Corning Glass Works.

17. Wilson-Powers B: Chemtempering photochromic lenses, Opt Manage 8(5):39, 1979.

18. Chase G: OLA Tech Topic 1993. (As quoted by Torgersen D: Impact resistance questions and answers, OLA Tech Topic p 4, 1998.)

19. F803-03, Standard specification for eye protectors for selected sports, West Conshohocken, Pa, ASTM International.

20. Classé JG: Legal aspects of sports vision, Optom Clin 3:27, 1993.

21. Classé JG: Legal aspects of sports-related ocular injuries, Int Ophthalmol Clin 28:213, 1988.

22. Woods TA: The role of opticianry in preventing ocular injuries, Intl Ophthalmol Clin 28:251, 1988.

23. Lee G: Sorting out those confusing ophthalmic lens options, Optom Manage 26:45, 1991.

24. Vinger PF: Prescribing for contact sports, Optom Clin, Sports Vis 3:129, 1993.

25. Classé JG: Prescribing for noncontact sports, Intl Ophthalmol Clin 3:111, 1993.

26. Gregg JR: Vision and sports: an introduction, Boston, 1987, Butterworth.

27. Breedlove HW: Prescribing for marksmen and hunters, Optom Clin, Sports Vis 3:77, 1993.

28. Legerton JA: Prescribing for water sports, Optom Clin, Sports Vis 3:91, 1993.

29. Doyle SJ: Acute corneal erosion from the use of anti-misting agent in swimming goggles, Br J Ophthalmol 8:419, 1994.

30. Bruneni J: What's driving high index to stand out? Eyecare Business p 31, 1998.

Proficiency Test

(Answers can be found in the back of the book.)

1. True or false? A −2.50 D high-index glass lens is heavier than a crown glass lens of equal thickness and power.

2. True or false? A high-index plastic lens is heavier than a lower index crown glass lens.

3. The purpose of blowing air against both sides of a glass lens after heating the lens in a thermal-hardening unit is:
   a. to create stress within the lens and increase impact resistance.
   b. to cool the lens quickly so that it can be put into the frame.
   c. to keep dust off the hot surfaces that otherwise might stick.
   d. to ensure that the lens cools evenly.

4. Arrange these new, unscratched lenses in order from the most to the least impact resistant. Assume that the test used for determining impact resistance uses a small, high velocity projectile.
   a. CR-39
   b. untreated crown glass
   c. chemically hardened crown glass
   d. heat-tempered crown glass
   e. polycarbonate

5. Arrange these materials in order from the material with lowest index of refraction to the material with the highest index of refraction.
   a. crown glass
   b. polycarbonate
   c. CR-39
   d. Corning Clears 16
   e. Trivex

6. Arrange these materials in order from the material with lowest density (weight per cubic centimeter) to the material with the highest density.
   a. crown glass
   b. polycarbonate
   c. CR-39
   d. Index 1.80 glass
   e. Trivex

7. True or false? Eyeglasses II no longer lists minimal information needed for a spectacle lens prescription as was found in Eyeglasses I.

8. What is the name of the instrument used to check to see if a glass lens has been heat treated?
   a. alphascope
   b. betascope
   c. colmascope
   d. deltascope

9. For lenses of equal powers and thicknesses, which lens material shows greater impact resistance when tested using a small, high velocity projectile?
   a. an untreated crown glass lens
   b. a chemically tempered crown glass lens
   c. a chemically tempered photochromic lens
   d. a CR-39 lens

10. For lenses of equal power and thickness, which lens material shows greater impact resistance when tested using a large, slow moving object?
    a. an untreated crown glass lens
    b. a chemically tempered crown glass lens
    c. a CR-39 lens

11. Given the following plano-powered lenses, which will be the most impact resistant?
    a. a 3-mm thick photochromic, chemically hardened glass lens
    b. a 2-mm thick polycarbonate lens
    c. a 3-mm thick heat-treated crown glass lens
    d. a 3-mm thick CR-39 lens

12. Which lenses do not have to be *individually* drop-ball tested? (There may be more than one correct response.)
    a. a −5.00 D single vision crown glass lens
    b. a +2.50 D single vision polycarbonate lens
    c. a −1.00 D single vision photochromic slab-off lens
    d. a +1.75 D Franklin-style (Executive) crown glass bifocal

13. True or false? Listing a lens material as part of an eyeglass prescription is inappropriate.

14. True or false? Because the laboratory takes full responsibility for the accuracy of safety and sports prescription eyewear, verification of lens thickness by the dispenser is unnecessary.

15. The correct ophthalmic terminology for eyewear that is used for everyday and not for sports or safety is:
    a. casual eyewear.
    b. everyday eyewear.
    c. formal eyewear.
    d. dress eyewear.
    e. standard eyewear.

16. What are the minimum thickness requirements mandated by the FDA for dress eyewear?
    a. 1.0 mm
    b. 1.5 mm
    c. 2.0 mm
    d. 2.2 mm
    e. There are no minimum thickness requirements.

17. When may retailers dispense prescription lenses that are not impact resistant?
    a. when the wearer signs a waiver accepting responsibility
    b. when no other types of impact-resistant lenses will fulfill the visual requirements of the wearer
    c. when the lenses are high-index glass and are unable to be either heat treated or chemtempered
    d. in any of the above circumstances
    e. in none of the above circumstances

18. What is the standard "referee test" for determining impact resistance suitable for dress ophthalmic lenses?
    a. a 1-inch steel ball dropped on the front surface of the lens from a height of 50 inches
    b. a 1-inch steel ball dropped on the front surface of the lens from a height of 52 inches
    c. a five-eighth-inch steel ball dropped on the front surface of the lens from a height of 50 inches
    d. a five-eighth-inch steel ball dropped on the front surface of the lens from a height of 52 inches
    e. a one-fourth-inch steel ball shot at the front of lens at a speed of 150 feet/sec

19. Which of the following lenses must be individually drop-ball tested and not just batch tested or exempted from testing?
    a. a stock high-index plastic antireflection coated lens
    b. a crown glass executive bifocal lens
    c. a fused flat-top 25 photochromic glass bifocal lens
    d. a glass slab-off lens
    e. All of the above must be individually drop-ball tested.
    f. None of the above must be individually drop-ball tested.

20. True or false? Plano sunglasses manufactured in quantity do not have to be impact resistant.

21. A wearer breaks his frames. You find a new frame, but the old chemically tempered glass lenses are too large.
    a. New lenses must be used in the new frame. Chemtempered lenses cannot be re-edged.
    b. The lenses can be re-edged and put back in the frame as is. The chemtempering is unaffected since the chemical change occurs on the surfaces of the lens.
    c. The lenses can be re-edged, but must be chemtempered all over again before being put into the new frame.
    d. The lenses can be re-edged, but must be chemtempered again and drop-ball tested again before being put into the new frame.

22. Which lens is most likely to break?
    a. an unscratched lens
    b. a lens that has been scratched on the front surface
    c. a lens that has been scratched on the back surface
    d. All lenses are equally likely to break.

23. The "duty to inform" someone of the safest options for their eyewear needs is:
    a. a legal responsibility.
    b. a professional responsibility.
    c. both a professional and a legal responsibility.

24. What are *basic-impact* safety eyewear minimum thicknesses?
    a. 2.0 mm
    b. 2.2 mm
    c. 3.0 mm (except +3.00 D and above, which have a minimum thickness of 2.5 mm)
    d. 3.2 mm (except +3.00 D and above, which have a minimum thickness of 2.8 mm)
    e. 3.2 mm (except +3.00 D and above, which have a minimum thickness of 2.5 mm)

25. What are the *high-impact* safety eyewear minimum thicknesses?
    a. 2.0 mm
    b. 2.2 mm
    c. 3.0 mm (except +3.00 D and above, which have a minimum thickness of 2.5 mm)
    d. 3.2 mm (except +3.00 D and above, which have a minimum thickness of 2.8 mm)
    e. 3.2 mm (except +3.00 D and above, which have a minimum thickness of 2.5 mm)

26. What is the standard "referee test" for determining impact resistance suitable for *basic-impact* prescription safety lenses?
    a. a 1-inch steel ball dropped on the front surface of the lens from a height of 50 inches
    b. a 1-inch steel ball dropped on the front surface of the lens from a height of 52 inches
    c. a five-eighth-inch steel ball dropped on the front surface of the lens from a height of 50 inches
    d. a five-eighth-inch steel ball dropped on the front surface of the lens from a height of 52 inches
    e. a one-fourth-inch steel ball shot at the front of lens at a speed of 150 feet/sec

27. How must a safety frame suitable for high-impact safety lenses be marked on the front and temples?
    a. size and manufacturer
    b. size, manufacturer and Z87
    c. size, manufacturer and Z87+
    d. size, manufacturer and Z87-2

28. True or false? Putting 2.0-mm thick CR-39 lenses in a safety frame, but not marking the lenses for safety, is acceptable if the person just wants the glasses for regular wear.

29. True or false? Putting 2.0-mm thick polycarbonate lenses in a safety frame, but not marking the lenses for safety, is acceptable if the person just wants the glasses for regular wear.

30. Which lens is the most impact resistant?
    a. a 2.2-mm thick crown glass lens that has been neither heat treated nor chemtempered
    b. a 2.2-mm thick crown glass lens that has been heat treated
    c. a 2.2-mm thick crown glass lens that has been chemtempered

31. True or false? A lens may be identified as having been chemically tempered by placing it in a colmascope. (A colmascope consists of two crossed polarizing filters that are back lighted.)

CHAPTER 24

How Lenses Are Edged

An optical laboratory may consist of two separate areas. One area creates the needed lens power. This is usually done by a process called *lens surfacing*, and the facility that does it is referred to as a *surfacing laboratory*.

The second area takes the correctly powered lens and finishes it. This is done by optically positioning the lens and grinding the edges so that the lens fits the shape of the chosen frame. The area where this occurs is known as the *finishing laboratory*. A finishing laboratory is also referred to as an *edging laboratory* because it is here that lenses are "edged" to the proper shape to fit the spectacle frame.

The processes that follow are an overview explanation of how edging is done. For a complete "how to" explanation on all aspects of an edging or finishing laboratory, see Brooks, *Essentials of Ophthalmic Lens Finishing*, published by Elsevier Inc.

SPOTTING OF SINGLE VISION LENSES WITHOUT PRISM

First, a lens is made ready for edging so that the refractive power and optical centration will be correct. For edging we should always be starting with a lens of a known power.

Power Verification and Spotting of Spheres

When the power of the lens to be verified is of known power, set the lensmeter for the expected sphere value. If the lens is a sphere, the target should be immediately clear, indicating a lens of the correct power.

Optically center the lens in the lensmeter by moving the lens until the center of the illuminated target crosses the center of the crosshairs in the lensmeter eyepiece or screen (Figure 24-1.) The marking device is then swung into position, and the front surface of the lens is spotted.

Power Verification and Spotting of Spherocylinders

When verifying spherocylinder lenses, the lensmeter power wheel is turned to the expected sphere power. The cylinder axis wheel is also turned to the axis of the prescription. The lens holding device is not allowed to touch the lens, and the lens is rotated until the sphere

lines of the lensmeter target are sharp and unbroken. When these lines are clear, the cylinder axis is correct.

With the lens correctly rotated for axis position, turn the lensmeter power wheel in the appropriate direction for checking the cylinder power.

Next carefully move the lens left, right, upward, or downward until the target is accurately centered. (Remember to pull the lens holding device away from the lens surface so that the lens will not get scratched.) When the target is accurately centered, the lens may be spotted (Figure 24-2).

The power verification in a spotting procedure for spherocylinder lenses is summarized in Box 24-1.

Marking the Lens for Right or Left

As soon as the lens is spotted, it should be removed from the lensmeter and marked for the right or left eye. Lenses are marked on the front surface with a wax pencil. The letter *R* or *L* in uppercase letters is written in the upper half of the lens above the three spots (see Figure 24-2).

SPOTTING OF SINGLE VISION LENSES WITH PRISM

The Optical Center of a Lens

When there is no prescribed prism in the prescription, the needed point of reference is the optical center (OC). The OC becomes the reference point. It is of major importance in aligning the lens. Therefore it is known as the *major reference point* or *MRP*. So *when there is no prism in the prescription, the OC is the MRP*.

When the Optical Center Is Not in the Line of Sight

Sometimes a prescription includes prescribed prism. The lens must be positioned so that the amount of prism called for will be in front of the wearer's pupil in the eye's line of sight. When prism is called for in the prescription, the point on the lens with the correct amount of prism becomes the point of reference. *When the prescription contains prescribed prism, the OC and MRP are two separate points.*

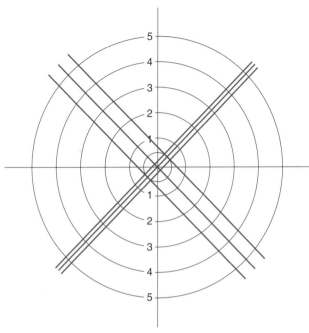

Figure 24-1. When both sphere and cylinder lines focus at the same time, the lens has a uniform power in all meridians and is spoken of as being spherical.

If the sphere and cylinder lines do not intersect at the center of the mires, the lens OC is not centered in front of the lensmeter aperture, and prism is being manifested.

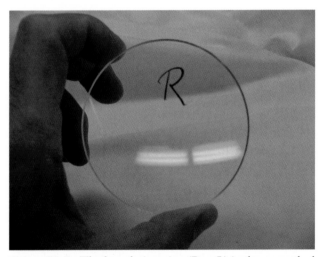

Figure 24-2. The lens designation (R or L) is always marked on the upper half of the lens so that the lens will not be blocked upside down. Though not as critical for nonprismatic finished single vision lenses, an inverted prism or an upside down multifocal would be worse than useless. (The lens is being viewed from the back side.)

There is a synonym for the MRP that is perhaps even more descriptive. That synonym is *"prism reference point"* or PRP. MRP and PRP are the same.

The procedure of spotting single vision lenses with prism is nearly identical to that of nonprism lenses. The only difference is in how the illuminated target is centered. Instead of placing the center of the illuminated

---

<table>
<tr><td>

BOX 24-1

How to Spot Single Vision Sphere or Spherocylinder Lenses Using a Standard Crossed-Line-Target Lensmeter

1. Dial in the lens sphere power and lens cylinder axis into the lensmeter.
2. Place the lens in the lensmeter.
3. Locate the MRP.
4. If the lens is spherical, spot the lens.
5. If the lens has a cylinder, rotate the lens until the sphere lines are clear.
6. If the lens has Rx prism, move the illuminated target until it is located at the position where the prism equals that called for in the prescription.
7. Spot the lens.

</td></tr>
</table>

target at the center of the crosshairs, the center of the illuminated sphere and cylinder target lines must be positioned to correspond to the location of the desired prismatic effect.

Example **24-1**

A right lens calls for 2.0Δ base-out prism. How would it be positioned for spotting?

Solution

To correctly position this lens:
- The center of the sphere and cylinder target intersection must be on the circular mire marked 2.0.
- Because the prism is horizontal, the illuminated target must be on the 180-degree line.
- Base out for the right eye is to the left. Therefore the center of the illuminated target must be on the 2Δ prism circle where it crosses the 180-degree line to the left.

When the lens is correctly positioned, the lensmeter target appears as shown in Figure 24-3.

Once this position is achieved and the cylinder axis is correct, the lens may be spotted. Figure 24-4 shows the lens spotted with the three lensmeter dots. The center lensmeter ink spot is no longer at the center of the uncut lens, but the center dot still indicates the location of the MRP.

When Prescribed Prism Includes Both Horizontal and Vertical Components

In a case in which both horizontal and vertical prisms are called for simultaneously in the same lens, the target must be moved both laterally and vertically until it reaches the desired position. That position is one where the target center is directly above (or below) the required horizontal prism reading. It is also exactly left or right of the required vertical prism reading.

Example **24-2**

A right eye requires 4.0Δ base out and 2.0Δ base up. How would the lens be positioned for spotting?

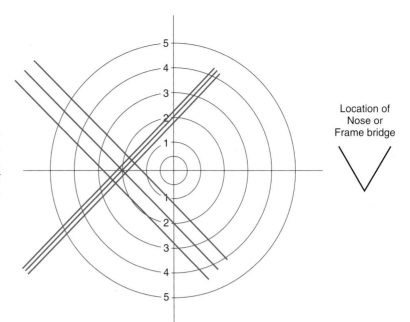

Figure 24-3. Prismatic effect can be created by decentering the lens in the lensmeter until the sphere and/or cylinder line intersection is positioned for the indicated amount. (Achievement of desired prism by decentration is limited by lens size and refractive power.)

Location of Nose or Frame bridge

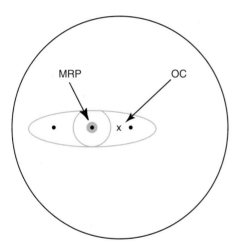

Figure 24-4. The MRP of a lens will ultimately be positioned before the wearer's pupil center. If prism is indicated in the prescription, the OC is displaced purposely. Therefore the point that will be important in centration and is consequently spotted is the MRP—not the OC.

Solution

To correctly position the lens, the target must be four full prism diopter units to the left of center *and* two full prism diopter units above center. This is shown in Figure 24-5.

SPOTTING OF FLAT TOP MULTIFOCALS

For multifocals the bifocal should be placed in the lensmeter like it will be when mounted in the frame. This means that for flat-top bifocals, the segment top should be horizontal. The sphere power is dialed into the lensmeter. If the lens has a cylinder component, the axis of the cylinder should be dialed in as well.

Next the MRP of the lens is located. When the lens is spherical, the lens may be spotted.

For multifocals with spherocylinder powers, the axis of the cylinder has been custom ground for that particular lens. The lensmeter is set for the axis ordered, and the lens rotated to the correct axis. With MRP and cylinder axis correct, the lens is spotted, just like a single vision lens. After the lens has been spotted, the three dots on the 180-degree line should be parallel to the upper edge of a flat-top segment (Figure 24-6, *A*). If they are not parallel to the top of the bifocal segment, the cylinder axis is off, and the lens was surfaced improperly.

To precheck the lenses as a pair, hold the lenses front to front with the segments overlapping (Figure 24-6, *C*). If there are not two different MRP heights or two different seg insets, the center spots of both lenses should be at the same place. If they are not, there is likely to be a problem with unwanted horizontal or vertical prism after the lenses are edged.

For a summary of spotting flat-top multifocals, see Box 24-2.

SPOTTING PROGRESSIVE ADDITION LENSES

Progressive addition lenses have certain "hidden" markings used in establishing lens orientation. Lenses coming from the surfacing laboratory are also marked with non-water-soluble ink. If the visible inked marks are correctly applied, there is no need to spot the lenses. However, they should be verified before edging.

Verifying Premarked Progressives

To check distance lens power, position the lens in the lensmeter to view through the circled area above the PRP. (The PRP usually comes marked with a

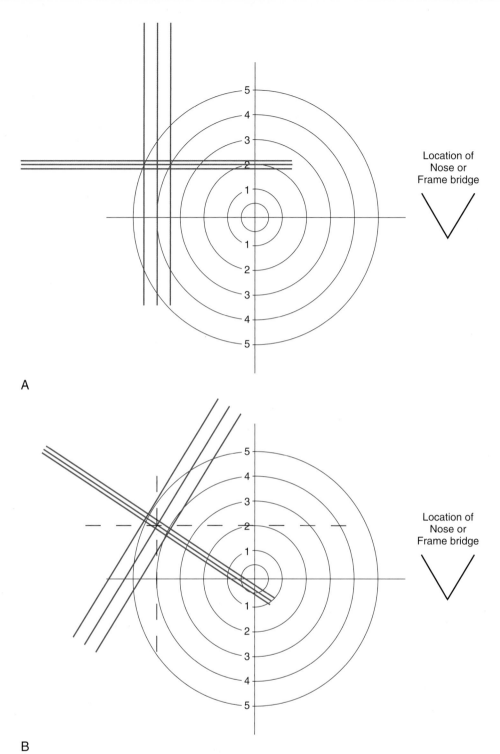

Location of
Nose or
Frame bridge

A

Location of
Nose or
Frame bridge

B

Figure 24-5. In positioning a prismatic lens, the only important reference is the center of the illuminated target. This is the place where the center sphere and cylinder lines cross each other. Where other parts of those lines may cross the circular mires is of no importance.

In the example shown, the sphere and cylinder line crossing point must be directly above or below the place where the 4.0Δ circle crosses the horizontal line farthest from the "nose." The sphere and cylinder line crossing point must simultaneously also be exactly at the same level as the top of the 2.0Δ circle. **A,** This is easy to see because the sphere and cylinder lines are aligned horizontally and vertically. However, if there is cylinder present at any axis other than 90 or 180, the lines will not look like this. Instead they may appear as shown in **(B).** The prismatic effect shown in **(B)** is exactly the same as in **(A).** Both are 4 base out and 2 base up.

It may be difficult to tell the exact position of the center of the illuminated target for a spherocylinder lens with an oblique axis. If you have difficulty, try this procedure. Temporarily turn the cylinder axis to 90 or 180 degrees. This will cause the illuminated target lines to be exactly horizontal and vertical. Now although the lines will be a bit blurred, they will duplicate the situation shown in **A** and make it easier to tell how much vertical and horizontal prism is present.

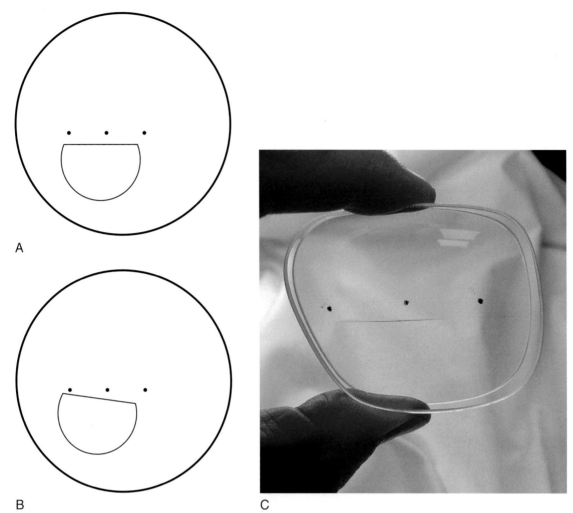

Figure 24-6. A, For spherocylinder lenses, the three dots should be parallel to the top of the segment. If they are not, the cylinder axis will be wrong. **B,** For spherical lenses, an angle between the three dots and the segment top is not a problem, even through it looks off. However, if the lens has a cylinder component, the axis of the cylinder will be wrong. **C,** Once flat-top bifocals have been spotted, they may be prechecked before edging. Hold the edged lenses front to front. They are held front to front because the segments and spots are closer to one another and will reduce the amount of parallax seen. Do not press the lenses into contact with one another to prevent scratching. Make sure the segments exactly overlap each other. With both lenses having equal seg insets and drops, the spots should also overlap as shown. If they do not overlap, there may be a problem with PDs being off or unwanted vertical prism.

dot.) This circled area used to locate the point for verifying distance power is called the *distance reference point* or *DRP* (Figure 24-7). Incidentally, remember that there will almost always be some prism at the DRP since the DRP of the lens is not the OC of the lens.

To check distance power, set the power wheel to the sphere power and the cylinder axis wheel to the ordered cylinder axis. Rotate the lens until the target lines are clear and unbroken. The non–water-soluble horizontal reference marks on the lens should be horizontally oriented and not tilted. If they are tilted, the axis of the cylinder is incorrect.

To check for prism, the lens is centered in the lensmeter at the PRP. (Remember, the PRP is the same as the *MRP*.)

Progressive lenses often come with equal amounts of vertical prism in both right and left lenses. This allows the lenses to be made thinner. Equal amounts of "yoked" vertical prism for "prism thinning" purposes are both allowable and usually expected. Both right and left lenses may read 1.5Δ base down at the PRP and are considered free of unwanted vertical prism.

As stated earlier, if the lenses are correct and have non–water-soluble progressive lens markings, there is no need to spot the lens. The existing markings will be used in the blocking process. If the lenses do not come with markings, or if it appears that the markings were inaccurately applied, then the markings must be reapplied.

When Progressive Lenses Are Not Premarked

In the event that a progressive addition lens has no visible markings, reconstruct the manufacturer's recommended system of identifying marks. This procedure was explained in Chapter 20.

PATTERNS

Pattern Measurements and Terminology

To allow the edger to shape the lens to fit the frame, a pattern is needed. That pattern can be a physical pattern made of plastic or an electronic pattern in the memory of a computer. Here are some specifics on pattern measurement and terminology.

The *mechanical center* of a pattern is the point on the pattern around which the pattern rotates. The mechanical center is easy to find since it is found in the middle of the large hole in the pattern (Figure 24-8).

Centration and Decentration

The process of moving a lens so that it will be in front of the eye is called *centration*. To center the lens in front of the eye, the lens must be moved *away* from a given reference point. When a lens is moved away from a given point, it is said to be *decentered* from that point. In this case the lens is moved away from or *decentered* from the location of the mechanical and boxing centers.

Pattern Making

Because of the vast number of available frame styles, it is impossible to have a complete library of patterns so that the correct pattern is available for every frame presented for lens fabrication. Ordering a pattern for every single frame that passes through the laboratory is totally impractical. The delays caused would not be acceptable to the wearer, not to mention the volume of paperwork that would be generated. For this reason, when running an edger that uses patterns, a system for making patterns is a necessity.

How the Pattern Is Placed on the Edger

By convention most people begin the edging process with the right eye. When the pattern is snapped into place on the edger, it will fit on the edger with either the front or the back of the pattern going on first. Going on one way will edge a right lens shape, whereas the other way will produce a left lens shape.

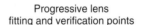

BOX 24-2

Spotting Flat-Top Multifocals

1. Dial the lens sphere power and lens cylinder axis into the lensmeter.
2. Place the lens in the lensmeter.
3. Locate the MRP.
4. If the lens is spherical, spot the lens.
5. If the lens has a cylinder, rotate the lens until the sphere lines are clear.
6. If the lens has Rx prism, move the illuminated target until it is located at the position where the prism equals that called for in the prescription.
7. Spot the lens.
8. For spherocylinder lenses and lenses with Rx prism, verify that the segment top and three lensmeter dots are parallel to one another.
9. When both lenses have been spotted, line up the lenses front to front to check for R-L spotting accuracy. The central spots should overlap.

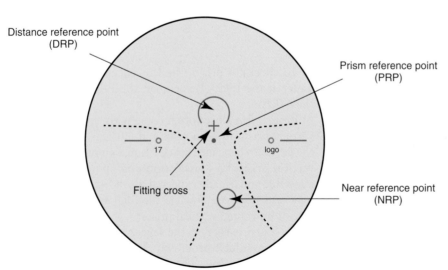

Progressive lens
fitting and verification points

Figure 24-7. Points of reference on a progressive addition lens.

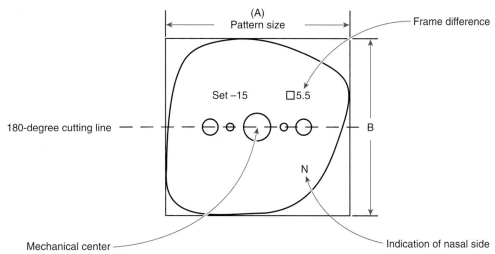

Figure 24-8. The same system of measurement that is used for frames and lenses is also used for patterns. Patterns do not come with A and B dimensions marked. But they do have a pattern set number to help in finding the correct edger setting. The "frame difference" helps in positioning MRP and multifocal heights when the laboratory does not have the frame.

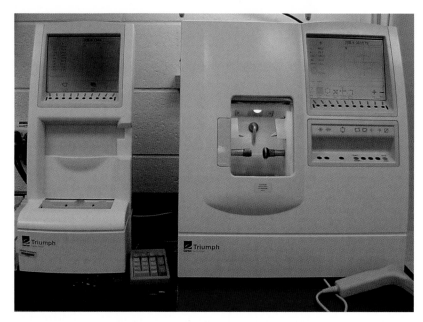

Figure 24-9. Here a tracer is next to the edger. It is electronically linked to the edger and has a screen to allow the traced shape to be viewed before edging.

USING A FRAME TRACER FOR PATTERNLESS SYSTEMS OF EDGING

Patternless edgers that do not use a physical pattern still need a shape to go by. This shape is given to the edger in digital form. Still to get a digital version of the shape, that shape must sooner or later be physically traced and transferred to the edger digitally.

A pattern shape is generated by using a frame tracer. A *frame tracer* is an apparatus that traces the shape of the frame's lens area and converts it into digital form.

A Frame Tracer Can Be Used in a Variety of Locations

A Tracer Can Be Situated Right Next to the Edger
When a tracer is situated right next to the edger, the person doing the edging has the frame in front of them

(Figure 24-9). The advantage to this setup is ease in visualizing what bevel placement will look best.

A Tracer Can Be a Part of the Edger
A tracer that is part of the edger has the advantage of requiring less working space (Figure 24-10).

A Tracer May Be Placed in the Order Entry Area of a Laboratory
When the tracer is placed in the order entry area of the laboratory, information is only entered once. The laboratory that has a tracer at "order entry" will be wired with a central laboratory computer.

A Tracer May Be Placed in a Remote-Site Dispensary
One of the biggest headaches for dispensers is the situation where a wearer wants to keep his or her old frame,

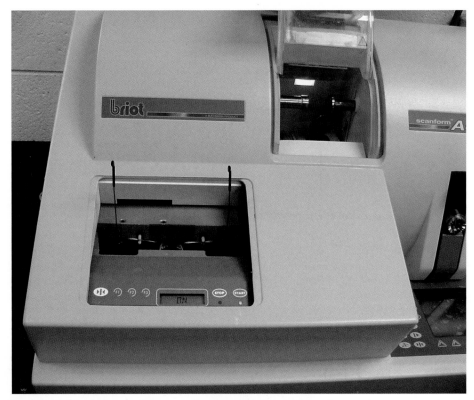

Figure 24-10. A frame tracer can be integrated into the edger and save space in the laboratory.

but cannot or will not give it up long enough to send it to the laboratory. If there is a frame tracer on site, the dispenser can remove one or both lenses, trace the shape, reinsert the lens or lenses, and give the spectacles back to the wearer (Figure 24-11).

The information is then sent to the laboratory electronically. It enters the computer system just as if it had been entered in the laboratory order entry area.

When the dispensary uses a frame tracer to send information, the laboratory can get a head start on any Rx before the new frame arrives. In the interest of time, the dispensary may choose to not send the new frame at all and insert the lenses themselves.

Tracers Can Transfer Data to a Surfacing Laboratory

For the surfacing laboratory to grind a lens to the optimum thickness, the laboratory needs accurate data. This is especially true for plus lenses. The size and shape the lens will have when edged is essential for calculating plus lens thickness. The more exact the data, the more precisely the thickness may be controlled. If the lens is traced, those tracing values may be sent to more places than just the edger. Values can be sent to a surfacing program that calculates lens curves and thickness, then controls the lens generator.

CENTRATION OF LENSES

Centration of Single Vision Lenses

During the edging process, the lens rotates around a central point while being ground to a specific shape to fit the frame. This central point of rotation corresponds to a hole in the pattern. This hole should always be in the middle of the pattern used on the edger to generate the shape. This middle point, the *geometric* or *boxing center* of the lens, is defined as being the center of the smallest rectangle that encloses the lens shape using horizontal and vertical lines.

For the MRP of the lens to be centered before the wearer's pupil, the lens must be moved, or *decentered*, away from the boxing center of the lens.

Distance Between Centers

For frames that conform to the boxing system of measurement, the distance between centers (DBC) is equal to the eye size (abbreviated A) plus the *distance between lenses* (DBL).

$$DBC = A + DBL$$

Decentration per Lens

Most commonly the wearer's PD will be less than the DBC. This will require that the lenses be decentered inward (nasally) toward the center of the frame. The amount of decentration per lens can be determined by

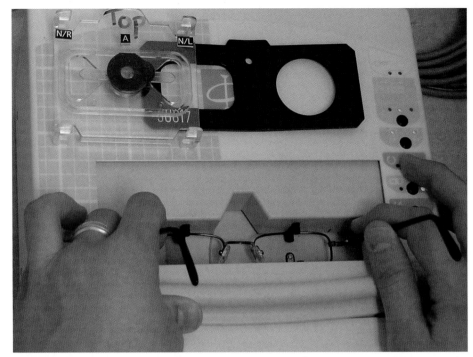

Figure 24-11. A frame tracer may be used at a remote, off-site location. This ensures that the frame dimensions as read at the dispensary are exactly what will be input into the edger.

subtracting the wearer's PD from the DBC (frame PD) and dividing by two.

$$\frac{DBC - \text{wearer PD}}{2} = \text{decentration per lens.}$$

Example **24-3**

A wearer's PD is 62 mm. The frame size has an A dimension of 48 mm and a DBL of 20 mm. What is the decentration per lens required?

Solution

To find decentration per lens, we use the formula

$$\text{decentration per lens} = \frac{DBC - PD}{2}$$

and since

$$DBC = A + DBL,$$
$$\text{decentration per lens} = \frac{A + DBL - PD}{2}$$

Then

$$\begin{aligned}
\text{dec. per lens} &= \frac{48 + 20 - 62}{2}\\
&= \frac{68 - 62}{2}\\
&= \frac{6}{2}\\
&= 3\,\text{mm}
\end{aligned}$$

So for the example, the decentration needed per lens is 3 mm inward.

Determining Decentration From Monocular PDs

When a prescription specifies the wearer's PD in reference to each eye individually, PDs are taken one eye at a time. This measurement is referred to as the *monocular PD*. For a monocular PD, the reference is basically from the center of the bridge of the nose to the center of the pupil. For example, if we have a more conventionally measured *binocular PD* of 64, we may have a right monocular PD of 31 and a left monocular PD of 33. This difference between left and right PDs is not unusual considering the asymmetry of facial features of many normal individuals.

For a monocular PD, decentration is determined by *first* dividing the distance between centers (DBC) of the frame by 2, *then* subtracting the monocular PD; thus

$$\text{decentration} = \frac{DBC}{2} - \text{monocular PD}$$

or

$$\text{decentration} = \frac{A + DBL}{2} - \text{monocular PD}$$

How to Calculate Vertical Centration

MRP height is the distance from the lower line of the box enclosing the shape of the lens up to the MRP loca-

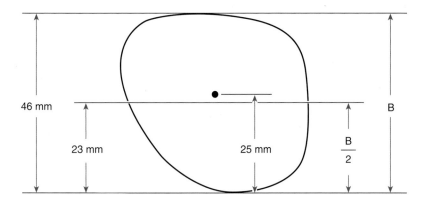

Figure 24-12. If the position of the MRP is given in terms of height from the lowermost portion of the shape, drop or raise can be calculated by subtracting one half of the B dimension from MRP height.

tion. The laboratory must convert from MRP height to MRP raise (or drop).

Example **24-4**

An order specifies an MRP height of 25 mm. The frame has a vertical dimension (B) of 46 mm. What will the MRP raise be?

Solution

Vertical decentration is calculated as

$$\text{vertical decentration} = \text{MRP height} - \frac{B}{2}.$$

In the example, since MRP height is 25 mm and the frame B is 46 mm, then

$$\begin{aligned}\text{vertical decentration} &= 25 - \frac{46}{2}\\ &= 25 - 23\\ &= 2\,\text{mm}\end{aligned}$$

It can be seen that since the MRP height is greater than half of the B dimension, the vertical decentration is positive, and the lens is moved up by 2 mm. The height above (or below) the horizontal midline of the lens may be visualized from Figure 24-12.

Steps in Centration of Single Vision Lenses

Here are the steps in using a centration instrument for single vision lenses:

Step 1: Spot the lens (as described earlier).

Step 2: If the instrument has blocking capabilities, stick a double-sided adhesive blocking pad on a lens block and mount the block on the instrument. Then peel the paper off the pad to expose the adhesive.

Step 3: Calculate the amount of horizontal decentration per lens required using the formula

$$\text{decentration per lens} = \frac{A + DBL - PD}{2}$$

Step 4: Determine if the lens must be decentered to the right or to the left. In most centering devices,

the lens will be face up. If the lens is a right lens and is facing up, decentration "in" is to the right. A left lens facing up would be decentered to the left.

Step 5: Adjust the position of the movable vertical reference line* in the instrument to the right or left by the amount of decentration calculated.

Step 6: Next place the right lens face up (front surface up) on the screen. Align the three spots on the lens with the horizontal line on the instrument screen.

Step 7: Place the center lens dot on the movable vertical reference line. (Remember, the position of this line corresponds to horizontal decentration.)

Step 8: When the MRP height is specified, decenter the lens up (or in rare instances down). The amount of decentration is according to the correct number of millimeters of MRP raise (or drop).

Step 9: Grasp the handle and swing it into place or press the button or foot switch. This will block the lens (Figure 24-13).

Example **24-5**

A frame has an eye size (A) of 54 mm and a DBL of 20 mm. The wearer's PD is 66 mm. The lenses are already spotted. How must the instrument be set and the lens placed to properly block the lens? Assume that the lens is a *left* lens.

Solution

Lens decentration is calculated as

$$\begin{aligned}\text{decentration per lens} &= \frac{A + DBL - PD}{2}\\ &= \frac{54 + 20 - 66}{2}\\ &= \frac{8}{2}\\ &= 4\,\text{mm}.\end{aligned}$$

---

*For single vision lenses, the movable vertical line is basically used as a place marker. When laying out single vision lenses, some people prefer not to use the movable vertical line at all. Instead they move the dot on the lens directly to the desired amount of decentration.

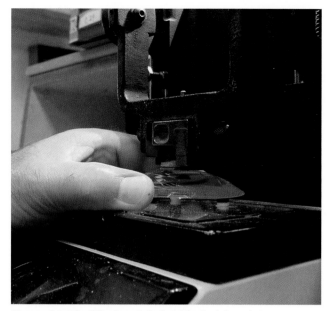

Figure 24-13. The lens is being blocked for edging.

To preset the movable vertical line in the instrument for the left lens, first recall in which direction the MRP should be moved. Because the wearer's PD is smaller than the frame's geometric center distance or "frame PD"*—the lenses will decenter nasally or inward. The lens is placed convex side up. Therefore the left lens is moved to the left so the movable vertical line is positioned 4 mm to the left of the central reference line.

Now place the lens face up in the instrument. Align it such that the central dot is at the intersection of the horizontal line and the movable vertical line, as shown in Figure 24-14. The other two dots must fall directly on the horizontal reference line.

Block the lens. The location of the center of the lens block will become the boxing center of the edged lens (Figure 24-15).

Centration of Progressive Lenses

The fitting cross is to be positioned exactly in front of the wearer's pupil and comes visibly marked on the lens. It is the only reference point for both horizontal and vertical lens positioning for the dispenser. It is also the primary reference point for both horizontal and vertical lens positioning for the edging laboratory.

In simplest terms, centration of a progressive addition lens is done as if the lens were a single vision lens. For single vision lenses, the MRP is placed at the correct monocular or binocular PD, depending upon how it is ordered. For a progressive lens, the fitting cross is placed at the correct monocular PD.

For a single vision lens, the MRP is placed on the horizontal midline of the lens, or at the specified MRP height, if one is ordered. For a progressive lens, the fitting cross is placed at the specified fitting cross height.

*"Frame PD" is equal to A + DBL.

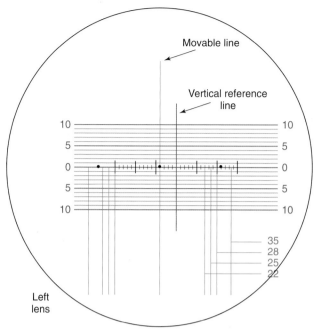

Figure 24-14. The movable line is preset to the correct decentration. The movable line helps to prevent the dot on the lens from getting "lost" on the grid. With the movable line pointing out the desired MRP location, the lens is positioned as shown.

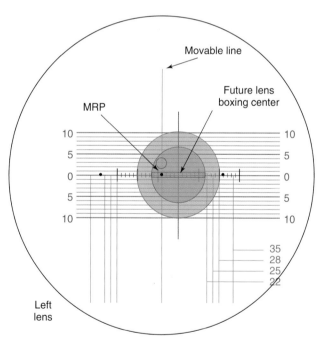

Figure 24-15. On the centration device, the block is always placed at the origin. The block center corresponds to the *future* geometric or boxing center of the *edged* lens.

Example **24-6**

A progressive addition lens is ordered as follows:

R: +3.00 − 1.00 × 070
L: +3.00 − 1.00 × 110
add +1.50

Monocular PDs are:

R: 33
L: 31

Vertical fitting cross heights are:

R: 25
L: 23

Frame dimensions are A = 50, B = 40, DBL = 20
Answer these questions.
1. How much horizontal decentration is required per lens?
2. How much fitting cross raise or drop is needed per lens?
3. How will the right lens appear on a centration device when correctly centered for blocking?

Solution

1. For a progressive lens, the horizontal decentration for a monocular PD is calculated in the same way as it is for a single vision lens. So in this example problem

$$\text{decentration} = \frac{(A + DBL)}{2} - \text{monocular PD}$$
$$= \frac{(50 + 20)}{2} - 33$$
$$= 2 \text{ mm.}$$

Therefore horizontal decentration for the right lens is 2 mm.
Horizontal decentration for the left lens is

$$\text{decentration} = \frac{(A + DBL)}{2} - \text{monocular PD}$$
$$= \frac{(50 + 20)}{2} - 31$$
$$= 4 \text{ mm.}$$

2. For the right lens the fitting cross raise or drop above or below the horizontal midline is calculated as follows:

$$\text{raise or drop} = \text{fitting cross height} - \frac{B}{2}$$
$$= 25 - \frac{40}{2}$$
$$= 25 - 20$$
$$= +5 \text{ mm.}$$

Therefore the fitting cross raise for the right lens is 5 mm. For the left lens, the fitting cross height is

$$\text{raise or drop} = \text{fitting cross height} - \frac{B}{2}$$
$$= 23 - \frac{40}{2}$$
$$= 23 - 20$$
$$= +3 \text{ mm.}$$

Therefore the fitting cross raise for the left lens is 3 mm.
3. The lens is positioned in the centration device using the fitting cross for reference.

BOX 24-3

Steps in the Centration of Progressive Addition Lenses

1. Find the location of the hidden circles on the front surface of the lens and dot the centers of the two hidden circles.
2. Place the lens on the manufacturer's lens blank chart. The dots must be on the indicated hidden circle locations. Verify the accuracy of the lens markings—especially the location of the fitting cross. If they are wrong, remove the old markings and redraw the marks on the lens.
3. Verify the lens by checking distance power at the DRP, prism power at the PRP, and near power at the NRP.
4. Calculate distance decentration per lens using monocular PDs.
5. Calculate fitting cross raise or drop.
6. Preset the movable line in the centration device for the distance decentration.
7. Place the lens face up in the centration device and position the fitting cross on the movable line.
8. Move the lens up until the fitting cross is at the fitting cross height.
9. Verify that the 180 markings on the lens are parallel to the horizontal lines in the centration device.
10. Block the lens for edging.

For a summary of how progressive addition lenses are positioned for edging, see Box 24-3.

Centration of Segmented Multifocal Lenses

The near-viewing segment area in conventional multifocal lenses has a clearly demarcated line that borders it. This can be used as a stable, convenient reference when positioning the lens for blocking.

The vertical location of the segment is measured for each wearer. The dispenser gives this vertical location in terms of segment height. This segment height must be converted to segment raise or drop.

The dispenser gives the horizontal location of the segment in terms of the wearer's distance and near PDs. This must be converted to segment inset relative to the boxing center of the edged lens.

The centration of standard flat-top bifocals is done as follows:
1. Verify the lens for power and MRP location. Spot the location of the MRP with the lensmeter.
2. Place the lens block in the instrument.
3. Determine the total seg inset required.

$$\text{total inset} = \frac{(A + DBL) - \text{near PD}}{2}$$

4. Determine if the lens must be decentered to the right or to the left. If the lens is convex side up, for a right lens decenter to the right; for a left lens, to the left.

5. Position the movable vertical line in the instrument to the right or left by the amount of decentration calculated.

6. Calculate the amount of seg drop or raise required.

$$\text{seg drop} = \text{seg height} - \frac{B}{2}$$

7. Place the lens face up in the instrument and align the segment between the segment border lines.

8. Move the lens up or down so that the segment top is at the seg drop or raise called for.

9. Grasp the handle of the instrument and swing it into place or press the button or foot switch. This will block the lens.

EDGING THE LENS

Edgers that require a physical pattern to guide the edger are often referred to as *patterned edgers.*

However, the template to produce a lens shape does not have to be something tangible, such as a plastic pattern. It can be a shape that is stored digitally. That electronic version can also guide the lens edger. Because this type of an edger works without a physical pattern, it is referred to as a *patternless edger.*

Edging With Patterns

Setting the Edger Size

If all lens patterns were exactly the same size as the required finished lens, then no size setting would be required. However, this would mean that instead of having one pattern for each frame shape, a separate pattern would be required for every available size.

This raises the question of pattern size. The "standard size" was set at 36.5 mm.

To Prevent Pattern Distortion, the Pattern is Made Larger

When a lens is edged to a shape that is 2 mm larger than the size of the pattern, the edger makes the lens a millimeter larger in every direction—nasally, temporally, upward, and downward. But in adding an equal amount of lens size to the original shape in every direction, the integrity of the original shape starts to be lost. To keep the shape from being distorted, the only feasible solution was to produce a pattern for larger style frames that was closer in size to the actual lens size being edged.

If the pattern is made larger than the standard 36.5-mm size, the lens will be too large. Without compensation, the lens will be edged larger than the frame eye size.

Example **24-7**

A pattern is supplied for a certain frame. This pattern measures 46.5 in its A dimension. Suppose the lens is to be edged for a 50-mm eye size. If the edger is calibrated for a pattern size standard of 36.5 mm, what size lens will be edged if the edger sizing dial is set for 50 mm?

Solution

For this edger, a 36.5-mm pattern will produce the lens size at which the dial is set. If a 50-mm lens is desired, the dial is set at 50 mm. However, since the pattern is 10 mm too large, the lens produced will also be 10 mm too large. Setting the edger at 50 mm in conjunction with this pattern will produce a lens having a 60-mm eye size.

Example **24-8**

In Example 24-7, what would the edger setting have to be to produce a 50-mm lens?

Solution

That pattern is 46.5 mm. This is 10 mm larger than the standard and will produce lenses 10 mm too large. Therefore 10 mm must be subtracted from the required eye size.

$$50 \text{ mm} - 10 \text{ mm} = 40 \text{ mm}.$$

To arrive at a 50-mm lens, the edger must be set for 40 mm.

Set Numbers

To make it easier to know how to compensate for a pattern that is larger than the 36.5-mm standard pattern size, frame manufacturers put a compensation number on the pattern. This compensating number is called the *set number.* Because patterns are almost always larger than the standard, this difference must be subtracted from the eye size. For this reason, set numbers are seen as negative numbers.

Patterns that accompany a manufacturer's frame in most cases have a set number stamped directly on the pattern. Knowing the eye size and pattern set number means the edger setting can be done without having to measure the pattern.

Example **24-9**

A lens is to be edged for a frame having an A dimension of 53 mm. The pattern is stamped "set-15."
1. What is the proper edger setting?
2. If measured, what would the expected A dimension of the pattern be?

Solution

1. "Set-15" means that we need to set the edger 15 mm less than the desired lens size. Therefore to find the edger setting, we use

$$\text{edger setting} = \text{eye size} + (\text{set number})$$

In this case that will be

$$\text{edger setting} = 53 + (-15)$$
$$= 38 \text{ mm}$$

So the edger is set for 38 mm.

3. Now what would the size of the pattern be? Set number is the difference between the standard sized pattern and the actual sized pattern. In other words,

$$\text{Set number} = \text{standard pattern size} - \text{actual pattern size}$$
$$= 36.5 - \text{actual pattern size}$$

In this case we know what the set number is, but not the pattern size. So changing the formula around algebraically results in

$$\text{Actual pattern size} = 36.5 - (\text{set number})$$

In this example, the numbers become

$$\text{actual pattern size} = 36.5 - (-15)$$
$$= 36.5 + 15$$
$$= 51.5 \text{ mm}$$

This pattern can be expected to have an A dimension of 51.5 mm.

What if the Pattern is the Same Size as the Frame's Eye Size? When an edger is calibrated for a standard size pattern whose A dimension is 36.5 mm, setting the edger at 36.5 mm will always produce a lens that is exactly the same size as the pattern. So if a pattern is made directly from a frame and duplicates the frame's eye size, then a 36.5-mm setting will give the correct lens size.

Some Patternless Edgers Do Decentration Calculations

Patternless edgers reduce the need for calculating edger setting numbers. This is because the digital "pattern" and the needed lens sizes are the same.* Some patternless edgers go further. Calculating lens decentration is not difficult. But like any simple arithmetic computation, it is easy to make a simple mistake.

It is not difficult for a patternless edger to do the decentration. When tracing both right and left lenses, the tracer also knows the DBL. The only thing that is not known is the wearer's PD. By asking for the PD, decentration can be easily given.

Some Edgers Do Both Calculations and Decentration. Even if the edger figures decentration, the person blocking the lens still has to first decenter, then block the lens.

Some patternless edgers are made to work with the blocker. If there is a direct interface between blocker and edger, the lens does not have to be decentered nasally by the operator. The operator just positions the spotted lens so that the OC (or MRP) is in the middle of the blocker grid as if there were no decentration at all. Then one of two things happens.

1. The blocker moves the lens block over to where it would normally be positioned.
2. The lens is blocked right in the middle, and the edger takes that factor into consideration when it is edging the lens.

---

*Sometimes it is necessary to trace a frame or pattern that is the same shape, but not the same size as the frame to be used. In this case size compensation in edger settings will be necessary.

Proficiency Test

(Answers can be found in the back of the book.)

1. True or false? Lenses are surfaced in a finishing laboratory.

2. Which type of lens has the same power over the entire lens?
   a. a single vision lens
   b. a segmented multifocal lens
   c. a progressive addition lens

3. What term is a synonym for a "finished lens"?
   a. single vision lens
   b. semifinished lens
   c. uncut lens
   d. progressive addition lens
   e. multifocal lens

4. A "frame tracer" is often used in conjunction with:
   a. a lensmeter.
   b. a lens blocker.
   c. a lens edger.

5. Of the steps in lens fabrication listed below, which process occurs last?
   a. blocking
   b. edging
   c. spotting

6. Arrange the steps in the edging process in their correct order.
   1. blocking
   2. centration
   3. edging
   4. finding lens axis and MRP location

   a. 2, 3, 1, 4
   b. 2, 4, 1, 3
   c. 1, 2, 3, 4
   d. 4, 2, 1, 3
   e. 4, 3, 2, 1

7. When spotting a single vision lens for edging, in reference to *edged lens orientation*, the lensmeter ink dots will be on:
   a. the sphere meridian.
   b. the cylinder meridian.
   c. the 180-degree meridian.
   d. the cylinder axis.

8. Which point should *always* appear either exactly in front of (or somewhat below) the wearer's pupil?
   a. OC
   b. DBC
   c. geometric center
   d. MRP
   e. DBL

9. If there is no prescribed prism in the prescription, all of these points except one are the same. Which one is not the same?
   a. OC
   b. MRP
   c. PRP
   d. NRP

10. For which of the following prescriptions is there a difference in the physical location of the OC and the MRP? (There may be more than one correct response.)
    a. −4.00 D sphere
    b. −4.00 − 2.00 × 180
    c. −4.00 D sphere with 0.5Δ base-in prism
    d. −4.00 − 2.00 × 180 with 0.5Δ base-up prism
    e. The OC and MRP are synonymous terms and hence are always at the same point on a lens.

11. A flat-top bifocal is spotted for the MRP, and it is immediately evident that the three dots are *not* parallel to the segment line. In which Rx is this of no consequence?
    a. It is always of consequence.
    b. −1.00 − 1.00 × 180
    c. pl −1.00 × 070
    d. −2.25 D sph

12. Horizontal and vertical prismatic effect for a progressive addition lens is verified at the:
    a. NRP.
    b. PRP.
    c. DRP.

13. True or false? Horizontal pattern size is measured horizontally through the central hole in the pattern.

14. A lens is to be edged for a frame with an A dimension equal to 48 mm and a DBL of 18 mm. If the wearer has a PD of 60 mm, what is the decentration per lens?
    a. 6 mm
    b. 5 mm
    c. 4 mm
    d. 3 mm
    e. 2 mm

15. Which is not a valid function for a frame tracer?
    a. to gather shape data to transfer to a patternless edger directly wired to that edger
    b. to gather shape data to transfer to a patternless edger to a remote location using phone lines
    c. to determine the DBL of the frame
    d. All of the above are possible functions of a frame tracer.

16. What is the DBC for a frame with the following dimensions?
    A = 47
    B = 39
    DBL = 20
    ED = 48

17. How much decentration per lens is required to correctly position these lenses for edging?
    R: +1.00 − 1.00 × 070
    L: −1.00 − 1.00 × 100
    A = 52
    B = 49
    DBL = 16
    PD = 70
    a. 1 mm in
    b. 1 mm out
    c. 1.5 mm in
    d. 2.0 mm in
    e. None of the above is correct.

18. How much decentration per lens is required for an Rx having the following specifications?
    A = 52
    B = 43
    ED = 54
    DBL = 18
    R monocular PD = 32
    L monocular PD = 33.5

19. How much decentration per lens is required for an Rx with these specifications?
    A = 48
    B = 38
    ED = 48
    DBL = 18
    R monocular PD = 31.5
    L monocular PD = 31.0

20. For this order, the wearer's PD is the same size as the (A) + (DBL) of the spectacle frame. The order specifies an MRP height of 23 mm for both lenses. If the frame has a vertical (B) dimension of 40 mm, how much vertical decentration is needed?

21. What vertical and horizontal decentration per lens is required for the following single vision Rx?
    $-1.25 - 0.75 \times 015$
    $-1.00 - 1.00 \times 162$
    height of MRPs: 26 mm
    PD = 66
    A = 53
    B = 48
    ED = 57
    DBL = 17

22. How much vertical and horizontal decentration of the MRPs of the lenses is required for the lenses that are to be placed in this frame?
    +3.00 D sphere with 2Δ base in
    +3.00 D sphere with 2Δ base in
    MRP height = 21 mm
    Wearer's PD = 61 mm
    A = 47
    B = 33
    DBL = 17

23. There are definite relationships between pattern size and edger setting. Assuming a standard pattern size of 36.5 mm, fill in the missing information for each of the lens size and pattern size combinations listed below.

Eyesize	Pattern Size	Set Number	Edger Setting
50	36.5	a	b
48	c	−10	d
45	e	f	37
g	44.5	h	44
50	36.5	i	j
k	l	−5	57
50	51.5	m	n
52	50	o	p

24. If a pattern is marked, "set-5," what is the pattern's A dimension?
    a. 37.5
    b. 41
    c. 45
    d. 41.5
    e. cannot be determined from information given

25. A pattern measures 56 mm. If the frame to be used has an A dimension of 58 mm and a DBL of 20 mm, what edger setting will result in a correctly edged lens, assuming a correctly calibrated edger?
    a. set at 36.5 mm
    b. set at 38.5 mm
    c. set at 54 mm
    d. set at 56 mm
    e. set at 58 mm

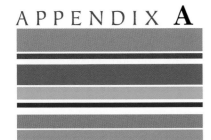

ANSI Z80.1 Prescription Ophthalmic Lenses— Recommendations

Before using the standards outlined in this section, one thing should be made clear. Unlike ANSI Standards for safety eyewear, standards for dress prescription eyewear are not requirements, but recommendations. They are completely voluntary. "The standard remains a recommendation. Therefore, it is the specific intent of the Z80 Committee that this standard not be used as a regulatory instrument."*

Each of the standards listed here are reliably achievable one at a time. The challenge of meeting all standards at the same time becomes more difficult, however. In fact, according to industry data, 25% of all spectacles made will fail in at least one of the areas listed.†

Therefore, these standards should serve as goals for excellence and a frame of reference. Ultimately, each person involved in the prescribing, dispensing, and manufacturing processes should have the visual well-being of the person who will be wearing the spectacles as their highest concern.

The information summarized here in tabular form is not meant to be all-inclusive. For complete information consult the original document. This is *Z80.1-2005 American National Standard for Ophthalmic—Prescription Ophthalmic Lenses—Recommendations.* This standard may be obtained from

> Optical Laboratories Association
> 11096 Lee Highway
> A101
> Fairfax, VA 22030-5039

*ANSI Z80.1-2005 American National Standard for Ophthalmic-Prescription Ophthalmic Lenses-Recommendations, Optical Laboratories Association, Fairfax, VA, 2006, p ii.
†ANSI Z80.1-2005, American National Standard for Ophthalmics-Prescription Ophthalmic Lenses-Recommendations. Fairfax, VA: Optical Laboratories Association, 2006; p. 1.

TABLE A-1
Distance Refractive Power Tolerances for Single Vision Lenses and Segmented Multifocals

	Power in Meridian of Highest Power	Tolerance on Meridian of Highest Power	Tolerance on Cylinder Powers of:		
			≥0.00 D, ≤2.00 D	>2.00 D, ≤4.50 D	>4.50 D
For single vision and segmented multifocals	From 0.00 up to ±6.50 D	±0.13 D	±0.13 D	±0.15 D	±4%
	Above ± 6.50 D	±2%	±0.13 D	±0.15 D	±4%

TABLE A-2
Distance Refractive Power Tolerances for Progressive Addition Lenses

	Power in Meridian of Highest Power	Tolerance on Meridian of Highest Power	Tolerance on Cylinder Powers of:		
			≥0.00 D, ≤2.00 D	>2.00 D, ≤3.50 D	>3.50 D
For Progressive Addition Lenses	From 0.00 up to ±8.00 D	±0.16 D	±0.16 D	±0.18 D	±5%
	Above ± 8.00 D	±2%	±0.16 D	±0.18 D	±5%

TABLE A-3
Tolerances for Cylinder Axis

Cylinder Power Stated Exactly	Cylinder Power Stated in Quarter Diopter Steps	Axis Tolerance in Degrees for the Stated Cylinder Power
Up to and including 0.25	0.25	±14
>0.25 up to and including 0.50	0.50	±7
>0.50 up to and including 0.75	0.75	±5
>0.75 up to and including 1.50	1.00, 1.25 and 1.50	±3
>1.50	1.75 and above	±2

When measuring for cylinder axis, the lens should be checked at the distance reference point. The distance reference point is that point on a lens where, according to the manufacturer, the distance power is to be measured. The distance reference point may not correspond to the prism reference point, as in the case of progressive addition lenses.

TABLE A-4
Addition Power Tolerances for Segmented Multifocals and Progressive Addition Lenses

Add Power	Tolerance
Up to and including 4.00	±0.12
>4.00	±0.18

TABLE A-5
Determining Unwanted Vertical and Horizontal Prism Tolerances Using the More Traditional Method: Single Vision and Segmented Multifocal Lenses Mounted in the Frame

	Tolerance
Vertical prism or PRP* placement	Within 1/3 prism diopter *or* within 1.0-mm difference between left and right PRP (prism reference point) heights in high-powered Rx with no prism ordered
Horizontal prism or PRP placement	Within 2/3 prism diopter (total from both lenses combined) *or* within ±2.5-mm variation from the specified distance PD for high-powered Rxs

*The prism reference point (PRP) is that point on a lens where prism power is to be verified. It has also been referred to as the major reference point (MRP).

TABLE A-6
Determining Unwanted Vertical and Horizontal Prism Tolerances Using the Power-Based Method: Single Vision and Segmented Multifocal Lenses Mounted in the Frame*

VERTICAL PRISM

For lenses of ±3.375 D or below in the vertical meridian . . .	unwanted vertical imbalance shall not exceed 0.33Δ
For lenses stronger than ±3.375 D in the vertical meridian . . .	the vertical differences between prism reference points may not be greater than 1.0 mm

HORIZONTAL PRISM

For lenses of ±2.75 D or below in the horizontal meridian . . .	unwanted horizontal prism for both eyes combined shall not exceed 0.67Δ
For lenses stronger than ±2.75 D in the horizontal meridian . . .	the horizontal difference from the ordered PD and the actual measured distance between the prism reference points shall not be greater than 2.5 mm

*Both the more traditional method and the power-based method yield exactly the same tolerance results.

TABLE A-7

Tolerances for Unwanted Vertical and Horizontal Prism:
Edged but Unmounted Single Vision and Segmented Multifocals and Uncut Multifocals

For both horizontal and vertical prism . . .	the tolerance must be within $\frac{1}{3}\Delta$ of the ordered prism power, *or* the PRP placement must be within ±1.0 mm of the ordered position

---

TABLE A-8

Tolerances for Progressive Addition Lens Fitting Cross (Fitting Point) Location

VERTICAL FITTING CROSS HEIGHTS

A single un-mounted lens	Actual fitting cross height must be within ±1.0 mm of the ordered fitting cross height
A pair of un-mounted lenses	*Also,* both fitting cross heights should be within 1 mm of each other relative to their ordered
A pair of mounted lenses	heights

HORIZONTAL FITTING CROSS LOCATION

A single un-mounted lens	Actual monocular interpupillary distance must be within ±1.0 mm from the monocular
A pair of un-mounted lenses	interpupillary distance specified.
A pair of mounted lenses	

HORIZONTAL TILT (AS MEASURED USING THE HIDDEN ALIGNMENT REFERENCE MARKINGS)

| Mounted lens | 2 degrees |

TABLE A-9

Unwanted Vertical and Horizontal Prism Tolerances for Progressive Addition Lenses

VERTICAL PRISM*

| For lenses of ±3.375 D or below in the vertical meridian . . . | vertical prismatic imbalance shall not exceed 0.33Δ[†] |
| For lenses stronger than ±3.375Δ in the vertical meridian . . . | the combined vertical variation from each prism reference point must not exceed 1 mm. |

HORIZONTAL PRISM

| For lenses of ±3.375 D or below in the horizontal meridian . . . | the combined unwanted horizontal prismatic effects at the prism reference points must not exceed 0.67Δ. |
| For lenses stronger than ±3.375 D in the horizontal meridian . . . | the horizontal variation from the ordered prism reference point location[‡] must not be greater than ±1.0 mm for either lens. |

---

*When prism thinning is used to reduce lens thickness, the vertical thinning prism is considered as if it were prescribed prism.

[†]For lens pairs with different cross heights, finding unwanted vertical prism is not as simple as dotting the stronger lens and sliding the spectacles across to read the other lens vertical prismatic effect. The second prism reference point will be at a different ordered height.

[‡]The horizontal prism reference point location is the same as the monocular PD.

TABLE A-10
Tolerances for Multifocal Segment Location and Tilt

Vertical segment heights	Tolerance
One unmounted lens	Actual height should be within ±1.0 mm from the ordered segment height
A lens pair (mounted or unmounted)	Actual height should be within ±1.0 mm from the ordered segment height *and* both lens segments in the pair should be within 1 mm of each other

Horizontal segment location* (Near PD)	Tolerance
Mounted lens pair	Near PD should be within ±2.5 mm of the ordered near PD. Inset should appear symmetrical and balanced unless specified monocularly

Segment Tilt (The amount the flat top of a segment line deviates from the horizontal)	Tolerance
Mounted lens	2 degrees

*For an E-line (Franklin style) bifocal, the center of the segment is located at the thinnest point on the segment ledge.

TABLE A-11
ANSI Z80.1-2005 Miscellaneous Tolerances

	Tolerance
Thickness (measured at the prism reference point)	±0.3 mm (when thickness is specified on the order)
Warpage	1.00 D (does not apply for points within 6 mm of the eyewire)
Base curve	±0.75 D (when specified on the order)
Impact resistance	Capable of withstanding the impact of a 5/8 inch steel ball dropped from 50 inches

WHAT IS THE MERIDIAN OF HIGHEST ABSOLUTE POWER?

To be able to understand the "meridian of highest absolute power" as referenced in Table A-1, consider the following:

- The power of one major meridian is the sphere power.
- The power of the other major meridian equals the sphere power plus the cylinder power.
- Of these two meridians, the meridian having the highest numerical value (plus or minus) is "the meridian of highest absolute power."

HOW TO DETERMINE IF REFRACTIVE POWER IS WITHIN TOLERANCE

Here is a cookbook method that may be used to see if the refractive power of a prescription is within ANSI standards.

Example A-1

Here is an example of a prescription where the meridian of highest absolute power is also the sphere power. Determine whether or not the prescription passes ANSI refractive power tolerances.

Methodology	Example
1. Note the refractive power of the ordered prescription.	1. $+4.25 - 1.75 \times 180$
2. Measure the refractive power of the ordered prescription.	2. $+4.37 - 1.62 \times 178$

3. Find the power in the meridian of highest absolute power for
  a. the ordered prescription and
  b. the measured prescription
	3.
	  a. $+4.25$
	  b. $+4.37$

4. Using Table A-1, determine:
  a. What is the tolerance for the meridian of highest absolute power?
  b. Is the meridian of highest absolute power within tolerance?
	4.
	  a. Tolerance for a 4.25 D power is ±0.13 D, giving a possible range of from $+4.12$ D to $+4.38$ D.
	  b. The $+4.37$ D measured power is within the tolerance range.

5. Using Table A-1 determine:
  a. What is the tolerance for the cylinder power?
 	
  b. Is the cylinder power within tolerance?
	5.
	  a. Tolerance for a 1.75 D cylinder is ±0.13 D, giving a possible range of from -1.62 to -1.88 D.
	  b. The -1.62 measured cylinder power is within the tolerance range.

6. Using Table A-3 determine:
  a. What is the tolerance for the cylinder axis?
 	
  b. Is the cylinder axis within tolerance?
	6.
	  a. Axis tolerance for a 1.75 D cylinder is ±2 degrees. This gives a possible range of between 178 and 2 degrees.
	  b. The measured axis is 178 degrees and thus within the tolerance range.
	  Conclusion: The prescription passes.

Example A-2

Here is an example of a prescription where the meridian of highest absolute power is not the sphere power. Determine whether or not the prescription passes ANSI refractive power tolerances.

Methodology	Example
1. Ordered power	1. $-5.00 - 2.00 \times 174$
2. Measured power	2. $-5.12 - 2.12 \times 174$

3. Power of meridian of highest absolute power for
  a. The ordered prescription
  b. The measured prescription
	3.
	  a. $\mid -5.00 - 2.00 \mid = 7.00$
	  b. $\mid -5.12 - 2.12 \mid = 7.24$

4.
  a. Tolerance for the meridian of highest absolute power.
  b. Is the meridian within tolerance?
	4.
	  a. 2% of 7.00 is $0.02 \times 7 = 0.14$ D. This gives a possible range of from -6.86 D to -7.14 D.
	  b. The measured power in this meridian is -7.24. This is well outside of ANSI standards.
	  Conclusion: The prescription does not pass.

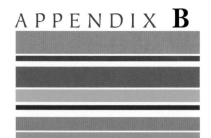

Special Purpose Frames

Clip-ons

Clip-ons are supplementary lenses in a mounting that fastens to the frame front of a conventional pair of spectacles. They fit on the outside of the front and may contain sun lenses, plus lenses for reading, prisms, or any other prescription desired for testing or visual training purposes.

Drop-ins

Drop-ins are supplementary lenses in a mounting that drops in behind the lenses of a conventional pair of spectacles. They are not always as practical as clip-ons because of their close proximity to the eyelashes. Here are two examples. Occasionally sun lenses in drop-in form are placed behind prescription eyewear. Also drop-in prescription lenses can be placed behind wraparound sunglass frames.

Entropion Spectacles

Entropion spectacles are equipped with an additional extension behind and roughly parallel to the lower eyewire, which is known as a crutch or gallery. The crutch supports the skin of the lower lid and prevents the lower lashes from turning in on the eye itself. Fortunately eyelid surgery is now able to reduce the need for entropion spectacles. (See also Ptosis Spectacles.)

Folding Frames

Folding frames are those with hinges placed at the bridge and halfway down each temple. This enables the glasses to be folded to a size equal to one half the width of the frame front. Such frames are popular for reading glasses and are often seen with over-the-counter readers.

Hemianopic Spectacles

Hemianopic spectacles are used by those with a homonymous hemianopia, which is a loss of vision on one side of the midline of the visual field. Such spectacles contain prism on one side of the lens with its base oriented toward the blind side. By glancing into the prism on the spectacles, the wearer is able to enlarge his or her visual field into the otherwise unseen area intermittently. The power of the prism used may vary, but is often on the order of 8∆. For more on this type of correction, see Chapter 17.

Hinged Front Spectacles

Hinged front spectacles are manufactured with two fronts. The frame front closest to the face is fixed, and the other is hinged and may be flipped down or up. The hinged front usually contains a near addition, although any type of lens could be mounted in the frame.

Lorgnettes

Lorgnettes are a specially designed frame front. Instead of temples there is a clip or stick with which the glasses may be held in front of the eyes. Lorgnettes are designed to be used for situations where vision at either distance or near must be corrected for short periods of time.

Makeup Spectacles

Makeup spectacles have independent rims that are hinged on the lower edge and may be tipped forward. Each lens may be used alone. When the right lens is tipped down, makeup may be applied to the right eye while viewing with the left and vice versa.

Monocle

A monocle is a single lens mounting held in place by being wedged between the cheek and upper eyebrow area.

Ptosis Spectacles

Ptosis spectacles are equipped with a crutch that is positioned behind and roughly parallel to the upper eyewire. The crutch supports the skin of the upper lid and prevents the lid from drooping closed. Metal frames can be fitted as ptosis spectacles using flexible wire as a mock-up to show the basic shape, then constructed from the model. Plastic frames can be mocked up using a thin card, then constructed in plastic or from a metal wire that has one end imbedded into the plastic of the upper rim of the frame.

Recumbent Spectacles

Recumbent spectacles are equipped with reflecting prisms that enable a person lying flat on his or her back to see straight ahead while looking straight up. These can be useful for those wishing to read while being required to remain on their backs for long periods of time. The prisms must be perfectly aligned or diplopia occurs, making wear impossible.

Reversible Spectacles

Reversible spectacles are only appropriate for an individual only able to use one eye, yet who needs different corrective lenses for distance and near. They can be used when multifocals are inappropriate or undesirable. Reversible spectacles are designed so that they may be worn upside down. Temples usually swivel at the endpiece so that the earpieces can be turned up or down. Alternate means of obtaining a reversal are also available.

Glossary

@ Symbol for at, or in the same meridian as.

Δ Symbol for *prism* power. When following a number, it denotes the units known as prism diopters. (See Diopter, prism)

∇ Symbol for *prism* power. When following a number, it denotes the units known as prism centrads. (See Centrad)

◯ Symbol for in combination with.

180-degree line A synonym for horizontal midline.

A

A The horizontal dimension of the boxing system rectangle that encloses a lens or lens opening.

Abbé value *See* value, Abbé.

aberration The resulting degradation of an image that occurs when a point source of light does not result in a single-point image after going through the lens or lens system.

aberration, chromatic The type of aberration that causes light of different wavelengths (colors) to be refracted differently through the same optical system.

aberration, lateral chromatic An aberration that produces images of slightly different sizes at the focal length of the lens, depending upon the color of the light. (Synonym: *chromatic power.*)

aberration, longitudinal chromatic Occurs when a point light source that is composed of several wavelengths (such as white light) forms a series of point images along the optical axis. Each of these images is a different color, and each has a slightly different focal length.

aberration, monochromatic An aberration that is present even when light is made up of only one wavelength (one color).

aberration, spherical An aberration that occurs when parallel light from an object enters a large area of a spherical lens surface, and peripheral rays focus at different points on the optic axis than do paraxial rays.

absolute refractive index *See* index, absolute refractive.

accurate sag formula *See* formula, accurate sag.

achromatic lens *See* lens, achromatic

actual power *See* power, actual.

add *See* addition, near.

add, nasal The modification of an existing spectacle lens shape for the purpose of creating a better frame fit by allowing more lens to remain in the inferior, nasal position after edging the lens than would be otherwise indicated by the original shape.

addition, near The plus power a multifocal lens segment has that is added to the power already present in the main portion of the lens.

age-related maculopathy *See* maculopathy, age-related.

alignment, horizontal The alignment of the right and left horizontal midlines in a pair of spectacles with a single horizontal plane (neither lens is higher than the other when viewed from the front).

alignment, standard An impersonal standard, independent of facial shape, for the alignment of spectacle frames.

alignment, vertical Lack of deviation of the two spectacle lenses from the vertical plane (one being neither farther forward nor backward than the other).

allowance, grinding Synonym for wheel differential.

allowance, vertex power The amount by which the front surface curvature of a lens must be flattened to compensate for a thickness-related gain in power.

American endpiece *See* endpiece, American.

American National Standards Institute An industry-based, nongovernmental standards-setting association. The American National Standards Institute is an agency that addresses standards throughout all of industry within the United States, of which the ophthalmic industry is only a small part. ANSI sets standards for aspects of the ophthalmic industry that includes lenses, frames, and contact lenses.

Amethyst Contrast Enhancer (ACE) A selectively absorbing glass developed by Schott that is said to enhance contrast and be advantageous for target and trap shooting, hunting, computer terminal viewing, skiing, and bird watching. The lens allows highest transmission around the blue, green, and red regions of the spectrum.

ametropia The refractive condition that occurs when parallel rays entering the eye do not focus on the retina when the eye is not accommodating.

ametropia, axial Ametropia that occurs because the eye is too long or too short.

ametropia, refractive Ametropia that occurs because the refractive elements (surfaces) of the eye are too strong or too weak.

analyzer, lens A trade name for an automated lensmeter.

angle of deviation The difference between the angle of incidence and the angle of refraction.

angle, apical The angle formed by the junction of two nonparallel prism surfaces.

angle, Brewster's The angle of incidence at which reflected light from a refracting surface is completely polarized.

angle, crest The angle from the tip to the top of the nose (between the eyes) compared with a vertical plane roughly parallel to the brows and cheeks.

angle, effective diameter The angle from the 0-degree side of the 180-degree line to the axis of the effective diameter. The angle is referred to by the letter *X* and is measured using the right lens.

angle, frontal 1. The angle with which each side of the nose deviates from the vertical. 2. The angular amount the nosepad face deviates from the vertical when the frame is viewed from the front.

angle, pantoscopic 1. In standard alignment: that angle by which the frame front deviates from the vertical (lower rims farther inward than upper rims) when the spectacles are held with the temples horizontal. 2. In fitting: that angle that the frame front makes with the frontal plane of the wearer's face when the lower rims are closer to the face than the upper rims (opposite-retroscopic angle). (Synonym: *pantoscopic tilt*.)

angle, retroscopic That angle that the frame front makes with the frontal plane of the wearer's face when the lower rims are farther from the face than the upper rims (opposite-pantoscopic angle). (Synonym: *retroscopic tilt*.)

angle, splay 1. That angle formed by the side of the nose with a straight anterior-posterior surface that would bisect it vertically (also called *transverse angle*). 2. The angle the face of a nosepad makes with a plane perpendicular to that of the frame front when viewed from above.

angle, temple fold The angle formed when a temple is folded to a closed position when viewed from the back.

angle, vertical When viewed from the side, that angle formed between the plane of the lenses and the long axis of the adjustable nosepads.

aniseikonia A relative difference in the size and/or the shape of the images seen by the right and the left eyes.

aniseikonia, anatomical When aniseikonia is caused by the anatomical structure, such as an unequal distribution of the retinal elements (rods and cones) of one eye compared with the other.

aniseikonia, asymmetrical A form of aniseikonia in which there is a progressive increase or decrease in image size across the visual field of one eye compared to the other.

aniseikonia, induced Aniseikonia that occurs when a size difference in right and left eye images is caused by an outside source, as from correcting ophthalmic lenses.

aniseikonia, inherent optical Aniseikonia that occurs when a size difference in right and left images is caused by the optics of the eye.

aniseikonia, meridional When one eye sees an image that is greater in size in one meridian than the corresponding image size for that same meridian in the other eye.

aniseikonia, symmetrical Aniseikonia in which one eye sees an image that is symmetrically larger than that of the other eye. One image is equally larger in every meridian compared with the image of the other eye.

anisometropia A condition in which one eye differs significantly in refractive power from the other.

ANSI Abbreviation for American National Standards Institute.

antireflection coating *See* coating, antireflection.

antiscratch coating *See* coating, antiscratch.

aperture 1. An opening or hole that admits only a portion of light from a given source or sources. 2. The central, optically correct portion of a lenticular lens.

aperture, lens The portion of the spectacle frame that accepts the lens. (Synonym: *lens opening*.)

apex The junction point at which the two nonparallel surfaces of a prism meet.

aphake A person whose crystalline lens has been removed and not replaced with an intraocular lens implant.

apical angle *See* angle, apical.

AR An abbreviation for antireflection coating.

arm Also called *bar, browbar*; in a semirimless mounting, the metal reinforcement that follows the upper posterior surface of a spectacle lens and joins the centerpiece to the endpiece.

arms, guard A synonym for pad arms.

arms, pad Metal pieces that connect adjustable nosepads to the front of a frame. (Synonym: *guard arms*.)

aspheric A nonspherical surface.

aspheric lens *See* lens, aspheric.

aspheric lenticular *See* lenticular, aspheric.

aspheric, full-field *See* lens, full-field asphoric.

astigmatic difference *See* difference, astigmatic.

astigmatism The presence of two different curves on a single refracting surface on or within the eye. This causes light to focus as two line images instead of as a single point.

astigmatism, marginal *See* astigmatism, oblique.

astigmatism, oblique 1. An astigmatic eye condition whereby the major meridians of the correcting lens are at an oblique angle, between 30 and 60 degrees or 120 and 150 degrees. 2. The lens aberration that occurs when rays from an off-axis point pass through a spherical lens and light focuses as two line images instead of a single point. (Synonyms: *radial astigmatism, marginal astigmatism*.)

astigmatism, radial *See* astigmatism, oblique.

ASTM American Society for Testing and Materials.

atoric lens *See* lens, atoric.

autolensmeter A lensmeter that measures the power and prismatic effect of the lens in an automated fashion.

axial ametropia *See* ametropia, axial.

axis meridian *See* meridian, axis.

axis of a cylinder An imaginary reference line used to specify cylinder or spherocylinder lens orientation and corresponding to the meridian perpendicular to that of maximum cylinder power.

axis, optical That line which passes through the center of a lens on which the radii of curvature of the front and back surfaces fall.

axis, prism The base direction of an ophthalmic prism, expressed in degrees.

B

B The vertical dimension of the boxing system rectangle that encloses a lens or lens opening.

back base curve *See* curve, back base.

back vertex power *See* power, back vertex.

bakelite One of the first plastics used to make frames. Bakelite is a synthetic resin invented around 1909 and was used for such items as pool balls, jewelry, buttons, radio cases, and lamps.

Balgrip mounting *See* mounting, Balgrip.

bar *See* arm.

barrel The housing for a screw on a pair of glasses.

barrel distortion *See* distortion, barrel.

base In a prism, the edge of maximum surface separation opposite the apex.

base curve *See* curve, base.

base down Vertical placement of prism such that the base is at 270 degrees on a degree scale.

base in Horizontal placement of prism such that the base is toward the nose.

base out Horizontal placement of prism such that the base is toward the side of the head.

base up Vertical placement of prism such that the base is at 90 degrees on a degree scale.

basic impact *See* impact, basic.

batch testing The practice of selectively testing a statistically significant number of lenses in a manufactured group.

BCD Boxing center distance. *See* distance, boxing center.

bent-down portion *See* earpiece.

best form lens *See* lens, corrected curve.

bevel The angled edge of the spectacle lens.

bevel, hidden An edged lens configuration that attempts to reduce the appearance of thickness by creating a small bevel with the rest of the lens edge remaining flat.

bevel, mini A lens edge configuration that has a bevel and an angled ledge.

bevel, pin Synonym for safety bevel.

bevel, safety 1. To remove the sharp interface between lens surface and bevel surface and the sharp point at the bevel apex. 2. The smoothed interface between lens surface and bevel surface and the smoothed lens bevel apex.

bevel, V A lens edge configuration having the form of a V across the whole breadth of the lens edge.

bicentric grinding *See* grinding, bicentric.

biconcave A term used to describe a lens that is inwardly curved on both surfaces.

biconvex A term used to describe a lens that is outwardly curved on both surfaces.

bifocal A lens having two areas for viewing, each with its own focal power. Usually the upper portion of the lens is for distance vision, the lower for near vision.

bifocal, blended A bifocal lens constructed from one piece of lens material and having the demarcation line smoothed out so as not to be visible to an observer.

bifocal, curved-top A bifocal lens having a segment that is round in the lower portion and gently curved on the top of the segment.

bifocal, Executive American Optical's trade name for the Franklin-style bifocal.

bifocal, flat-top A bifocal with a segment that is round in the lower half, but flat on the top.

bifocal, Franklin A bifocal having a segment that extends the entire width of the lens blank.

bifocal, minus add A bifocal with a large, round segment at the top of the lens. The segment is powered for distance viewing and the rest of the lens for near viewing. (Synonym: *minus add bifocal*.)

bifocal, Panoptik A bifocal lens resembling a flat-top bifocal, but having a segment that has a slightly curved upper edge with rounded corners.

bifocal, Rede-Rite *See* bifocal, minus add.

bifocal, ribbon A bifocal with a segment that resembles a circle with the top and bottom removed.

bifocal, round seg A bifocal with a segment that is perfectly round. The width of the segment is normally 22 mm, 25 mm, or 38 mm.

bifocal, upcurve *See* bifocal, minus add.

binocular PD *See* PD, binocular.

bitoric lens *See* lens, bitoric.

blank geometrical center *See* center, blank geometrical.

blank seg drop *See* drop, blank seg.

blank seg inset *See* inset, blank seg.

blank, finished lens A lens that has front and back surfaces ground to the desired powers, but not yet edged to the shape of the frame.

blank, pattern A predrilled, flat piece of plastic from which a pattern may be cut.

blank, rough A thick, round "lens" with neither side having the finished curvature. Both sides must yet be surfaced to bring the lens to its desired power and thickness.

blank, semifinished lens A lens with only one side having the desired curvature. The second side must yet be surfaced to bring the lens to its desired power and thickness.

bleaching, optical The lightening of a photochromic lens from exposure to red light or IR radiation.

bleaching, thermal The lightening of a photochromic lens from exposure to heat.

blended bifocals *See* lens, blended bifocal.

blended myodisc *See* lens, blended myodisc.

block That which is attached to the surface of a lens to hold it in place during the surfacing or edging process.

blocker The device used to place a block on the lens to hold the lens in place during the surfacing or edging process.

blocker, layout A centering device with the capability of also blocking the lens. The layout blocker does not mark the lens first, but blocks it immediately after centration.

blocking, finish The application of a holding block to an ophthalmic lens so that it may be edged to fit a frame.

blocking, surface The application of a holding block to an ophthalmic lens so that one side may be ground to the correct curvature and polished.

Boley gauge *See* gauge, Boley.

box, light A box with a white, translucent piece of plastic on top and a full spectrum bulb inside. When used in the optical laboratory, the white, illuminated background serves as a backdrop for comparison of two lens colors.

boxing center *See* center, boxing.

boxing center distance *See* distance, boxing center.

boxing system *See* system, boxing.

Box-o-Graph A flat device containing grids and slides, used in the measurement of pattern and edged lens size.

Brewster's angle *See* angle, Brewster's.

bridge The area of the frame front between the lenses.

bridge, comfort A clear plastic saddle-type bridge that is used on a metal frame.

bridge, keyhole The top, inside area of a keyhole bridge is shaped like an old-fashioned keyhole. From the top, it flares out slightly, resting on the sides of the nose, but not on the crest of the nose.

bridge, metal saddle A metal bridge for a spectacle frame that arches across in a thin band, sitting directly on the crest of the nose. (Synonym: *W bridge.*)

bridge, pad The bridge commonly used in metal frames having adjustable nosepads.

bridge, saddle A frame bridge that is shaped like a saddle in a smooth curve and follows the bridge of the nose smoothly.

bridge, semisaddle A bridge that looks much the same as a saddle from the front, but has permanent, nonadjustable nosepads attached to the back of the bridge. (Synonym: *modified saddle bridge.*)

bridge, skewed That misalignment that occurs when one lens in a pair of spectacles is higher than the other yet neither lens is rotated.

bridge-narrowing pliers *See* pliers, bridge-narrowing.

bridge-widening pliers *See* pliers, bridge-widening.

browbar *See* arm.

buildup pads *See* pads, buildup.

bushing A small, hollow cylindrical sleeve that fits into the hole in the lens through which a screw passes. Its purpose is to prevent stress and abrasion.

C

C The horizontal width of a lens or lens opening as measured at the level of its geometrical center. (Synonym: *datum length.*)

C size The circumference of an edged lens.

cable temple *See* temple, cable.

caliper, vernier A hand-held width measuring device with a short graduated scale that slides along a longer graduated scale allowing a measure of fractional parts or decimals.

carbon fiber A material made from strands of carbon fibers combined with nylon. When used for spectacle frames, it is thin, strong, but not adjustable.

carrier The outer, nonoptical portion of a lenticular lens.

cataract A loss in clarity of the crystalline lens of the eye, which results in reduced vision or loss of vision.

cellulose acetate A material extracted from cotton or wood pulp and used extensively for making spectacle frames.

cellulose acetopropionate *See* Propionate.

cellulose nitrate *See* zylonite.

cement lens *See* lens, cement.

center, blank geometrical The physical center of a semifinished lens blank or an uncut finished lens blank. The blank geometrical center is the center of the smallest square or rectangle that completely encloses the lens blank.

center, boxing The midpoint of the rectangle that encloses a lens in the boxing system.

center, cutting Synonym for mechanical center.

center, datum The midpoint of the datum length (C dimension) of a lens as measured along the datum or horizontal midline.

center, edging Synonym for mechanical center.

center, geometrical 1. The boxing center. 2. The middle point on an uncut lens blank.

center, mechanical The rotational center of a pattern found at the midpoint of the central pattern hole. (Synonyms: *cutting center, edging center*)

center, optical That point on an ophthalmic prescription lens through which no prismatic effect is manifested.

center, reading That point on a lens at the reading level that corresponds to the near PD.

center, rotational The point on a pattern around which it rotates during edging.

center, seg optical That location on the segment of a bifocal lens that shows zero prismatic effect when no refractive power is in the distance portion of the lens.

centerpiece The portion of a rimless mounting consisting of bridge, pad arms, pads, and strap area.

Centrad ∇ A unit of measurement of the displacement of light by a prism. One centrad is the prism power required to displace a ray of light 1 cm from the position it would otherwise strike on the arc of a circle having a 1-m radius.

centration The act of positioning a lens for edging such that the lens will conform optically to prescription specifications.

chamfering The word *chamfer* means to bevel. In lens finishing, chamfering is taken to mean the act of smoothing off or safety beveling the sharp edges of a hole, slot, or notch drilled in a spectacle lens to prevent the chipping of the hole, slot, or notch, when the spectacles are worn. *Note: Chamfering* and *safety beveling* are synonymous.

chassis The portion of the frame that includes the eyewire and center or bridge section. Commonly refers to the metal eyewire and bridge of a combination frame.

chemical tempering *See* tempering, chemical.

chemtempering *See* tempering, chemical.

chord A straight line that intersects two points of an arc.

chord diameter *See* diameter, chord.

chromatic aberration *See* aberration, chromatic.

chromatic power *See* aberration, lateral chromatic.

circumference gauge *See* gauge, circumference.

clock, lens *See* measure, lens.

clock, seg Designed like a conventional lens clock (lens measure) except that the three points of contact are closely spaced. Now most lens clocks also have narrowly spaced contact points so that there is little if any difference between a newer lens clock and a seg clock.

coating, antireflection A thin layer or series of layers of material applied to the surface of a lens for the purpose of reducing unwanted reflections from the lens surface and thus increasing the amount of light that passes through to the eye.

coating, antiscratch A thin, hard coating applied to plastic lens surfaces to make them more resistant to scratching.

coating, color A coating applied to the surface of a lens for the purpose of reducing light transmission.

coating, dielectric A mirrorlike coating that reflects certain wavelengths selectively.

coating, edge Application of color to the edge of a lens for the purpose of decreasing edge visibility.

coating, flash A metalized lens coating that absorbs light and has only a hint of reflectance.

coating, metalized A thin layer of metal on the front of the lens to both absorb and reflect light.

coating, mirror A coating applied to a lens causing it to have the same properties as a two-way mirror.

coating, scratch resistant A synonym for antiscratch coating.

collar *See* shoe.

colmascope An instrument that uses polarized light to show strain patterns in glass or plastic lenses. (Synonym: *polariscope*.)

color coating *See* coating, color.

color, reflex The residual color of an antireflection-coated lens.

coma The lens aberration that occurs when the object point is off the axis of the lens. Instead of forming a single, point image off the optic axis, the image appears shaped like a comet or ice cream cone.

combination frame *See* frame, combination.

comfort bridge *See* bridge, comfort.

comfort cable temple *See* temple, cable.

compensated power *See* power, compensated.

compensated segs *See* segs, R-compensated.

compounding (of prism) The process of combining two or more prisms to obtain the equivalent prismatic effect expressed as a single prism.

concave An inward-curved surface.

conditioner, lens A specially formulated solution into which a plastic lens is immersed before being tinted. The purpose of lens conditioner is to prepare the lens for a fast and even uptake of dye.

conjugate foci *See* foci, conjugate.

contour plot *See* plot, contour.

convergence 1. An inward turning of the eyes, as when looking at a near object. 2. The action of light rays traveling toward a specific image point.

convertible temple *See* temple, convertible.

convex An outward-curved surface.

coolant A liquid used to cool and lubricate the lens-grinding wheel interface during the grinding process.

coquille The thin nonpowered demonstration lens that comes in a spectacle frame to hold the shape of the frame as intended and to more realistically simulate the appearance of the frame for the prospective wearer. (Synonyms: *dummy lens, demo lens*.)

Corlon lens *See* lens, Corlon.

corrected curve lens *See* lens, corrected curve.

corridor, progressive The area of a progressive-addition lens between the distance and near portions where the power of the lens is gradually changing.

cosine For a right triangle, the ratio of the side adjacent to the angle considered, to the hypotenuse.

$$\text{Cosine} = \frac{\text{Adjacent}}{\text{Hypotenuse}}$$

cosine-squared formula *See* formula, cosine-squared.

countersink curve *See* curve, countersink.

cover lens *See* lens, cover.

CR-39 A registered trademark of Pittsburgh Plate Glass Co. for an optical plastic known as Columbia Resin 39. It has been the standard material from which conventional plastic lenses are made.

crazed The cracked appearance of a lens with a damaged or defective coating.

crest The highest and centermost part of the bridge of a spectacle frame.

crest angle *See* angle, crest.

cribbing The process of reducing a semifinished lens blank to a smaller size to speed the surfacing process or reduce the probability of difficulty.

cross curve *See* curve, cross.

cross, fitting A reference point 2 to 4 mm above the prism reference point on progressive-addition lenses. The fitting cross is positioned in front of the pupil.

cross, power A schematic representation on which the two major meridians of a lens or lens surface are depicted.

crown glass *See* glass, crown.

curl *See* earpiece.

curvature The reciprocal of the radius of curvature of a curved surface, quantified in reciprocal meters (m^{-1}), and abbreviated by R.

curvature of field The lens aberration that causes the spherical power of the lens to be off in the periphery when compared with the center of the lens. For a flat object, this results in a curved image. (Synonym: *power error.*)

curve, back base The weaker back-surface curve of a minus cylinder-form lens. When the lens is a minus cylinder-form lens, the back base curve and the toric base curve are the same.

curve, base The surface curve of a lens that becomes the basis from which the other remaining curves are calculated. In the United States and most other parts of the world, this is usually the front surface spherical curve of the lens.

curve, countersink For the manufacture of fused-glass semifinished bifocal and trifocal lenses, the countersink curve is that curve that is ground into the main lens in the area where the segment is to be placed. The countersink curve matches the back curve of the bifocal or trifocal segment. When the segment is placed on the countersink curve of the main lens, the two may then be fused together.

curve, cross The stronger curve of a toric lens surface.

curve, nominal base A 1.53-index-referenced number assigned to the base curve of a semifinished lens. For moderately powered crown-glass lenses, the needed back surface tool curve may be found by subtracting the nominal base curve from the prescribed back vertex power.

curve, tool The 1.53-index-referenced surface power of a lap tool used in the fining and polishing of ophthalmic lenses.

curve, true base Synonym for true power.

cut, nasal The removal of an inferior, nasal portion of the lens shape to create a better frame fit.

cutting line *See* line, cutting.

cylinder A lens having a refractive power in one meridian only and used in the correction of astigmatism.

D

D An abbreviation for diopter of refractive power. *See* diopter, lens.

datum center *See* center, datum.

datum center distance *See* distance, datum center.

datum line *See* line, datum.

datum system *See* system, datum.

DBC Distance between centers.

DBL Distance between lenses.

DCD Datum center distance.

decentration 1. The displacement of the lens optical center or major reference point away from the boxing center of the frame's lens aperture. 2. The displacement of a lens optical center away from the wearer's line of sight for the purpose of creating a prismatic effect.

decentration, effective The distance from the axis of a decentered cylinder to the point from which decentration began.

degression The decrease in plus power measured from the lower viewing area to the upper viewing area of an occupational progressive addition lens.

demand, dioptric The inverse of the reading distance in meters, independent of actual bifocal addition power.

demo lens *See* coquille.

depth, middatum The depth of an edged lens measured through the datum center.

depth, reading The vertical position in the lens through which the wearer's line of sight passes when reading.

depth, sagittal (sag) The height or depth of a given segment of a circle.

depth, seg The longest vertical dimension of the lens segment before the lens has been edged.

deviation, angle of *See* angle of deviation.

diameter, chord The length of the chord of an arc or circle. When processing spectacle lenses, this diameter is equal to the minimum blank size required for cutting a lens, but does not include the 2-mm safety factor for lens chipping that is included in the MBS formula.

diameter, effective Twice the longest radius of a frame's lens aperture as measured from the boxing center. Abbreviated ED.

dielectric coating *See* coating, dielectric.

difference, astigmatic The linear distance between the two line foci that occurs in the lens aberration called *oblique astigmatism*. When expressed in diopters, this difference is called the *oblique astigmatic error*.

difference, frame In the boxing system, the difference between frame A and frame B dimensions, expressed in millimeters. Synonym: *lens difference*.

difference, pattern In the boxing system, the difference between pattern *A* and *B* dimensions, expressed in millimeters.

differential, wheel The difference in millimeters between the size of the lens produced in roughing and finishing operations during edging.

diopter, lens (D) Unit of lens refractive power, equal to the reciprocal of the lens focal length in meters.

diopter, prism (Δ) The unit of measurement that quantifies prism deviating power; one prism diopter (1Δ) is the power required to deviate a ray of light 1 cm from the position it would otherwise strike at a point 1 m away from the prism.

dioptric demand *See* demand, dioptric.

disability glare *See* glare, disability.

discomfort glare *See* glare, discomfort.

dispersion, mean The quantity $(n_F - n_C)$-the index of blue light minus the index of red light-that helps to define the chromatic nature of a lens material.

dispersive power *See* power, dispersive.

dissimilar segs *See* segs, dissimilar.

distance between centers (DBC) In a frame or finished pair of glasses, the distance between the boxing (geometrical) centers. (Synonym: *geometrical center distance*.)

distance between lenses (DBL) In the boxing system, the distance between the two boxed lenses as positioned in the frame. It is the shortest distance between a lens pair measured from the inside nasal eyewire grooves across the bridge area at the narrowest point (usually synonymous with *bridge size*).

distance reference point *See* point, distance reference.

distance, boxing center Synonym for distance between centers.

distance, datum center The distance between the datum centers in a frame or pair of glasses as used in the older datum system of measuring frames and lenses.

distance, frame center Synonym for distance between centers.

distance, geometrical center The distance between the boxing (geometrical) centers of a frame.

distance, interpupillary (PD) The distance from the center of one pupil to the center of the other when either an infinitely distant object is being viewed (distance PD) or a near object is being viewed (near PD).

distance, near centration The distance between the geometrical centers of the near segments.

distance, vertex The distance from the back surface of the lens to the front of the eye.

distometer The instrument used to measure vertex distance.

distortion The lens aberration that results when image magnification changes from the center to the edge of the image resulting in either a barrellike minification or pincushion-like magnification when compared with the object.

distortion, barrel The type of distortion normally caused by a minus lens that results in the image of a square object taking on a smaller barrel-shaped appearance.

distortion, pattern The loss of correct edged lens shape resulting from use of a pattern that is too large or small in comparison with the lens size being edged.

distortion, pincushion The type of distortion normally caused by a plus lens that results in the image of a square object taking on a larger pincushion-shaped appearance.

divergence The action of light rays going out from a point source.

double gradient tint *See* tint, double gradient.

double-D lens *See* lens, double-D.

double-segment lens *See* lens, double-segment.

doublet *See* lens, achromatic.

dress eyewear *See* eyewear, dress.

dress To reshape the cutting surface of a grinding wheel.

drop-ball test *See* test, drop-ball.

drop, blank seg The vertical distance from the blank geometrical center to the top of the multifocal segment.

drop, seg 1. The vertical distance from the major reference point (MRP) to the top of the segment when the segment top is lower than the MRP. 2. The vertical distance from the horizontal midline to the top of the segment when the segment top is lower than the horizontal midline (laboratory usage). (Antonym: *seg raise*.)

DRP An abbreviation for distance reference point. *See* point, distance reference.

dummy lens *See* coquille.

E

ear That portion of the strap area on a classic or antique type rimless mounting that extends from the shoe, contacting the surface of the lens. (Synonym: *tongue*.)

earpiece That part of the temple that lies past the temple bend. (Synonym: *curl*.)

ED Effective diameter.

edge coating *See* coating, edge.

edge, rolled A lens edge configuration that reduces minus lens edge thickness by rounding out the back surface edge of the lens.

edger The piece of machinery used to physically grind the uncut lens blank to fit the shape of the frame.

edger, hand A grinding wheel made especially for changing a lens shape or smoothing a lens edge by hand.

edger, patterned A lens edger that uses patterns to produce the correct lens shape.

edger, patternless An edger that uses an electronic tracing of a lens shape, rather than a physical pattern to produce the correct lens shape.

effective decentration *See* decentration, effective.

effective diameter *See* diameter, effective.

effective diameter angle *See* angle, effective diameter.

effective power *See* power, effective.

eikonometer, space An instrument used to quantitatively measure image size differences between right and left eyes.

electrometallic wheel *See* wheel, electrometallic.

electroplated wheel *See* wheel, electroplated.

ellipse, Tscherning's The elliptical-shaped graph that shows the best lens form(s) a lens can have for eliminating oblique astigmatism.

emmetrope A person without refractive error.

emmetropia The absence of refractive error.

endpiece angling pliers *See* pliers, endpiece angling.

endpiece One of the two outer areas of the frame front to the extreme left and right where the temples attach.

endpiece, American An older classification of a spectacle frame's metal endpiece that has a stop protruding from the single barrel on the temple, preventing the temple from opening out too far.

endpiece, butt-type A spectacle frame endpiece construction in which the front is straight and the temple butt is flat, and both meet at a 90-degree angle.

endpiece, English An older classification of a spectacle frame's metal endpiece that has a "stop" or "knuckle" that comes out around the hinge barrels and prevents the temples from opening out too widely.

endpiece, French An older classification of metal endpiece in which the temple is slotted between the two barrels, and the stop is on the frame front as an extension of the single barrel.

endpiece, mitre-type A spectacle frame endpiece construction in which the frame front contact area and temple butt meet at a 45-degree angle.

endpiece, turn-back A spectacle frame endpiece design in which the frame front bends around and meets the temple end to end.

English endpiece *See* endpiece, English.

equation, Fresnel The formula for determining the amount of light that will be reflected from an uncoated lens surface, based on the index of refraction of the lens material.

Equithin A term used by the Varilux Corporation when referring to the use of yoked prism for thickness reduction on a pair of progressive-addition lenses. *See also* prism, yoked.

equivalent, spherical The sum of the spherical component and one half of the cylinder component of an ophthalmic lens prescription.

equiconcave lens *See* lens, equiconcave.

equiconvex lens *See* lens, equiconvex.

error, image shell A quantitative measure of the lens aberration called curvature of field or power error. The image shell error is the dioptric difference between the place where the peripheral image actually focuses and where it should focus.

error, oblique astigmatic The "astigmatic difference" that occurs in the aberration of oblique astigmatism as expressed in diopters.

error, power *See* curvature of field.

Executive bifocal *See* bifocal, Executive.

extractor, screw A device that resembles a screwdriver, but has a barbed tip instead of a blade. The barbed tip digs into a damaged screw head or the remaining tip of a broken-off screw and is turned to remove the damaged or broken screw.

eyesize In the boxing system, the A dimension. (The horizontal dimension of the lens opening of a frame, which is bounded by two vertical lines tangent to the left and right sides of that lens opening.)

eyewear, dress Eyewear designed for everyday use.

eyewear, safety Eyewear designed to be worn in situations that could be potentially hazardous to the eyes and thus must meet higher standards of impact resistance than conventional eyewear.

eyewear, sports Eyewear designed to protect the eyes and/or enhance vision in specific sports situations. What is appropriate will vary dramatically, depending upon the sport.

eyewire The rim of the frame that goes around the lenses.

eyewire forming plier *See* plier, eyewire forming.

eyewire shaping plier Eyewire forming plier.

F

F Often used in equations to denote lens refractive power in diopters. Alternative symbol for F is D.

face form *See* form, face.

facet An edge configuration resembling the appearance of beveled glass that is sometimes used with high-minus lenses to reduce edge thickness and weight.

factor, power That part of spectacle magnification that is determined by the power and position of the lens.

factor, shape That part of spectacle magnification that is determined by the shape of the lens, including front curve, refractive index, and lens thickness.

farsightedness *See* hyperopia.

FDA Food and Drug Administration.

figure-8 liner *See* liner, figure 8.

file, pillar A general purpose file used in dispensing.

file, rat-tail A file that is used in dispensing on drilled lenses, to (1) reduce lens thickness in an area to allow for proper lens strap grasp or (2) to smooth the edges of the drilled lens hole.

file, ribbon *See* file, slotting.

file, riffler Spoon-shaped file used in dispensing, good for getting at small, hard-to-reach areas.

file, slotting Used for reslotting screws or making a slot where none previously existed.

file, zyl Used in dispensing to file plastic parts of a frame.

finger-piece pliers *See* pliers, finger-piece.

fining In surfacing the process of bringing a generated lens surface to the smoothness needed so that it will be capable of being polished.

finished lens *See* lens, finished.

finishing The process in the production of spectacles that begins with a pair of uncut lenses of the correct refractive power and ends with a completed pair of spectacles.

first focal length *See* length, first focal.

first principal focus *See* focus, first principal.

fitting cross *See* cross, fitting.

flash Synonym for swarf.

flat surface touch test *See* test, flat surface touch.

flat-top bifocal *See* bifocal, flat-top.

focal point *See* point, focal.

focal power *See* power, focal.

foci, conjugate Object and image points for a lens or lens system that correspond. In simplified terms, light rays originating at one point will be focused at the other.

focimeter Synonym for lensmeter.

focus, first principal The point at which parallel light rays entering the back surface of a lens are brought to a focus. For positive lenses this is a real focal point, for negative, virtual. (Synonym; primary focal point.)

focus, second principal That point at which parallel light rays entering the front surface of a lens are brought to focus. For positive lenses the focal point is real, for negative, virtual. (Synonym; secondary focal point)

fork, centering A forklike device that was used to hold a lens in position for blocking or for placing a lens in an older style edger at a specific orientation.

form, face An expression of the extent to which the curve in the frame front varies from the classical four-point touch position, taking on the curved form of the face.

form, minus cylinder The form a spectacle lens prescription takes when the value of the cylinder is expressed as a negative number.

form, plus cylinder The form a spectacle lens prescription takes when the value of the cylinder is expressed as a positive number.

former British equivalent of *pattern*.

formula, accurate sag The formula used to find sagittal depth, which states that where *r* is the radius of curvature of the surface and *y* is the semidiameter of the chord.

formula, cosine-squared A formula used to obtain the "power" of an oblique cylinder, usually in the 90-degree meridian.

formula, lensmaker's A formula used to find the dioptric power of a surface or radius of curvature. The formula states that where *F* is the lens refractive power in diopters, n′ is the refractive index of the lens, and *n* is the refractive index of the media surrounding the lens.

formula, sine-squared A formula used to obtain the "power" of an oblique cylinder, usually in the 180-degree meridian.

four-point touch *See* touch, four-point.

frame center distance *See* distance, frame center.

frame center distance *See* distance, geometrical center.

frame difference *See* difference, frame.

frame PD Synonym for distance between centers or geometrical center distance.

frame tracer *See* tracer, frame.

frame, combination 1. A frame having a metal chassis with plastic top rims and temples. 2. A frame having some major parts of plastic construction and some of metal.

frame, nylon cord A frame that holds the lenses in place by means of a nylon cord that fits into a groove around the edge of the lens.

frame, shell An older expression referring to a plastic frame. Derived from when tortoise shell was used as a frame material.

frame, string mounted *See* frame, nylon cord.

Franklin bifocal *See* bifocal, Franklin.

French endpiece *See* endpiece, French.

Fresnel equation *See* equation, Fresnel.

Fresnel lens *See* lens, Fresnel.

Fresnel prism *See* prism, Fresnel.

front That portion of the spectacles that contains the lenses.

front vertex power *See* power, front vertex.

front, wave The outer border formed by light rays diverging from their point of origin.

frontal angle *See* angle, frontal.

front-to-bend (FTB) Temple length expressed as the distance from the plane of the frame front to the bend of the temple.

FTB *See* front-to-bend.

full-field aspheric *See* aspheric, full-field.

fused multifocals *See* multifocals, fused.

G

galalith One of the first plastics used to make spectacle frames. Galalith was developed in 1897 from casein (a milk protein) and formaldehyde and used initially for buttons and jewelry. It fell from use after World War II.

gauge, Boley A measuring gauge that may be used to measure the width of lenses or frame lens apertures.

gauge, circumference A device used to measure the distance around the outside of a previously edged lens or a coquille for the purpose of more accurately duplicating the size of an existing lens when edging a new lens.

GCD Geometrical center distance.

generating The process of rapidly cutting the desired surface curvature onto a semifinished lens blank.

geometrical center See center, geometrical.

geometrical center distance See distance, geometrical center.

geometrically centered pattern See pattern, geometrically centered.

German silver See nickel silver.

glare control lenses See lenses, glare control.

glare, disability Glare that reduces visual performances and visibility and may be accompanied by discomfort.

glare, discomfort Glare that produces discomfort, but does not necessarily reduce visual resolution.

glass, crown A commonly used glass lens material having an index of refraction of 1.523.

glazed lens See lens, glazed.

glazing 1. The insertion of lenses into a spectacle frame. 2. The clogging of empty spaces between the exposed abrasive particles of an abrasive wheel, resulting in reduced grinding ability.

GOMAC system See system, GOMAC.

GOMAC Groupement des Opticiens du Marche Commun. (A committee of Common Market opticians formed for the purpose of establishing European optical standards.)

gradient lens See lens, gradient.

gradient tint See tint, gradient.

grayness A lens surface defect caused by incomplete polishing.

grind, bicentric Synonym for slabbing-off.

grinding allowance Synonym for wheel differential.

grinding, bicentric Grinding a portion of a lens so as to add a second optical center. It is often used to create vertical prism in the lower portion of one lens for the purpose of alleviating vertical imbalance at near. (Synonym: *slabbing-off*.)

groover, lens The piece of equipment used to place a groove around the outer edge of a spectacle lens for the purpose of holding the lens in the frame with a nylon cord or thin metal rim.

guard arms See arms, pad.

H

half-eyes Frames made especially for those who need a reading correction, but no correction for distance. They are constructed to sit lower on the nose than normal and have a vertical dimension that is only half the size of normal glasses.

hand edger See edger, hand.

hand stone See stone, hand.

HAZCOM Hazard Communication Standard (HCS). The Occupational Safety and Health Administration's *Hazard Communication Standard* requires all employers to provide their employees with information and training about any possible exposure to hazardous chemicals in the workplace. Information is to be in written form and should explain workplace policy on protection from hazards.

heat treating See treating, heat.

height, seg The vertically measured distance from the lowest point on the lens or lens opening to the level of the top of the segment.

Hide-a-Bevel Originally a trade name for an edge-grinding system that produces a shelf effect behind the bevel on thick-edged lenses. Now Hide-a-Bevel refers to this type of lens edge configuration in general.

high impact See impact, high.

high-index lens See lens, high-index.

high mass impact test See test, high mass impact.

high velocity impact test See test, high velocity impact.

hinge The part of the frame that both holds the temple to the front and allows the temple to fold closed.

hollow snipe-nosed pliers See pliers, hollow snipe-nosed.

horizontal alignment See alignment, horizontal.

horizontal midline See midline, horizontal.

hyperope A person with hyperopia.

hyperopia The refractive condition of the eye whereby light focuses behind the retina. Plus lenses are required to correct for hyperopia. (Synonyms: *hypermetropia* and *farsightedness*.)

I

Ilford mounting See mounting, Balgrip.

image jump See jump, image.

image, real An image formed by converging light.

image shell error See error, image shell.

image, virtual An image formed by tracing diverging rays that are leaving an optical system back to a point from which they appear to originate.

imbalance, vertical A differential vertical prismatic effect between the two eyes. At near this can be induced by right and left lenses of unequal powers when the wearer drops his or her eyes below the optical centers of the lenses.

impact, basic The ANSI requirements for impact resistant safety eyewear that include a minimum thickness requirement of 3.0 mm unless lenses are +3.00

D of power or higher in the highest plus meridian. In this case a 2.5-mm minimum edge thickness is permissible. Glass lenses are permissible. Lenses must be capable of withstanding the impact of a 1-inch steel ball dropped from 50 inches.

impact, high The ANSI requirements for impact resistant safety eyewear that allows a minimum thickness of 2.0 mm when the lens material is capable of withstanding both the impact of a 1-inch steel ball dropped from 50 inches and the impact of a $1/4$-inch steel ball traveling at 150 feet/sec.

implant, intraocular lens A plastic lens placed inside the eye as a replacement for the eye's natural crystalline lens. An intraocular lens implant is commonly used to replace a crystalline lens that has lost its clarity because of a developing cataract.

impregnated wheel *See* wheel, impregnated.

index, absolute refractive The ratio of the speed of light in a vacuum to the speed of light in another medium.

index, refractive The ratio of the speed of light in a medium (such as air) to the speed of light in another medium (such as glass).

index, relative refractive The ratio obtained by dividing the speed of light in a certain medium (usually air) by its speed in another medium.

index, UV A measure of the amount of ultraviolet radiation present on a given day.

infrared Invisible rays having wavelengths longer than those at the red end of the visible spectrum yet shorter than radio waves.

inset The amount of lens decentration nasally from the boxing center of the frame's lens aperture. (Antonym: outset.)

inset, blank seg The horizontal distance from the blank geometrical center to the center of the multifocal segment.

inset, geometrical The lateral distance from the distance centration point to the geometrical center of the segment. (Synonym: *seg inset*.)

inset, net seg The amount of additional seg inset (or outset) required to produce a desired amount of horizontal prismatic effect at near, added to the normal seg inset required by the near PD.

inset, seg The lateral distance from the major reference point to the geometrical center of the segment.

inset, total The amount the near segment must move from the boxing center to place it at the near PD (near centration distance).

intermediate The area of a trifocal lens between the distance viewing portion and the near portion.

interpupillary distance *See* distance, interpupillary.

intraocular lens implant *See* implant, intraocular lens.

invisible bifocals *See* lens, blended bifocal.

iseikonic lenses *See* lenses, iseikonic.

isocylinder line *See* line, isocylinder.

J

jig Also called "third hand." A jig consists of adjustable clips mounted on a base. It is used to hold a frame in place while soldering.

jump, image The sudden displacement of image as the bifocal line is crossed by the eye.

K

keyhole bridge *See* bridge, keyhole.

kevlar A nylon based frame material.

Knapp's law *See* law, Knapp's.

knife-edge A plus lens ground to an absolute minimum thickness, such that the edge of the lens is so thin that it has a knifelike sharpness to it; that is, an edge thickness of zero.

L

Lambert's law of absorption *See* law, Lambert's.

laminated lens *See* lens, laminated.

lap A tool having a curvature matching that of the curvature desired for a lens surface. The lens surface is rubbed across the face of the tool and, with the aid of pads, abrasives, and polishes, the lens surface is brought to optical quality.

lateral chromatic aberration *See* aberration, lateral chromatic.

law, Knapp's When an eye is axially ametropic, Knapp's law states that a correctly positioned, refractively correct spectacle lens will return the size of the retinal image to the same size as that produced by an emmetropic eye.

law, Lambert's Lambert's law of absorption predicts how the amount of light transmitted will change based on a change of thickness of the absorbing material.

law, Malus' A law of physics that predicts how much polarized light will be transmitted by an obliquely oriented polarizing filter.

law, Snell's An equation that predicts the refraction of light as it passes from one medium to another by stating that $n \sin i = n' \sin i'$ where n and n' are the refractive indices of the two materials, i is the angle of incidence, and i' is the angle of refraction.

layout blocker *See* blocker, layout; marker/blocker.

layout The process of preparing a lens for blocking and edging.

LEAP A 3M Company adhesive pad blocking system.

length, datum The horizontal width of a lens or lens opening as measured along the datum line.

length, first focal For a thin lens, the distance from the lens to the first principal focus.

length, overall temple The length of a spectacle lens temple as measured from the center of the hinge barrel, around the temple bend, to the posterior end of the temple.

length, second focal For a thin lens, the distance from the lens to the second principal focus.

length-to-bend (LTB) Temple length measured from the center of the hinge barrel to the middle of the bend.

lens analyzer *See* analyzer, lens.

lens conditioner *See* conditioner, lens.

lens groover *See* groover, lens.

lens measure *See* measure, lens.

lens opening *See* opening, lens.

lens protractor *See* protractor, lens.

lens size *See* size, lens.

lens washer *See* washer, lens.

lens, achromatic A lens considered to be without chromatic aberration because selected wavelengths toward either end of the visible spectrum focus at one point. Synonym: *achromatic doublet.*

lens, aspheric A lens whose surface gradually changes in power from the center to the edge for the purpose of optimizing the optical quality of the image or reducing the thickness of the lens.

lens, aspheric lenticular A lenticular lens whose optically usable central portion has a front surface with a gradually changing radius of curvature. The farther from the center of the lens, the longer the front surface radius of curvature becomes.

lens, atoric A lens with a cylinder component whose surface gradually changes in power from the center to the edge. Each of the two major meridians changes in power by different amounts based on the cylinder power of the lens and for the purpose of optimizing the optical quality of the image in both meridians.

lens, best form *See* lens, corrected curve.

lens, bitoric A lens with toric surfaces on both the front and the back.

lens, blended bifocal Bifocal lenses with a segment area that is not visible to the observer. Blended bifocals are usually round-segment lenses that have the demarcation line between the distance portion and the bifocal portion smoothed away.

lens, blended myodisc A minus lens, lenticular in design, with the edges of the bowl blended so as to improve the cosmetic aspects of the lens.

lens, cement Custom-made lenses that have a small segment glued onto the distance lens.

lens, corrected curve A lens whose surface curvatures have been carefully chosen with the intent of reducing those peripheral lens aberrations that are troublesome to the spectacle lens wearer. (Synonym: *best form lens.*)

lens, cover A thin lens that is temporarily glued to the surface of a semifinished blank to protect the surface of the lens and facilitate accurate grinding, as in the case of a slab-off grind on a glass lens.

lens, demo *See* coquille.

lens, double-D A multifocal lens with a flat-top bifocal-style segment in the lower portion of the lens and an inverted flat-top bifocal-style segment in the upper portion of the lens.

lens, double-segment A multifocal lens that has two segments, one in the lower and one in the upper portion of the lens.

lens, dummy *See* coquille.

lens, equiconcave A lens that is inwardly curved on both front and back surfaces with both inward curves having the same minus power.

lens, equiconvex A lens that is outwardly curved on both front and back surfaces with both outward curves having the same power.

lens, finished A spectacle lens that has been surfaced on both front and back to the needed power and thickness. A finished lens has not been edged for a spectacle frame, but is still in uncut form.

lens, Fresnel A lens made from a thin flexible plastic material, having concentric rings of ever-increasing prismatic effect that duplicate the refractive effect of a powered spectacle lens.

lens, full-field aspheric An aspheric lens that continues in its asphericity in an optically usable manner all the way to the edge of the lens blank.

lens, glare control Present usage of the term denotes a lens that absorbs wavelengths toward the blue end of the spectrum in an attempt to reduce glare and increase contrast.

lens, glazed 1. A prescription or nonprescription lens mounted in a frame. 2. The thin plastic demonstration lens that comes in a pair of spectacle frames. (Synonyms: *dummy lens, coquille.*)

lens, gradient A lens having a tinted upper portion that gradually lightens toward the lower portion of the lens.

lens, hand-flattened lenticular A negative lenticular lens with the lenticular produced on a hand edger and hand polished.

lens, high-index A lens with an index of refraction that is at the upper end of the range of available indices of refraction for lenses, yielding a lens that is thinner than other lenses of the same size and power.

lens, laminated An ophthalmic lens that is made up of more than one layer. One example is a polarized lens.

lens, lenticular A high-powered lens with the desired prescription power found only in the central portion. The outer carrier portion is shaped to reduce edge thickness and weight in minus prescriptions and center thickness and weight in plus prescriptions.

lens, meniscus A lens having a convex front surface and a concave back surface.

lens, mineral Synonym for glass lens.

lens, minus cylinder form A lens ground such that it obtains its cylinder power from a difference in surface curvature between two back surface meridians.

lens, minus lenticular A high-minus lens that is lenticular in design, having a central area containing the prescribed refractive power and a peripheral carrier with a different power chosen to reduce edge thickness.

lens, multidrop A high-plus, full-field aspheric lens in which the surface power drops rapidly as the edge of the lens is approached.

lens, multifocal A lens having a sector or sectors where the refractive power is different from the rest of the lens, such as bifocals or trifocals.

lens, myodisc 1. Traditional definition: a high-minus lens that is lenticular in design, having a central area containing the prescribed refractive power and a peripheral carrier that is plano in power. The front curve is either plano in power or very close to plano. 2. General usage: any high-minus lens that is lenticular in design.

lens, negative lenticular A high-minus lens that has had the peripheral portion flattened for the purpose of reducing weight and edge thickness. (General usage synonym: *myodisc*.)

lens, occupational progressive A progressive addition lens that is prescribed and/or designed for specialized tasks and will not be used for full-time generalized wear.

lens, Percival form A lens design that concentrates on the elimination of power error instead of oblique astigmatism.

lens, photochromic A lens that changes its transmission characteristics when exposed to light.

lens, planoconcave A lens that is plano (flat) on one surface and inwardly curved on the other surface.

lens, planoconvex A lens that is plano (flat) on one surface and outwardly curved on the other surface.

lens, plus cylinder form A lens ground so that it obtains its cylinder power from a difference in surface curvature between two front surface meridians.

lens, point focal A lens design that concentrates on the elimination of oblique astigmatism instead of power error.

lens, polarizing A lens that blocks light polarized in one plane, such as light reflected from a smooth, nondiffusing surface.

lens, prism segment A 10-mm deep ribbon-style segment containing a prismatic effect for near. The ribbon segment extends to the nasal edge of the lens blank.

lens, progressive-addition A lens having optics that vary in power, gradually increasing in plus (or decreasing in minus) power from the distance to near zones.

lens, quadrafocal A multifocal lens that has a flat-top trifocal segment in the lower portion of the lens and an inverted flat-top bifocal-type segment in the upper portion of the lens.

lens, reverse-slab A slab-off lens that has base-down prism below the slab line, instead of base up.

lens, single-vision A lens with the same sphere and/or cylinder power throughout the whole lens, as distinguished from a multifocal lens.

lens, size *See* lens, iseikonic.

lens, spheric lenticular A lenticular lens whose optically usable central portion has a front surface that does not vary in curvature, but is entirely spherical.

lens, stock A lens that is premade, does not have to be custom surfaced, and is ready to edge.

lens, uncut A lens that has been surfaced on both sides, but not yet edged for a frame.

lens, X-Chrom A red contact lens worn on only one eye in an attempt to improve color vision for certain red-green color defectives.

lens, Younger seamless Trade name for a blended bifocal made by Younger Optics.

lenses, iseikonic A lens pair with their curvatures and thicknesses specially chosen to produce a difference in image magnification between the left and right eyes for the purpose of correcting image size differences between right and left eyes. Also known as *size lenses*.

lensmaker's formula *See* formula, lensmaker's.

lensmeter The instrument used for finding power and prism in spectacle lenses.

lensometer A trade name for a type of lensmeter.

lenticular A high-powered lens with the desired prescription power found only in the central portion. The outer carrier portion is ground so as to reduce edge thickness and weight in minus prescriptions and center thickness and weight in plus prescriptions.

lenticular lens *See* lens, lenticular or lenticular.

lenticular, aspheric A lenticular lens whose optically usable central portion has a front surface with a changing radius of curvature.

lenticular, hand-flattened A negative lenticular lens with the lenticular portion produced on a hand edger and hand polished.

lenticular, negative A high-minus lens that has had the peripheral portion flattened for the purpose of reducing weight and edge thickness. (Synonym: *myodisc*.)

lenticular, spheric A lenticular lens whose optically usable central portion has a front surface that does not vary in curvature, but is entirely spherical.

let-back *See* spread, open-temple.

level, reading A synonym for reading depth. *See* depth, reading.

library temple *See* temple, library.

light box *See* box, light.

line, cutting A term that was used for the 180-degree line that used to be hand marked or stamped on a lens after it had been properly positioned for cylinder axis orientation and decentration. It was used as a reference line in blocking and edging a lens.

line, datum A line drawn parallel to and halfway between horizontal lines tangent to the lowest and highest edges of the lens. (Synonyms: *horizontal midline, 180-degree line*.)

line, isocylinder One of the lines on the contour plot of a progressive-addition lens denoting the location of unwanted cylinder of a given dioptric power.

line, mounting 1. The horizontal reference line that intersects the mechanical center of a lens pattern. 2. Historical usage: On metal or rimless spectacles, the line that passes through the points at which the pad arms are attached and that serves as a line of reference for horizontal alignment.

line, 180-degree A synonym for horizontal midline.

liner, figure-8 A liner that fits into the top eyewire channel of some nylon cord frames.

longitudinal chromatic aberration *See* aberration, longitudinal chromatic.

LTB The length-to-bend measure of a frame temple.

M

maculopathy, age-related A degeneration of the sensitive macular area of the retina. Also called *macular degeneration*.

magnification difference *See* difference, magnification.

magnification, relative spectacle (RSM) The amount of magnification produced by a given eye, relative to that of a standard eye.

magnification, spectacle (SM) The difference in the size of an image seen by a spectacle lens corrected eye compared with the size of the image seen by the same eye without a spectacle lens correction.

Malus' law *See* law, Malus'.

major reference point *See* point, major reference.

marginal astigmatism *See* astigmatism, oblique.

marker An older style centering device used to accurately position a lens and stamp it with the horizontal and vertical reference lines used for reference in lens blocking.

marker/blocker A device used to accurately position a lens and then either (1) stamp it with horizontal and vertical reference lines for use in later lens blocking, or (2) block it directly while still in the device.

material safety and data sheet A single sheet of paper containing information about a potentially hazardous chemical found in the workplace. MSDS sheets should include physical and chemical characteristics, known acute and chronic health effects, exposure limits, precautionary measures, and emergency and first-aid procedures.

MBL Minimum between lenses.

MBS Minimum blank size. *See* size, minimum blank.

mean dispersion *See* dispersion, mean.

measure, lens A small, pocket-watch-sized instrument for measuring the surface curve of a lens. Also called a *lens clock* or *lens gauge*.

memory plastic A plastic material that can be bent or twisted and still return to its original shape.

meniscus lens *See* lens, meniscus.

meridian, axis The meridian of least power of a cylinder or spherocylinder lens; for a minus cylinder the least minus meridian, for a plus cylinder the least plus meridian.

meridian, major One of two meridians in a cylinder or spherocylinder lens. These meridians are 90 degrees apart and correspond to the maximum and minimum powers in the lens.

meridian, power The meridian of maximum power of a cylinder or spherocylinder lens; for a minus

cylinder the most minus meridian, for a plus cylinder the most plus meridian.

metal bonded wheel *See* wheel, metal bonded.

metal saddle bridge *See* bridge, metal saddle.

metalized coating *See* coating, metalized.

middatum depth *See* depth, middatum.

midline, horizontal In the boxing system of lens measurement, the horizontal line halfway between the upper and lower horizontal lines bordering the lens shape. (Synonym: *180-degree reference line*.)

minibevel A lens edge configuration that has a bevel and an angled ledge.

minimum between lenses The datum system equivalent of the boxing system's distance between lenses (DBL).

minus add bifocal Bifocal, minus add.

minus cylinder form *See* form, minus cylinder.

minus cylinder form lens *See* lens, minus cylinder form.

minus lenticular lens *See* lens, minus lenticular.

mirror coating *See* coating, mirror.

Monel A whitish, pliable, nicely polishing metal frame material that is made from nickel, copper, and iron; it also contains traces of other elements.

monochromatic aberration *See* aberration, monochromatic.

monocular PD *See* PD, monocular.

monovision A refractive correction in which one eye is used for distance and the other eye for near viewing.

mounting 1. The name for a spectacle lens frame when the lenses are held in place without the aid of an eyewire as with rimless or semirimless mountings. 2. The attaching of lenses to a rimless or semirimless spectacle frame.

mounting line *See* line, mounting.

mounting, Balgrip A mounting (frame) that secures the lens in place with clips attached to a bar of tensile steel that fits into a nasal and a temporal slot on each side of the lens.

mounting, Ilford Synonym for Balgrip mounting.

mounting, Numont A lens mounting that holds the lenses in place only at their nasal edge. The lenses are attached at the bridge area and the temples are attached to a metal arm that extends along the posterior surface temporally. Thus each lens has only one point of attachment.

mounting, rimless A mounting that holds the lenses in place by some method other than eyewires or nylon cords. Usually the method of mounting is by screws or posts through the lenses. (Synonym: *three-piece mounting.*)

mounting, semirimless Mountings similar to rimless, but with the addition of a metal reinforcing arm, which follows the upper posterior surface of the lens and joins the centerpiece of the frame to the endpiece.

mounting, 3-piece *See* mounting, rimless.

mounting, Wils-Edge A lens mounting (frame) that secures the lens in place by means of a grooved arm that grips the top of the lens.

MRP An abbreviation for major reference point. *See* point, major reference.

MSDS Abbreviation for material safety and data sheet.

multidrop lens *See* lens, multidrop.

multifocal A lens having a sector or sectors where the refractive power is different from the rest of the lens, such as bifocals or trifocals.

multifocals, fused Glass multifocal lenses in which the segment cannot be felt because it is fused into the distance portion.

multifocals, occupational Any segmented or progressive-addition lens that is designed or chosen by careful forethought and positioned for a specialized viewing situation.

multifocals, one-piece Multifocal lenses that are made of one material with any change in power in the segment portion of the lens the result of a change in the surface curvature of the lens.

multifocals, segmented Multifocal lenses having a visible, clearly demarcated bifocal or trifocal area. Nonsegmented multifocals would be progressive-addition lenses.

myodisc *See* lens, myodisc.

myope A person with myopia.

myopia The refractive condition of the eye whereby light focuses in front of the retina. Minus lenses are required to correct for myopia. (Synonym: *nearsightedness.*)

N

n An abbreviation for refractive index.

nasal The side of a lens or frame that is toward the nose (inner edge).

nasal add *See* add, nasal.

nasal cut *See* cut, nasal.

NBC The abbreviation for nominal base curve.

near power *See* power, near.

near reference point *See* point, near reference.

near Rx The net lens power resulting from the combination of the add power and the distance power.

nearsightedness *See* myopia.

net seg inset *See* inset, net seg.

neutralize To determine the refractive power of a lens. Most often this is done with the aid of a lensmeter.

neutralizer A solution used to reduce the color in or remove the color from a previously tinted lens.

nickel silver A whitish-appearing metal frame material containing more than 50% copper, 25% nickel, and the rest zinc. (Synonym: *German silver.*)

nominal base curve *See* curve, nominal base.

normal A line perpendicular to a reflecting or refracting surface at the point of incidence of an incoming ray of light.

nosepads Plastic pieces that rest on the nose to support the frame.

NRP An abbreviation for near reference point. *See* point, near reference.

number, set The compensating number used with a pattern to arrive at a compensated eyesize setting for the edger.

Numont mounting *See* mounting, Numont.

Numont pliers *See* pliers, Numont.

nystagmus A condition characterized by a constant, involuntary back-and-forth movement of the eye.

O

oblique astigmatic error *See* error, oblique astigmatic.

oblique astigmatism *See* astigmatism, oblique.

OC Optical center.

occupational multifocals *See* multifocals, occupational.

Occupational Safety and Health Administration The U.S. government agency responsible for setting workplace safety policy and ensuring worker safety.

OD Latin, oculus dexter (right eye).

OLA Abbreviation for the Optical Laboratories Association.

one-piece multifocals *See* multifocals, one-piece.

open temple spread *See* spread, open temple.

opening, lens The portion of the spectacle frame that accepts the spectacle lens. (Synonym: *lens aperture.*)

OPL An abbreviation for occupational progressive lens. *See* lens, occupation progressive.

optical axis *See* axis, optical.

optical bleaching *See* bleaching, optical.

optical center *See* center, optical.

Optical Laboratories Association A professional association of optical laboratories.

optically centered pattern *See* pattern, optically centered.

Optyl The trade name for an epoxy resin material used to make spectacle frames.

OS Latin, oculus sinister (left eye).

OSHA Occupational Safety and Health Administration.

outset The amount of lens decentration temporally from the boxing center of the frame's lens aperture. (Antonym: *inset.*)

overall temple length *See* length, overall temple.

P

pad arms *See* arms, pad.

pad-adjusting pliers *See* pliers, pad-adjusting.

pad bridge *See* bridge, pad.

pads, buildup Small nosepad-shaped pieces of plastic applied to the frame bridge and used to alter the fit of the bridge.

PAL An abbreviation for progressive addition lens. *See* lens, progressive addition.

Panoptik *See* bifocal, Panoptik.

pantoscopic angle or tilt *See* angle, pantoscopic.

pantoscopic angling pliers *See* pliers, pantoscopic angling.

parallax The apparent change in position of an object as the result of a change in viewing angle.

paraxial rays *See* rays, paraxial.

pattern difference *See* difference, pattern.

pattern A plastic or metal piece having the same shape as the lens aperture for a given frame. Used in lens edging as a guide for shaping the lens to fit the frame.

pattern, geometrically centered A pattern with mechanical and geometrical centers on the same horizontal plane.

pattern, optically centered A pattern with its mechanical center above boxing center.

patterned edger *See* edger, patterned.

patternless edger *See* edger, patternless.

PD An abbreviation for interpupillary distance (*See* distance, interpupillary.).

PD, binocular The measured distance from the center of one pupil to the center of the other pupil without regard to how each eye may vary in its distance from the center of the bridge of the frame.

PD, distance The wearer's interpupillary distance specified for a situation equivalent to when the wearer is viewing a distant object.

PD, frame Synonym for geometrical center distance or distance between centers.

PD, monocular The distance from the center of the frame bridge to the center of the wearer's pupil measured for each eye separately.

PD, near The interpupillary distance as specified for a near viewing situation.

peening The act of putting a rivetlike head on the end of the posts (rivets) on so-called "riveted hinges" or on the tip of a frame screw.

peening pliers *See* pliers, peening.

Percival form lens *See* lens, Percival form.

peripheral rays *See* rays, peripheral.

phoria The direction of the line of sight of one eye with reference to that of the partner eye when fusion is interrupted, as when one eye is covered.

photochromic lens *See* lens, photochromic.

photometer An instrument for measuring brightness. When used with lenses, the percent transmission of the lens is measured in a given spectral area or areas.

pillar file *See* file, pillar.

pincushion distortion *See* distortion, pincushion.

planes, variant A form of vertical misalignment of a spectacle frame in which the lens planes are out of coplanar alignment (one lens is farther forward than the other).

plano (pl) A lens or lens surface having zero refracting power.

planoconcave lens *See* lens, planoconcave.

planoconvex lens *See* lens, planoconvex.

pliers, bridge-narrowing Used to narrow the bridge of a plastic frame.

pliers, bridge-widening Used to widen the bridge of a plastic frame.

pliers, chipping Pliers that were primarily used to chip or break away the outer portions of an uncut or semifinished glass lens to either reduce its size or bring it into the rough shape needed to approximate the finished shape.

pliers, endpiece angling Pliers used in the adjustment of older style rimless mountings.

pliers, eyewire-forming Pliers with horizontally curved jaws used to shape or form the upper and lower eyewires of a metal frame to match the meniscus curve of the edged lens.

pliers, fingerpiece Pliers used for adjustment of the temple-fold angle of plastic frames. Fingerpiece pliers have parallel jaws and were originally designed for adjusting fingerpiece mountings. Also called *Fits-U pliers.*

pliers, hollow snipe-nosed Thin-nosed pliers with a hollowed-out central jaw area.

pliers, Numont Holding pliers specially designed for use with Numont mountings. Numont pliers serve the same purpose for Numont mountings as endpiece angling pliers do for older style rimless mountings.

pliers, pad-adjusting These pliers have one cupped jaw to conform to the face portion of an adjustable nosepad; the other jaw is shaped to allow the back of the pad to be held securely while being angled.

pliers, peening Pliers with a round cupped edge for placing a rivetlike head on the end of a screw.

pliers, punch Pliers with a fine, rounded, rodlike projection that is placed against the filed end of the rivet to punch it out of a plastic frame. Also used to punch out damaged frame screws.

pliers, rimless adjusting Pliers used to grasp a rimless mounting at the point of attachment between lens and mounting.

pliers, snipe-nosed Pliers that taper to a small tip on both jaws, allowing use in tight places. Often used in the adjustment of pad arms.

pliers, square-round Used to adjust pad arms, these pliers have a small round section on one jaw and a squared off section on the other.

pliers, strapping Pliers having two flat jaws. One jaw extends beyond the other and then overlaps it. Used to adjust straps of an antique rimless or semirimless mounting.

plot, contour A line diagram used to plot the areas of unwanted cylinder or spherical equivalent power over the viewing areas of a progressive-addition lens.

plus cylinder form *See* form, plus cylinder.

plus-cylinder–form lens *See* lens, plus cylinder-form.

point One tenth of a millimeter of lens thickness.

point, distance centration The British equivalent of the major reference point.

point, distance reference (DRP) That point on a lens where, according to the manufacturer, the distance power is to be measured. Distance power consists of sphere, cylinder, and axis. The DRP may not correspond to the prism reference point (PRP), as with progressive-addition lenses.

point, focal A point to or from which light rays converge or diverge.

point focal lens *See* lens, point focal.

point, major reference (MRP) The point on a lens where the prism equals that called for by the prescription.

point, near reference (NRP) That point on the lens where, according to the manufacturer, the power of the near addition is to be measured.

point, prism reference (PRP) The point on a lens where prism power is to be verified. Also referred to as the *major reference point*.

polariscope *See* colmascope.

polarizing lens *See* lens, polarizing.

polyamide A strong, nylon-based frame material that allows a frame to be made thinner and lighter.

polycarbonate A 1.586-index lens material known for its strength.

power cross *See* cross, power.

power factor *See* factor, power.

power meridian *See* meridian, power.

power, actual Synonym for true power.

power, back vertex The reciprocal of the distance in air from the rear surface of the lens to the second principal focus. Is used when measuring spectacle lenses.

power, chromatic *See* aberration, lateral chromatic.

power, compensated In surfacing, back vertex power that has been converted to a 1.53-index frame of reference. Used for the purpose of finding a 1.53-index-referenced tool curve for a lens with a different index of refraction.

power, dispersive The following quantity $\dfrac{n_F - n_C}{n_D - 1}$ used for quantifying chromatic aberration of a given material. Dispersive power is abbreviated as the Greek letter omega, or ω.

power, effective 1. The vergence power of a lens at a designated position other than that occupied by the lens itself. 2. That power lens required for a new position that will replace the original reference lens and yet maintain the same focal point.

power, focal A measure of the ability of a lens or lens surface to change the vergence of entering light rays.

power, front vertex The reciprocal of the distance in air from the front surface of a lens to the first principal focus.

power, near The sum of the distance power and the near add. (Synonym: *near Rx*.)

power, nominal An estimate of total lens power, calculated as the sum of front and back surface powers. (Not to be confused with nominal base curve.) Synonym: *approximate power*.

power, prism The amount light is displaced in centimeters at a distance 1 m away from the lens or prism.

power, refractive The dioptric value that accurately describes the ability of a lens or lens surface to converge or diverge light. For a lens surface in air, the refractive power is expressed as $F = \dfrac{n-1}{r}$ where n is the refractive index of the lens material and r is the radius of the surface expressed in meters.

power, true The 1.53-index-referenced curvature of the base curve of a lens. True power is found by using a lens clock or sagometer (sag gauge) that is 1.53-index referenced.

precoat A spray or brush-on liquid that when applied to a lens, protects the surface during processing, and/or makes the adhesion of a block to the lens possible.

Prentice's Rule *See* Rule, Prentice's.

Prep, Lens A trade name for lens conditioner.

presbyopia The refractive state in which the crystalline lens within the eye becomes nonelastic as a result of the aging process.

pressure, lateral The pressure of the temples against the sides of the head just above the ears.

prism Two nonparallel, transparent surfaces that cause entering light to change direction as it exits.

prism axis *See* axis, prism.

prism diopter *See* diopter, prism.

prism power *See* power, prism.

prism reference point *See* point, prism reference.

prism, Fresnel A prism made from thin flexible material and consisting of small rows of equal-powered prisms resulting in the same optical effect as that of a conventional ophthalmic prism.

prism, Risley's An application of obliquely crossed prisms in which two equally powered prisms are placed one on top of another and can be rotated from bases in the same direction to bases in completely opposite directions resulting in variable prism power. Also called *rotary prism*.

prism, Rx Prism in an ophthalmic lens prescription that has been called for by the prescribing physician.

prism, yoked Vertical prism of equal value ground on both right and left lenses of a progressive or Franklin-style lens for the purpose of reducing lens thickness.

progressive-addition lens *See* lens, progressive-addition.

progressive corridor *See* corridor, progressive.

propionate The common name for the frame material cellulose acetopropionate. Propionate has many of the same characteristics as cellulose acetate and is better suited for injection molding.

protractor, lens A millimeter grid on a 360-degree protractor used in the lens centration process for both surfacing and finishing.

PRP An abbreviation for prism reference point. *See* point, prism reference.

pseudophake A person who has had their crystalline lens removed and replaced with an intraocular lens implant.

pterygium A growth of tissue that begins on the white of the eye and extends onto the cornea.

punch pliers *See* pliers, punch.

Q

quadrafocal *See* lens, quadrafocal.

R

radial astigmatism *See* astigmatism, oblique.

raise, seg 1. The vertical distance from the major reference point to the top of the seg when the seg top is higher than the MRP. 2. The vertical distance from the horizontal midline of the edged lens to the top of the seg when the seg top is higher than the horizontal midline (laboratory usage). (Antonym: seg drop.)

rat-tail file *See* file, rat-tail.

rays, paraxial Those rays of light that pass through the central area of the lens.

rays, peripheral Those rays of light that enter the lens nearer the edge than the center.

R-compensated segs *See* segs, R-compensated.

reading center *See* center, reading.

reading depth *See* depth, reading.

reading level *See* level, reading.

real image *See* image, real.

Rede-Rite bifocal *See* bifocal, minus add.

reduced thickness *See* thickness, reduced.

reference point, distance *See* point, distance reference.

reference point, near *See* point, near reference.

reference point, prism *See* point, prism reference.

reflex color *See* color, reflex.

refraction 1. The bending of light by a lens or optical system. 2. The process of determining the needed power of a prescription lens for an individual.

refractive ametropia *See* ametropia, refractive.

refractive index *See* index, refractive.

refractive power *See* power, refractive.

relative refractive index *See* index, relative refractive.

relative spectacle magnification *See* magnification, relative spectacle.

resolving (of prism) The process of expressing a single prism as two prisms whose horizontal and vertical base directions are perpendicular to each other, but whose combined effect equals that of the original prism.

retroscopic angle or tilt *See* angle, retroscopic.

reverse-slab lens *See* lens, reverse-slab.

ribbon bifocal *See* bifocal, ribbon.

ribbon file *See* file, slotting.

riding-bow temple *See* temple, riding-bow.

riffler file *See* file, riffler.

rim *See* eyewire.

rimless Having to do with frames (mountings) that hold lenses in place by some method other than eyewires. Most rimless mountings have two points of attachment per lens.

rimless mounting *See* mounting, rimless.

Rimway mounting *See* mounting, semirimless.

Risley's prism *See* prism, Risley's.

rolled edge *See* edge, rolled.

rolling A pulling of the eyewire such that it covers less of the front of the lens bevel than back or vice versa.

round-seg bifocal *See* bifocal, round-seg.

Rule, Prentice's A rule that states that the decentration of a lens in centimeters times the power of the lens is equal to the prismatic effect: $\Delta = cF$

rule, three-quarter The three-quarter rule states that for every diopter of dioptric demand, the optical center of each reading lens or the geometrical center of each bifocal addition should be inset 0.75 (three-quarters) mm.

Rx prism *See* prism, Rx.

S

saddle bridge *See* bridge, saddle.

safety bevel *See* bevel, safety.

safety eyewear *See* eyewear, safety.

sag A synonym or abbreviation for sagittal depth. *See also* depth, sagittal.

sagittal depth *See* depth, sagittal.

scratch A furrowed-out line that has jagged edges.

screw extractor *See* extractor, screw.

second focal length *See* length, second focal.

second principal focus *See* focus, second principal.

seg *See* segment.

seg clock *See* clock, seg.

seg depth *See* depth, seg.

seg drop *See* drop, seg.

seg height *See* height, seg.

seg inset *See* inset, seg.

seg optical center *See* center, seg optical.

seg width *See* width, seg.

segment (seg) An area of a spectacle lens with power differing from that of the main portion.

segment, prism *See* lens, prism segment.

segmented multifocals *See* multifocals, segmented.

segs, dissimilar A method of correcting vertical imbalance at near that uses different bifocal segment styles for the right and left eyes.

segs, R-compensated A method for correcting vertical imbalance at near that uses ribbon-style bifocal segments that have been modified so that the segment optical center for one lens is high in one segment and low in the other.

semidiameter Diameter divided by 2. In ophthalmic optics, semidiameter refers to half of the chord for the arc of a given surface and is used in calculating the sagittal depth of the surface.

semifinished blank *See* blank, semifinished.

semifinished lap tool *See* tool, semifinished lap.

semirimless mountings *See* mountings, semirimless.

semisaddle bridge *See* bridge, semisaddle.

set number *See* number, set.

shaft The portion of the temple between the butt end and the bend.

shank *See* shaft.

shape memory alloy (SMA) The name applied to a titanium alloy made with 40% to 50% titanium and the rest nickel. It is very flexible and returns to its original shape. Synonym: *memory metal*.

shell frame *See* frame, shell.

shield On a plastic frame, the metal piece to which rivets are attached to hold the hinge in place.

shields, side Protective shields attached to the spectacle frame at the outer, temporal areas to protect the eyes from hazards approaching from the side.

shoe That part of the strap area of a mounting that contacts the edge of the lens, bracing it. Also called *shoulder* or *collar*.

shop, back Synonym for surfacing laboratory.

shop, front Synonym for finishing laboratory.

shoulder *See* shoe.

side shields *See* shields, side.

sine For a right triangle, the ratio of the side opposite the angle considered, to the hypotenuse:

$$\text{Sine} = \frac{\text{Opposite}}{\text{Hypotenuse}}$$

sine-squared formula *See* formula, sine-squared.

single-vision lens *See* lens, single-vision.

size lenses *See* lenses, iseikonic.

size, lens In the boxing system, the A dimension of a lens or lens opening.

size, minimum blank The smallest lens blank that can be used for a given prescription lens and frame combination.

sizer A frame chassis or frame front used exclusively for checking edged lens size accuracy.

skewed bridge *See* bridge, skewed.

skull temple *See* temple, skull.

slab-off Grinding a portion of a lens so as to add a second optical center. Often used to create vertical prism in the lower portion of one lens for the purpose of alleviating vertical imbalance at near.

sleek A furrowed-out line on a lens, which resembles a scratch, but whose edges are smooth instead of jagged.

slotting file *See* file, slotting.

smoothing, edge The process of bringing the bevel surfaces of an edged lens to a finer, smoother finish.

Snell's law *See* law, Snell's.

snipe-nosed pliers *See* pliers, snipe-nosed.

solid tint *See* tint, solid.

space eikonometer *See* eikonometer, space.

spectacle magnification *See* magnification, spectacle.

spectrophotometer A device used to measure the transmission of each wavelength of light across the spectrum.

sphere (sph) A lens having a single refractive power in all meridians.

spheric lenticular *See* lenticular, spheric.

spherical aberration *See* aberration, spherical.

spherical equivalent *See* equivalent, spherical.

spherocylinder The combination of sphere and cylinder powers into a single lens.

splay angle *See* angle, splay.

sports eyewear *See* eyewear, sports.

spotting The placing of spots on a lens with a lensmeter in such a manner that the lens will be oriented correctly for axis and positioned for major reference point and horizontal meridian locations.

spread, open temple That angle an open temple forms in relationship to the front of the frame (also called *let-back*).

square-round pliers *See* pliers, square-round.

SRC An abbreviation for scratch resistant coating.

staking tool A multipurpose tool used to apply concentrated force to parts of a frame, such as when punching out damaged hinge rivets.

standard alignment *See* alignment, standard.

stars Microchips at the lens surface-lens bevel interface.

stock lens *See* lens, stock.

stock, lens 1. An inventory of lenses. 2. The material from which a semifinished blank is made. When the surface of a lens is ground, *lens stock* is removed from the semifinished blank to bring the lens to its needed thickness.

stone 1. An abrasive grinding wheel. 2. To sharpen the cutting ability of a grinding wheel by honing it with an abrasive stick.

stone, hand Synonym for hand edger.

strabismus The condition whereby one eye is pointed in a different direction than the other eye.

straight-back temple *See* temple, straight-back.

strap An old-style mechanism for holding drilled lenses in an antique rimless or semirimless mounting.

strapping pliers *See* pliers, strapping.

stria A streak seen in a lens caused by a difference in the refractive index in the material. The streak causes a distortion in the object viewed and is not a physical streak, such as a mark on or in the lens. (The plural of stria is striae.)

surfacing The process of creating the prescribed refractive power, prism, and major reference point location on a lens by generating the required curves and bringing the surface to a polished state.

swarf Fibrouslike lens material resulting from the grinding process for certain types of lens material, such as polycarbonate.

system, boxing A system of lens measurement based on the enclosure of a lens by horizontal and vertical tangents to form a box or rectangle.

system, datum A system of lens measurement that defines the lens or eyesize as being the width of the lens along the datum line and the bridge size as the width of the bridge at the level of the datum line.

system, GOMAC A European Economic Community standard for measuring lens and frame dimensions incorporating portions of both the boxing and datum systems.

T

tables, sag A set of tables used for finding sagittal depth when surface power and lens diameter are known.

tables, surfacing Tables supplied by a lens manufacturer for the purpose of helping the surfacing laboratory accurately determine the tool curves and lens thicknesses needed to grind lenses to the specified back vertex power. Surfacing tables are now largely replaced by computer software programs.

tangent For a right triangle, the ratio of the side opposite the angle considered to the side adjacent: $\text{Tangent} = \dfrac{\text{Opposite}}{\text{Adjacent}}$

tap Consists of a chuck on a handle in which threaders of varying size may be placed. It is used to restore threading that has been damaged.

tempering, chemical The process of increasing the impact resistance of glass lenses by immersing them in a bath of molten salt. (Synonyms: *chemtempering, chem hardening.*)

temple The part of a pair of spectacles that attaches to the frame front and hooks over the ears to hold spectacles in place.

temple, cable Cable temples are of metal construction with the curl, or postear portion, constructed from a flexible coiled cable. The postear portion follows the crotch of the ear where the ear and the head meet and extends to the level of the earlobe. (Old synonym: *Relaxo temple.*)

temple, comfort cable *See* temple, cable.

temple, convertible Temples that are straight through their entire length, but are designed to be bent down to take on the form of a skull temple.

temple, library The type of spectacle frame temple that begins with average width at the temple butt and increases in width toward the posterior end of the temple. Library temples are practically straight and hold the glasses on primarily by pressure against the side of the head. (Synonym: *straight-back temple.*)

temple, riding-bow Plastic temples with thin, round postear portions that curve around the ear, following the crotch of the ear where the ear and the head meet and extend to the level of the earlobe. They often are used in children's and safety frames and are the plastic version of the metal comfort cable temple.

temple, skull The type of spect frame temple that bends down behind the ear and follows the contour of the skull, resting evenly against it.

temple-fold angle *See* angle, temple-fold.

temporal The area of a lens or frame that is toward the temples (outer edge).

test, drop-ball A test to determine impact resistance of ophthalmic lenses whereby either a $5/8$- or 1-inch steel ball is dropped onto the front surface of the lens from a height of 50 inches.

test, flat surface touch A test for temple parallelism in which the spectacles are positioned upside down on a flat surface with temples open.

test, high mass impact A pointed, conical-tipped projectile weighing 17.6 oz is dropped from 51.2 inches through a tube and onto the eyeglasses. The lens must not break, nor come out of the frame. (Note: A proposed change to this test modifies the distance from 51.2 to 50 inches.)

test, high velocity impact This test simulates a high-velocity, low-mass object. In the high velocity impact test for frames, a series of $1/4$-inch steel balls traveling at 150 feet per second are directed at 20 different parts of the frame with lenses in place. A new frame is used for each impact. Neither the frame nor the lens can break. Nor can the lens come out of the frame. The same test is used for high impact safety lenses. The lens must withstand a single high velocity impact.

thermal bleaching *See* bleaching, thermal.

thermoelastic A term used to describe a material that will bend when heated and will return to its original shape when reheated.

thermoplastic A term used to describe a material that will bend when heated, but does not return to its original shape when reheated because it does not have a "plastic memory."

thickness, reduced The thickness of an optical medium divided by its refractive index.

three-quarter rule See rule, three-quarter.

tint, double gradient A lens tint that has two colors, one at the top and a second at the bottom. The color at the top is darkest at the top and fades out toward the middle of the lens. The color at the bottom is most intense at the bottom and lightens toward the middle.

tint, gradient The variation in light transmission of a lens from a low transmission (dark) to high transmission (light) from one area of the lens to another. Usually the lens is dark at the top and lightens at the bottom.

tint, solid A tint that has the same color and light transmission over the entire lens.

tint, triple gradient A lens with three colors. The color at the top is darkest at the top and fades out toward the middle of the lens. The color at the bottom is most intense at the bottom and lightens toward the middle. The third color is in the middle of the lens.

tongue See ear.

tool, lap A tool used for fining and polishing lens surfaces. The tool used must have a surface identical in curvature to that of the lens for which it is to be used (i.e., if the lens surface is convex, the tool must be concave and both must have the same curvature).

toric A surface having separate curves at right angles to one another.

toric base curve See curve, toric base.

toric transposition See transposition, toric.

total inset See inset, total.

touch, four-point A check for vertical alignment carried out by placing a straight edge so that its edge goes across the inside of the entire front of the spectacles below the nosepad area.

tracer, frame An instrument used to physically trace the inside groove of a frame's lens opening or the outside edge of a lens for the purpose of creating a digitized shape. That shape is then transmitted to a patternless edger so that the shape can be duplicated when the lens is edged.

Transitions A trade name for a brand of plastic photochromic lenses.

transmission The percent of light passing on through a lens and out the back surface, compared with the amount of light incident upon the first surface.

transposition, toric The process of transposing a prescription from the form in which it is written to another form, such as from a plus to a minus cylinder form.

treating, heat The process of hardening a glass lens by first heating it in a kiln, then quickly cooling by blowing forced air against both front and back surfaces. (Synonyms: *air hardening, heat hardening, heat tempering.*)

trifocals Lenses having three areas of viewing, each with its own focal power. Usually the upper portion is for distance viewing, the lower for near, and the middle or intermediate portion for distance in between.

triple gradient tint See tint, triple gradient.

Trivex The brand name for a PPG Industries plastic lens material known for its high impact resistance and ability to be processed in a manner similar to that of other plastic lenses.

true 1. To bring a pair of glasses into a position of correct alignment. 2. To reshape the cutting surface of a worn grinding wheel so that it cuts at the angles and in the manner originally intended. 3. In surfacing when using a hand pan, a step following roughing and smoothing, using a somewhat finer grade of abrasive to bring the lens to an exact curve.

true base curve See curve, true base.

true power See power, true.

trueing See true.

Tscherning's ellipse See ellipse, Tscherning's.

turn-back endpiece See endpiece, turn-back.

U

ultraviolet Rays having a wavelength somewhat shorter than those at the violet end of the visible spectrum.

uncut A lens that has been surfaced on both sides, but not yet edged for a frame.

upcurve bifocal See bifocal, minus add.

UV index See index, UV.

V

value, Abbé The most commonly used number for identifying the amount of chromatic aberration for a given lens material. The higher the Abbé value, the less chromatic aberration present in the lens. Abbé value is the reciprocal of ω (dispersive power) and is symbolized by the Greek letter nu, or ν. In other words:

$$\frac{1}{\omega} = \nu$$

(Synonyms: *nu value, constringence.*)

variant planes See planes, variant.

V-bevel See bevel, V.

vertex distance See distance, vertex.

vertex power allowance See allowance, vertex power.

vertical alignment See alignment, vertical.

vertical angle See angle, vertical.

vertical imbalance See imbalance, vertical.

Vertometer Trade name for a type of lensmeter.

virtual image See image, virtual.

W

W bridge *See* bridge, metal saddle.

washer, lens Also called *lens liner*, a plastic material that is inserted between a loose lens and the eyewire.

wave A defect in lens surface curvature causing a localized irregular variation in lens power.

wave front *See* front, wave.

wheel differential *See* differential, wheel.

wheel, electrometallic Synonym for electroplated wheel.

wheel, electroplated An abrasive wheel made by electrolytically depositing metal on the wheel in such a manner as to encompass diamond particles. This type of wheel is often used to grind plastic lenses

wheel, finishing The wheel used in edging to bring the lens edge to its final configuration.

wheel, hogging Synonym for roughing wheel.

wheel, impregnated Synonym for a metal-bonded wheel.

wheel, metal-bonded Abrasive wheels made by mixing diamond material with powdered metal that is heated in a mold until fusion of the metal occurs.

wheel, roughing An edger wheel that rapidly cuts a lens to near its finished size.

width, seg The size of a bifocal or trifocal segment measured horizontally across its widest section.

Wils-Edge mounting *See* mounting, Wils-Edge.

X

X-Chrom lens *See* lens, X-Chrom.

X-ing A vertical misalignment evidenced by a twisting of the frame front such that the planes of the lenses are out of coincidence with each other.

Y

yoked prism *See* prism, yoked.

Younger seamless *See* lens, Younger seamless.

Z

Z80.1 The identification number for the American National Standard for Ophthalmics-Prescription Ophthalmic Lenses-Recommendations.

Z87 The identification number for the American National Standard Practice for Occupational and Educational Eye and Face Protection, denoting safety lenses and frames.

zero inset method *See* method, zero inset.

zone, blended The blurred area between distance and near areas on an "invisible" bifocal. (Not to be confused with the progressive zone of a progressive-addition lens.)

zone, progressive That portion of a progressive-addition lens between the distance and near portions where lens power is gradually increasing.

zyl file *See* file, zyl.

zyl An abbreviation for the frame material zylonite. Often used to refer to plastic frames in general.

zylonite An early frame material that accepts a good polish, but is flammable at high temperatures.

Proficiency Test Answer Key

Chapter 1

1. c
2. d
3. e
4. b
5. a
6. d
7. h
8. a
9. f
10. c
11. b
12. g
13. i
14. e
15. d
16. c
17. b
18. e
19. a
20. b
21. f
22. g
23. c
24. h
25. e
26. d
27. b
28. f
29. a
30. c
31. b
32. c
33. a

Chapter 2

1. False
2. True
3. a. Yes
   b. No
   c. Yes
4. No
5. a
6. c
7. e
8. d
9. c
10. d, e
11. c
12. b, e
13. a
14. c
15. d
16. b
17. a
18. c
19. e

Chapter 3

1. False
2. a, b, c, d, e
3. b
4. True
5. False
6. e
7. No
8. 2.5 mm per lens
9. c
10. 3.75 mm per lens
11. a
12. 58.03 mm (or 58 mm, to the nearest 0.5 mm)
13. c
14. The dioptric demand is 1/0.20 or 5 D. Using the 3/4 rule, the inset per eye is 3/4 × 5, or 3.75 mm, and the near PD would be 64 − (2) × (3.75) = 56.5 mm. Using Table 3-1, the inset per eye is 4 mm, so the near PD would be 64 − (2 × 4) = 56 mm.
15. 55 mm. This was found using Table 3-2.
16. 59 mm. This was found using the 3/4 rule.
17. R: 30.5 mm
    L: 32.0 mm

    These were found using Table 3-2.

Chapter 4

1. d, e
2. b, f
3. c
4. a
5. a
6. c
7. a, b
8. d
9. a
10. b
11. False
12. True
13. False (The color will draw attention to the "salt" component, but should not necessarily be avoided. It depends upon the preference of the wearer.)
14. False
15. a
16. b
17. a
18. c
19. b
20. b
21. c
22. Nasal cut
23. d
24. b
25. c
26. Less because of the magnification effect of the lenses
27. b
28. False
29. Use antireflection coating
30. Solid construction, adjustable nosepads, comfort cable temples, light frame, small lens size, small ED
31. b
32. False
33. False
34. d

Chapter 5

1. False
2. c
3. a
4. b

5. True

6. d

7. a

8. c (Remember, it is not advisable to move an MRP height below the horizontal midline of the glasses unless the lenses are intended exclusively for near work.)

9. d

10. b

11. c

12. a

13. b (One diopter change in base curve changes vertex distance by approximately 0.6 mm. Of course if the eye size is small, the vertex distance will be smaller than 0.6 and vice versa.)

14. e

15. e

16. c

17. b

18. d

19. b

20. e
  or f [44 − (21 + 14)] = 9
  or [44 − (21 + 13)] = 10

21. e

22. d

23. b

24. True

25. d

26. a

27. c

28. c

29. e

30. b

31. True

32. False

Chapter 6

1. The Rx was written in reverse and should appear as:

O.D. −4.50 Sphere

O.S. −4.25 − 0.75 × 010

2. Carry components to 2 decimal places: +4.50 − 1.00 × 017

3. Leave degree sign off axis reading

4. Use a prefatory zero before the cylinder value: +2.00 − 0.75 × 033

5. False, the original examination form or prescription should be used

6. b, c

7. b

8. a. plus
  b. minus
  c. sphere
  d. sphere and axis, +2.00 and 015
  e. minus, cylinder, −2.00
  f. minus

9. b

10. a. a
  b. −2.50 −0.50 × 110

11. True

12. d

13. +1.75

14. b

15. False

16. True

17. d

18. False

19. False

20. a

21. d

22. a

23. b

24. b

25. b

26. b

27. e

28. b

29. a

30. a

31. a

32. b

33. a

34. a

35. a

36. a

37. a

38. a

39. d

40. c

41. e

42. c

43. a. +3.00 −2.00 × 180
  b. −5.00 +2.00 × 090
  c. +5.00 −2.00 × 090
  d. −3.00 +2.00 × 180

Chapter 7

1. False

2. True

3. c

4. a, b

5. d

6. b

7. b, e

8. a

9. a, c, d

10. c, d

11. True

12. b

13. d

14. e

15. c

16. False

17. b

18. a

19. d

20. a

21. False

22. A rolled eyewire

23. A spherical lens

24. A lens edged off axis

25. Heat the frame and plunge it into cold water

26. Use a straight edge and hold it along the top of both multifocal segments. Both seg tops should be parallel to the straight edge.

Chapter 8

1. True

2. False

3. b

4. a

5. c

6. e

7. d

8. b

9. a. True
  b. False
  c. False
  d. true

10. b

11. a

12. a. True
  b. True
  c. True
  d. True

13. b

14. a

15. c

16. e

17. True

18. e

19. a

20. False

21. False

22. b

23. b

24. c

25. c

26. a

27. b

28. b

29. a

30. c

31. e

32. a

33. c

34. c

Chapter 9

1. e

2. b

3. b

4. b

5. c

6. d

7. d

8. c

9. c

10. False

11. False

12. b

13. d

14. True

15. True

16. c

17. c

18. d

19. True

20. True

21. a

22. a

23. b

24. c

25. c

26. c

27. b

28. False

29. c

Chapter 10

1. False

2. True

3. True

4. True

5. True

6. False

7. True

8. b

9. True

10. a

11. b

12. c

13. b

14. False

15. c

16. d

17. True

18. d

19. e

20. c

21. True

22. True

23. True

24. a

25. False

26. False

27. b

28. False

29. c

30. e

31. a

32. True

33. c

34. b

35. False

Chapter 11

1. c

2. d

3. c

4. e

5. a. $a = 7$
  b. $a = 20$
  c. $a = \dfrac{19}{4}$
  d. $a = 11$
  e. $a = \dfrac{23}{7}$
  f. $a = \dfrac{4b + 3}{4}$
  g. $a = \dfrac{12 + 8b}{b}$
  h. $a = 4b - 2bc$
   or
   $a = 2b(2 - c)$

6. b

7. a. .05
  b. 1
  c. 0.25
  d. 0.01
  e. 2
  f. 4
  g. 8
  h. $^4/_3$ or 1.33

8. a. 100
  b. 4
  c. a · a (or simply a²)
  d. 49
  e. 144
  f. 225

9. a. 11
  b. 8
  c. 22
  d. b
  e. 2
  f. 5a

10. a. 343
  b. 3
  c. 10
  d. 1
  e. 100
  f. a
  g. 16

11. 16.18 m

12. 2.96 m from the ground

13. a. 2 m
  b. 3.46 m

14. a. 8.544 units
  b. 20.556 degrees

15. (−6, +10.39)

16. 128.024 km

17. a. 77.16 m long
  b. 90 degrees
    7.1 degrees
    18.9 degrees

18. c

19. a. 207 lbs
  b. 58 degrees

20. a. approximately 281 lbs
  b. 12 degrees

Chapter 12

1. d

2. d

3. c

4. a

5. b

6. b

7. c

8. b

9. e

10. d

11. c

12. a

13. a

14. b

15. d

16. a

17. c

18. a

19. b

20. d

21. e

22. c

23. a

24. a. +2.25 + 1.25 × 102
b. +0.50 −1.00 × 165
c. −0.50 × 165/+0.50 × 075

25. d

26. c

27. +1.25 − 4.25 × 075
−3.00 + 4.25 × 165

28. −0.50 + 125 × 103
+ 0.75 × 103/−0.50 × 013

29. b

30. a

Chapter 13

1. c

2. a

3. c

4. a

5. False

6. True

7. e (depending on whether the lenses were made up in plus or minus cylinder form)

8. True

9. b

10. a. F_1 at 90 = +8.00 D
b. F_1 at 180 = +10.00 D
c. F_2 = −8.75 D

11. d

12. *a.* F_1 at 90 = +8.00D
F_1 at 180 = +6.00D
F_2 = −6.75D
b. F_1 = +6.00D
F_2 at 90 = −4.75D
F_2 at 180 = −6.75D

13. b

14. +0.75 −1.12 × 100

15. +2.00 −1.00 × 020

16. 0.06424 meters or 64.24 millimmeters

17. 0.08970 meters or 89.70 millimeters

18. +11.52 D

19. −2.64 D

20. a. Actual front surface power in 90-degree meridian = +6.00 D
Actual front surface power in 180-degree meridian = +5.00 D

b. Value of the cylinder = 1.00 D

21. a. +4.00 −3.00 × 090
b. +3.70 −2.78 × 090

22. d

23. Nominal power is +8.25 D
True power is +8.17 D
Refractive power is +10.79 D

24. b

25. e

26. d

27. False

28. True

29. e

30. e

31. e

32. b

33. e

34. c

35. c

36. a. Complete answer is −3.75 −1.75 × 034.

37. a

38. d

39. c

40. a

41. a

42. b

43. c

44. b

45. a

46. a

47. a

48. d

49. e

Chapter 14

1. +11.37 D

2. O.D. −25.40 D sphere
O.S. −22.39 D sphere

3. b

4. +8.75 D

5. b

6. d

7. b

8. d

9. b

10. e, or using accurate formula, +14.23 D

11. +7.00 D

12. a. +10.00 D
b. +10.26 D

13. −10.21 D

14. b

15. c

Chapter 15

1. a

2. b

3. d

4. b

5. c

6. a

7. d

8. b

9. b

10. a

11. c

12. e

13. c

14. b

15. a. (3)
b. (4)

16. a

17. 4.5 Base 207
4.5 Base 27 DN

18. 3.25 Base 107 DN

19. 1.50 Base 181

20. 5.38 Base 158

21. 3.35 Base 153

22. a. 4 Base at 150 down
2 Base down and 3.5 Base in

b. 4 Base at 150 down
2 Base down and 3.5 Base out

23. 3.90 Base 140 UP
3.90 Base 140
3.90 Base 40 UP
3.90 Base 40

24. 2.50 Base 53 DN
2.50 Base 233
2.50 Base 127 DN
2.50 Base 307

25. 7.81 Base 140 UP
7.81 Base 140
7.81 Base 140 DN
7.81 Base 320

26. 5.00 Base 127 UP
5.00 Base 127
5.00 Base 127 DN
5.00 Base 307

27. 5.4 Base 146 DN
    5.4 Base 326
    4.1 Base 101 DN
    4.1 Base 281

28. 5.6 Base 10 DN
    5.6 Base 190
    4.6 Base 60 DN
    4.6 Base 240

29. 4.24 Base 45 DN
    4.24 Base 225
    4.24 Base 45 UP
    4.24 Base 45

30. 2.61 Base 107 DN
    2.61 Base 287
    2.61 Base 107 UP
    2.61 Base 107

31. 4.93 Base 60 DN
    4.93 Base 240
    4.70 Base 115 UP
    4.70 Base 115

32. 1.82 Base 74 UP
    1.82 Base 74
    1.82 Base 74 DN
    1.82 Base 254

33. 4.07 Base 11 UP
    4.07 Base 11
    4.32 Base 10 DN
    4.32 Base 190

34. 4.70 Base 25 UP
    4.70 Base 25
    4.25 Base 28 DN
    4.25 Base 208

35. 5.25 Base 31 UP
    5.25 Base 31
    5.25 Base 49 DN
    5.25 Base 229

36. 1.25 Base 53 DN
    1.25 Base 233
    1.25 Base 101 DN
    1.25 Base 281

37. 1.50 Base 149 DN
    1.50 Base 329
    1.50 Base 135 UP
    1.50 Base 135

38. 3.25 Base 171 UP
    3.25 Base 171
    3.37 Base 153 DN
    3.37 Base 333

39. a. True
    b. False
    c. False

40. b

41. 5.00 Δ Base at 143

42. b

43. a. 6 Δ Base Up
       6 Δ Base 90
    b. 0.5 Δ Base up and
       0.5 Δ Base In
       0.71 Δ Base 135
    c. 4.00 Δ Base down
       and 5.00 Δ Base In
       5.39 Δ Base 338.2

44. a. 3.76 Δ BD OD
       3.76 Δ BU OS
    b. 3.42 Δ BD OD
       3.42 Δ BU OS

45. c

Chapter 16

1. 1.20Δ Base in

2. –7.00 D

3. a

4. d

5. c

6. e

7. 4.375Δ Base out (or
   2.188Δ Base out O.D.
   and 2.188Δ Base out
   O.S.)

8. 2.60Δ Base out (total)
   (or 1.00Δ Base out
   O.D. and 1.60Δ Base
   out O.S.)

9. 2.75Δ Base in

10. 3.00Δ Base in

11. 2.30Δ Base in

12. b

13. c

14. b

15. a. (1) Base in
    b. (2) Base out, (3) Base
       up

c. Base (40+90), or
   Base 130
d. (1) Base in, (4) Base
   down
e. (1) Base in, (3) Base
   up

16. a

17. There is a total of
    0.074Δ Base in prism
    (0.037Δ base in per
    eye). There is a net
    vertical prismatic
    effect of 0.00Δ. (This
    is because 0.14Δ of
    Base-down prism is
    present in front of
    both left and right
    eyes, giving a net
    difference of zero.)

18. 0.44Δ Base up and
    1.63Δ Base out

19. 1.60Δ Base in and
    0.28Δ Base down

20. 1.26Δ Base in and
    0.36Δ Base up

21. 2.86Δ Base in and
    0.64Δ Base down O.D.
    or Base up O.S.

22. a. no power
    b. –2.00 D
    c. –0.24 D
    d. –1.77 D
    e. –3.00 D
    f. –1.50 D

23. a. –4.875 D
    b. 1.95Δ Base out (or
       Base 180)

24. a. +3.82 D
    b. 0.76Δ Base in (or
       Base 0)

25. $P = \dfrac{100g(n-1)}{d}$
    $= \dfrac{100(1)(0.8)}{54} = 1.48$

26.
$$P = \frac{100g(n-1)}{d}$$
$$= \frac{100(7.8-5.4)(1.66-1)}{40}$$
$$= \frac{100(2.4)(0.66)}{40}$$
$$= 3.96\Delta \text{ Base } 180$$
(or 4Δ Base Out)

Chapter 17

1. b

2. False

3. False

4. c

5. d

6. a

Chapter 18

1. a

2. False

3. Coma

4. b

5. c

6. Lens power and lens
   front curve

   or

   Lens power and lens
   back curve

7. b

8. d

9. b

10. b

11. + 9.00 D

12. + 9.75 D

13. + 7.75 D

14. + 4.00 D

15. + 5.25 D

16. + 4.43 D

17. + 3.94 D

18. + 3.00 D

19. True

20. a, b, c

21. b, c

22. c

23. d

24. False

25. False

Chapter 19

1. b

2. e

3. b

4. e

5. c

6. a

7. b

8. a

9. False

10. a. 3

b. 1

c. 4

d. 2

e. 1

11. e

12. c

13. b

14. a

15. d

16. True

17. d

18. c

19. b

20. a

21. a

22. e

23. e

24. d

25. b

26. b

27. c

28. d

29. 4.51 D

30. c

31. a. 9.5 mm

b. 35 mm is both the theoretical and available segment size.

32. a

33. c

34. b

35. d

36. c

37. d

38. a

Chapter 20

1. e

2. c

3. e

4. False

5. False

6. True

7. False

8. c

9. True

10. True

11. a

12. True

13. a

14. a, b

15. True

16. b

17. True

18. c

19. True

20. False

21. d

22. a

23. a

24. a

25. b

26. e

27. e

28. False

29. b

30. e

31. +0.50 +0.75 × 090

32. c

33. False

34. False

35. a. 1.50 Δ Base down

b. No prism thinning required

36. b

37. e

38. R: 21 mm
L: 19 mm

39. R: 31.5 mm
L: 31.5 mm
The prism amount would not need to be changed.

40. a. Yes. Both monocular PDs should be changed to 32 mm.

b. Yes. Reduce the prism to 2.5Δ base in per eye.

Chapter 21

1. e

2. a. SM = 7.67%

b. SM = 1.63%

c. 6.04%

3. True

4. b

5. True

6. c

7. b

8. d

9. b

10. d

11. c

12. b

13. a

14. c

15. a. 3

b. 2

c. 4

d. 2

e. 1

f. 1

g. 1

h. 1

16. False

17. c

18. True

19. c

20. d

21. b

22. b

23. d

24. c

25. a. 2

b. 2

c. 1

26. a. 6.00 × 0.6 = 3.60Δ

b. 1

27. a

28. a

29. R Power in 90 is –1.25.
L Power in 90 is –9.56.
Imbalance is (8.3 × 1.1) = 9.13Δ

30. c

31. d

32. b

33. a. 2

b. no

34. True

35. True

36. b

37. d

38. c

Chapter 22

1. False
2. False
3. False
4. False
5. True
6. True
7. True
8. False
9. False
10. True
11. False
12. True
13. True
14. False; because so much incoming light is absorbed by the lens itself, the amount of light internally reflected from the back surface of the lens is small compared with the amount reflected from the front surface. This means the percentage increase in overall transmission will not be much. However, the bothersome reflections seen from behind the wearer that are reflected off the back surface of the lens and appear relatively bright compared with the attenuated image coming through the tinted lenses will be eliminated.
15. False
16. False
17. False
18. a
19. False
20. False
21. True
22. False
23. False
24. False
25. e
26. c
27. a
28. c
29. d
30. c
31. e
32. a
33. b
34. d
35. a
36. c
37. e
38. a
39. a
40. a
41. a
42. b
43. e
44. c
45. d
46. d
47. a
48. b
49. e
50. b
51. e
52. a, d
53. 1.288
54. 20%
55. 86.21%

Chapter 23

1. True
2. False
3. a
4. e, a, c, d, b
5. c, a, e, b, d
6. e, b, c, a, d
7. True
8. c
9. d
10. b
11. b
12. b, c, d
13. False
14. False
15. d
16. e
17. b
18. c
19. c
20. False
21. d
22. c
23. b
24. c
25. a
26. a
27. d
28. False
29. False
30. c
31. False

Chapter 24

1. False
2. a
3. c
4. c
5. b

6. d
7. c
8. d
9. d
10. c, d
11. d
12. b
13. False
14. d
15. d
16. 67 mm
17. b
18. R: 3 mm in
    L: 1.5 mm in
19. R: 1.5 mm in
    L: 2 mm in
20. +3 mm
21. 2 mm in and 2 mm up
22. 1.5 mm in and 4.5 mm up
23. a. 0
    b. 50
    c. 46.5
    d. 38
    e. 44.5
    f. −8
    g. 52
    h. −8
    i. 0
    j. 50
    k. 62
    l. 41.5
    m. −15
    n. 35
    o. −13.5
    p. 38.5
24. d
25. b

Index